Clinical Laboratory and Diagnostic Tests

Significance and Nursing Implications

Third Edition

Kathleen Morrison Treseler, R.N., M.S.N.
Professor Emeritus
School of Nursin
Seattle Universit
Seattle, Washingt

APPLETON & LANGE
Norwalk, Connecticut/San Mateo, California

Notice: The author and the publisher of this volume have taken care that the
information and recommendations contained herein are accurate and compatible
with the standards generally accepted at the time of publication. Nevertheless,
it is difficult to ensure that all the information given is entirely accurate
for all circumstances. The publisher disclaims any liability, loss, or damage
incurred as a consequence, directly or indirectly, of the use and application of
any of the contents of this volume.

Copyright © 1995 by Appleton & Lange
A Simon & Schuster Company
Copyright © 1988, 1982 by Appleton & Lange

All rights reserved. This book, or any parts thereof, may not be used or
reproduced in any manner without written permission. For information,
address Appleton & Lange, 25 Van Zant Street, East Norwalk, Connecticut 06855.

96 97 98 99 / 10 9 8 7 6 5 4 3 2

Prentice Hall International (UK) Limited, *London*
Prentice Hall of Australia Pty. Limited, *Sydney*
Prentice Hall Canada, Inc., *Toronto*
Prentice Hall Hispanoamericana, S.A., *Mexico*
Prentice Hall of India Private Limited, *New Delhi*
Prentice Hall of Japan, Inc., *Tokyo*
Simon & Schuster Asia Pte. Ltd., *Singapore*
Editora Prentice Hall do Brasil Ltda., *Rio de Janeiro*
Prentice Hall, *Englewood Cliffs, New Jersey*

Library of Congress Catalog Card Number 94–72994

ISBN 0-8385-1373-5 NBZI

90000

9 780838 513736

Aquisitions Editor: David P. Carroll
Production Service: Tage Publishing Service, Inc.

PRINTED IN THE UNITED STATES OF AMERICA

DEDICATION

This edition is dedicated to my family: my husband, our children, their spouses, and *their* children, in thanks for all the support and assistance they have given throughout the production of this edition. The support was essential, not only in the writing process, but especially in day-to-day living.

Family, you bring love, laughter and a sense of continuity and enrichment to each day. To each one of you goes my thanks and my love.

Kathleen M. Treseler

CONTENTS

FIGURES AND TABLES

FIGURES

TABLES

PREFACE

This Third Edition of the text began, primarily, as a simple updating of the work. It ended as a fairly thorough rewrite, of multiple additions, and deletion/replacement of a number of tests no longer, or rarely in use. The scope and techniques of both test sections (clinical laboratory and diagnostic) have undergone remarkable change in a fairly short period of time. While test names may be the same the test process or use may be very different. Or the name may change without change in the test. Many "old faithful" tests have been virtually replaced by new, more accurate tests. Some diagnostic tests can now be used together, one modality supporting or extending the other.

The term *Diagnostic Modalities*, as used in this text, differentiates between diagnostic tests that are performed in the clinical laboratory on samples from the patient (e.g., blood, tissue, urine, or other specimens), categorized as Clinical Laboratory tests, from the tests that require the presence of the patient during the testing process, categorized as Diagnostic Modalities.

The text does not attempt to cover *all* tests in either of the two categories. Selection of tests to be included was based on those most frequently used in local laboratories, or those just recently placed in use. Since the laboratories being used for reference include free standing, as well as hospital-centered, laboratories, many with markedly different populations, the scope is to be broad-based. This text attempts to include tests most frequently used in the above settings.

Nursing makes use of these data as important assessment information for planning, implementing, and evaluating nursing care. Perhaps, even more important, the data can be invaluable in patient education before, and after the test in question. It can assist the client and her or his family to understand, and cooperate with the purpose and process of the test, as well as indicate the impact of the findings on the medical diagnosis, nursing needs, treatment plan, and ultimate recovery. Lack of knowledge can increase anxiety about what can be a frightening experience, especially if the test process is an unknown. Fear, or lack of understanding can decrease the ability of the client to cooperate fully, which may well increase the need for test repetition.

Notable changes/additions from the previous edition in terms of placement and/or depth of coverage are to be found in Chapters 6, 15 and 16.

Chapter 6, now titled *Infectious and Sexually Transmitted Disease*, has been extensively updated and revised (e.g., immunization schedules for children and adults; infection control procedures based on CDC requirements (hospital and home); revision of a great many of the previous tests for sexually transmitted diseases, as well as many figures and tables. Infections and sexually transmitted diseases are areas of continuing change and the reader needs to be aware of this.

Chapter 15 previously limited to *Pregnancy* has been enlarged and titled *Reproductive System*. It now incorporates "Tests for Risk Populations" (primarily the fetus or infant) which includes new tests, as well as updated material previously included in Chapter 1 (i.e., prenatal and newborn screening tests; tests related to preeclampsia; and tests related to gonadal function (male and female).

A completely ***new*** addition, *Tests to Monitor Cancer: Tumor Markers*, immediately precedes the section on Diagnostic Modalities and covers Carcinoembryonic Antigen test (CEA); Serum Acid Phosphotase (SAP); Prostate Specific Antigen (PSA); Alphafetoprotein (AFP) as a tumor marker; Papanicolaou Smear (PAP); and HCG-Beta Subunit, used for detection/follow-up of gestational trophoblastic neoplasms, e.g., choriocarcinoma. Some user-helpful additions include such things as a clear definition of the DNA (Nucleic Acid) Probe and an appendix addition of terminology and definitions related to recent testing methods (e.g., recombinant DNA).

If introduced early, and selectively, in the nursing curriculum, this book will help students understand the relationship of a test to clients' medical problems and help them to make useful observations. The overview of physiology in the screening test section will reinforce learning from courses in anatomy and physiology; the brief pathophysiological explanations in the same section recall and supplement course material from pathophysiology and medical-surgical nursing. The *Implications for Nursing* are, for the most part, medical-surgical concepts, and support information about general patient care for the physical disorders most frequently related to the test being discussed. The role of the nurse as teacher is reinforced throughout the text, and principles of teaching and learning are consistently reinforced.

The organization of the book remains constant, as seen in previous editions:

1. *An outline format* is used wherever feasible to provide quick retrieval of specific information about the test in question.
2. *Implications for nursing* remain a major part of almost every test in order to assist the reader to apply the information provided.
3. *Extensive use of lists, tables, and figures* are included to help the reader find material rapidly and see the relationship of one set of facts to another.
4. *Current information* is given about the tests, as well as an evlauation providing information on the present use of the test itself, and the usefulness of the information provided, where indicated.
5. *Reference range of normal variation in test results for different age groups* (senior adult, adult, young adult and specific age levels for pediatric clients) are given when available.
6. *Causes for variations in reference norms* related to age and/or physiological differences are provided; in depth when indicated.
7. *Cross-referencing* is provided within the body of the text, using the "decimal" or "scientific" numbering system which clearly indicates the location of the reference.

Each *diagnostic test* is placed within a category (e.g., X-ray) and a subcategory (e.g., Contrast Studies) in which terms are defined and information applicable to *all* such tests is given (e.g., in the case of contrast studies, reaction to contrast media is discussed). The specific test is explained in terms of the purpose, procedure, and contraindications, if any, and the nursing implications spell out whether a permit is usually required; the physical preparation needed prior to the test; the patient/family education usually needed (which includes what the nurse must, or may, do before and after the test); and finally, the length of time usually needed for the test to be accomplished. For convenience in locating specific tests, the tests have been placed in categories that generally reflect the type of diagnostic modality to be used (e.g., ultrasound, electrodiagnostic) rather than the part of the body or body system to be examined as with clinical laboratory tests. Each diagnostic test lists as many synonyms for the test as could be found.

The book is divided into five parts: Part I, *Multisystem Screening Tests*, includes tests for blood chemistry, hematology, coagulation and urinalysis.

Part II discusses the *Diagnosis of Infectious Diseases* and focuses on patient care, teaching and specifics of a wide variety of infectious diseases. There is particular emphasis on sexually transmitted disease and a strong focus on both AIDS and hepatitis.

Part III, *Laboratory Tests of Specific Body Systems*, looks at each system: endocrine, renal, gastrointestinal, respiratory, cardiovascular, collagen-vascular, hematologic, neurologic, reproductive (which covers both male and female reproductive systems with a heavy emphasis on pregnancy) and includes identification of nursing diagnoses that are applicable when a specific body system malfunctions.

Part IV discusses most diagnostic tests and related nursing actions in the commonly used (and some uncommon) x-ray studies, angiograms, nuclear diagnostic tests, magnetic resonance imaging (MRI), and tomography (PET and Spect).

Part V focuses on testing for acceptable levels of therapeutic and/or potentially toxic drugs.

Part I

MULTISYSTEM SCREENING TESTS

Screening tests increase the reliability and precision of the diagnostic process, often provide an indication of the initial severity of a disease process, and are one of the more reliable indicators that treatment is effecting desirable change.

At one time, with the appearance of automated analyzers, screening tests were expanded to large batteries of tests (multiphasic screening) because automation provided multiple determinations at low cost. Because of the cost of the subsequent follow-up on false, or nonpathological, positive or negative findings, however, and the increasing reluctance of insurance carriers to cover such costs, this wholesale approach is much less in evidence today (Harvey et al., 1991).

The term *screening test* still implies to many the idea of a large group of tests done together to investigate a full system or total body function. Such a group of tests is perhaps better termed a *profile*—an in-depth investigation. As used here, screening test means just that—a singular test that can give information about a fairly broad area of body function and that detects the most characteristic signs of a disorder that may require further investigation.

Through visual, tactile, auditory, and verbal investigation of an individual, a diagnostician can frequently, but not always, gather sufficient clues to make suspect a specific disease process. If there are several possible causes, the diagnostician must seek specific data for each possible diagnosis from clinical laboratory tests or the other diagnostic testing tools available (e.g., x-ray, computed tomography [CT scan], echography, ultrasound, exercise testing, pulmonary function tests). This process works well when there are overt signs or symptoms evident in the initial observations. In many pathological states, however, no overt clues are present until the condition is fairly well established or advanced. Because of this, screening tests are used to assist the diagnostician in determining the state of health, by supporting the presence of a disorder or ruling it out. Screening tests make it possible to decrease risks. For example, the person undergoing surgery will face fewer chances of having a heretofore unknown disorder cause serious complications when met with the stress of

1

surgery. Screening tests also guide the practitioner in the provision of preventive measures or teaching, which can keep the disorder from further development. Still another use of such tests is the reinforcement of the diagnostician's initial considered hunch as to the presence of a physiological dysfunction.

Just as a person's blood pressure is taken routinely on a visit to a physician or during a stay in the hospital—in the absence of hypertension or even a family history of increased blood pressure—screening tests can be done without clinical indication to detect abnormalities having a high incidence in the general population. It is evident then that screening tests will vary with the population served. Not all hospitals or physicians, even in the same given area, will use the same tests for screening purposes. The information gathered from screening tests forms part of the "data base" for problem-oriented medical and nursing practice.

According to Collins (1975), a test must meet five criteria to qualify as a screening test. It must be:

1. Simple to perform and inexpensive
2. An accurate procedure with few false positives or negatives
3. Capable of being performed completely by laboratory or nursing personnel
4. Harmless and relatively painless
5. Used for the purpose of uncovering a serious or common disease that is treatable

An additional criterion, directed at the diagnostician—whether physician, nurse, laboratory technologist, or other member of the health care team—should be the presence of the necessary knowledge and understanding of human physiology and the test in question to interpret the results in relation to what is known of the history and present status of the person tested. This implies, as well, an understanding of the interrelationships among the screening tests and common, nonpathological variations in the results. Fundamental to this criterion is the diagnostician's knowledge and understanding of the scope of his or her own discipline's practice in the management of abnormalities and the scope of practice of other members of the health care team so that collaboration and cooperation will exist among those members in managing patient care. The focus of this text is to help the nurse meet this criterion.

ONE

BLOOD CHEMISTRY SCREEN

The term *blood chemistry screen* involves analysis of the major chemical constituents of the blood. The laboratory processes that can be used for this are many and varied. The purpose of this chapter is not to look at the laboratory procedure per se, though attention is paid to specific steps in the collection of specimens that could alter the results of those laboratory procedures, but to help the practitioner know and understand what can be learned from the outcomes of the test for a given individual. The practitioner can then more adequately inform the person having the test about what is being done and why. The nurse can also alter nursing care on the basis of the findings to better meet the client's needs.

An important factor related to the type or method of testing used in a given laboratory is that each type or method used will produce varied policies, procedures, and *reference values*. Because of the variety of testing methods, the time needed to obtain results also varies. (A report may also be delayed because the outcomes are equivocal and had to be checked and rechecked.) Therefore, the practitioner should not try to apply policies, procedures, or in particular, *reference values* from one laboratory to another.

Of the blood chemicals analyzed in the blood chemistry screen, many have a direct or indirect influence on body fluid balance (e.g., sodium, albumin, glucose). The practitioner then needs to be able to interpret the results in terms of body fluid changes as well as changes in the concentration of the chemical itself within that fluid.

Body fluid is primarily water and is found in the body cells (*intracellular*), in the space between cells but outside the vascular system (*interstitial*), and in the vascular system (*intravascular*). Interstitial and intravascular body fluid is often discussed as one entity—*the extracellular fluid compartment*—as opposed to that body of fluid found in the *intracellular compartment*. (The interstitial space is often only a potential space.) Water moves among these three areas both passively (without using energy) and actively (using energy) depending on the comparative increase or decrease in osmotic pressure among the three areas. (*Osmotic pressure* is defined as the relative number of particles in a solution on either side of a membrane.) Osmotic pressure is maintained at equilibrium between the body spaces by a delicate balancing act using diffusion, osmosis, and filtration. Disruption of this balance, also known as chemical equilibrium, occurs most readily in infants, the frail elderly, and obese individuals. The nurse needs to be especially alert to changes in those substances that help maintain the equilibrium. Alterations in sodium intake or elimination are the most common causes of body fluid alterations, but increased glucose levels (which increase body fluid loss) and decreased concentrations of serum total proteins (especially albumin because it is the predominant intravascular protein), which influence movement of fluid out of the vascular and into the interstitial and intracellular spaces, can also be major contributors to fluid imbalances.

Some terms with which the nurse needs to be familiar in the management of body fluid imbalances are as follows:

- **Colloid.** A gelatinous substance that does not pass through a membrane
- **Colloidal Solutions.** Usually intravenous solutions made up of fluids and particles (e.g., blood, plasma, dextran) that are not capable of passing through a semipermeable membrane. Used to maintain circulating fluid volume in the vascular system and prevent shock. Often used after severe hemorrhage
- **Crystalloid Solutions.** Solutions containing dissolved ions that can pass through a semipermeable membrane
- **Diffusion.** The spontaneous mixing of molecules or ions of two or more substances, which is rate-dependent on the concentrations of the substances (an increased concentration increases the rate), the temperature of the solutions (an increased temperature increases the rate), the size of the molecules (smaller molecules move faster), and the size of the chamber (the rate increases with increased chamber size)
- **Filtration.** Passive transport of a fluid by hydrostatic pressure (the force exerted by the weight of a solution)
- **Osmolality.** The number of dissolved solute particles in a solution (see also 7.2.2A.B "Serum and Urine Osmolality")
- **Osmolality (Serum).** A measure of the number of dissolved particles per unit of water in the serum
- **Osmolarity.** The concentration of a solution in terms of osmoles of solute per liter of solution
- **Osmole.** A unit of osmotic pressure equivalent to the amount of solute substances that dissociate in solution to form 1 mol of particles
- **Osmosis.** The diffusion of water across a cell membrane; the passage of a pure solvent from a solution of lesser concentration to one of greater solute concentration when the two solutions are separated by a membrane that selectively prevents the passage of solute molecules but is permeable to the solvent
- **Osmotic Pressure.** The amount of pressure necessary (i.e., the number of particles in solution) to stop the flow of water across the membranes
- **Plasma.** The fluid portion of the blood
- **Serum.** The fluid portion of the blood from which fibrinogen has been separated

1.1 SERUM SODIUM

Synonym: Plasma sodium

Normal Ranges (mEq/L)

Adult	136–145
Senior adult	
Male	134–147
Female	135–145

Pediatric	
Premature (cord)	116–140
Newborn (cord)	126–166
Newborn (to 7 days)	135–145
Infant	139–146
Child	138–145

Definition. The serum sodium test is a measurement of the major cation (electrolyte, positive charge) in the vascular space, part of the extracellular fluid (ECF).

It should be considered a ratio measurement, the ratio between sodium and water, rather than a direct measure of the total body sodium. Serum sodium levels reflect the balance of water to sodium. There is no laboratory test that can measure the sodium concentration of the total body; however, one can look at the size of the extracellular space (by looking at postural blood pressure, edema, and neck vein distension, for example) and gain an estimation of the total body sodium because water and sodium imbalances coexist.

The sodium bicarbonate buffer system is one of the major renal controls of hydrogen levels, which makes sodium an important cation in maintaining the body's acid-base balance as well as in maintaining fluid distribution in the body.

1.1.1 Hypernatremia

Synonyms: Increased serum osmolality, water deficit, hypertonic dehydration

Definition. Hypernatremia literally means an excess of sodium in the blood, thus an increase in its measurement; it is usually indicative of water loss in excess of sodium loss.

Physiology. Hypernatremia is a fairly rare occurrence. It is seen most often in the elderly, in patients in critical care settings, or in populations with neurological defects. An increase in the serum sodium level suggests a loss of body water in excess of sodium loss or an increase in sodium intake in excess of water intake. True sodium excess (also called absolute sodium excess) is almost always accompanied by edema because of the corresponding excess of water. The dilution within the intravascular space is the probable cause of normal or low sodium values when, in fact, the total body sodium is elevated.

An increased sodium concentration involves the total ECF very early because water will diffuse across the vascular membranes in an effort to dilute the intravascular solution and reestablish an isotonic solution. The total ECF will ultimately contain a high solute load that produces large urine volumes, further depleting the water stores of the body and increasing the solute concentration. If free water is not given, increased serum osmolality results.

During the process the body attempts to compensate by:

1. Suppression of aldosterone secretion by the adrenal gland
2. An increase in sodium excretion in the urine
3. A release of antidiuretic hormone (ADH) by the pituitary in response to increased osmolality of the ECF

If compensation fails before water is pulled from the intracellular space, cellular dysfunction will occur (see "Pathophysiology").

Pathophysiology. Hypernatremia is much less common than hyponatremia, but it is considered one of the most dangerous of all body fluid dysfunctions. When the compensatory mechanisms listed in "Physiology" are not adequate, or if free water is not given, signs and symptoms become obvious. When severe, a finding of altered sensorium is expected. (Signs and symptoms also include agitation; flushed appearance; fever; a dry, sticky mouth; increased and then decreased urine output; complaints of thirst; decreased deep tendon reflexes; increased pulse, respiration, and blood pressure; and variation in serum sodium levels [usually increased but could be normal—see discussion of volume excess, "Pathophysiology"].) Hypernatremia (increased osmolality) can occur with both extracellular volume deficit or extracellular volume excess. Increased osmolality with an ECF volume deficit usually is related to loss of transcellular fluids (i.e., gastrointestinal fluids, sweat). Despite being ECFs, they are hypotonic when compared to serum so that the patient will have a postural drop in blood pressure, yet also have an increased plasma sodium.

When hypernatremia (increased osmolality) occurs with volume excess, it usually relates to too severe an imposition of free water restriction for the patient being treated for increased osmolality with ECF volume deficit (Rokosky & Shaver, 1982, p. 93).

SERUM SODIUM LEVELS INCREASED IN:

1. Conditions causing water loss
   a. Severe, prolonged vomiting due to any cause, but especially pyloric obstruction
   b. Nasogastric suctioning, which removes more water and chloride than sodium
   c. Some infectious diseases such as tracheobronchitis in which more water is lost than electrolytes because of deep, rapid respirations and fever. (The rate of insensible water loss is greatly increased with fever)
   d. Profuse, watery diarrhea from any cause when electrolyte and fluid replacement is absent or is inadequate. Diarrhea in infants and senior adults is more likely to lead to a hyperosmolar state than in older children and adults. The thirst stimulus may not be intact in the elderly, or they may be confused and unaware of thirst or unable to respond to it appropriately. Therefore, lost fluids would not be replaced adequately. Infants, having higher metabolic rates than adults, require more water. The greater relative skin surface area, which includes the gastrointestinal membranes until the age of 3, results in greater relative fluid losses from both the gastrointestinal tract and the outer skin surfaces, especially if fever is present (Metheny & Snively, 1983)
   e. Diabetes insipidus because of decreased secretion or the total absence of secretion of ADH, which leads to a decrease in reabsorption of water by the distal and collecting kidney tubules. Sodium continues to be reabsorbed as the aldosterone mechanism still functions. An extremely low urine-specific gravity will be noted (Sabiston, 1981)
   f. Primary aldosteronism, although debated in the literature and felt by many to involve consistent reabsorption of more sodium than water, because of the increased reabsorption of sodium in exchange for potassium and hydrogen in the kidney. Serum concen-

trations are almost always above 140 mEq/L and can be above 144 mEq/L despite water reabsorption. This may be due to the polyuria accompanying the disease (Sodeman & Sodeman, 1982)

2. Conditions causing sodium increase
   a. Inadequate intake of free water, probably the most frequent cause of hypernatremia. This may be due to an inability to perceive thirst or an inability to respond to thirst. Such problems can be found in the unconscious person, the person with clouded sensorium (stroke, cerebral edema), or the elderly (see item 1d), the person with food or water restriction (n.p.o.) for prolonged periods in preparation for diagnostic tests or surgery, and the infant whose needs are misinterpreted
   b. High-solute feedings such as high-protein tube feedings or formulas with a high salt content (rare now with commercial formula preparation). Infants are at particular risk because of their immature renal function. The high-solute load acts as an osmotic diuretic, removing water from the body in a dilute urine
   c. There are many conditions in which the total body sodium is increased but the increase is not reflected in the sodium value because of *water retention,* which follows salt retention and produces serum levels within normal limits (see Table 1–1)

1.1.2 Hyponatremia

Synonyms: Decreased serum osmolality, water excess, hypotonic dehydration, low-sodium syndrome

Definition. Hyponatremia can be defined as a deficiency of sodium in the blood or salt depletion, usually indicative of water increase in excess of sodium increase (i.e., when excessive electrolyte-free water has been ingested and retained).

TABLE 1-1. COMPARISON OF SERUM SODIUM LEVELS WITH TOTAL BODY SODIUM

Condition	Serum Sodium	Total Body Sodium
Edema (cardiac, renal, hepatic disease)	Low (hyponatremia)	High
Prolonged sweating	Low	Low
Diuretics and low-sodium diets	Low	Low
Addison's disease	Low	Low
Edema (cardiac, renal, hepatic disease)	Normal	High
Excretion of dilute urine, early stages of GI sodium loss	Normal	Low
Excess oral or intravenous sodium intake	High (hypernatremia)	High
Water and sodium loss with water loss greater than sodium loss	High	Low

Note that a low or high serum level does not necessarily correspond with the total body sodium. From Soltis, B. (1979). Fluid and Electrolyte Imbalance. In W. J. Phipps, B. C. Long, N. F. Woods (eds.). *Medical-Surgical Nursing: Concepts and Clinical Practice.* St. Louis: C. V. Mosby, with permission.

Physiology. When a condition of decreased serum osmolality occurs, the body's compensatory mechanisms are as follows:

1. An increased secretion of aldosterone by the adrenal gland that is stimulated by the renin-angiotensin mechanism (which in turn is triggered by the decrease in renal arterial pressure). The result is twofold
   a. Increased reabsorption of sodium by the kidney and
   b. Increased absorption of sodium from the gut
2. A decrease in the amount of sodium eliminated in perspiration
3. Inhibited ADH secretion so that less fluid is reabsorbed by the kidney—the mechanism thought to be a response to the swelling of cells when ECF hypoosmolality occurs

Pathophysiology. The usual cause for excessive retention of electrolyte-poor or, free fluid by the body involves an impairment of the kidneys' ability to excrete it, as in end-stage renal failure. However, any disease that impairs the function of any of the compensatory mechanisms can also be a causative agent (e.g., ADH-secreting tumors, severe stress, tumor of the hypothalamus).

When ECF hypoosmolality occurs, cells swell. Water diffuses into the interstitial (intracellular) space as osmolality between all compartments is attempted. In response to this, potassium—the major intracellular cation—moves out of the cell and is usually lost in the urine.

Rapid changes in osmolality may induce seizure activity. Because of this, the use of hypertonic solutions to treat hypoosmolar states is usually reserved for emergency situations.

It is also possible for an individual to experience a volume deficit and decreased osmolality (hyponatremia) together, for instance, when a volume deficit is treated with only electrolyte-free fluid.

SERUM SODIUM LEVELS DECREASED IN:

1. Conditions causing sodium loss
   a. Diarrhea or vomiting because of sodium loss in excess of water loss (as well as water loss in excess of sodium loss [see "Serum Sodium Levels Increased in," item 1]. Isotonic loss can occur as well and depletes both sodium and water equally). Sodium loss in excess of water loss is more likely to occur in
      (1) Diarrhea occurring in an ileostomate
      (2) Prolonged vomiting involving a loss of intestinal as well as gastric fluids
      (3) Infants who are at particular risk for sodium loss as well as fluid loss because they tend to lose large amounts of sodium through their skins even when well and their kidneys do not concentrate urine well (Phipps et al., 1983)
   b. Draining intestinal fistulas
   c. Prolonged use of diuretics with inadequate electrolyte replacement or replacement with water only
   d. Addison's disease because of a loss of mineral corticoids secretion (aldosterone) with a subsequent loss of the reabsorptive mechanism for sodium in the kidney
   e. Chronic renal insufficiency with acidosis, the so-called salt-wasting disease, because of an inability of the kidney to conserve sodium and the excretion of maximal amounts of salt

2. Conditions causing water excess
   a. Abnormal water retention
      (1) Liver disease with ascites because of a consistently reduced excretion of both water and sodium coupled with renal failure that causes poor water excretion of even that diminished amount in the glomerular filtrate
      (2) Congestive heart failure with edema (dependent or pulmonary) because of decreased cardiac output, which decreases the glomerular filtration rate (GFR)
      (3) Renal insufficiency with urinary suppression
      (4) Elevated serum glucose levels because of the increased osmotic pull of glucose as seen in poorly controlled diabetes mellitus
   b. Excessive water intake and inadequate salt replacement (water intoxication)
      (1) Overheating of the body because of strenuous exercise, high fever, or sudden increases in ambient temperature
      (2) Individuals taking diuretics
      (3) Individuals who are vomiting
      (4) Some mental aberrations characterized by excessive intake of water
      (5) Some elderly persons whose thirst satisfaction requires excess water (Metheny & Snively, 1983; Ravel, 1989)
3. Conditions causing both water excess and sodium loss. The syndrome of inappropriate ADH (SIADH) causes both water excess and sodium loss. SIADH occurs as a complication of many conditions and should be considered when low sodium levels are reported with cancer of the lung, head trauma, myxedema, tuberculosis, or meningitis. The water excess is secondary to inappropriate release of ADH. A decrease in aldosterone secretion occurs secondary to the plasma dilution and increased GFR, and sodium is excreted. In this condition, therefore, the serum sodium level is decreased by two mechanisms: dilution by water retention and excessive urinary sodium losses (Sodeman & Sodeman, 1982)

IMPLICATIONS FOR NURSING IN IMBALANCES OF WATER: HYPER- AND HYPOOSMOLALITY

1. Determine patients at risk for water imbalances by
   a. Noting the written medical history and by direct patient assessment. Check for conditions that may lead to or enhance water imbalance (e.g., heart disease, inadequate liver function; see previous section for others)
   b. Expecting a change in the plasma sodium level immediately after most surgery. This change is generally due to the rapid administration of intravenous fluids (a plasma sodium decrease) or the tendency of the body to conserve extracellular fluid postoperatively (an increase). Serum sodium levels usually return to normal limits in 24 to 72 hours. Intravenous injections generally contain sodium, which fosters sodium excretion. Care must be taken not to swamp the postoperative patient with sodium and water loads that are hypotonic at a time when ADH levels are high (e.g., 5 percent dextrose in water (D_5W), D_5 and 0.45 mEq normal saline (NS), any saline solution less than 0.9 mEq/L). Fluid overload can cause dilutional hypoproteinemia and lead to congestive heart failure, pulmonary edema, tissue edema of the brain, and (particularly) peripheral areas of the body (Sabiston, 1981).
2. Before working with an individual at risk, increase your own knowledge of sodium concentrations in the diet to help the person adapt his or her dietary selections to prevent the occurrence of imbal-

ance. Collaboration with the physician and dietician is encouraged in order to facilitate and reinforce their plans of care

3. General implications for persons with a water imbalance
   a. All individuals with actual or potential water imbalances should receive strict intake and output measurements and daily weight checks as independent nursing actions
   b. All persons with actual or potential water imbalances should have urine-specific gravity tested at least once daily as an independent nursing measure. If the ability of the kidney to concentrate is of particular concern, the first voiding in the morning should be tested
   c. In the presence of a water imbalance of unknown origin, check for the present use and possible abuse of diuretics. Early physiological response to diuretics is the loss of extracellular water primarily. With prolonged use and replacement of the water loss only, actual plasma sodium depletion can occur
   d. Be aware of how long a patient has been kept with nothing by mouth (n.p.o.), especially those persons at risk for water imbalance. Monitor baseline data (items a and b), and inform the physician when the data indicate a developing water imbalance
   e. Any patient who is dehydrated, whatever the imbalance causing the problem, should receive mouth care for comfort and to prevent tissue damage. The nurse should also consult with the physician to provide adequate hydration consistent with the patient's physical problems. Hydration must be undertaken with caution to prevent fluid overload. This is particularly true for the older adult and both infants and young children because of the immaturity of the homeostatic mechanisms in the young or the increased length of time needed for these mechanisms to work in the older adult. It is also true for the person with cardiac or renal dysfunction since both affect renal body fluid regulation

4. Nursing implications with saline imbalance (loss of proportional amounts of water and sodium—isotonic dehydration, isotonic saline loss)
   a. Baseline laboratory data to be monitored include red blood cell count (RBC) and hematocrit. Urinary sodium levels are of value as well (see Chapter 4). Serum protein and lipid levels are affected by too many variables to be useful as baseline data for evaluation. If a recent RBC and hematocrit are not available, an order might be requested from the physician.
      Compare the RBC and hematocrit with the serum sodium concentration. If the serum sodium is within normal limits and the RBC and hematocrit values are elevated, isotonic saline loss probably exists, a state of true sodium and water deficit. (Patients with polycythemia will show this without saline depletion)
   b. Monitor patients with or at risk of saline imbalance for signs of circulatory overload or collapse
      (1) Check vital signs at least every 4 hours during the day, noting especially changes in blood pressure and pulse
      (2) Inspect neck veins in both the supine position and with the head of the bed elevated at 45°
      (3) Note the quality and rate of vein filling of the hands. The normal filling rate is 3 to 5 seconds
      (4) Weigh daily, same time, same clothing
      (5) Listen to the lungs for rales
      (6) Check for dependent edema: the ankles in ambulatory persons or those up in a chair, the sacrum in the person on bed rest. Measure the ankle circumference for baseline data, and record
      (7) Take patients' blood pressure when they are lying down, sitting, and standing for postural changes

5. Nursing implications related to decreased plasma sodium levels because of excess water
   a. The nurse can confirm excess water (dilutional hyponatremia) by checking characteristic laboratory evidence and comparing with data from the patient's history and physical. Laboratory data suggesting or confirming the presence of excess water are as follows
      (1) Serum osmolality decreased to less than 274 mOsm/kg plasma water. If a serum osmolality test has not been done, the serum sodium concentration can be used as a fairly accurate estimation. Use the following equation (Groer & Shekleton, 1983) to get a rough but adequate measurement of serum osmolality:

Serum osmolality = Plasma sodium [Na+] × 2

        (2) Serum sodium levels decreased to less than 130 mEq/L (can be decreased to less than 115 mEq/L)

        (3) Serum potassium levels decreased or within normal limits

        (4) Serum urea nitrogen (BUN) levels decreased or within normal limits

        (5) Hemoglobin and hematocrit values decreased

        (6) Mean corpuscular volume (MCV) increased or within normal limits

        (7) Mean corpuscular hemoglobin concentration (MCHC) decreased. The changes in the blood indices—hemoglobin, hematocrit, MCV, and MCHC—are due to the swelling of the RBCs together with all other body cells

  b. With a drop in the serum sodium level to 125 mEq/L or lower, observe the patient for signs and symptoms of water excess: behavioral changes of inattention, confusion, drowsiness, delirium; weight gain; increased rate and depth of respiration; neuromuscular changes of muscle cramping after use; and isolated muscle twitching, weakness, headache, incoordination; and signs of increased intracranial pressure (increased blood pressure, slowed pulse rate, slowed respirations, projectile vomiting, papilledema). Symptoms of water excess are not usually significant until the 125-mEq/L level has been reached. This complication is frequently called water intoxication.

      Observation for these symptoms is especially important in the person with SIADH because the onset is very rapid, often bypassing the earlier symptoms of changes in sensorium and drowsiness and presenting with far advanced symptoms (i.e., delirium, psychotic behavior, or convulsions). Treatment must be rapid to prevent coma or even death from occurring; therefore, changes should be reported as soon as identified and with adequate emphasis and follow-up to elicit an immediate response on the part of the physician

  c. With falls in serum sodium levels, an error still seen is an attempt to replace the sodium by giving broth or some other high-sodium food. Because the concentration of total body sodium is not known, all that the nurse can be sure of is the presence of excess water, and treating excess water with sodium chloride is inappropriate

6. Nursing implications related to decreased serum sodium levels resulting from sodium loss

  a. Ensure that any patient having nasogastric or intestinal suction is receiving not only ounce-for-ounce water replacement but also milliequivalent-for-milliequivalent electrolyte replacement

  b. Irrigate any nasogastric or intestinal tubes with normal saline solution only. The individual at risk for water imbalance can be pushed into excess by irrigation with water

7. Teaching needs for persons at risk for or diagnosed as having fluid imbalance depend on the diagnosis, current status, previous knowledge, and ability to learn. Some content areas concerning prevention are as follows

  a. Determine the individual's previous level of knowledge about the prevention or self-care of fluid imbalances

  b. Determine whether the client is ready or able to learn. Identify a support person who may be ready and able to learn if the client is not, and start with information the learner wants to learn

  c. Correct misconceptions and reinforce the correct information

  d. The following is a list of probable learner populations for information about sodium and water

        (1) Instruct those persons who will be involved in active sports, who will begin work in a hotter environment, or who will be moving to a hotter climate, to replace salt lost in perspiration by the judicious use of salt together with fluid replacement. (Caution: hypernatremia can occur with the use of salt tablets.) Taking fluids containing sodium or salty foods such as potato chips should be recommended and warning given against drinking only water to slake thirst

        (2) Teach individuals who will be taking diuretics at home the signs and symptoms of a sodium deficit and excess as well as a water excess and deficit. Stress the need to take medication only as prescribed, without variation. Teach those signs and symptoms that should be reported to the physician as well as what steps the individual can take independently to prevent imbalance (as given earlier). A family member or responsible home caretaker should be included in all teaching

(3) Teach the patient, family, home caretaker to read the labels on all foods and medications for sodium content

(4) Instruct patients receiving a low-sodium diet which foods to avoid, those to be used in moderation, and those low enough in sodium to be used freely. (The American Heart Association has free booklets available that describe mild, moderate, and strict sodium-restricted diets. They are usually distributed through physicians, dieticians, or nurses. The nurse giving diet-related instruction should acquire copies of the booklet for distribution.) The following is a list of some frequently used foods that are high in sodium

    (a) Meat: bacon, luncheon meats, frankfurters, ham, kosher meats, sausages, salt pork

    (b) Vegetables: sauerkraut and other vegetables prepared in brine or with salt added during or after cooking

    (c) Fish: sardines

    (d) Miscellaneous: processed cheese, meat tenderizers, relish, horseradish, bouillon cubes, peanut butter, catsup, mustard, olives, pickles, Worcestershire sauce, potato chips, pretzels

(5) Instruct the person about the high sodium content of ingestates other than food, for example, toothpastes or powders, certain drugs (laxatives, pain relievers, sedatives, cough syrups, even some antibiotics), and chewing tobacco or snuff

1.2 SERUM CHLORIDE

Synonym: Plasma chloride

Normal Ranges (mEq/L)

Adult	95–110
Senior adult	Not available, could be assumed to mirror sodium concentration changes
Pediatric	
Cord	96–104
Newborn	98–104 (to 7 days)
Infant	95–110
Child	101–105

Definition. Serum chloride is the most abundant extracellular anion; yet, it may be one of the least important electrolytes to measure, particularly in a screening procedure. Often, an emergency study will omit the chloride measurement. Its frequent use may be more a factor of historical interest or its inclusion in the automated electrolyte series. Serum chloride was the first electrolyte that could be easily measured, and clinical laboratories established and used chloride tests long before sodium, potassium, or pH measurements were available. Emphasis on the "chloride shift" as a discrete, physiological, compensatory measure rather than using the shift of other ions (i.e., hydrogen, sodium, potassium) is based on that fact. It must, however, be included in electrolyte studies if the purpose is to detect the presence of unmeasured anions (the "anion gap"; see Appendix A). Even though measurement of serum chloride levels may not be essential, it is not unimportant, particularly when assessing acid-base balance.

    Chloride is the most plentiful of the extracellular anions. Eighty percent of the total body chloride is in the ECF, and chloride constitutes two thirds of the anions in the plasma; however, its actual concentration is greater in the lymph and interstitial fluid than in the plasma. Although its intracellular amount is very low, it is believed to be significant because it is found in highly specialized cells (e.g., nerve cells) (Stroot et al., 1984). The body does not produce any chloride. It is fully derived from exogenous sources, yet increased amounts ingested will affect the serum levels only slightly (Howard & Herbold, 1982). Dietary sources of chloride include dairy products, meat, and some vegetables and fruit. The food content of chloride is roughly proportional to the sodium content. Foods high in sodium are also high in chloride. Exact daily minimum requirements of chloride have not been established, but the normal adult usually takes in from 60 to 100 mEq daily.

Chloride and sodium usually vary proportionally in the plasma of a healthy person. Serum concentrations of chloride do not vary markedly during development from infant to adult, the highest concentrations being found in the first few months of life. There is no difference between the sexes.

Physiology. Once ingested, chloride appears to be absorbed in the ileum and, in even greater amounts, in the colon in exchange for bicarbonate. The net absorption of chloride from the colon exceeds that of sodium. Absorption is not an active process. Chloride seems to be absorbed as a paired ion with sodium. Absorption of ingested chloride is almost total (Tietz, 1990). If there is inadequate chloride available, bicarbonate will be absorbed with sodium. Chloride's functions in the body include a principal role, with sodium, in the regulation of osmotic pressure and water distribution. One of its major solo functions is as an integral part of the production of hydrochloric acid for digestion. The serum level will actually decrease about 2 mEq/L at the height of gastric secretion. Almost twice the amount of chloride found in the serum is actually secreted for this purpose only, and then it is reabsorbed. Chloride plays a role in acid-base balance because it combines with sodium in competition with bicarbonate. It also acts as a coenzyme for digestive amylases (Howard & Herbold, 1982).

Chloride is regulated secondarily to the sodium concentration. Usually, about 90 percent is excreted in urine, the rest in feces and sweat. The rate at which it is excreted depends on the amount ingested and the presence of adequate fluid. It is reabsorbed in the renal tubules under the indirect control of aldosterone and in response to the pH of the ECF—chloride being excreted and bicarbonate reabsorbed when the pH is low and vice versa.

Pathophysiology. Changes in chloride concentration, when proportionate to changes in Na^+ concentrations, indicate variations in fluid balance. (The pathophysiology is discussed with plasma sodium.) When chloride concentrations change independently of the serum sodium content, the situation is usually one of acid-base imbalance. A loss of chloride requires an increase in serum bicarbonate to maintain the total concentration of anions in the ECF and to combine with sodium. (The total anions of the ECF must always equal the total cations.) This state is called hypochloremic metabolic alkalosis. Increased retention or ingestion (as with chloride-based drugs) of chloride ions leads to a commensurate excretion of bicarbonate in the urine, which in turn leads to a decrease in the concentration of the base bicarbonate and a state of hyperchloremic metabolic acidosis.

In hypochloremia, greater amounts of sodium are reabsorbed secondary to increased aldosterone concentrations in the tubules (decreased chloride levels assumes decreased sodium because they are usually paired). Bicarbonate is reabsorbed with the sodium in the absence of chloride, which increases the base content of the body—metabolic alkalosis. Sodium will be reabsorbed in preference to potassium or even hydrogen, despite the increasing alkalosis. If the serum potassium concentration is low, the hydrogen ion is the major cation excreted, potassium being given priority for reabsorption. This leads to an acidic urine with hypokalemic, hypochloremic alkalosis. The renal compensatory mechanism does not function. Excretion of chloride decreases when serum levels are decreased unless aldosterone secretion has not been simulated, as in adrenal cortical insufficiency. Respiratory compensation for metabolic alkalosis attempts to increase the hydrogen concentration by retaining carbonic acid through decreasing the rate and depth of respirations.

SERUM CHLORIDE LEVELS DECREASED IN:

1. Conditions causing respiratory acidosis such as pulmonary emphysema, pneumonia, pneumothorax, pulmonary edema, and hypoventilation secondary to poliomyelitis, anesthesia, or other restrictive conditions. The decrease is due to increased excretion of chloride to compensate for increased anion levels in the serum (bicarbonate)
2. Conditions causing a decreased intake of chloride such as starvation or a severely restricted intake of sodium chloride in the treatment of heart, kidney, or liver disease
3. Conditions leading to an increased loss of chloride such as
   a. Vomiting, especially in the case of pyloric obstruction
   b. Nasogastric suctioning. As in item a, gastric secretions are lost that contain much greater concentrations of chloride than sodium because of the loss of hydrochloric acid
   c. Diarrhea secondary to bacterial infections, which decreases the transit time of nutrients in the colon and thus decreases the absorption of the major part of ingested chloride
   d. Diarrhea secondary to either congenital (rare) or acquired chloridorrhea. It is thought that the accompanying potassium deficit in chloridorrhea may affect the permeability of the intestinal mucosa and interrupt the chloride bicarbonate exchange. The acquired form of chloridorrhea is characterized by an inability to absorb chloride adequately. The increased concentration of chloride in the feces further increases the diarrhea because it acts as an osmotic cathartic (Sodeman & Sodeman, 1982)
   e. Excessive use of diuretics (mercurial or chlorothiazide), which act to reduce sodium reabsorption and, indirectly, chloride reabsorption (Collins, 1975)
   f. Addison's disease, with a marked decrease during addisonian crisis because of the loss of aldosterone stimulation of sodium reabsorption and with it the indirect stimulation of chloride reabsorption
   g. Primary aldosteronism because of an increase in serum bicarbonate levels secondary to the increase in sodium retention and the resultant metabolic alkalosis
   h. Chronic pyelonephritis because of a lack of tubular reabsorption despite a serum deficit of chloride. (All conditions listed thus far can lead to metabolic alkalosis)
   i. Diabetic ketoacidosis, even in the face of hemoconcentration, because of chloride loss in osmotic diuresis, vomiting, gastric dilation, paralytic ileus, and the return of sodium to the blood as sodium bicarbonate rather than as sodium chloride in an attempt to maintain acid-base balance. In other metabolic acidotic states the chloride level may be

lower than would be expected because other negative ions, acetate, phosphate, or lactic acid are present

4. Hypokalemic metabolic alkalosis. A severe decrease in the serum chloride content itself can lead to or maintain a hypokalemic alkalosis as well as follow it. A decrease in the availability of chloride ions to pair with sodium as anions leads to a decrease in sodium reabsorption. The compensatory mechanism causes an increase in the excretion of potassium in the urine in exchange for sodium with bicarbonate reabsorption (Jones et al., 1982)

5. Conditions leading to the retention of fluid in the vascular space, which causes a dilutional rather than an actual decrease (see "Serum Sodium Levels Decreased In" in Section 1.1). Conditions such as acute renal failure with urine suppression and congestive heart failure are examples

SERUM CHLORIDE LEVELS INCREASED IN:

1. Conditions leading to intravascular fluid decrease with a relative rather than an actual increase in chloride levels in the serum (see "Serum Sodium Levels Increased In" in Section 1.1)

2. Some forms of metabolic acidosis such as that secondary to drug poisoning (salicylate) or renal tubular acidosis because of a primary deficiency of the base bicarbonate

3. Excessive treatment with chloride medication such as ammonium chloride

4. Primary hypoparathyroidism (40–50 percent of cases) in the absence of vomiting, diarrhea, or diuretic use (Ravel, 1989).

IMPLICATIONS FOR NURSING: SERUM CHLORIDE

1. Prevention of metabolic alkalosis is frequently possible, and therefore identification of individuals at risk for hypokalemia or hypochloremia is an important first step (see "Implications for Nursing" in Section 1.3). Any patient who has a nasogastric tube in place and functioning, has been vomiting, has a dietary restriction in sodium and thereby is restricted in chloride intake, has diarrhea, is receiving diuretics that are not potassium sparing and is not receiving supplemental potassium, or has an adrenal dysfunction, should be considered at risk for hypochloremia and thus at risk for metabolic alkalosis

2. Closely monitor the plasma potassium and CO_2 content (or combining power or venous CO_2 direct measurement), indicating bicarbonate or base concentrations, for a possible decrease, and compare them to serum chloride levels in the populations at risk. Arterial blood gases are not routinely ordered and are usually not necessary to monitor these individuals adequately

3. Check for signs and symptoms of metabolic alkalosis
   a. Complaints of circumoral numbness and tingling
   b. Hypertonicity of musculature
   c. Decreased rate and depth of respirations
   d. Alkaline urine (other causes for alkalinity must be taken into account such as immobility or the tendency toward sodium conservation and thus extracellular alkalosis after surgery)
   e. Complaints of nervousness or other signs of central nervous system stimulation
   f. Indications of tetany resulting from the binding of calcium to protein in metabolic alkalotic states
      (1) Trousseau's and Chvoestek's signs: carpopedal spasm with constriction of the upper arm musculature as with a tourniquet; twitching of the facial muscles in response to a tapping of the seventh cranial—the facial—nerve at the angle of the jaw in front of the ear

       (2) Complaints of numbness or tingling of the extremities

4. Ensure replacement of chloride as well as potassium in preventative electrolyte therapy for risk populations or when metabolic alkalosis is present. Potassium chloride can be given. Small amounts are effective.
   a. Call attention to the need for chloride if it is not being given
   b. If the individual is allowed oral intake and sodium chloride is not contraindicated, provide salty foods to replace chloride by diet. Recall that most of the chloride ingested is absorbed
5. After treatment for metabolic alkalosis the nurse should assess for laboratory outcomes indicating success; for example, serum chloride and potassium levels increase to within normal limits, the venous CO_2 concentration decreases to within normal limits, urine pH becomes acid (i.e., 6 or lower). Recall, however, that urine pH is not a good indicator of response in hypokalemic metabolic alkalosis. It may be acid even at the height of alkalemia. Response to therapy would be indicated by an initial increase in pH as the bicarbonate begins to be excreted
6. Any person at risk for or diagnosed as having a fluid imbalance is equally at risk for chloride imbalance. The nursing implications are identical (see "Implications for Nursing" in Section 1.1)
7. In children a positive serum chloride balance is particularly important to expand the ECF compartment. Therefore, all children should be considered risk populations for chloride imbalance
8. Mature adults and the aged should be considered risk populations because
   a. Renal response to pH changes is less precise and imbalances occur more rapidly
   b. Anemia is a frequent accompaniment of age (for many reasons) and thus a major buffering system would be depleted (i.e., the chloride shift of hemoglobin)
   c. Pulmonary function is frequently compromised in the elderly and this will interfere with both carbon dioxide elimination and the ability to maintain adequate oxygen blood levels, which would seriously interfere with respiratory compensation for metabolic alkalosis
9. Patient teaching about specific preventative measures in risk populations is an important and often neglected nursing responsibility. Content, including appropriate electrolyte replacement in conditions causing chloride loss, and assessments the individual can make to check the effectiveness of electrolyte replacement should be covered

1.3 SERUM POTASSIUM

Normal Ranges (mEq/L)[a]

Adult	3.5–5.5
Senior adult	
Male	3.5–5.6
Female	3.5–5.2
Pediatric	
Premature (cord)	5.0–10.2
to 7 days	3.5–6.0
Premature (48 hr)	3.0–6.0
Newborn (cord)	5.6–12.0 (3.5 to 6.0 to 7th day after birth)
Newborn	5.0–7.7
Infant	4.1–5.3
Child	3.5–4.7
Thereafter	3.4–5.6

[a]Levels in serum tend to be 0.4–0.5 mEq/L higher than whole blood or plasma (Ravel, 1989).

Definition. The screening test for potassium (the major intracellular cation) measures the concentration of potassium in the plasma. Sampling of plasma rather than serum is recommended by many laboratories because there is a release of potassium during blood clotting and the serum potassium level will be falsely elevated. Plasma potassium is more stable and used for plasma determinations. Potassium is the major cation of the intracellular fluid (ICF); close to 90 percent of total body potassium is in the ICF. Potassium plays an essential role in maintenance of excitability in both nerve and muscle tissue. A proper balance among potassium, sodium, and calcium is highly important for all muscular function but imperative to cardiac muscle function.

Potassium exerts effects on almost all cellular metabolism. In carbohydrate metabolism, a decreased potassium level causes a decrease in glucose uptake in the liver. In protein metabolism, growth retardation occurs secondary to decreased potassium levels because there is a potassium-dependent step in protein synthesis. Enzyme reactions of adenosine triphosphate (ATP), coenzyme A, and adenosine diphosphate (ADP) all depend on potassium for part of their activation.

Potassium must be ingested daily because the body does not store it in any large amounts. Either an increase or a decrease in potassium levels may precipitate physiological problems.

1.3.1 Hyperkalemia

Definition. Hyperkalemia is defined as a plasma level of greater than 5.5 mEq/L. With adequate renal function it is virtually impossible to maintain a state of hyperkalemia because potassium is so readily excreted by the kidney (Stroot et al., 1984). A significant potassium increase is found primarily in severe renal failure with azotemia. Increased plasma levels of potassium occur much less frequently than do decreased levels (Sodeman & Sodeman, 1982).

Physiology. There is a constant exchange between extracellular sodium and intracellular potassium. With an increase in extracellular potassium levels, the membrane potential is decreased, and the cell becomes highly excitable. As a result, there is increased irritability of all nerve and muscle cells. This is not a steady state, and in a short time the cell activity is exhausted, thereby resulting in muscle weakness and flaccid paralysis.

The compensatory mechanism to increased extracellular potassium levels is increased renal excretion and decreased reabsorption of potassium in the colon, both in response to aldosterone. An increase in the extracellular potassium content promptly stimulates aldosterone release so that more sodium and less potassium will be reabsorbed by the kidney. The ratio of reabsorption of sodium and potassium is usually 2:1 in favor of sodium (Swedish Hospital Medical Center [SHMC], 1984).

SERUM POTASSIUM LEVELS INCREASED IN:

1. Any condition causing severe oliguria or anuria, for example, states of renal failure with azotemia. A not uncommon cause of death in renal failure is potassium intoxication (potassium levels above 7 mEq/L) leading to cardiac arrest (Sodeman & Sodeman, 1982). Even with no potassium intake, it is probable that potassium levels will increase secondarily to tissue catabolism in renal failure. Congestive heart failure with decreased cardiac

output is a frequent cause of prerenal kidney failure and results in oliguria and increased plasma potassium levels

2. Chronic adrenal insufficiency (Addison's disease) with a diminished aldosterone output can lead to increased serum potassium levels. Untreated adrenal insufficiency is a contraindication for giving potassium

3. In the first 24 hours after severe burns, hyperkalemia is marked because of the release of large amounts of potassium into the circulation from burned tissue. This situation is reversed in the next stage of the burn injury course, that of diuresis as edema fluid is remobilized into circulation. Crushing injuries increase serum potassium levels in much the same way

4. Excess administration of potassium, especially with an inadequate urinary output, can lead to hyperkalemia. Excess ingestion may be due to a lack of knowledge on the part of the person taking potassium-containing medications. Too rapid or an excess intravenous administration of potassium is a fairly frequent cause of increased levels

5. A transitory state of hyperkalemia occurs after strenuous exercise. Potassium leaves the cell after muscle use because of the sodium-potassium exchange in cellular contraction. This plus lactic acidosis is believed to be the cause of muscular fatigue and pain (Kee, 1990). A similar process may account for the transitory increase in potassium levels found after convulsions

6. Defective potassium secretion resulting from tubular defects has been found to occur at times with pyelonephritis

7. Overuse of aldosterone antagonist diuretics (e.g., spironolactone) can lead to a hyperkalemic state because of increased reabsorption of potassium by the kidney

8. False increases in plasma potassium levels can occur and are related to states of venous stasis resulting from a combination of tourniquet compression and muscular activity before venipuncture (repeated fist clenching to "bring up the veins"). False increases are also found in patients with thrombocytosis or leukemia. This increase is thought to be due to the release of potassium from platelets or white blood cells (WBCs) in the clotting process after the blood is removed from the body

1.3.2 Hypokalemia

Definition. Hypokalemia is defined as a serum level of less than 3.5 mEq/L. Syndromes of potassium deficit are relatively common. If potassium deficiency is sufficiently severe, both functional and actual structural changes occur in the kidney (Sodeman & Sodeman, 1982), which perpetuate fluid, electrolyte, and acid-base imbalances.

Physiology. When serum potassium is depleted for whatever cause, the resting cell membrane potential is increased. During excitation, potassium should move out of the cell to replace the deficit, and sodium should move inward to maintain the electrolyte balance, thus depolarizing the membrane. But because of the decrease in extracellular potassium levels, the resting membrane potential (the ratio between intracellular and extracellular potassium) is increased, and the cell is less excitable. Muscular weakness and atony are hallmarks of potassium deficit.

Even with serum potassium depletion, however, the ratio between intracellular and extracellular potassium is not always out of balance, and the classic signs and symptoms may not occur. Slowly developing potassium depletion may allow time for both compartments to experience commensurate drops, and the resting potential of the cell membrane would be close to normal.

Mechanisms to compensate for potassium depletion are not fully known, but suppression of renal tubular cell secretion is thought to occur. This mechanism is less prompt and certainly less effective than the mechanism for sodium control. In part, this decrease in effectiveness is due to the fact that conditions leading to a potassium deficit often stimulate aldosterone secretion, which causes potassium loss (Sodeman & Sodeman, 1982). Even when the potassium intake is reduced to nothing, the urine excretion of it will still be at least 5 to 20 mEq over 24 hours. Therefore, potassium depletion will occur if its intake is less than 5 to 20 mEq/day or when potassium losses occur from extrarenal sources (e.g., excessive loss in feces). Potassium excretion varies with diet but usually ranges between 26 and 123 mEq/24 hr. The amount would be higher in infants because the immaturity of their kidneys would result in decreased reabsorption.

Alkalotic states tend to perpetuate potassium deficits because potassium is excreted in exchange for hydrogen in the kidney and potassium shifts into the cell in exchange for hydrogen.

Periods of stress favor excretion of potassium secondary to the increased secretion of steroids, notably aldosterone and cortisone.

SERUM POTASSIUM LEVELS DECREASED IN:

1. Diarrhea states. Potassium is normally secreted into the colon in large quantities. The amount of this unbound potassium that will be reabsorbed depends on (a) the rapidity with which it transits the colon; and (b) the amount of aldosterone activity, since the colon is sensitive to steroid hormones in a manner similar to the kidney. A frequent cause of diarrhea in older adults has been laxative abuse. In children the more frequent cause is infection, viral or bacterial
2. Large losses of gastrointestinal fluids. This may be due to prolonged vomiting, gastrointestinal suctioning (primarily intestinal), a fistula, or ileostomy drainage
3. Massive diuresis or continuous, prolonged diuresis. Potassium is lost in proportion to the diuresis. Diuresis occurs for a number of reasons
   a. Administration of diuretics over a prolonged period without adequate follow-up to determine electrolyte levels or without adequate electrolyte replacement. This can occur because of a lack of knowledge on the part of the patient about the need for potassium replacement in the diet or a lack of follow-through on the part of the health care team
   b. Glycosuria with concomitant, obligatory loss of water and electrolytes
   c. The diuretic stage of burns (usually 24 to 48 hours after the injury)
   d. The diuretic phase of acute renal failure
4. Postoperative patients with multiple losses of potassium. Potassium deficits can occur secondary to cellular trauma with the loss of intracellular potassium (surgical trauma); increased catabolism of cells for nutritional needs that is due, in part at least, to the n.p.o. state of most surgical patients; gastrointestinal surgery in which patients frequently encounter stress postoperatively; and nasogastric suction, causing alkalosis, which favors potassium loss
5. Patients after treatment for diabetic ketoacidosis. The administration of insulin drives glucose and potassium into the cell. Usually, this has been preceded by a loss of potassi-

um in osmotic diuresis that is secondary to an increase in extracellular potassium in exchange for hydrogen at that time

6. Stress response. An increased secretion of steroid hormones is a major part of the stress response. Steroids favor sodium retention to serum chloride levels in the populations at risk. Test for blood and potassium loss, as discussed. Vomiting, diarrhea, or anorexia can also occur secondarily to stress (see Appendix B)

7. Lack of an adequate intake of potassium (anorexia, lack of potassium-rich foods in the diet, starvation). This can occur as a response to illness or as an effect of inadequate finances. Patients at risk include the unconscious patient

8. Endocrine diseases such as Cushing's syndrome and primary aldosteronism. The increase in corticosteroid production favors potassium loss

9. Malabsorption syndromes where the gut is not able to absorb nutrients. Malabsorption occurs in cystic fibrosis and adult-onset sprue as well as many other conditions

10. Inappropriate use of enemas. This has not been a frequent cause of potassium loss in recent years, but it cannot be overlooked. The use of multiple enemas before diagnostic procedures (enemas until clear), particularly in a patient at risk for electrolyte imbalance, could induce rather rapid hypokalemia. Enema fluid, if not expelled from the body, can be absorbed through the bowel wall, thereby diluting the potassium in the interstitial space and ultimately all ECF. Hypertonic enemas can damage bowel mucosa and lead to an increased potassium loss in feces

---

IMPLICATIONS FOR NURSING: SERUM POTASSIUM

1. The nurse can make a most useful contribution to community health by helping to prevent the occurrence of potassium imbalances because many if not most are preventable
2. Prevent hyperkalemia by
   a. Identifying persons at risk (see "Serum Potassium Levels Increased in")
   b. Preventing false increases by discouraging the "hand pump" method of vein distention for venipuncture. Use warm arm or hand packs instead
   c. Ensuring that patients receiving glucocorticoid therapy (e.g., those with Addison's disease) do not abruptly discontinue the use of drugs
   d. Ensuring that persons receiving potassium supplements have plasma levels checked appropriately, perhaps once a month if they are otherwise stable
   e. Monitoring both potassium and sodium levels in the patient at risk for potassium imbalance
   f. Teaching high-risk patients self-care by
      (1) Identifying and correcting their lack of knowledge about potassium-rich foods
      (2) Providing information about the approximate potassium content of such foods
      (3) Helping the patient and home caretaker to plan the diet by calculating the proper potassium intake so as not to exceed the personal intake limit
   g. Protecting any patient receiving intravenous potassium from hyperkalemia. Administer slowly, never in undiluted or concentrated form, at no more than 20 mEq/hr unless by direct, written physician order and, even then, not unless the patient has a cardiac monitor. Usually, only peripheral lines are used for potassium infusion. If a central line is used, monitoring of administration is particularly important, since there is less opportunity for dilution of the potassium. Plasma potassium levels exceeding 7 mEq/L may cause fatal arrhythmias as they reach the heart (Luckmann & Sorensen, 1987). Slow or discontinue the potassium infusion if redness, swelling, or a complaint of burning occurs at the infusion site. Never "speed up" a potassium infusion, ex-

cept by direct written order. The urine output must be at a minimum of 30 ml/hr for 24 hours for potassium administration

h. Placing any patient at risk for potassium imbalance on strict intake and output

i. Observing for and preventing metabolic acidosis

3. Protect patients with hyperkalemia by

a. Providing monitoring (cardiac), if possible

b. Observing for pulse irregularity or slowing (bradycardia)

c. Observing for electrocardiographic (ECG) changes. The following depicts the progression of changes that may be found in untreated hyperkalemia

    (1) The amplitude (vertical) of T waves increases with a narrowed base and peaking (commonly occurs in humans when the plasma K^+ reaches about 7 mEq/L)

    (2) The amplitude of R and S waves increases

    (3) Atrioventricular and intraventricular block occurs

    (4) Loss of P waves—atrial arrest at a plasma K^+ of about 9 mEq/L

    (5) Depression of the ST segment (obliteration of the segment with the T wave originating from the S)

    (6) Spread of QRS and T waves into a smooth biphasic curve (sine wave) (plasma K^+ level about 10 mEq/L or above [Sodeman & Sodeman, 1982])

d. Assessing for ascending muscular weakness, which can progress to flaccid quadraplegia

e. Being alert for complaints of dyspnea (air hunger), which signifies respiratory paralysis

f. Providing fresh blood, if possible, for transfusions. The breakdown of older blood cells releases potassium

g. Ensuring that patients in acute renal failure are adequately and promptly dialyzed. Sudden death occurs frequently in patients with anuria of 1 week's duration because of potassium intoxication and cardiac arrest (Sodeman & Sodeman, 1982)

h. Teaching the patient/family/home caretaker the purpose of medical treatment to decrease anxiety and increase cooperation and compliance

    (1) The physician may opt to use calcium infusions as rapidly effective therapy in emergency situations where the sine wave has appeared and there is no time to decrease the potassium level. Increased calcium levels antagonize the effects of hyperkalemia on the cardiac membrane. Hypocalcemia intensifies the problem

        (a) This therapy should not be used in patients taking digitalis, since digitalis intoxication can be precipitated with even a moderate reduction in the serum potassium concentration

        (b) Once begun, the treatment with calcium must be continued until the potassium imbalance has been corrected (Brunner & Suddarth, 1988)

    (2) Intravenous glucose with insulin is often given as a treatment in moderately severe hyperkalemia that does not warrant calcium. Potassium will shift into the cells with the glucose and insulin, and plasma potassium levels will decrease by as much as 1 to 2 mEq/L. This decrease will persist for several hours. Nondiabetic patients may not require insulin

    (3) Hypertonic sodium, such as in the form of sodium bicarbonate with isotonic saline, is given intravenously to patients with hyperkalemia to increase the renal excretion of potassium and cause alkalosis, which drives potassium into the cells. Potassium levels will be decreased because of dilution as well as the increased renal excretion of potassium. Lactate or bicarbonate may be given if the hyperkalemia exists concurrently with acidosis

    (4) Polystyrene sulfonate (hypertonic kayexalate) can be given by mouth or as a retention enema for the patient unable to take oral fluids. Kayexalate is an exchange resin that removes excess potassium from the blood through the colon in exchange for sodium and hydrogen. The patient will need to be encouraged to retain the enema fluid. Many kits come equipped with a flanged tube that, when blocked after administration of the enema, helps retain the solution in the patient who is unable to do so

    (5) Debridement of necrotic tissue such as after a burn or crushing injury may be necessary to decrease the amount of potassium being released into the system from the injured and

dead cells. Measures to prevent decubitus should be undertaken to prevent necrosis and increased potassium release

4. Prevent hypokalemia by
   a. Identifying persons at risk (see "Serum Potassium Levels Decreased in")
   b. Assessing for signs and symptoms of a deficit, with particular attention to the sequence of occurrence in an attempt to help differentiate from long-term hyperkalemia. Hypokalemia causes the following problems not seen in prolonged hyperkalemia: complaints of muscle pain, hyporeflexia, fairly early nausea and vomiting, paralytic ileus, and orthostatic hypotension
   c. Monitoring intake and output
   d. Checking serum potassium levels frequently. If the patient has several risk factors (e.g., receives diuretics, has intestinal drainage, is n.p.o., and is without replacement of electrolytes), at least weekly levels should be available. If not, collaborate with the physician
   e. Being aware of potassium available in foods and teaching the patient/family/home caretaker in menu planning to include foods high in potassium (see item 2f)
   f. Checking whether a salt substitute is made with potassium for a patient who is also receiving a low-salt diet. If not, check with the physician as to the advisability of change
   g. Being aware of the availability of potassium-sparing diuretics (spironolactone [Aldactone], triamterene [Dyrenium]) that can be used in place of or in conjunction with thiazide diuretics
   h. Monitoring other electrolyte levels important in the maintenance or assessment of potassium levels; for example, chloride, because a decrease in chloride levels perpetuates the potassium deficit; serum sodium, because decreased levels foster potassium loss; and urinary potassium to evaluate the effectiveness of interventions. A return to normal concentrations of potassium in a 24-hour urine specimen indicates successful treatment
   i. Requesting ounce-for-ounce and milliequivalent-for-milliequivalent replacement for any losses through gastric or intestinal suction
   j. Collaborating with the physician or x-ray department to find alternatives to multiple enemas before diagnostic testing in the patient at risk for hypokalemia or making sure that serum levels are monitored
   k. Being alert for signs and symptoms of metabolic alkalosis that could cause or be due to decreased potassium levels

5. Protect the patient with hypokalemia by
   a. Observing closely for signs of digitalis intoxication in the hypokalemic patient taking the drug. Even a moderate decrease in potassium levels can enhance the effect of digitalis and precipitate a toxic state
   b. Checking serum digitalis levels if available and assessing for signs and symptoms of digitalis intoxication. These are not unlike symptoms of hypokalemia, so it is necessary to be alert for complaints of vision changes—colored vision—which are symptoms more specific to digitalis intoxication. Pure glycosides are thought to produce fewer of the early gastrointestinal symptoms and thus give less warning of intoxication
   c. Instructing the patient on oral potassium supplements concerning side effects and measures to be taken to alleviate or prevent the side effects. The major side effect is gastric irritation
      (1) Prevention
         (a) With the exception of "controlled-release" preparations such as Slow-K, which should not be dissolved, dilute with cold water or orange juice any potassium, whether liquid, powder, or effervescent tablet. Dissolve completely
         (b) Instruct the patient to sip slowly and to take the medication either with meals or immediately after meals
      (2) Symptoms to be reported to physician
         (a) Abdominal pain
         (b) Nausea, vomiting
         (c) Distention
         (d) Evidence of gastrointestinal bleeding (tarry stools, hematemesis)

1.4 SERUM GLUCOSE

Synonyms: Blood glucose or sugar, plasma glucose or sugar

Normal Ranges (mg/dl)[a]

Adult	
1 hour p.c.	60–140 mg
Younger than 50 (fasting for 2 hours p.c. and random)[b]	60–110
Older than 50 (fasting for 2 hours p.c. and random)	60–125
Senior adult (fasting for 2 hours p.c.)	
Male	52–135
Female	58–135
Pediatric (fasting for 2 hours p.c.)	
Premature	20–60
Newborn	20–110
Child	60–100

[a]Normal ranges for tests done on whole blood as opposed to serum or plasma will vary, usually being somewhat lower.
[b]p.c.: "postcibum"—after eating.

Definition and Physiology. Glucose is the principal body fuel and is obtained primarily from the diet but can be produced by the body's own metabolism. Sugars other than glucose are usually converted to glucose within the body, as are most carbohydrates that are ingested. Simple sugars such as glucose are used quickly, but other nutrients such as proteins, when ingested in greater quantity than needed, are gradually converted to glycogen and stored in the liver to be used to maintain normal serum glucose levels between meals. The maintenance of normal fasting serum levels depends on the interaction of a number of body structures, among them the liver, peripheral tissues, and hormones, all of which act to raise or lower serum glucose levels. The kidneys are also capable of gluconeogenesis. They can synthesize up to 10 percent of the liver's capability. Because serum glucose levels generally become abnormal only when there is a serious disruption of this interaction, checking the serum glucose level helps evaluate the function and integrity of this system. Two measurements of serum glucose, the *fasting glucose test* and the *2-hour postprandial test* (after meals, or *postcibum*, after eating, usually written as serum glucose 2-hr p.p. or p.c.), have been found to be most useful as screening tests and will be discussed here. A third, *random glucose measurement,* which is done without any preparation of the individual being tested, has been found to be of little value clinically because the results may vary so widely, depending on the intake or lack of intake of food before obtaining the blood sample.

The **fasting glucose test** roughly evaluates the body's ability to regulate glucose and provides information about the kind of abnormality, if one occurs. No food or drink, other than water, is given for 8 hours before the blood sample is taken.

The **2-hour p.c. test** is a simple screening test to demonstrate the ability of the body to adjust to and dispose of a glucose load. A fasting blood sample is usually drawn first. The person is then given approximately 100 g of glucose by diet or in a solution, and a second blood sample is drawn exactly 2 hours later. If both values are within the normal limits, the mechanism is considered normal. If the blood value has not returned to the upper limit of normal in the 2-hour p.c. sample, the mechanism is considered abnormal, and further testing may be necessary to identify the precise nature of the problem. Some authorities feel that the use of an intravenous glucose load is more accurate than oral administration and that indications for the oral test are few (Scipien & Barnard, 1983).

1.4.1 Hyperglycemia

Definition. Hyperglycemia is defined simply as an excess of glucose in the blood above the upper range of normal for a given age. Although increases in fasting serum glucose levels are most frequently related to the presence of diabetes mellitus, the number of diseases and physiological conditions that can result in major increases is vast, and the nurse should be alert to the need to assess for cause. Also, it is well for the nurse to be aware that although a normal fasting blood glucose level rules out an active and acute diabetic problem, it does not rule out the diagnosis of diabetes mellitus. Only 30 to 40 percent of diabetics can be diagnosed by fasting serum glucose levels. The 2-hour p.c. test is an excellent screening test for diabetes, however, with levels above 160 mg/dl usually being considered diagnostic. (The glycosylated hemoglobin level frequently replaces the 2-hour p.c. glucose level as the most useful screening test. See Section 7.4.2.)

Physiology. Serum glucose levels are maintained by several different processes in the body. Absorption of all sugars from the small intestine is rapid, with glucose being immediately available in the bloodstream. The liver is extremely important in the control of blood glucose levels. It synthesizes glucose to glycogen and fat when uptake is excessive (glycogenesis), or when the supply is low, the liver can convert the glycogen to glucose (glycogenolysis) as well as synthesize glucose from some of the amino acids or from the glycerol of fat breakdown (gluconeogenesis).

The liver also converts other forms of sugar to glucose, as does the intestine. Glucose is preferred to fat or protein for energy supply, but when insulin is insufficient, fat is mobilized. The action of liver regulation is influenced by several hormones, including and primarily insulin. These are thyroid, adrenocortical hormones (glucocorticoids in particular), epinephrine, and glucagon. Glucagon promotes glucose production and control of glucose storage, which includes both stimulation of glucose synthesis in the liver (glucogenesis) and the breakdown of glycogen to glucose (glycogenolysis). Measurement of glucagon is important in the diagnosis of alpha cell tumors of the pancreas.*

To be properly used, glucose must enter the cell, and for this, insulin is required. Normally, very little glucose is excreted in the urine, usually a maximum of 0.5 to 0.75 g over 24 hours. If serum glucose levels exceed 170 mg/dl, the level of the renal threshold for glucose, excretion increases. Table 1–2 gives a brief overview of the roles played by hormones in glucose regulation. All of these roles can be triggered by physiological activities such as exercise or nervous excitement.

SERUM GLUCOSE LEVELS INCREASED IN:

1. Stress response: potential result of acute trauma, anoxia, hypoglycemia, severe exercise, hemorrhage, severe pain, emotional excitement, or exposure to extreme heat or cold. In

---

*Glucagon normal serum levels, plasma (pg/ml): Healthy adults (fasting): 50–150; hypoglycemia: two- to threefold increase; hyperglycemia: decrease of 50% from normal; pancreatic alpha cell tumor: 900–7800 (Henry, 1991, p. 174).

TABLE 1-2. ROLES OF HORMONES IN GLUCOSE REGULATION

Hormone	Action	Result
Insulin	Facilitates transfer of glucose across cell membrane for all cells except brain cells	Decreases blood glucose
Thyroid[a]	Stimulates intestinal and renal absorption of glucose	Increases blood glucose
	Increases metabolic rate, thus increasing utilization of glucose in the periphery	Decreases blood glucose
Glucocorticoids	Mobilize protein and fat stores and influence hepatic gluconeogenesis; thought to decrease the cell's ability to use glucose	Increase blood glucose Increase blood glucose
Epinephrine	Influences conversion of glycogen to glucose in both liver and muscle (glycogenolysis); blocks insulin release	Increases blood glucose
	Increases glucose uptake in tissue cells	Decreases blood glucose
Glucagon	Promotes conversion of glycogen to glucose in the liver	Increases blood glucose
Growth hormone	Believed to reduce the rate of glucose utilization in the cells	Increases blood glucose
	May also increase insulin resistance of cells and lead to destruction of beta cells of the pancreas (this is not well understood)	Increases blood glucose

[a]The two responses given are dependent on the concentration of hormone in the serum.
Data from Carnevali & Patrick, 1979; Collins, 1975; and Sabiston, 1981.

the first few hours of stress response, liver glycogen is broken down to glucose, which is released to the blood and raises the serum glucose concentration. The rate of glucose production is usually increased, and hyperglycemia results. With continued stress and in the absence of an adequate intake of glucose to meet metabolic needs, fat is mobilized from depot stores and converted by hydrolysis to free fatty acids (FFAs) and glycerol. Finally, protein is oxidized when glycogen stores are depleted. The rise in serum glucose levels is unaccompanied by an appropriate rise in insulin, probably related to the concomitant rise in epinephrine production in response to stress (Sabiston, 1981), which maintains the hyperglycemia. Increased serum glucose levels that are secondary to stress can be seen in myocardial infarct, cerebral infarct, some malignancies, gestational diabetes (carbohydrate metabolism would be normal between pregnancies; the increase in glucose during pregnancies may be totally stress related), after acute injury and fright, as in automobile accidents, and with surgery. Levels as high as 400 mg/dl have been found in some individuals during anesthesia despite normal carbohydrate metabolism (Laboratory of Pathology, 1991); see Appendix B

2. Cushing's disease or any condition that will increase glucocorticoid secretion due to increased gluconeogenesis and decreased peripheral use of glucose. All the eleven oxygenated adrenocortical hormones act in a manner directly opposite to that of insulin

3. Diabetes mellitus, usually because of a lack of insulin, but can be due to a lack of effective insulin (insulin resistance). Fasting blood glucose levels over 150 mg/dl are highly suggestive of diabetes mellitus. Levels found in diabetic ketoacidosis/coma are usually between 400 and 800 mg/dl. Values higher than 800 mg/dl are suggestive of concomitant renal failure (Laboratory of Pathology, 1991)

4. Acromegaly because of insulin resistance and decreased cellular use of glucose. Usually, both the fasting and the 2-hour p.c. values are increased

5. Hyperthyroidism because of increased absorption of glucose and other carbohydrates from the gut. Peripheral use of glucose is increased, which leads to a normal serum glucose concentration in some individuals, but the 2-hour p.c. level will be increased (see Table 1–2)

6. Pheochromocytoma because of the increased secretion of epinephrine in which insulin release may be blocked and glucogenolysis increased. Again, the fasting value of glucose may be normal, but the 2-hour p.c. test result will be elevated

7. Chronic pancreatitis, an unusual finding, however, because of a reduction in insulin production secondary to destruction of the islet cells of the pancreas. There may also be a slight decrease in glucose uptake in the liver and decreased cellular use

8. Administration of some drugs (e.g., the chlorothiazide diuretics) because of the suppression of insulin release—mechanism unknown—and (dilantin) because of a membrane-stabilizing effect on the pancreas, inhibits effective insulin release (Govoni & Hayes, 1985)

9. Postsurgical patients temporarily, partially because of the hyperglycemic properties of the stress response (see item 1), but frequently resulting more directly from the intravenous infusion of dextrose, which is often run rapidly in an attempt to replace lost fluid volume and depleted stores of glucose, thereby causing a slight, temporary increase in serum concentrations

10. Nonketotic, hyperosmolar coma, which usually occurs in the insulin-dependent diabetic because of inadequate insulin secretion for peripheral use of glucose but with adequate secretion to prevent fat breakdown. Serum glucose can reach levels as high as 1000 mg/dl with minimal or negative ketones. This condition is usually triggered by body water loss. Marked hypernatremia is a helpful diagnostic sign

1.4.2 Hypoglycemia

Definition. Hypoglycemia is a disorder characterized by a fasting serum glucose level below the lower range of normal for the age group—less than 46 mg/dl (previously 60 mg/dl) in the adult and an associated group of symptoms that can be relieved by ingesting food or carbohydrates of some form. Symptomatic hypoglycemia usually does not occur until the serum glucose level is 50 mg/dl or lower or when the serum glucose level drops rapidly. Documented, significant hypoglycemia is distinctly uncommon except in certain patient populations. In many instances there seems to be no demonstrable cause for the deficit. The serum glucose level falls after eating (reactive hypoglycemia) and may do so several hours after a meal or exercise. Hypoglycemia may also be symptomatic of a variety of disorders. Newborns frequently show a low serum glucose concentration, which may be asymptomatic unless extremely low. Infants are especially susceptible to hypoglycemia because of their extremely high metabolic rate. Newborns who are not fed by mouth during the first few hours of life are at particular risk. Hypoglycemia also occurs in more than half of the newborns of diabetic mothers and is a frequent cause of seizures in the infant, as are elevated temperature and hypocalcemia. The frequency of its occurrence increases with premature or low-birthweight infants. The stressed infant is also at risk (sepsis, respiratory distress syndrome) (Scipien & Barnard, 1983). The largest population of persons with hypoglycemia, however, are those with no demonstrable cause, so-called functional hypoglycemia (Henry, 1991).

As can be seen by reviewing the physiology of the regulation of serum glucose concentrations, the mechanisms tend to foster increased serum glucose levels.

Physiology. Symptoms of acute hypoglycemia reflect the widespread response in the body as the sympathetic nervous system is activated. Influenced by epinephrine, glycogenolysis is stimulated by a low serum glucose concentration as a compensatory mechanism. When the hypoglycemia is corrected and serum glucose levels rise to the upper range of normal, secretin is released, which in turn stimulates the islet cells of the pancreas to increased insulin production, and the liver output of glucose is inhibited. Again, the carefully integrated mechanism discussed previously for control of the serum glucose concentration is totally involved. If there is pathology of any of the mechanism's areas, an imbalance will occur.

Although glucose is added to the blood from only three sources (intestinal absorption, glycogenolysis, and gluconeogenesis), it is removed from the blood in innumerable ways, all the reductions being essential to the function of the part and the body as a whole. Only when glucose is stored as adipose tissue or lost in the urine is its removal not essential to body function. Levels of urine glucose are usually not indicative of hypoglycemia. The amount found in urine does not correspond in any ratio to the serum level of glucose.

In summary, hypoglycemia occurs in response to both lack of food and ingestion of it, particularly ingestion of high-carbohydrate meals (Sodeman & Sodeman, 1982).

1.4.3 Definitions of Diabetes by Type

Diabetes (General definition): a term referring to a variety of disorders characterized by excessive urination (polyuria), for example:

1. *Brittle diabetes:* Diabetes that is difficult to control and tends to oscillate between hypoglycemia and diabetic ketoacidosis.
2. *Gestational diabetes:* Recognition of impaired glucose tolerance occurring during pregnancy.
3. *Diabetes insipidus:* Urinary output of 2 to 10 liters per day with an increased intake that does not match urine output.
4. *Diabetes insipidus*
   a. *Central (or pituitary):* A metabolic disorder secondary to neurohypophyseal injury which limits the quantity of antidiuretic hormone (ADH/Vasopressin) produced, or released; in turn causing failure of tubular reabsorption of water in the kidney. Causes include infection, neoplasm, trauma, or radiation injuries to the posterior lobe of the pituitary gland. It is also believed to be inherited.
   b. *Diabetes insipidus, nephrogenic:* A rare congenital and familial form of diabetes mellitus, due to the failure of renal tubules to reabsorb water. ADH levels are excessively high but the renal tubules do not respond to it.
5. *Diabetes mellitus:* A group of syndromes having in common a disturbance in oxidation and utilization of glucose which is secondary to a malfunction of the beta cells of the pancreas (beta cell function is the production and release of insulin) (Miller & Keane, 1983, p. 311).

There are at least two major types (and several sub-types) of diabetes mellitus, that is *insulin dependent diabetes mellitus* (IDDM) and *non-insulin-dependent diabetes mellitus*

(NIDDM). (See Table 1.4) In the past these types were referred to by rather misleading titles, that is, "juvenile onset" and "maturity onset." While IDDM is more likely to develop early in life, and NIDDM later in life, they can, and do occur in both the very young and the very old.

SERUM GLUCOSE LEVELS DECREASED IN:

1. Liver disease because of impaired gluconeogenesis and depleted glycogen stores in advanced liver disease, often manifestated by confusion
2. Islet cell adenoma because of excessive and unregulated insulin release. Islet cell hyperplasia, carcinoma, and retroperitonal sarcoma can also be sources of increased production of insulin
3. Addison's disease because of impaired gluconeogenesis or panhypopituitarism due to decreased glucocorticoid production and decreased intestinal absorption. In panhypopituitarism (anterior pituitary insufficiency), hypothyroidism probably adds to the problem, as may the decrease or absence of growth hormone
4. Malnutrition because of decreased intake, which leads to depletion of the liver stores of glycogen
5. Postgastrectomy because of a rapid passage of glucose to the intestine, which sharply increases insulin production and the rapid depletion of serum glucose (tachyalimentation of glucose)
6. Impaired glucose tolerance (IGT), also known as subclinical diabetes mellitus or prediabetes, because of a delayed but excessive insulin secretory response to the carbohydrate intake. Hypoglycemia occurs 3 to 5 hours after eating
7. Excessive administration of insulin in a diabetic patient because of an improper insulin regimen, dietary omission, or excessive physical activity (insulin reaction). (See Fig. 1–1)
8. Functional or spontaneous hypoglycemia, with the cause or mechanism unknown (strenuous exercise to the point of exhaustion can cause hypoglycemia in healthy individuals)
9. Alcohol intake in the fasting state
   a. In prediabetic individuals (impaired glucose tolerance) because of an impairment in gluconeogenesis-depleted glycogen
   b. In individuals with inadequate liver function (e.g., cirrhosis)
10. Rare instances by the intake of certain commonly prescribed drugs other than known hypoglycemic drugs taken for that purpose (e.g., salicylates, haloperidol [Haldol], propoxyphene [Darvon]) (Jones et al., 1982)
11. Infants born to diabetic mothers, probably because of maternal hyperinsulism or hyperglycemia. As mentioned, the incidence of hypoglycemia is increased in premature, low-birthweight infants and is not an uncommon finding in any stressed infant because of rapid depletion of glucose stores
12. Sudden removal of intravenous glucose in an infant because of increased levels of insulin secreted in response to the available glucose
13. Hereditary reactive hypoglycemias such as leucine sensitivity, fructose intolerance and galactosemia, all usually diagnosed in infancy or early childhood.
    Serum glucose levels are sharply decreased in:

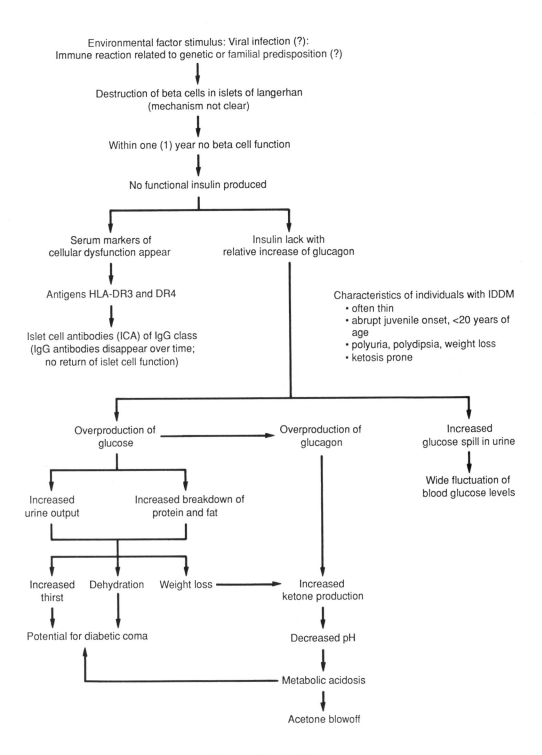

Environmental factor stimulus: Viral infection (?):
Immune reaction related to genetic or familial predisposition (?)

↓

Destruction of beta cells in islets of langerhan
(mechanism not clear)

↓

Within one (1) year no beta cell function

↓

No functional insulin produced

Serum markers of
cellular dysfunction appear

↓

Antigens HLA-DR3 and DR4

↓

Islet cell antibodies (ICA) of IgG class
(IgG antibodies disappear over time;
no return of islet cell function)

Insulin lack with
relative increase of glucagon

Characteristics of individuals with IDDM
• often thin
• abrupt juvenile onset, <20 years of
  age
• polyuria, polydipsia, weight loss
• ketosis prone

Overproduction of
glucose

Overproduction of
glucagon

Increased
glucose spill in urine

↓

Wide fluctuation of
blood glucose levels

Increased
urine output

Increased breakdown of
protein and fat

Increased
thirst

Dehydration

Weight loss

Increased
ketone production

↓

Potential for diabetic coma

Decreased pH

↓

Metabolic acidosis

↓

Acetone blowoff

Figure 1-1. Type I: Insulin dependent diabetes mellitus (IDDM).

a. *leucine sensitivity:* Leucine provokes an exaggerated insulin secretory response (symptomatic hypoglycemia) to protein food intake, with reactive hypoglycemia; the first reaction usually occurring early in the first year of life.

b. *hereditary fructose intolerance and/or galactosemia:* Occurs secondary to an inherited deficiency of a hepatic enzyme, causing acute inhibition of hepatic glucose output with the ingestion of fructose or galactose (Merck Manual, 1992, pp. 1127–1128).

IMPLICATIONS FOR NURSING: SERUM GLUCOSE

1. Patient preparation for the test
   a. Patients should be kept n.p.o. except for water for 8 hours before the test
   b. Insulin should be withheld for any diabetic having blood drawn for glucose determinations. Give insulin promptly after blood is taken and ensure that food is given within 2 hours thereafter
2. Identify individuals at risk for glucose imbalance
   a. Extremes of age: the very young and the very old, are always a high-risk group, if only because of a lack of an intact system for integrating blood glucose regulation
   b. Recent studies indicate that babies born to mothers over age 25 and with fathers, rather than mothers, who have insulin-dependent diabetes mellitus (IDDM), may be at a greater risk for developing diabetes ("Older Maternal Age May Reduce Risk for IDDM," 1992) (See Fig. 1–2.)
   c. Children exposed to IDDM in utero are no longer considered immune to it for their first 20 years; rather, they may have a slightly decreased risk if born after the mother developed IDDM ("Older Maternal Age May Reduce Risk for IDDM," 1992).
3. Protect the patient at risk by
   a. Knowing and assessing for early signs and symptoms of glucose imbalance in persons at risk. Recall that the onset is more rapid in infants and children and profound changes can occur with great speed; therefore, frequent observations are necessary
      (1) Hypoglycemia—signs and symptoms. The sequence given is typical, but the pattern varies
          (a) Mild/early: hunger, tremor, perspiration, weakness, blurred vision, impaired mentation, headaches, feelings of anxiety
          (b) Moderate: mental confusion, neuromuscular function impairment—staggering gait; irrational, hostile behavior (often misinterpreted as drunkenness)

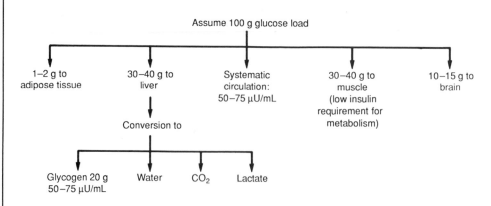

Figure 1–2. Normal distribution of glucose metabolism.

(c) Profound: coma, epileptoid seizures. Permanent brain damage or death will occur if untreated

(d) Mental retardation in the infant or young child. In the infant, signs and symptoms are similar to those of seizure activity (e.g., jittery, listless, yet hyperirritable and restless)

(e) Assess the neonate for hyperbilirubinemia and hypoglycemia, both possible effects of maternal IDDM.

(f) Remember that hypoglycemia may occur when the cord is cut if the pancreas continues to secrete.

(g) Be aware of increased risk for patients with high insulin levels, dyalipidemia (especially low levels of HDL cholesterol and high levels of triglycerides), hypertension and type-II (non-insulin-dependent diabetes mellitus (NIDDM), sometimes called *syndrome X*, and monitor for indicators. (See Fig. 1–3 and Tables 1–3 and 1–4.) Also, some hypertensive

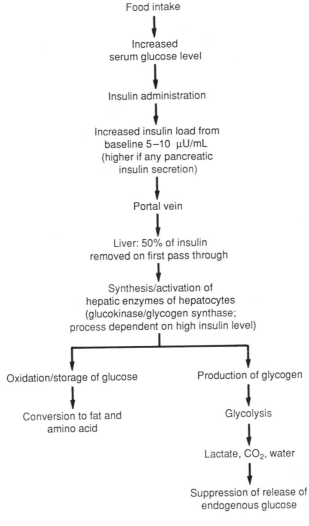

Figure 1-3. Diabetic response to increased insulin level.

TABLE 1-3. FACTORS CONTRIBUTING TO NON-INSULIN-DEPENDENT DIABETES MELLITUS (NIDDM)

Genetic Factors	Metabolic Factors	Age-Related Factors	Life-style
Obesity (?) (80 percent of NIDDM patients are obese)	Pregnancy (increased metabolic workload and decreased insulin resistance) Emotional/physical stress causing gluconeogenesis and increased secretion of catecholamines Pharmacological (e.g., hyperglycemia due to administration of nicoticinic acid, some diuretics)	Decreased beta cell function (decreased number and weight per cell) leading to decreased synthesis of insulin	Sedentary life-style (tending to increase obesity) High caloric intake (Repeated demands for insulin production leading to beta cell exhaustion [?])

   medications have been found to increase insulin resistence (e.g., thiazides; beta block-ers); other improve insulin sensitivity (e.g., alpha blockers, angiotension converting en-zyme inhibitors) and should be used (Haffner et al., 1992, pp. 141, 145)

(2) Hyperglycemia—signs and symptoms

 (a) Mild: increased thirst, increased intake of fluids, increased appetite, polyuria, loss of weight because of the catabolism of muscle cells and a loss of body fluid, decrease in muscle mass, fatigue

 (b) Precoma: drowsiness, dryness of skin, increased rate of respiration, nausea, vomiting, abdominal pain, acetone breath (may occur now or later)

 (c) Coma: Kussmaul's respiration; weak, thready pulse; decreased temperature (unless in-creased because of dehydration) and blood pressure; loss of consciousness

b. Awareness of factors that vary the need for glucose and the need for or use of insulin in those persons at risk for glucose imbalances (e.g., changes in diet, amount of exercise, presence of infection, other stressors) (see Appendix B)

c. Placing all persons at risk for blood glucose imbalance on a regimen of strict intake and output recording

d. Assessing for signs, symptoms, and history of both hyper- and hypoglycemia, bear in mind the possibility of nonketotic hyperosmolar coma. Foremost in the risk group for this pathology is usually a diabetic with IDDM in the upper age group who has some cardiovascular or renal com-plications and a recent history of acute infection or other acute stress. Obtain as detailed a record of the individual's intake and output of fluids as possible

e. Acquiring accurate knowledge of the possible and planned medical treatment to provide antici-patory teaching for the patient and family, to help reinforce any teaching done by the physician, and to ensure decreased anxiety as well as knowledgeable compliance with the medical plan of care by the family and patient

4. Prevent hyperglycemia by

a. Adequate and knowledgeable blood (fingerstick) and urine testing and recording to provide baseline data about glycosuria and ketonuria. Significant hyperglycemia must be present to pro-duce glycosuria in most cases (see "Physiology" in Section 1.4.1). Urinary TMs vary with peo-ple, and glucosuria is not a true indicator of serum levels. Therefore, compare urine findings with the serum glucose level

TABLE 1-4. COMPARISON OF DIABETES MELLITUS

TYPE I: Insulin-Dependent Diabetes Mellitus (IDDM)	TYPE II: Non-Insulin-Dependent Diabetes Mellitus (NIDDM)

Synonyms

Brittle diabetes; idiopathic diabetes; juvenile diabetes; juvenile-onset diabetes	Adult-onset diabetes; ketosis-resistant diabetes; maturity-onset diabetes; stable diabetes

Characteristics

Abrupt symptom onset Age-related, usually < 30 years old; peak 10–13 years Genetic relationship(?): more common in white race Pancreatic islet cells decreased in size Insulin dependent Ketoacidosis prone Locale: higher incidence in northern hemisphere Viral relationship? Onset often in conjunction with viral infections. Cause: autoimmune reaction? Weather relationship? Incidence increased in northern hemisphere and in autumn/winter	Increased incidence in groups encountering a new environment, e.g., migrant groups; most common among Pima indians after migration to northern hemisphere Insulin resistence over time Ketone free except when under great stress Patients may maintain normal weight or become obese; obesity a major risk factor and a familial pattern Most diabetics are included in this type Occurrence of nonspecific pancreatitis related to increased serum lipids; fatty atrophy of pancreas and liver with increased liver size Onset in individuals >40 years; primarily males; familial pattern; inherited susceptibility Rare islet cell antibodies, incidence less than for type I Weight loss occurs in some, cause unclear

Pathophysiology

Destruction of 80–90 percent of islets of Langerhan insulin–secreting beta cells (ultimately all cells destroyed) Atrophy of functioning cells with fibrosis, decreased size Presence of islet cell antibodies (IgC) to human leukocyte antigen D and DR (HLA-D; HLA-DR) in 85% of newly diagnosed cases; ultimately antibodies disappear Inherited susceptibility not as strong as type-II diabetes Usually not insulin resistent	Nonspecific pancreatic changes Uneven hyalinization of islet-typical lesion of pancreas Fatty infiltration of pancreatic and hepatic tissues with atrophy May be caused by gene-environmental interaction Decreased liver uptake and metabolism of glucagon Mechanisms of development unclear; reduced by weight loss

Data from McCance & Huether, 1990, pp. 613–619.

(1) Research types of testing materials available and those being used. It is important to know what a given method actually tests for and what false positives or negatives are possible

(2) Follow directions exactly as provided with the test being used. Always use the color scale that is provided with the test being used

(3) Some controversy surrounds the need to use only second voidings (double-voided specimen) for urine testing, but such a procedure is followed in many places in expectation of more accurate results. The presence of acetone with sugar may indicate impending diabetic

ketoacidosis; check for adequate food intake and an acetone odor of the urine. If present, inform the physician of the appearance of ketones

    (4) Fingerstick blood glucose monitoring done by the nurse or patient requires extreme care. Instructions provided by the manufacturer should be followed carefully. The expiration date on the test material container should be checked before use. When frequent fingersticks are necessary, the nurse or the patient should be sure that different sites are selected on the sides of the fingers each time

    (5) Teaching Self-testing. Become familiar with how the monitor to be used functions and

        (a) Provide adequate verbal and hands-on instruction in checking blood glucose levels to the client and an assistant who will be available in the home if needed. Each should be comfortable with and accurate in following the process. This includes doing a fingerstick test that provides adequate whole blood for the test but without too much blood flow. Use of the nondominant hand is usually recommended for the fingerstick test.

        (b) Read the findings according to the manufacturer's ranges of normal needs to include information as to the difference in normal ranges for whole blood (used in this test) and the normal ranges for most other blood testing in the hospital, which is based on either serum or plasma for glucose testing. The normal range for whole blood vary with changes in hematocrit:

            Decreased hemoglobin = Increased aqueous content of blood

        (RBCs contain 73 percent water; plasma contains 93 percent water.) (Lewis & Collier, 1992, pp. 1298–99). For example, given a hematocrit at 45 percent and whole-blood glucose at 100 mg/dl, an increase in hematocrit to 60 percent will change whole-blood glucose to 104 mg/dl. The reverse is also true: with a decrease in hematocrit to 20 percent, whole-blood glucose would change to 91 mg/dl. (Whole blood is also used with bedside continuous glucose monitors) (Henry, 1991, p. 175)

b. Giving insulin or oral hypoglycemic medication as prescribed, carefully noting and reporting the response. Several kinds of insulin pumps have been tested with good to excellent results, but at present implantable pumps are available in the United States only on clinical trials. Such pumps are felt to be a possibility only for patients who are highly motivated as installation of a pump requires surgery as well as blood glucose monitoring at least four times a day. There are two types of pumps. One is implanted into the peritoneal cavity with a catheter attached to a controlled pump. The other is a patient-controlled device subject to limits set by the physician. It is a radio-controlled pulsatile mechanism with a handheld programmer. Very few pump failures or need for catheter replacements have occurred (Insulin Pumps, 1992, p. 42)

c. Storing medication properly between uses to help maintain its effectiveness

d. Applying a sound knowledge base concerning dietary needs in helping the patient select a diet he or she can live with, thereby increasing the probability of compliance to the dietary plan

e. Using testing agents other than Clinitest for pregnant women, nursing mothers, or patients taking large doses of ascorbic acid, when testing urine glucose yourself, or teaching the process. Clinitest reacts to lactose as well as glucose, and these populations tend to spill lactose. Use of the cephalosporin antibiotics (Keflin, Keflex) will also produce false positives for urine glucose when tested by Clinitest. Ingestion of large doses of aspirin has the same effect

f. Teaching the patient and home caretaker all of the foregoing precautions, providing a rationale, and also including necessary information about weight reduction, when indicated. The signs and symptoms of imbalance must also be taught and the steps that should be taken immediately upon the occurrence of an imbalance. The diabetic also needs to be made aware of the possibility of sugar in items other than food such as medications. Teaching must be tailored to the level of the learner and his or her ability to learn. Techniques can be adapted for many physical and mental deficits so that self-care is possible and error free. For instance, special materials are available for people with vision problems. The reader is referred to the many excellent resources available for preparation in teaching diabetics

5. Assess hyperglycemia and prevent complications by
   a. Notifying the physician at the first indication of hyperglycemia so that adequate insulin and glucose coverage can be instituted and an adequate number of serum glucose determinations made
   b. Observing for any changes in the level of consciousness
   c. With increases in insulin dosage, observing for signs and symptoms of hypoglycemia
   d. Checking plasma potassium levels in any patient with hyperglycemia or after administering large doses of insulin. Because the cells cannot use glucose without insulin, cellular catabolism occurs, and potassium is released from the cell to be excreted in the urine. Excessive amounts may be excreted because, in the presence of increased serum glucose levels, there is an accompanying increase in serum osmolality and an osmotic diuresis and hypokalemia result. It is important, however, to recall that total body potassium is not always reflected in the plasma levels, so it is necessary to assess for signs and symptoms of a potassium deficit as well. Hypokalemia can also occur after the administration of large doses of insulin because of K^+ entering the cells
   e. Checking the urine for glucose and acetone at least four times during the day. The presence of acetone without glycosuria is usually indicative of inadequate food intake, primarily of carbohydrates
   f. With an increase in blood glucose levels, or with a repeated pattern of glucosuria in the first urine check of the day before the administration of insulin, in the face of previous increases in dosage to rectify the problem, checking the serum CO_2 content, if available (or any *venous* CO_2 measurement; a decrease in the venous CO_2 concentration usually indicates a metabolic, acidotic state because it is a measure of the bicarbonate reserves of the body). If the venous CO_2 content remains within normal limits, the cause of the glycosuria may be an actual overdosage of insulin rather than a lack of insulin. The condition is called the *Somogyi reaction* (see Appendix H). This reaction is a fairly common occurrence in teenagers (Price & Wilson, 1992) and, unfortunately, not that uncommon in adults. A nurse aware of this possibility will apply a high index of suspicion in assessing the "hard-to-control" or "brittle" diabetic. Taking a thorough history will help identify the presence of the reaction. Provide an adequate care plan that will document data necessary for identification
6. Prevent hypoglycemia by
   a. Being especially alert for signs and symptoms of the condition in all infants, especially newborn, premature, and low-birthweight children
   b. Becoming acquainted with the expected time of the peak effect of the type of insulin in use for diabetic patients and observing carefully at that time for any signs or symptoms of hypoglycemia
   c. Providing distribution of food throughout the day
      (1) Provide to coincide with the peak effect of the hypoglycemia agents; frequently the third hour after meals is a critical time
      (2) Balance exercise, rest, sleep, and food intake
      (3) Check the actual dietary intake to ensure ingestion of adequate CHO (50 to 60 percent of the total calories) containing a high proportion of complex carbohydrates and fiber while avoiding simple sugars. Ensure that the fat intake (preferably unsaturated or red fish saturated oil/fat) is no more than 35 percent of the total calories and that the protein intake is sufficient to meet body needs (usually 25 percent or less of the total calories) (Patrick et al., 1986)
      (4) If appropriate, plan with the physician, dietician, and patient to have simple sugar food immediately on hand for use with early signs and symptoms of hypoglycemia. Hard candies, orange juice, lump sugar, or a candy bar are all good possibilities. A candy bar with nuts is preferable because this will not only supply the quick glucose needed but will also provide some protein to help maintain increased glucose levels
      (5) Be alert for hypoglycemia in the risk population during the early morning hours because it typically occurs after an 8- or 9-hour fast
   d. Noting early evidence of confusion that might be due to hypoglycemia in patients with liver disease. To differentiate from other possible causes of confusion, it is helpful to keep records of dietary intake on these patients

e. Observing the patient at risk for hypoglycemia during sleep and checking for restlessness and diaphoresis, which can indicate a serum glucose deficit

f. Teaching the patient and family the purpose for and administration of glucagon for emergency use in case of hypoglycemia if it has been ordered for the patient

g. Seeking alternatives to prolonged periods n.p.o. for individuals at risk for hypoglycemia. Discuss this with the physician or laboratory personnel

7. Validate the presence of hypoglycemia as opposed to hyperventilation by

   a. Questioning as to the presence of numbness or tingling of the fingertips and the circumoral area, complaints of dyspnea, or evident shortness of breath

   b. Observing for frequent deep sighs or sighing respirations

   c. Being aware that hyperventilation occurs more frequently in females than in males. (If hyperventilation appears to be the causative factor for signs and symptoms, teach rebreathing by using a paper bag; use any available, appropriate measures to reduce anxiety and relax tension, thereby slowing the respiratory rate)

8. Treat hypoglycemia reactions by

   a. Taking seizure precautions for individuals with confirmed hypoglycemia or with fragile compensatory responses to changes in serum glucose levels. This is especially pertinent in the care of infants

   b. Keeping a record of the time of day the hypoglycemia reaction occurs. This can help provide clues to the underlying cause if unknown

   c. Getting a history of nutritional intake before the attack to help identify precipitants

   d. Providing high-carbohydrate foods with or without a direct order from the physician as soon as hypoglycemia has been validated. Follow through after the attack by collaborating with other members of the health team to prevent yet another reactive hypoglycemic episode secondary to the high-carbohydrate intake given to treat the original episode. Glucose is rapidly assimilated, and in individuals capable of producing their own insulin, insulin production will increase. In the person not able to produce insulin, the glucose may well not use up all the administered insulin and cause a second drop in the serum glucose concentration once the glucose is assimilated. Providing a balanced diet (i.e., adequate complex carbohydrates and fiber [see item 6]) and instituting measures to prevent hypoglycemia directly and through patient–family teaching may help accomplish some control

   e. If the individual is unconscious, administering glucagon subcutaneously or intramuscularly, if available. If not available immediately, contact a physician and request a stat order for the drug. It is possible to provide some immediate glucose to the unconscious person if a high-carbohydrate substance such as a sugar cube is placed in the buccal cavity. Absorption is fairly rapid in this area; however, this should only be done if there is no possibility of the individual aspirating. Usually, the glucagon dose can be repeated once or twice if the original dose was not adequate. The person should awaken 10 to 20 minutes after receiving the glucagon. If not, repeat the dose

   f. Starting an intravenous line at the to-keep-open (TKO) rate if the patient is unconscious or at risk of unconsciousness. Also, prepare and have ready for administration 1 L of intravenous glucose 5% in water or saline, depending on the problems other than glucose concentration that the patient is facing

   g. Providing oral carbohydrate intake as soon as the patient awakens

   h. If residual signs and symptoms persist, reassuring the patient and family that it is not unusual to continue to feel weak, have a headache, or be nauseated. At the same time, take what measures are available to diminish such discomforts. Because the patient will be weak and may be confused, it is imperative to provide for his or her safety

9. Protect patients in any imbalance by providing a safe environment. Some decrease in mentation or alertness accompanies both hypo- and hyperglycemia, and visual disturbances are a frequent accompaniment. Persons with hyperglycemia are also poor risks in dealing with infections. Hypoglycemia states foster accidents resulting from weakness or dizziness.

1.5 PLASMA CREATININE

Synonyms: Blood creatinine, serum creatinine (see also "Creatinine Clearance Test" in Section 8.1)

Normal Ranges (mg/dl)

Adult	0.7-1.5
Senior adult	0.6-1.2
	Within lower range of adult normal values
Newborn	0.4–1.2
0–4 yr	0.1–0.7
4–10 yr	0.2–0.9
10–16 yr	0.3–1.1

Definition. Creatinine is the least variable of the nonprotein nitrogen (NPN) substances in the serum and is a sensitive indicator of renal function. It is an end product of muscle metabolism that is liberated from the muscle and excreted in the urine at a virtually constant rate. Therefore, the serum level is also constant in the healthy person. Of all the NPN substances, only creatine—which is the precursor of creatinine—is used by the body. It is stored for energy in muscle metabolism.

Creatinine is correlated with changes in the serum urea nitrogen (BUN) for diagnostic purposes but is more accurate as an index of the glomerular filtration rate (GFR) because it is produced in amounts related to muscle mass, which changes very little while the BUN level rises in response to many factors (see Section 1.6). It is therefore used as an indicator with known renal disease or in those instances where the cause of an elevated BUN value is uncertain.

Creatinine is a relatively unstable compound, especially in urine, and prevention of some destruction is accomplished in the laboratory by freezing separated serum or urine. The clinical use of serum creatinine measurement increased with the introduction of rapid automated methods.

Physiology. Creatine, an amino acid of nonprotein base, is an ingredient of muscle tissue that is formed through the action of creatine phosphokinase (CPK) when energy is needed for metabolic processes. When used for energy, it forms the inactive metabolite creatinine, which is liberated from the muscles into the blood at a constant rate. Higher levels are produced in males than in females because of their greater muscle mass. The glomerulus of the kidney filters the creatinine, and it is not reabsorbed by the tubules. Thus the rate of excretion in the urine is also constant. Blood levels appear to fluctuate even less than do urinary levels, perhaps because of the ability of the tubules to secrete creatinine in the presence of increased serum levels. Creatinine is excreted unchanged in the urine because it is little modified in its passage through the nephron. It is more readily excreted by the kidneys than is urea or uric acid.

SERUM CREATININE LEVELS DECREASED IN:

- Any severe muscle-wasting process such as muscular dystrophy because of a reduction in the total body muscle mass and, hence, the amount of creatine converted to creatinine each day. Decreases may be found as well in myasthenia gravis for much the same reasons

SERUM CREATININE LEVELS INCREASED IN:

1. Chronic renal insufficiency (uremia) secondary to chronic glomerulonephritis, diabetic nephrosis, polycystic kidney, nephrosclerosis, chronic pyelonephritis, and gout, to name a few, because of the inability of the kidneys to excrete creatinine. Serum creatinine levels may be normal in some cases of *acute* uremia or *mild* chronic renal disease because it takes 7 to 10 days for plasma creatinine level to stabilize when GFR decreases (McCance & Huether, 1990). An elevated serum creatinine level indicates severe, long-standing renal impairment. An increase of over 4 to 5 mg/dl is evidence of marked impairment. Chronic nephritis with uremia can produce levels as high as 20 to 30 mg/dl (Laboratory of Pathology, 1991).
2. Obstructive uropathy of long standing, which can occur in prostatic hypertrophy, bilateral ureteral stricture, and renal calculi because of the compromise of free urine flow and the GFR. Renal clearance is depressed.
3. Chronic decreases in the GFR because of prerenal causes, as seen in chronic congestive heart failure.
4. False values reported in some methods of testing (original Jaffe test) that produce secondary interference because of the reaction of materials other than creatinine (Krupp et al., 1987).
5. Some people with a remarkably enlarged muscle mass, which produces increased amounts of creatinine. The elevation is usually slight.
6. Some instances of acromegaly because of an increased muscle mass. Again, the serum value will show only slightly increased levels.
7. Diabetic ketoacidosis because of a falsely elevated reading caused by the increase of ketones in the serum.
8. Rejection of a kidney transplant because of decreasing filtration of waste products by the failing kidney. In such cases serial determination of the serum creatinine level may be the more sensitive indicator of renal function (Luckmann & Sorensen, 1987).

IIMPLICATIONS FOR NURSING: SERUM CREATININE

1. There may be no patient preparation for testing serum creatinine levels. It is preferable, however, that the person be without food and drink other than water for 8 hours before having the blood sample drawn
2. The nurse can be instrumental in the prevention of some types of damage to the renal system and thereby help prevent renal insufficiency characterized by increased creatinine levels in the serum. Identifying the population at particular risk (prolonged bed rest coupled with decreased self-movement, ketonuria secondary to diabetes mellitus, lupus erythematosus or other collagen disorders, or those with a history of urinary tract infections, to list a few only) is important. Providing adequate fluid intake (minimum of 30 to 50 ml/hr for 24 hours) and maintaining an acid urine help prevent stone formation in the urine with the probable superimposed infection. Meticulous technique in dealing with urinary catheterization is imperative
3. Prevention of renal impairment is part of the nurse's responsibilities when giving nephrotoxic drugs. A thorough knowledge of the side effects of drugs to be administered is the minimal acceptable base for patient care. Observe for increases in the serum creatinine and BUN levels when these drugs are being given. Any person with a history of renal impairment, regardless of

the present level of renal function, should be safeguarded particularly diligently and alternate non-nephrotoxic medication substituted when at all possible. Collaborate with the physician. (A few drugs found to be highly nephrotoxic yet quite frequently used include gentamicin, the cephalothins as a group, colchicine, and kanamycin)

4. The patient in early renal failure with only slight if any increases in creatinine levels has a decreased ability to concentrate urine. Note changes in the urine concentration by doing daily specific gravity determinations on patients at risk for or in early renal failure. As it advances, the specific gravity tends toward 1.010—isosthenuria. Observe these individuals for nocturia, polyuria, and polydipsia. Note changes in the urine color

5. With increased serum creatinine levels, bear in mind that this measurement is considered the most specific test of renal function, and all other parameters of renal function should be assessed. All parameters should be looked at for interrelationships so as to validate the finding of the elevated creatinine level and begin the task of preventing complications. Other parameters include
   a. Strict intake and output recording
   b. Daily weights, same time, same clothing
   c. Observations of blood pressure—sitting and lying down—pulse, and neck vein distention for potential fluid overload or deficit
   d. Serial assessments for fluid retention in edema—periorbital and pulmonary

6. Monitor BUN levels and compare with creatinine levels. The BUN level rises and falls more rapidly than does the creatinine level. One could expect the BUN increase to precede an increase in serum creatinine levels in early failure. If there is no increase in the creatinine levels, other possibilities should be explored to explain the elevated BUN level (see Section 1.6)

7. Check the RBC count and the other blood indices. Almost all persons with chronic renal failure (indicated by an increased serum creatinine level) become anemic

8. Observe for easy bruising or oozing from mucous membranes. This is more likely to occur in the individual who has advanced renal insufficiency such as uremia. Provide for protection from injury: shoes while up and about to prevent slipping, oral medications whenever possible, and the use of the smallest possible gauge needle for injections when they cannot be avoided (see Section 3.12 or "Implications for Nursing" in Section 2.3.2 for more precise suggestions)

9. Prevent infection by all means available that are consistent with the person's individual needs when serum creatinine levels are increased. The person with uremia is particularly susceptible to infection, and infection is difficult to treat because of the altered antibiotic metabolism (Hekelman & Ostendarp, 1979). Infection also tends to increase the severity of the azotemia (presence of urea or other nitrogenous substances in the blood) because of the increase in cellular catabolism. Observe the person with elevated serum creatinine levels for signs and symptoms of infection to include observations more than for increased temperature and white blood count. The individual in end-stage renal failure may have a low body temperature in face of an infection or may have an increased white blood count without an infection being present (Harvey et al., 1991)

10. Observation of the serum creatinine level is imperative for the person who has had a kidney transplant. If all data suggest a rejection, the nurse should of course report the information immediately and prepare to take whatever isolation precautions are used in the facility housing the patient. Observations that indicate rejection include a decreased urine output, increased specific gravity of urine, increased blood levels for BUN and serum creatinine, and the appearance of protein in the urine

11. Patients receiving chronic dialysis are often dialyzed on the basis of changes in creatinine levels. BUN, because of its more rapid change, is preferable in determining the effectiveness of dialysis. Serum creatinine levels of 8 to 15 mg/dl have been given as an indicator for dialysis in end-stage renal disease; however, such criteria vary depending on the physician and the institution involved

12. Because an elevation of the serum creatinine level is usually accompanied by an elevation of the BUN level, nursing implications for azotemia apply (see "Implications for Nursing" in Section 1.6)

13. Any drug that remains in the plasma in solution will be filtered at the glomerulus, as is creatinine. The dosage of such drugs is usually modified by the physician in cases of impaired renal function, and dosage must be adapted to the age-related changes in creatinine clearance as well. The nurse should know how the drugs given are excreted and should observe the individual for evi-

dence of overdosage or prolonged effect if the medication is excreted through the kidney (e.g., penicillin). Many drugs require dosage adjustment depending on renal function in creatinine clearance. Extreme caution in the administration of drugs is imperative. If the person will be administering any drug himself or herself, adequate understanding of the possible side effects and what actions to be taken in the face of their occurrence is needed by that person and a responsible family member. Instruction by the nurse must be thorough and well evaluated for adequate learning on the part of the person or family

14. Persons with renal insufficiency and increased serum creatinine levels require more than the usual attention paid to getting adequate rest; it must be balanced with enough exercise to maintain muscle tone and circulation. An increase in physical exercise does not usually increase serum creatinine levels in the healthy individual, although it may increase the BUN level because of increased cellular catabolism; however, exercise should be done with caution because of the related problems of elevated BUN levels causing changes in awareness and judgment and because of the weakness that is associated with anemia

15. Because creatinine is produced only within the body, there are no dietary restrictions related to it; however, the person with renal insufficiency is likely to have some fluid or dietary restriction with which the nurse should be conversant to provide teaching and oversee intake

1.6 SERUM UREA NITROGEN

Synonyms: BUN, blood urea nitrogen (see also "Urea Nitrogen" in Section 8.1.4)

Normal Ranges (mg/dl)

Adult	4–22
Senior adult	8–18
Pediatric	<20
Newborn/infant	8–28
Thereafter	10–20

Definition. Urea is one of the more abundant nonprotein nitrogen (NPN) constituents in the body. Besides urea, these constituents include creatinine, uric acid, ammonium, and amino acids. At one time all constituents were measured together (NPN test), but because testing for individual compounds is fairly simple and yields more precise data, the NPN test has been almost completely replaced by the individual tests.

Urea is the major nitrogenous waste product of protein catabolism and is produced solely in the liver. In the United States urea is commonly measured as urea nitrogen, whereas in Europe the measurement is expressed as urea only. Urea is found in equal concentrations in all body fluids, with the exception of whole blood because of a difference in the percent concentration of serum and erythrocytes. Therefore, serum or plasma is preferred to whole blood for urea nitrogen analysis.

Determinations of serum urea nitrogen and serum creatinine are the two most commonly ordered tests to detect the kidney's ability to excrete metabolic waste. Increases in these values are used, among others, as indicators for the need for dialysis in chronic kidney failure patients. Interpretation of urea nitrogen values requires a knowledge of exogenous protein intake, fluid intake, and conditions that can increase endogenous production (e.g., muscular activity, trauma, infection, strict dieting/fasting/starvation). Any of these variables can cause increased concentrations in blood or urine that are not a true reflection of renal clearance of urea per se.

The two tests can be used, with the foregoing precautions in interpretation, as crude indicators of improvement or deterioration of the individual's kidney function.

Although the urea nitrogen determination is much less specific than is that for serum creatinine, it is widely used—particularly in pediatrics, as a screening test for kidney function and as one that tells something of the individual's state of hydration. Lesser degrees of renal impairment require more sophisticated testing such as clearance tests (Scipien & Barnard, 1983).

Physiology. Urea is produced through a process of protein degradation: protein is transformed from amino acids to ammonia (oxidated deamination) as an end product and thence to urea (ornithine cycle) within the liver. Because the body does not use urea, it is carried in the blood from the liver until excreted in the urine. Levels vary physiologically, depending directly on the protein intake in diet (exogeneous) and the state of hydration (the ratio of solute to solvent in the body) or indirectly on the rate of tissue catabolism (rapid cellular breakdown causing increased nitrogenous waste) or the rate of tissue anabolism (decrease in levels because of the increased rate of tissue building such as occurs in pregnancy, growth spurts, or convalescence) (Guyton, 1982). Urea is excreted in the glomerular filtrate and reabsorbed (probably through diffusion) in the nephron tubule. Only a fraction of all waste material contained in the glomerular flltrate is excreted, but because urea is poorly reabsorbed by the tubules, little urea is reabsorbed, a beneficial effect.

SERUM UREA NITROGEN LEVELS DECREASED IN:

(Little clinical significance is attached to decreased levels of urea nitrogen, as it is not a substance necessary for body function. Decreased values are seen less frequently than increased values. It has been suggested that a low urea nitrogen level may well be a good prognostic sign, because it indicates good renal function with adequate output.)
1. Any condition with increased secretion of androgen hormones or growth hormones, probably because of the anabolic effect of these hormones
2. Normal pregnancy related to
   a. Increased renal plasma flow (RPF) and GFR secondary to expansion of plasma volume
   b. The anabolic state of the body
3. Severe hepatic insufficiency, particularly that associated with the obstruction of portal vein flow, because of the inability of the liver to convert ammonia to urea. A concomitant rise in blood ammonia levels would be expected
4. Rapid changes in hydration such as in
   a. Rapid rehydration when no nitrogenous compounds have been added to the intravenous solution
   b. The individual who has been overhydrated and then subjected to rapid diuresis. The decreases in urea nitrogen levels associated with rapid changes in hydration are in themselves temporary and are usually of academic interest only

Azotemia. Before examining the conditions in which serum urea nitrogen levels are increased, we need to discuss azotemia, that is, an excess of urea or other nitrogenous products in the blood. Consistent elevations of urea nitrogen levels occur only when the renal function, specifically the GFR, is reduced by 40 to 60 percent. The GFR can be altered not only by renal disease but also by prerenal deviation of water (loss of circulating volume for whatever cause), which leads to an increase in the urea nitrogen retained. Azotemia occurs generally because of a loss of circulating volume, excessive protein catabolism, or impairment of renal function. Interpretation of increases in urea nitrogen levels depends on knowledge of both renal and extrarenal factors and their relative importance.

SERUM UREA NITROGEN LEVELS INCREASED IN:

1. Renal failure, second stage (renal insufficiency) and third stage (end stage or uremia), because of the inability of the diseased kidneys to excrete urea. Temporary increases in urea nitrogen levels can occur in the first stage of renal failure (decreased renal reserve) if the renal mechanism is stressed. Therefore, increases could be expected in chronic glomerulonephritis, diabetic nephrosis, polycystic kidney, nephrosclerosis, and chronic pyelonephritis, all of which exhibit parenchymal kidney damage of some type
2. Dehydration because of a decreased circulating plasma volume
3. Water or saline losses in children, particularly infants. The urea nitrogen rise is often spectacular because of the infant's proportional increased amount of body water compared with adults
4. Starvation because of increased protein catabolism and hypoproteinemia. This situation is also seen temporarily in long-term, high fevers
5. Bleeding gastric ulcer because of an increased production of urea from the breakdown products of blood (protein) dumped into the gastrointestinal tract. There is also an accompanying decrease in circulating volume that may be of more importance than the increase in protein catabolism
6. Congestive heart failure because of retention due to decreased cardiac output, which results in a decrease in renal blood flow and a decreased GFR. A serum urea nitrogen value is usually determined in general cardiac assessment to learn whether or not kidney function has been disturbed
7. Shock (hypovolemic, cardiogenic, vasomotor collapse, septic) because of the accompanying decrease in GFR. Adequate kidney perfusion is mandatory for excretion of urea
8. Obstructive uropathy, which usually must be severe and bilateral because of the remarkable reserves available for kidney function. An increased urea nitrogen concentration is due to a decrease in the renal clearance of urea. This occurs in conditions such as prostatic hypertrophy, bilateral ureteral strictures, renal calculi, and arteriosclerosis or thrombosis of the renal vasculature
9. Ingestion or inhalation of nephrotoxic substances such as carbon tetrachloride or heavy metals such as mercury because of damage to the kidney parenchyma. Because damage to the liver often occurs first, especially when the substance is ingested, signs and symptoms of liver damage (jaundice) may precede the elevation of the urea nitrogen level (Hahn et al., 1982)
10. Thyrotoxicosis because of excessive protein catabolism. Increased protein catabolism may also lead to an increase in urea nitrogen levels in uncontrolled diabetes mellitus, adrenocortical hyperfunction, and some neoplastic diseases
11. Rejection of a kidney transplant because of decreasing urine output
12. Athletes after extraordinary activity because of excessive muscle breakdown

13. Intestinal obstruction because of a loss of circulating plasma volume by "third spacing" of fluids into the gut

---

IMPLICATIONS FOR NURSING: INCREASED SERUM UREA NITROGEN LEVELS

1. Preparation for having a blood sample taken for urea nitrogen determination is usually minimal; however, in the person to whom it is particularly important that the test reflect the actual urea nitrogen levels as closely as possible, intake should be restricted to water only for 8 hours before taking the blood sample. Most laboratories do not require this restriction, although it is the preferable procedure (see also item 2d[2])

2. The amount of the rise in the BUN level can provide clues as to the probable cause, which in turn will assist the nurse in planning care
   a. In true hypernatremia (increased ratio of salt to water in the ECF) the BUN can be three to four times the normal level
   b. Hospitalized persons' normal levels are slightly higher than those seen in active "normal" adults, possibly because of an increased catabolic state
   c. Although BUN values can go as high as 400 mg/dl, they usually do not exceed 200 mg/dl, which is the level one would expect in the person with severe kidney disease and with coma or stupor. In any case, levels in excess of 100 mg/dl are usual in severe kidney disease
   d. With values above 40 mg/dl in the adult, in the absence of dehydration the nurse should initiate the following observations
      (1) Individuals with increased urea nitrogen levels should have careful records kept of fluid intake and output. This is particularly important in the care of infants and children or those adults with a history of renal dysfunction
      (2) A history of food intake should be taken for the 24 hours before the blood test
      (3) Eliminate the presence of dehydration as a probable cause of increased serum urea nitrogen levels by checking the hematocrit level and the urine-specific gravity. They will be increased if dehydration resulting from a saline deficit is present. The urine output will also be decreased unless severe diuresis is occurring because of renal disease or the second stage of response to a burn

3. Increases in serum urea nitrogen levels frequently cause lethargy and confusion. Adequate nursing care would include maintaining the safety for the individual (creating a safe environment and preventing injury) by providing supervision over self-care and restriction of activity, providing psychological security through reality orientation and realistic reassurance as to the reason for the changes and the possibility of improvement, and assessing for change in intellectual function. This last can be done by instituting a daily repetition of some intellectual task with which the individual's normal mental ability can be determined (e.g., mathematical problems or riddles that require clarity of thought)

4. Prevent further increases in urea nitrogen levels by the prevention of avoidable stress such as infection, great increases in muscular activity, or psychological stresses, whatever they may be, as identified for the individual

5. An increase in serum urea nitrogen levels not resulting from dehydration may be treated by a decrease in dietary protein by the physician, and in the absence of the physician, the nurse can do no harm by restricting protein intake until such time as the physician may be consulted

6. Persons with high levels of serum urea nitrogen who are undergoing hemodialysis, particularly for the first time, should be monitored closely for the occurrence of a syndrome known as dialysis disequilibrium. This is demonstrated by the occurrence of nausea, vomiting, mental confusion, hallucination, or convulsions about 2 hours after start of dialysis. The responsibility of the nurse is to identify the syndrome correctly and report the fact immediately. Dialysis may be discontinued depending on the standing procedure of the unit involved (see Appendix C for more information on this syndrome)

7. In any person who has had a serum urea nitrogen determination taken when not in the fasting state described earlier, the nurse should obtain and record a history of food and drink intake for the 8-hour period before testing

8. Check for an increase in serum ammonia levels in the person with liver disease and increased BUN levels. This is particularly important when there have been changes in the level of consciousness or mentation. Treatment for hepatic encephalopathy should not be omitted because the mental confusion or decreased level of awareness is thought to be due only to the increased BUN concentration

9. Plasma potassium levels should be noted in the person with known renal dysfunction and an increased BUN content. The nurse should also monitor the individual for signs and symptoms of hyperkalemia (see Section 1.3.1)

10. Compare BUN with serum creatinine levels for a more accurate interpretation. A person with a low protein intake may well have a normal BUN value even in the face of severe renal impairment. An elevated BUN with a normal serum creatinine level would indicate probable intestinal bleeding or another protein increase

11. Note the RBC count for the appearance of anemia. Increased serum urea nitrogen levels over 200 mg/dl reduce the life span of RBCs to about half of normal, and in some patients anemia is also secondary to decreased erythropoietin production

12. Observe for signs and symptoms of pericarditis if the serum urea nitrogen level remains elevated above 100 mg/dl

1.7 SERUM URIC ACID

Synonym: Serum urate

Normal Ranges (mg/dl)

Adult	
Female	2.7–7.3
Male	4.0–8.5
Senior adult	
Female	2.4–7.2
Male	2.9–8.8
Child (up to 15 yr, then elevates sharply to adult levels)	
Female	2.0–7.3
Male	2.0–8.5

Definition. Uric acid is another of the nitrogenous waste products found in the blood. It is derived from the breakdown of purines from the nucleic acids of cells and from xanthines. (Xanthines are purine compounds found in most body tissues). It is one means of quantifying the nuclear metabolic process. The test is a fairly simple determination that can be used for the identification of certain diseases, gout being the primary example, and is helpful in differentiating among several diseases.

There are numerous foods that add an exogenous source of purine and thus uric acid production. Ingestion of those foods tends to influence the amounts of uric acid excreted daily more than the serum levels, given normal kidney function. Normal serum levels tend to increase with age, and normal values are consistently higher in males than in females after the age of 4. It is now known that urate production and/or synthesis is accomplished by using multitude simple body compounds (e.g., carbon dioxide, glycerine, and ammonia) as well as purines, making dietary management of hyperuricemia less important, though still useful.

Pathological conditions related to increases or decreases in serum uric acid levels are confined to adults for the most part. Responses to myeloproliferative disease or its treatment and genetic abnormalities are the major causes of increases in children.

Physiology. The physiological process of uric acid production is that of catabolism of purine nucleotides from organs having a high metabolic rate, such as the liver, bone marrow, and possibly muscle, as well as conditions in which excessive cellular breakdown takes place (McCance & Huether, 1990; Laboratory of Pathology, 1991). Purines that are ingested as complex proteins are degraded in the intestine and absorbed into the blood where they are carried to the liver and catabolized into the waste product uric acid. Once formed, uric acid is not catabolized further but joins the "uric acid pool" of the body. Approximately 50 to 75 percent of this pool is excreted from the body daily. Uric acid is totally filtered and excreted at the glomerulus and then totally reabsorbed in the proximal tubule. The filtrate is then actively secreted in the distal tubule, which is responsible for total urinary urate. Blood and urine levels vary with purine ingestions as well as protein and caloric intake. A second avenue of excretion is by way of the intestinal lumen. As much as one third of the total amount of uric acid lost daily is thought to be lost by this route.

Pathophysiology of Hyperuricemia (Gout). An excessive accumulation of uric acid occurs in the blood with overproduction of uric acid (hyperuricemia), increased cell destruction, defect in the purine biosynthetic enzyme, and/or defect in uric acid excretion. The presence of excessive uric acid formation or retention causes Gout, which occurs in two forms. *Primary gout* is related to enzyme defects and occurs only in men, causing increased purine synthesis and overproduction of uric acid. *Secondary gout* occurs as a result of an acquired chronic disease, such as chronic glomerular nephritis or because of the use of a drug that interferes with the normal balance between production and excretion of uric acid, such as diuretics.

Uric acid crystals do not precipitate until serum levels exceed 6.5 mg/100ml. The crystals collect largely in the synovial fluid of the joints. A rapid inflammatory process occurs in a matter of hours, with leukocytic phagocytosis of the crystals followed by a release of lysosomal enzymes that cause injury and inflammation as well as great pain. Because of this metabolic activity, the synovial fluid can become more acidic, which fosters further urate crystal formation and an extension of the inflammatory process. Urate crystals are deposited in relatively avascular tissues such as tendon and cartilage as well as the synovial fluid and in the interstitial tissues of the renal pyramid. With recurrent attacks, additional areas of the body will be included and damaged. Accumulations in tissue such as cartilage are called tophi. Tophi are hard, translucent swellings that can be noted frequently in the helix of the ear. The presence of increased levels of urate in the urine has a high potential for the development of uric stones, particularly in acid urine, that ultimately cause renal damage. Some 10 to 20 percent of individuals with hyperuricemia develop urate stones—renal calculi.

SERUM URIC ACID LEVELS DECREASED IN:

1. Conditions that have been treated with specific drugs
   a. Large doses (4 to 6 g/24 hr) of salicylates. Salicylates have a paradoxical, dose-related effect on uric acid retention and excretion. A low dosage blocks the distal tubule secretion of uric acid, whereas high doses block reabsorption from the proximal tubule. Salicylate is one of a number of *uricosuric drugs* with this dose-related response
   b. Phenylbutazone (Butazolidin) and oxyphenbutazone (Tandearil)
   c. Probenecid (Benemid)
   d. Allopurinol (Zyloprim)
   e. Corticosteroids
   f. Coumarin compounds
   g. Sulfinpyrazone (Anturane)
2. Massive hepatic necrosis because of the diminished ability of the liver to catabolize purine. Serum levels are greatly depressed
3. Fanconi's syndrome (a familial, slowly progressive kidney disease with progressive degeneration of the renal parenchyma and metabolic disorders) because of the lack of tubular reabsorption of uric acid
4. Wilson's disease (hepatolenticular degeneration) because of the lack of tubular reabsorption of uric acid

SERUM URIC ACID LEVELS INCREASED IN:

1. Gout because of varying causes that are not fully understood. The primary form is thought to be due to a metabolic defect in purine metabolism that causes increased production of uric acid or a defect in uric acid excretion. Secondary gout occurs in a variety of diseases associated with the overproduction and destruction of cells (see "Pathophysiology"). The total urate pool may be increased from 3 to 25 times normal
2. Starvation because the increase in cell turnover (catabolism) coupled with decreased excretion, probably related to the accompanying metabolic acidosis, which favors urate stone formation
3. Lesch–Nyhan syndrome, a congenital form of gout. It is associated with mental retardation, compulsive self-mutilation, and neurological problems similar to cerebral palsy and is first identified in childhood
4. High-fat diet and nondiabetic ketosis because of the depletion of hepatic glucogen. This causes gluconeogenesis, which in turn increases the formation of purine breakdown products (Henry, 1991)
5. Some instances of renal disease such as chronic glomerulonephritis because of a decreased renal clearance and tubular secretion. A similar picture occurs in other obstructive or suppressive urinary flow problems
6. Eclampsia (toxemia of pregnancy) because of a decreased renal clearance of uric acid, the mechanism of which is not understood. With eclampsia the BUN concentration is within normal limits, which helps in the differential diagnosis among other toxic or inflammatory conditions
7. Leukemia because of an increased production and destruction of WBCs that results in an increased rate of turnover of the nucleic acid of those cells and leads to increased purine

catabolism. Increased uric acid levels are also found in polycythemia vera, multiple myeloma, lymphoblastoma, lobar pneumonias, and remission stages of pernicious anemia because of this same augmentation of nuclear catabolism

8. Diabetic glomerulosclerosis and some collagen disorders when renal function has been compromised, which leads to a decrease in the renal clearance and tubular secretion of uric acid

9. Renal hypertension—when the BUN level rises above 25 mg/dl, there is a sharp rise in uric acid levels

10. Psoriasis and sarcoidosis as well as other diseases that may cause joint pain and swelling. Uric acid increases in these situations are due to renal retention of uric acid

11. Individuals who are receiving long-term diuretic therapy. The effect is believed to be due to inhibition of the tubular secretion of uric acid

12. Conditions that have been treated with specific drugs

   a. Small doses of salicylate (less than 2 g/24 hr) (see "Serum Uric Acid Decreased in," item 1a)

   b. Thiazide diuretics (see item 11)

   c. Acetazolamide (Diamox). Can actually cause an increase or decrease in uric acid secretion. The increase is due in part to the drug's ability to increase the alkalinity of the urine

   d. Spironolactone (Aldactone)

   e. Methyldopa

IMPLICATIONS FOR NURSING: SERUM URIC ACID

1. Patient preparation for a serum uric acid test includes prohibiting intake of food or drink other than water for 8 hours before the test. There is no special preparation necessary for testing urine uric acid levels

2. With any increase in serum uric acid levels, gout is suspected and must be ruled out before proceeding with other diagnoses. The nurse should collect significant data to facilitate this process

   a. A detailed family history for the incidence of gout is important because of the strong familial factor in its incidence

   b. Age. Its occurrence is almost nonexistent before puberty. An increased incidence is seen in early middle age and on into the fifth decade. Tophi formation can occur earlier, however

   c. Sex. Rare in females, especially before menopause. Tophi formation is also rare in females

   d. Laboratory data. Check indicators of acute gout other than increased serum uric acid, which is essential for the diagnosis of gout

      (1) WBC count for leukocytosis

      (2) Erythrocyte sedimentation rate for an increase

      (3) Increase in urinary uric acid levels in a 24-hour specimen

         In *chronic* gout, the laboratory changes listed before would be present in a variable degree. Not all persons with increased serum uric acid will overexcrete. Indicators to be checked include

         (a) BUN for evidence of increased nitrogenous waste retention, which could indicate an inadequate blood flow to the kidney rather than increased uric acid because of gout

         (b) Plasma creatinine for evidence of kidney damage, possibly related to gouty nephropathy, or other causes of renal destruction

e. Question for a history of "arthritis" symptoms, particularly involving the lower extremities. Check for a history of or the presence of exquisite pain, usually in a joint, redness, and swelling, all of which are characteristic of gouty arthritis

f. Check the helix of the ears for the presence of a tophaceous deposit

g. Report increased uric acid levels found in infants and children not having known malignancies or treatment for malignancy. Assess for signs of Lesch–Nyhan syndrome, which includes failure to thrive at about 6 months and orange urate crystals on the diaper. Although no treatment has been found for the neurological disorders, the extent of renal damage can be reduced by giving allopurinol, which reduces the formation of uric acid. This drug is useful in all patients with increased uric acid levels and renal disease. It does not produce its effect in the kidney, as do the uricosuric drugs (probenecid, Anturane). Rather, it blocks the metabolic pathway of uric acid production

3. Prevent increased uric acid levels and the possible occurrence of acute gout in susceptible individuals by

a. Preventing the occurrence of precipitants of acute gout or hyperuricemia when logical or feasible. Precipitants include trauma; certain drugs (see "Serum Uric Acid Increased in," item 12); possibly overeating, especially of foods with a high purine content (organ meats such as liver, heart, kidney; wild game; goose; anchovies; herring; sardines; mackerel; scallops; and meat extracts, broth, and gravy); minor or major surgical procedures; ingestion of beer, wine, or ale; sudden weight loss; and a high-fat diet

b. If not preventable, making certain that the physician is aware of the possibility of hyperuricemia so that colchicine can be prescribed and administered prophylactically. Usually, a serum uric acid level greater than 9 mg/dl is one of the major indications for beginning a preventative program

c. Assisting the individual in selecting an optimum diet. Exclusion of all purine foods is rarely done and rarely satisfactory when done, but elimination of the high-purine-content foods listed earlier is feasible. A high-carbohydrate diet tends to increase uric acid excretion

d. Observing for evidence of prodromal symptoms and signs of an acute attack: diuresis, probably resulting from increased levels of urinary solutes; mood changes, possibly caused by increased retention of nitrogenous waste; and increased pain or discomfort in affected joints

e. Teaching affected individuals and home caretakers the precautions given above as well as the necessity of taking maintenance medication exactly when, in what amounts, and for as long as directed by the physician. The action of uricosuric drugs is dose-dependent (see "Serum Uric Acid Levels Decreased in," item 1a). Colchicine and allopurinol produce a cumulative dosage effect, and probenecid may be given on a lifelong schedule

4. Prevent the development of complications or modify the severity of the complications by

a. Observing the response of the individual in an acute gouty attack to the administration of colchicine or other gout medications

(1) Colchicine relieves the pain resulting from gout only. It has no effect on pain caused by other joint inflammations. The specific pain relief is helpful in establishing a diagnosis or supporting one

(2) Report the lack of pain relief. The drug is usually administered every hour or 2 hours until the pain is relieved or gastrointestinal side effects occur. Pain and swelling should subside within 8 to 12 hours and disappear in 24 to 72 hours (Berkow, 1992)

(3) By itself colchicine does not reduce serum urate levels. It can be given in combination with probenecid (Colbenemid), which has a uricosuric effect (excretion of uric acid in the urine). Given alone, probenecid aggravates acute gout and increases serum uric acid levels

(4) Monitor serum uric acid levels. The goal of treatment is usually 6 mg/dl, preferably less

b. Keeping accurate intake and output records. The daily output should be from 2000 to 3000 ml/d at a minimum. A high fluid intake helps minimize uric acid precipitation, thereby preventing the formation of urate stones and kidney damage. Excellent hydration is imperative when uricosuric therapy is used, at least 3000 ml/day, unless contraindicated by poor cardiac or kidney function, in which case collaboration with the physician over methods to maintain kidney function is imperative. Since gout is a fairly chronic condition with remissions and exacerbations, the affected individual should be taught this process and its rationale. Monitor serum creatinine as well as BUN levels for evidence of renal damage

c. Testing urine pH with a pH-sensitive strip, such as Nitrazine paper, and teaching the procedure to the affected person and home caretaker. Urate stones form best in acid media, so a urine pH of 7.0 (alkaline) is optimal (reference range 4.5–8.0). Urine acidity will increase with the onset of an acute attack. The physician may order sodium bicarbonate, sodium citrate, or other medications such as Diamox to help alkalinize the urine. Any indication of heart disease, hypertension, or renal insufficiency should be reported before beginning this therapy because they could be contraindications to the increased sodium intake

d. Providing alkaline ash foods when not otherwise contraindicated to assist in urine alkalinization. Although not vital if medication is being given, such intervention can be of use. Alkaline ash foods include most fruits and vegetables with the exception of corn, lentils, plums, prunes, and cranberries, which are acid ash

e. Ensuring that acetaminophen (Tylenol) is given in the place of aspirin, particularly when uricosuric medications are in use (Benemid, Anturane), because salicylates nullify the action of these drugs. Check urinary uric acid levels, if available, for an increase when uricosuric drugs are being given. Twenty-four-hour specimens give the most reliable data. An increase indicates effective drug action

f. Monitoring serum glucose levels of individuals receiving oral hypoglycemic agents and Anturane or Benemid at the same time. These drugs have hypoglycemic qualities that potentiate the antidiabetic medication. False-positive Clinitest reactions occur with Benemid as well

g. Monitoring the complete blood count, hemoglobin, and platelets of individuals receiving colchicine and allopurinol because of the potential for bone marrow depression. If possible, periodic checks during therapy should be evaluated against a baseline determination done before initiation of the medication

h. Monitoring the prothrombin time of persons receiving oral anticoagulants and allopurinal for increased levels because of an increase in the half-life of the anticoagulant in the face of allopurinal administration

1.8 SERUM TOTAL PROTEIN

Synonyms: Total protein, TP

Normal Ranges (g/dl)

Adult	6.0–8.2
Senior adult	6.0–7.8
Pediatric	
Premature	4.3–7.6
Newborn	4.6–7.6
Infant	6.0–6.7
Child	5.5–8.2

Definition. The term plasma protein is often used interchangeably with serum or total protein, but there is a difference. Plasma protein contains the coagulation factor fibrinogen, but serum protein does not. Reliable measurements can be made on either plasma or serum, but serum protein is the measurement most used. Plasma proteins as a group include fibrinogen, hormones, serum enzymes, and conjugated proteins (lipoproteins, glycoproteins, and metal binding proteins). They account for the major part of the solids in plasma. Interstitial fluid is very similar to plasma. It is the presence of albumin, globulin, fibrinogen, and prothrombin that differentiates the two. These proteins in plasma exert the colloid osmotic pressure that maintains equilibrium in the capillaries, one of the major functions of plasma protein. Besides maintaining the normal distribution of water between blood and tissues, another major function of plasma protein is as a transport agent to cells; many vital metabolites, metal ions, hormones, and lipids are bound to and carried by specific proteins (Tietz, 1990). Plasma proteins are also concerned with nutrition, acid-base balance (serum proteins are amphoteric and can combine with acids or bases—given a normal range of blood pH, protein acts as an acid and will combine with cations), immunity, and enzyme action. Serum protein, or total protein (TP), is a measurement of albumin and of the many different globulin fractions only. Serum and plasma proteins are the most conveniently available body protein for examination and measurement.

Because total protein determination represents several different proteins, it is not a good indicator of change in any one individual fraction. Changes in TP concentration occur in many disease states, and information about these changes is of clinical value in evaluating the course of disease or response to treatment, although rarely of assistance in diagnosis. Changes in TP may occur in one, several, or all fractions. Changes can occur in different directions in different fractions without changing the TP concentration itself. In the past, for more definitive information the physician would order testing of TP, serum albumin, globulin, and an albumin/globulin ratio (A/G ratio). Although these tests are still in use, a more valuable and accurate examination of the protein fractions is that of protein electrophoresis.

Physiology. Proteins are taken into the body in the diet. Many research experiments have shown a direct relationship between the formation of plasma protein, to include antibody formation, and the amount and quality of dietary protein ingested. Almost all of the protein taken in food is fully digested to amino acids in the small intestine. According to Howard and Herbold (1982), "If the dietary protein lacks even one of the essential amino acids, the body reacts as if all essential amino acids are deficient," and unless all are available at much the same time, complete protein utilization does not occur. Amino acids are transported to the liver by the bloodstream where albumin, the alpha and beta globulins, prothrombin, and fibrinogen are synthesized exclusively. Gamma globulins are produced by B lymphocytes and carried out primarily in plasma cells and lymphoid tissue. The plasma cell is the end-stage production and storage cell. Once synthesized, plasma proteins are released into the bloodstream. All body proteins form a large pool that can be drawn on by any tissue that needs protein. The protein pool is in dynamic equilibrium. For instance, a single molecule, synthesized in the liver and released into the plasma pool, may make up a part of an enzyme of some cell, yet eventually be incorporated into the hemoglobin in an erythrocyte. All body cells contain protein that can be used to meet caloric requirements when dietary protein is unavailable. Amino acids are used for energy or to form substances such as the aforementioned enzyme, hormones, or any other of the many protein substances essential to the body. Approximately 15 to 20 g of plasma proteins, about one tenth of the circulating plasma proteins, are formed daily from this protein pool, and an equal amount is broken down by complete degradation daily. A marked elevation of total protein levels occurs rarely. Slight elevations are not uncommon. When there is an increase in the level of a protein, particularly one of low molecular weight, large amounts are excreted. Evidently, having passed through the glomerular sieve of the kidney, the protein saturates the reabsorptive capacity of the tubule.

The ultimate fate of protein is not clear. Any albumin that seeps into the ECF is returned to the blood via the lymph. The body protein reserve is well assimilated, and only a very small portion is excreted. The protein that is filtered through the glomerulus is almost totally reabsorbed—it is assumed by the proximal tubules. Only about 1 percent of the albumin filtered is excreted in urine. Plasma proteins are destroyed by way of the digestive tract as well as the kidney and by catabolism in tissue cells, particularly in the liver. Amino acids are liberated by catabolism in tissue cells, particularly in the liver. Amino acids liberated by catabolism and leaked into the gastrointestinal tract are presumed to be reabsorbed into the portal circulation and reused in protein synthesis.

Regulation of protein synthesis is also unclear. It seems obvious that an equilibrium exists among protein synthesis, catabolism, and dietary intake, with the body constituents being replaced rapidly at a constant rate. As noted, the quality and quantity of amino acids available in the diet influence the rate of synthesis. Also affecting protein synthesis is the metabolic rate of the body and the action of certain hormones. Growth hormone, androgens, and insulin increase protein synthesis. Protein catabolism increases in response to glucocorticoids and high concentrations of thyroid. If these hormones are present at physiological levels, however, there is an anabolic effect on protein metabolism.

When there is a limited intake or supply of carbohydrates, adipose tissue—followed by the nonnitrogen fraction of protein—is used for energy. An ample supply of carbohydrate allows conservation of body stores of protein for tissue maintenance and growth. Thus carbohydrate has a protein-sparing action.

Pathophysiology. The TP concentration will decrease in several conditions, which is almost always a reflection of a decrease in the albumin fraction. Globulins, most frequently the alpha globulin fraction, usually increase at the same time, and the result may be a TP concentration that is within normal limits. Edema almost invariably occurs when the TP concentration falls below 5.3 g/dl, which is considered the critical level. Hypoproteinemia occurs slowly and insidiously in many unrelated disease states. It can occur secondary to an inadequate intake of protein—to include the lack of one or all essential amino acids—and impaired absorption, secondary to inadequate protein synthesis within the body (as in liver disease or genetic disorders), or secondary to an increased loss of protein that occurs with renal dysfunction or pathological states that increase the amount of low-molecular-weight proteins in the circulation that can be filtered and lost (intravascular hemolysis). Loss also occurs because of increased protein catabolism (cachectic wasting in malignancies), increased levels of catabolic hormones, or in gastrointestinal enteropathies.

Hyperproteinemia usually occurs secondary to pathological loss of fluid or a marked decrease in water intake. The absolute amount of serum proteins is unchanged, but there is an increase in concentration resulting from the loss of solvent water. An absolute increase in serum protein levels is seen in multiple myeloma, which is discussed later.

SERUM TOTAL PROTEIN LEVELS INCREASED IN:

*1. States of severe fluid loss such as in severe vomiting, diarrhea, Addison's disease, diabetic acidosis, or early stages of burns. In burns of highly vascular tissue a great fluid shift occurs by extravasation into deeper tissues and dehydration of the nondamaged tissue occurs. More fluids and sodium are lost initially than is protein. Later, hypoproteinemia can occur as protein is lost into the burned area

*2. States of prolonged, inadequate fluid intake. Without adequate water intake, dietary protein cannot be properly metabolized, and water is drawn from the interstitial and intercellular spaces to supply the necessary volume to excrete the increased solute load. Eventually, without replacement, the total body water stores will be depleted, and the serum TP concentration will rise

*3. Therapy using albumin infusion. Transient increases in the TP concentration have been shown

*4. The condition known as multiple myeloma. This is considered an immunoproliferative disease—a plasma cell tumor that produces excessive amounts of abnormal immunoglobins (gamma globulin). The serum albumin concentration is often decreased. Abnormal proteins that sometimes appear in the urine are called Bence Jones proteins, which are light chains from immunoglobulin molecules. Serum hyperviscosity can occur. Bence Jones proteins are almost entirely secreted in the urine 12 hours after synthesis, which can cause an excretion of as much as one half of the daily nitrogen intake (Henry, 1991). Quantities of serum proteins other than gamma globulin are unaltered except for a decrease in the serum albumin content, which is not characteristic of the disease. More likely it reflects malnutrition related to the increased protein demand of a malignant process or renal loss when the kidney is affected by the myeloma

SERUM TOTAL PROTEIN LEVELS DECREASED IN:

1. Conditions causing impaired utilization or synthesis such as
   a. Potassium deficit. Potassium is an essential element in protein synthesis. Any person with a prolonged disturbance in body fluids can be at risk for a protein deficit since the causes of abnormalities in body fluids are often causes of protein deficit as well
   *b. Chronic liver disease. A lack of adequately functioning hepatocytes causes a decreased production of albumin, primarily in conditions such as portal cirrhosis. There is often a simultaneous increase in globulin, which may cause a TP concentration that is within the normal range, or in a less frequent occurrence the TP level is increased. Changes in serum proteins are important in the diagnosis and evaluation of liver disease because so many are formed there
   c. Pancreatic insufficiency, as with chronic pancreatitis, because of the impaired digestion or absorption consequent to the inadequate amounts or total absence of proteolytic enzymes produced in the pancreas
   d. Idiopathic steatorrhea. There is impaired absorption from the intestine of not only protein but also carbohydrate and fat, which causes the use of plasma protein for energy, which further diminishes the serum TP concentration. There is a decrease in albumin and all globulin fractions. Other malabsorption syndromes may cause similar problems (e.g., cystic fibrosis, adult-onset sprue*).

---

*In these lists, asterisks indicate states in which changes in albumin concentration parallel serum protein changes.

2. Conditions causing increased protein loss such as

   *a. Inflammatory gastrointestinal disease as with ulcers or colitis. The rate and amount of protein leakage into the gastrointestinal tract is increased, which significantly increases the amount of protein lost in the feces. Ordinarily, amino acids are reabsorbed and reused

   *b. Nephrotic syndrome. The glomerulus becomes increasingly permeable, which allows greater amounts of protein, usually albumin, to be filtered out and excreted in the urine. The syndrome can occur secondary to glomerulonephritis, amyloidosis, lupus erythematosus, or Kimmelstiel-Wilson disease. Both albumin and gamma globulin fractions are decreased. There is protein loss from the body of more than 50 to 70 mg/kg/day. The total protein pool is greatly decreased with the loss of albumin, and its rate of synthesis as well as catabolism increases. A *reduction* in the synthesis rate sometimes occurs and may be due in part to the usually poor protein–calorie nutritional state of the individual (Henry, 1991, pp. 400–403)

   c. Hemorrhage. A loss of large portions of intravascular components, both water and solute, stimulates the release of ADH and water conservation. Replacement of the circulating volume is primarily with water, and the TP concentration is decreased

   *d. Acute and chronic infections, primarily bacterial. Infections, particularly those accompanied by fever, tend to reduce the appetite, especially for protein foods, and decrease the absorption rate from the gastrointestinal tract. The increased metabolic rate resulting from fever increases the caloric need, and protein catabolism can occur in the absence of adequate carbohydrate intake or fat stores. A negative nitrogen balance ensues. The major decrease is in albumin. A concomitant rise in both alpha and gamma globulin may produce a TP that is within the normal range

   e. Burns (see "Serum Total Protein Levels Increased in," item 1)

*3. Conditions related to inadequate intake lead to varying degrees of malnutrition, so-called protein–calorie malnutrition. There is a decreased synthesis of all plasma proteins, even alpha globulin, which is usually raised in hypoproteinemias, and an increased use of plasma protein for energy. Fasting alone results in a decrease in albumin synthesis of 30 to 40 percent (McCance & Huether, 1990, p. 62). Concentrations of nitrogenous waste products in the plasma (BUN, urea, creatinine) usually decrease as well. Protein deficits occur slowly, so any decrease in total plasma protein levels indicates prolonged protein deprivation. The causes of malnutrition are extensive. Some causes include the inability to eat because of a decreased level of consciousness or anorexia nervosa; decreased ability to chew secondary to myotonia or the loss of molars; incomplete protein intake, lack of one or more of the essential amino acids secondary to fad diets, or cultural or economic strictures; increased metabolic requirements secondary to malignancy or hyperthyroidism; or inadequate intake of carbohydrates to spare protein for growth and metabolism

4. Conditions causing dilution and a relative decrease in serum protein concentrations such as

   a. Excessive administration of water and sodium after acute trauma (e.g., surgery). The basic drive of the body after acute trauma is to retain water. Aldosterone is stimulated to conserve sodium, which in turn helps to conserve water, and there is a loss of potassium to conserve sodium. The body can then be easily overwhelmed by fluid (Sabiston, 1981), and total protein levels appear depressed because of increased solvent in the extracellular space

*b. Transudation of plasma protein, particularly albumin, into ascitic fluid
*c. Early phase of pregnancy in which hydration changes occur

---

IMPLICATIONS FOR NURSING: SERUM TOTAL PROTEIN

Prevention of malnutrition and of protein deficiency is a major need that can be accomplished by the nurse, both in the hospital and in the community. Oddly enough, deficiency states are more frequently encountered in the hospital in the United States. Nursing actions to meet this need may include any or all of the following.
1. Patient preparation. No food or drink other than water for 8 hours before the test is preferred, although not essential. In some instances dietary intake of fat may be limited
2. Education of all clients in the elements of basic nutrition regardless of diagnosis, educational level, occupation, or setting in which they are met. Such education may be sorely needed not only by the health care consumer but also by many health care providers
3. Acquisition of knowledge of the essential amino acid content of foods so that diet planning will include adequate combinations of foods to provide all essential amino acids despite dietary restrictions. Vegetarian diets can include all essential protein, but not without great care in planning
4. Identification of risk populations in which a detailed nutritional assessment must be carried out
    a. Nutritional screening and assessment should be done for all pregnant women on the initial visit if possible. Risk factors to look for relate to age, socioeconomic status, and past history of medical or obstetric problems
    b. Persons with renal disease, especially if on protein restriction
    c. Persons with chronic liver disease
    d. Persons presenting with anemia, cause unknown
    e. Persons with pathology that causes increased metabolic demands (e.g., acute infections, malignancy, hyperthyroidism)
    f. Persons with decreased intestinal absorptive function (e.g., chronic diarrhea, acute diarrhea in children, colitis, adult-onset sprue, cystic fibrosis, and new ileostomates)
    g. Persons not receiving food by mouth (e.g., n.p.o., postsurgical, unconscious, on tube feedings)
    h. Persons with chronic illnesses of any kind
    i. Teenage females (high incidence of anorexia nervosa, bulimia, unbalanced intake of "junk food")
    j. Poor, unemployed, or underemployed individuals
    k. Persons unable to meet their own nutritional need because of physical or mental difficulties (e.g., the frail elderly, the handicapped person, the confused person, the mentally ill person)
5. Assessment of the nutritional status
    a. Check the height and weight. Compare the height for age and the weight for height. This will give more useful information about the nutritional status than does weight for age. A height deficit could be present because of chronic malnutrition. The height-for-age and weight-for-height approach is especially useful in children because they may be both wasted and stunted. In the adult, determining the height of parents and siblings is helpful. Also useful in the adult is determining the weight at age 25 as a baseline for comparison. Assess for recent changes
    b. Check for the presence of edema, skin lesions, dullness, dryness, and the loss of hair. Prolonged protein malnutrition decreases the tissue turnover rate and body surface temperature (by 1 to 2 degrees), which alters skin and nail growth and appearance. Edema can occur both because of decreased production of albumin and inadequate cardiac function
    c. Check for a history of change in affect (increasing apathy?), frequent infections (there is an increased susceptibility to infection with malnutrition because of depression of the immune defense system), or a history of delayed wound healing (inadequate protein synthesis)
    d. Check and record muscle mass daily by using the same muscle each time at the same area, preferably of a limb that is in use for activities of daily living (ADLs) at least

    e. Check pertinent laboratory data when available. If not available and other assessment data indicate malnutrition, request that tests be performed

        (1) TP. Will have normal or decreased levels with a decreased concentration of albumin, which is the protein primarily responsible for colloid osmotic pressure and probably is the primary nutritional source of body tissues

        (2) RBC count. May be decreased because of a lack of available protein for production; because of a lack of iron absorption, which will cause a hypochromic, microcytic anemia; or because of a lack of vitamin B_{12} absorption, which will cause a macrocytic, normochronic anemia

        (3) Blood indices

           (a) Hemoglobin levels may decrease because of iron or protein deficiency

           (b) MCV: decreased with hypochromic microcytic anemia; increased with hyperchromic, macrocytic anemia

           (c) MCHC: decreased with hypochromic, microcytic anemia; increased with hyperchromic, macrocytic anemia (rarely seen)

        (4) WBC count. Polymorphonuclear leukocytes (neutrophils) will increase in the presence of acute infection; check the lymphocyte count in children with a history or the presence of infection. If less than 6300/mm³ (the average for a 2-year-old), it could indicate an impaired defense against infection. This can lead to further difficulties in assessment (e.g., false negative on a tuberculin skin test) (Howard & Herbold, 1982)

        (5) Plasma potassium. Potassium is essential for protein synthesis and is decreased in malnutrition states

        (6) BUN, urea clearance, creatinine. Decreased levels occur in long-term malnutrition. (Other laboratory values may be decreased secondary to the decrease in protein. Chemicals such as calcium are transported in the blood by being bound to protein. Therefore, a decrease in available protein will cause a decrease in circulating calcium)

    f. Note the presence or absence of teeth and any prosthesis. Determine whether prostheses are usually worn. Persons with partial lower molar dentures frequently leave them out, thereby decreasing their ability to chew and increasing the probability of selecting soft, easily masticated foods. This can eliminate many good sources of protein

6. For the individuals identified at risk for protein deficiency or so diagnosed, the nurse can help ensure adequate intake and use of all essential amino acids

    a. The greater the amount of protein intake, the greater the water requirement. This need is especially important in the person receiving tube feedings, with a fever, with a high catabolic rate, or who has a decreased ability to concentrate urine. Elderly persons may require an increased water intake even without an increase in protein intake because of the frequent occurrence of impaired renal function in the elderly. With ingestion of a high-protein diet, urine volumes will be increased, even if no extra fluids are given. This can lead to excessive saline loss and dehydration. Fluids are therefore imperative with a high-protein diet

    b. Individuals who are nutritionally depleted and have nonelective surgery that necessitates prolonged periods n.p.o. should be closely monitored when returned to a diet to ensure an adequate and complete protein intake. Anorexia is one of the symptoms of malnutrition that makes the process of encouraging protein intake particularly challenging for the nurse. Malnutrition is more common in the elderly than in young adults in the United States and requires special awareness with this population

    c. It is well to remember that there is a starvation effect in the first few days postsurgery for almost all ill persons. A weight loss of 0.5 lb/day in the adult is not unusual. Weight loss may be thought of as a benefit for the obese individual, but the obese person can be and usually is malnourished despite an excessive intake of food. Check for dilutional hypoproteinemia before instituting measures to replace protein (see "Serum Total Protein Levels Decreased in," item 4)

    d. Measurement of muscle mass is helpful in determining the protein loss, but without exercise such measurement is of no value in checking the effectiveness of protein replacement. Without exercise, body protein may continue to be lost despite adequate intake. Provision of active and passive bed exercises (described in "Implications for Nursing: Platelet Count," item 6, in Section 3.11) and early ambulation may assist the nutritional status as well as improve the appetite.

Teach the patient and family members the rationale for exercise to increase their compliance with the action and independent effort on their part

e. Obtain a diet history to determine what types of protein would be most acceptable to the individual and his or her frequency of eating. Provide these choices if possible

f. Provide foods with adequate potassium to ensure protein synthesis

g. Provide adequate carbohydrate in the diet, especially in the presence of fever, to spare protein from being used for energy. Minimum daily requirements of carbohydrates have not been established. The general rule is 100 g/day, 150 g/day if fasting, to prevent muscle breakdown (Howard & Herbold, 1982)

h. Protect the individual who is malnourished from exposure to infection because such individuals have an increased risk secondary to decreased antibody production and decreased lymphocyte proliferation (Lewis & Collier, 1992)

i. When protein intake is restricted, as in some types of renal disease, about 70 to 75 percent of the allowed protein in the diet should be from foods with high biologic value, that is, containing complete amino acids and able to assimilate readily. Fresh and dried beef serum and lactalbumin (milk protein) are most effective, followed by egg white, beef muscle, liver casein, and gelatin (Harper et al., 1979)

7. The person with hypoproteinemia, because of the nephrotic syndrome, may lose large amounts of clotting factor IX and must be monitored for bleeding tendencies. Conversely, the plasma levels of fibrinogen and other coagulation factors may be increased so that some authors feel there is an increased frequency of thrombosis in these individuals (Frolich, 1980). Observation of peripheral circulation, the use of antithromboembolic hose (i.e., TED hose), and early ambulation can be helpful

8. The average daily protein requirements of infants can be more than three times those of adults (2 to 3.5 g/kg of infant weight; 1.0 g/kg of adult weight) and increases markedly during illness. Absorption is less than in adults because food is propelled very rapidly through the digestive tract because of that system's immaturity (Whaley & Wong, 1991). Therefore, malnourishment in the infant tends to be even more serious and have more permanent outcomes than in the adult. Frequent nutritional assessment should be carried out in the infant and growing child, and parents should be taught the process as well as its importance

1.9 SERUM PROTEIN FRACTIONS

1.9.1 Serum Albumin

Synonym: Plasma albumin

Normal Ranges (g/dl)

Adult (>15 yr)	3.3–5.0
Senior adult	3.2–4.5 (salt fractionation)
Pediatric	
Newborn infant	2.9–5.5
Child to age 3	3.8–5.4
Child/adolescent to age 15	3.3–5.5

Definition. Albumin is a plasma protein synthesized in the liver and the major constituent of the serum protein. It can be directly measured and alterations in its serum concentration parallel many alterations in the serum total protein (see abnormalities indicated by an asterisk under

"Serum Total Protein Levels Increased in" in Section 1.8). Albumin has a half-life of approximately 30 days and is considered a reliable index of the severity and prognosis in patients with chronic hepatic disease (Henry, 1991). Those patients showing a rise in the serum albumin content have a more favorable prognosis than those who do not. Albumin measurement is not as useful as the measurement of fibrinogen or prothrombin in dating the onset of liver cell failure because its half-life is much longer (Sodeman & Sodeman, 1982).

Physiology. Albumin is the most important serum protein in maintaining intravascular oncotic pressure. Should it decrease, edema results. Albumin is considered the primary nutritional source for body tissue. Serum albumin is important in transport, being the major vehicle for calcium, magnesium, bibirubin, and fatty acids transport as well as the transport of many drugs. Effective blood levels of such drugs are altered by a decrease in the serum albumin concentration. There is some evidence that the production of albumin may be regulated by osmotic effects rather than—or as well as—the change in serum albumin concentration itself, but the rate of snythesis usually increases when serum levels are decreased. Synthesis occurs in the liver. With a failure in dietary intake of protein such as in fasting, there is a marked decrease in synthesis. The liver is believed to be responsible for about 10 percent of the normal albumin catabolism (Sodeman & Sodeman, 1982).

Pathophysiology. In disease states affecting protein concentrations, serum albumin levels tend to decrease or remain the same and do not rise above normal except with hemoconcentration or dehydration. A decrease in the albumin concentration frequently is associated with an increase in globulin levels (see "Pathophysiology" in Section 1.9.2). Albumin is lost in pathology by extravasation (burns, ascites), in urine with tubular dysfunction (nephrosis), nephrotic syndrome, or by increased leakage into the gut (colitis). Synthesis of albumin is decreased in conditions causing a lack of protein intake or absorption (liver disease). Decreases in serum albumin levels usually lead to edema because of the loss of intravascular oncotic pressure. [Complete absence (analbuminemia) is very rare and, surprisingly causes only mild edema]

For conditions in which the albumin concentration increases or decreases, see serum TP increases and decreases in Section 1.8.

IMPLICATIONS FOR NURSING: SERUM ALBUMIN

See "Implications for Nursing: Serum Total Protein" in Section 1.8.

1.9.2 Serum Globulin

Synonym: Plasma globin

Normal Ranges (gm/dl)

Adult   2.3–3.5

Senior adult (g/dl)

Male	3.1–3.4
Female	2.8–3.2[a]
Infant	No specific variation from adult

[a]Computed from total protein and albumin ranges as given in Carnevali and Patrick (1979).

Definition. Serum globulin is the major constituent, after albumin, of the TP or serum protein. The TP measurement can be used to estimate globulin concentration. The globulin concentration is the remainder when albumin—corrected for NPN—is measured directly and subtracted from the total protein concentration. The globulin fraction of the serum protein is a very complex mixture, with functions that are also multiple, complex, and not fully understood. The serum globulin is a relatively imprecise measure and gives little or no specific information for diagnosis. It is rarely reported separately. The rapid increase in knowledge of the molecular structure of proteins has outdated much terminology used in protein classification—even terms such as albumin and globulin (Harper et al., 1979). Generalizations about serum globulins are of even less value than those about albumin because of the complexity of the group of proteins given this name, both in function and molecular structure. The one feature they all share is their insolubility in water and concentrated salt solutions and their solubility in weak, neutral salt solutions (Henry, 1991). Globulin fractions are usually classified as alpha, beta, or gamma, and subclasses have been defined for each fraction. See 4.8.2 Protein Electrophoresis, Urine.

Physiology. Serum globulins are produced at several sites in the reticuloendothelial system of the body. Most of the alpha and beta globulins originate in the liver, but gamma globulins are produced from plasma cells and lymphoid tissue and are made up of amino acids only (Harvey et al., 1991). The antibody activity of the plasma, interstitial fluid, and body secretions is associated with the gamma globulin fraction, called immunoglobulins, the symbol for which is Ig. The collective group of immunoglobulins has been defined and is known as G, M, A, D, and E (e.g., IgG, IgM). They provide protection against bacterial and viral infection, parasites, allergens, and malignancy. Distinct function specialization has been described for some of the Ig subclasses. The alpha and beta globulins are made up principally of mucoproteins and glycoproteins. Beta globulin is also made up of lipoproteins. Transport is a major function of these globulin fractions, and beta provides a vehicle for transport of fat in plasma. Transferrin, a beta globulin, is one of the many metal-binding globulins that provides transport for copper and iron. Both alpha and beta globulins transport fat-soluble vitamins and certain hormones, for example, corticosteroid-binding globulin (CBG), thyroid-binding globulin (TBG), and antihemophilic globulin (AHG) or factor VIII, a protein involved in the clotting process. Cryoglobulins are cold-precipitable gamma globulins (Henry, 1991).

The human fetus is capable of forming antibodies, but the greatest amount of immunity of an infant is that obtained through the placenta from the mother. This is usually IgG, which makes up 75 to 85 percent of the Ig function (Frolich, 1980). By the end of his or her first year, the infant is able to produce adult concentrations of immunoglobulin.

The protein from which both albumin and globulin are made is found in the "protein pool," described with serum proteins, and the same general processes of formation and degradation apply. Little is known, however, about the regulation of globulin production other than its response to antigen stimulation. Although the area is currently under intensive study, much is still theoretical or totally unknown.

Pathophysiology. Very few generalizations can be made about globulin response in disease. In acute infections a slight increase, particularly of gamma globulin levels, reflects the synthesis of antibodies to the infecting agent. A greater rise occurs in chronic infections (Tietz, 1990). When there is a state of hypoproteinemia in the body, the alpha globulin concentration increases, which is thought to reflect an increase in glycoprotein and lipoprotein levels (plus C-reactive protein). This is seen frequently in advanced metastatic cancer, but no diagnostic pattern has been noted (Henry, 1991). Acute cellular necrosis is also frequently accompanied by an increase in the alpha globulin alpha. This globulin, however, has been seen to have decreased levels in acute hepatocellular necrosis, so the generalization is not always true. Beta globulins have not been associated with specific disease processes with any regularity. Changes in transferrin concentrations are reflected by changes in beta globulin, and increases in accumulation of lipids are reflected by increases in beta globulin. The possible relationship as a cause of atherosclerosis is being studied.

In many diseases there is a constant association between a decreased albumin concentration and an increased level of alpha globulins (nephrosis, cirrhosis, acute infections), but little is known of the process.

Decreases in the immunoglobulins produce, not surprisingly, an increased susceptibility to infections because humoral immunity, as opposed to cellular immunity, is immunity resulting from circulating antibodies in the gamma globulin fraction of the plasma protein.

SERUM GLOBULIN LEVELS INCREASED IN:

1. Familial idiopathic dysproteinemia because of a genetic effect causing an increased production of globulin in relation to albumin
2. Diseases associated with continuing cell necrosis or tissue destruction
   a. Viral hepatitis because of the immunologic response to the virus and to the necrotic process in the liver cells as well as to proliferation of reticuloendothelial cells in the liver. All globulin fractions increase. The increase begins before the onset of jaundice, peaks in 8 to 10 days, and does not return to normal for an extended time, 3 to 4 months. Increases are also seen in diffuse hepatocellular diseases such as cirrhosis and chronic active hepatitis. The liver is often infiltrated with plasma cells and lymphocytes
   b. Acute febrile disease because of increased tissue breakdown
   c. Cancer because of tissue wasting
   d. Advanced tuberculosis, also probably because of tissue wasting
3. Multiple myeloma because of a gamma globulin increase secondary to production of the abnormal immunoglobulin (monoclonal or M protein). The alpha and beta fractions occasionally increase. Ultimately, in some cases a secondary decrease in gamma globulin production can occur and cause hypogammaglobulinemia or agammaglobulinemia
4. Nephrotic syndrome because of the loss of gamma globulin in the urine. Concentrations of alpha and beta globulin increase

SERUM GLOBULIN LEVELS DECREASED IN:

1. Hypogammaglobulinemia because of the decreased production of gamma globulin, cause unknown

2. Agammaglobulinemia, whether congenital, physiological, idiopathic, or acquired secondary to conditions such as multiple myeloma, leukemia, or Hodgkin's disease because of a marked decrease or total absence of gamma globulin production

---

IMPLICATIONS FOR NURSING: SERUM GLOBULIN

1. Any individual with either a decrease or an increase in globulin content can be expected to exhibit some degree of immunologic deficiency specific to the person. Therefore, a nursing history should be taken when changes in globulin concentrations occur to determine the
   a. Frequency of occurrence of infections
   b. Evidence of chronic infection
   c. Failure to recover from infections
   d. Frequent reinfection
   e. Infection with unusual agents (history may reveal no logical source of infection)
   f. Familial history of deficiency
2. Observation of infants with a familial history of immunoglobulin deficiency for evidence of the disease process may not be fruitful until around 3 months of age because of the maternal transfer of immunoglobulins. Observe for
   a. Validating laboratory findings: decreased serum lymphocyte count and a lack of increase in lymphocytes in response to antigens; bone marrow showing a lack of plasma cells
   b. Evidence of graft-versus-host response (fever, skin rash, alopecia, hepatosplenomegaly, diarrhea, and ulceration of the mucous membrane of the gastrointestinal tract, mouth, and anus) 7 to 20 days after the administration of any blood supplements or other foreign tissues.
        Immunodeficient infants have a poor prognosis. A histocompatible bone marrow transplant is the only effective treatment, although injections of gamma globulin provide a passive immunity that is transitory. A very few infants have been kept alive by provision of a totally sterile environment, but to be effective, this environment must be provided before the infant has any infection
3. Nursing care of immunodeficient infants consists of
   a. Assisting in preventing infection and teaching family members the process (isolation, skin and mouth care)
   b. Providing support to the family in the care of a fatally ill child
   c. Providing family support against feelings of guilt and impotency in the very likely occurrence of chronic fungal infections of the mouth and nails despite the family's vigorous efforts to prevent or treat such infections
   d. Providing access to genetic counseling for the family (Whaley & Wong, 1991)
   e. The infant may exhibit symptoms similar to rheumatoid arthritis as one form of allergic manifestation. The reader is referred to Scipien & Barnard, 1983, for nursing care
4. Acquired forms of hypogammaglobulinemia or agammaglobulinemia should be suspected in persons with malabsorption syndromes because of the possibility of a defective synthesis of globulin. A high index of suspicion should be held also for any adult with a malignancy, particularly those involving the lymphatic or reticuloendothelial systems. Any individual with such a diagnosis should be carefully guarded against infection and a thorough history taken of types of infections to which the person has been particularly susceptible
5. The most common secondary immunodeficient state includes not only exaggerated susceptibility to infection but also thrombocytopenia. This implies the need for observation of unusual bleeding tendencies and nursing measures to protect the person from bleeding (see "Implications for Nursing: Platelet Estimation" in Section 2.3.2; "General Implications for Nursing Related to Problems in Coagulation" at the end of Chapter 3; and "Implications for Nursing: Serum Total Protein," item 7, in Section 1.8).

1.9.3 A/G Ratio

Synonyms: Albumin/globulin ratio, plasma A/G ratio

Normal Ranges (gm/dl)

Albumin
Less than 15 years	3.3–5.5
15 years or more	3.3–5.0
Globulin	2.3–3.8
A/G ratio	1.0–2.0

Definition. The A/G ratio is an expression of the ratio of albumin to globulin in the blood or urine. It is used to express protein changes in disease. It is computed by dividing the albumin concentration by the globulin concentration. Before the advent of electrophoresis and immunophoresis techniques, the A/G ratio was the best indicator available for looking at the component parts of serum total proteins, for in any one individual the A/G ratio is quite constant.

In several disease states there is a fairly constant relationship between the increase in globulin and the decrease in albumin levels (e.g., cirrhosis, nephrosis, acute infections, pneumonia, rheumatic fever, typhus), and following the A/G ratio was one of the best tools available for watching the response to treatment. Generally, the albumin concentration tends to decrease in abnormal conditions, and globulin exhibits a simultaneous increase. Both the albumin and the globulin fractions can be measured reliably in either plasma or serum.

The A/G ratio is now felt to have little significance, especially if absolute values are available (Widmann, 1983). As far back as 1969 the A/G ratio was felt to be of little importance, awkward, imprecise, and with no real clinical application (Henry, 1991), and one authority felt that the analysis of disease states would be enhanced if it were abandoned (Tietz, 1990). Despite its lack of "clinicopathologic significance" (SHMC, 1984), its use persists.

Physiology. See "Physiology" in Section 1.8.

A/G RATIO DECREASED IN:

- Any condition that decreases the albumin fraction of TP (see Sections 1.8 and 1.9.1)

A/G RATIO INCREASED IN:

- Any condition that increases globulin over albumin (see Sections 1.8 and 1.9.2).

IMPLICATION FOR NURSING

No food or drink for 8-12 hours prior to the test

1.9.4 Serum Prealbumin

Synonym: Tryptophan-rich prealbumin

Normal Range: 10–40 mg/dl

Prealbumin has a very high tryptophan content. Tryptophan is an amino acid thought to play a crucial role in protein synthesis control (SHMC, 1985). Prealbumin also functions as a dual-carrier protein: a "backup" carrier of thyroxine and a carrier protein for the retinal-binding protein (RBP) complex with vitamin A, although its carrier function is thought to be a very minor one.

Testing for prealbumin became a fairly routine laboratory procedure with the advent of total parenteral nutrition (TPN, hyperalimentation), although the substance has been known and testable for some time. Prealbumin is usually measured—along with some or all of the following tests: complete blood count (CBC), differential, prothrombin time, calcium, phosphorus, magnesium, glutamic oxalic transaminase/aspartate aminotransferase (GOT/AST), bilirubin, electrolytes, BUN, glucose, and albumin—to assess the adequacy of TNP.

It is also used to indicate the severity of acute liver disease (viral and toxic hepatitis) by its reflection of hepatic synthesis. Measurement of this substance is most useful in assessing the nutritional status of the individual receiving TPN for several reasons. It has a much shorter half-life (only 2 days) than does serum albumin; therefore, its measurement is indicative of a more recent nutritional status. It can also be used for checking individuals with low oncotic pressure who receive albumin concentrates, the administration of which will invalidate serum albumin levels.

PREALBUMIN LEVELS INCREASED IN:

- Administration of corticoids (Henry, 1991)

PREALBUMIN LEVELS DECREASED IN:

1. The neonate, in whom the level rapidly rises to the normal range within the first few weeks of life
2. Liver disease because of a decreased ability of the liver to synthesize prealbumin/albumin
3. Malnutrition for whatever cause (e.g., cachexia of malignancy, ulcerative colitis)

1.10 TOTAL SERUM BILIRUBIN

Synonyms: Total bilirubin, total plasma bilirubin

Normal Ranges (mg/dl)

Age	Total	Direct
0–1 day	0–6	0–1.5
1–2 days	0–8	0–1.5
3–5 days	0–12	0–1.5
6 days—adult	0.1–1.2	0–0.3
Senior adult: as for adult		

Definition. Bilirubin is one of two substances making up the bile pigments, biliverdin being the other. Approximately 85 percent of the bilirubin formed is derived from conversion of the heme from hemoglobin. The total bilirubin test can be done equally well on either serum or plasma and is one of the tests included in a "liver profile"; it is a test based on the secretory and excretory functions of the liver and therefore is of major importance in the profile. In itself it is not specific for any one disease but is extremely helpful in sorting out liver or biliary dysfunction when correlated with a thorough history and physical examination. Total serum bilirubin is useful in measuring the depth and progress of jaundice and is of considerable value in detecting "latent" jaundice (serum levels greater than 2 mg/dl) (see "Pathophysiology," the next section). Serum bilirubin, of all the tests included in a liver profile, is probably the most informative. Knowledge of bilirubin metabolism has increased the knowledge and understanding of liver physiology. Its estimation has immense importance in the newborn where it serves as a prime index of exchange transfusion necessity and effectiveness in the prevention of kernicterus.

Total bilirubin and the direct-reacting (conjugated, water-soluble) fraction can be accurately measured, but the indirect-reacting (unconjugated, water-insoluble) fraction is inferred by subtracting the direct from the total. The total bilirubin value represents the sum of both conjugated and unconjugated bilirubin. Bilirubin is destroyed by exposure to white light, artificial light, or sunlight. Although a breakdown of bilirubin into its fractions is helpful in the differential diagnosis of jaundice, total bilirubin determination is an excellent screening test to indicate hyperbilirubinemia, whatever the cause.

Physiology. The mechanism of bilirubin metabolism is complex and not completely understood (see Fig. 1–4). Approximately 6 to 8 g of hemoglobin is released each day, and some 263 mg of bilirubin are produced daily in the normal adult—with 5 L of blood and a hemoglobin concentration within normal limits. Many molecules share the same binding site on the albumin molecule with bilirubin and, when present in large numbers, will compete for binding. With even a slight decrease in available albumin, the binding sites may become inadequate, and bilirubin or other molecules will appear in increased concentrations in the serum. The compensatory mechanism for increased concentrations of bilirubin is an increased rate of excretion of the conjugated fraction or an increased rate of binding or conjugation, when possible, of the unconjugated fraction. When the hepatic reserve is exceeded, the indirect (unconjugated, water-insoluble) bilirubin value rises, and a pathological state exists. This provides a rationale for the pale jaundice seen in advanced malnutrition.

Enzymes needed for bilirubin conjugation mature late in fetal development and are not fully developed until the tenth month after conception. Therefore, all premature and some obstensibly full-term, but physically immature, low-birthweight newborns will have impaired conjugation in differing degrees of severity (Sodeman & Sodeman, 1982). This, coupled with excessive RBC breakdown because of the change from the hypoxic uterus to the air at birth, causes what is termed *physiological hyperbilirubinemia.* The liver "learns" to conjugate bilirubin within 3 to 5 days, and serum bilirubin levels return to normal in most instances.

Bilirubin metabolism provides the only source of endogenous carbon monoxide, and measurements of its production rate are used in some testing methods to determine the rate of heme product catabolism and thereby infer the rate of hemolysis (Sodeman & Sodeman, 1982).

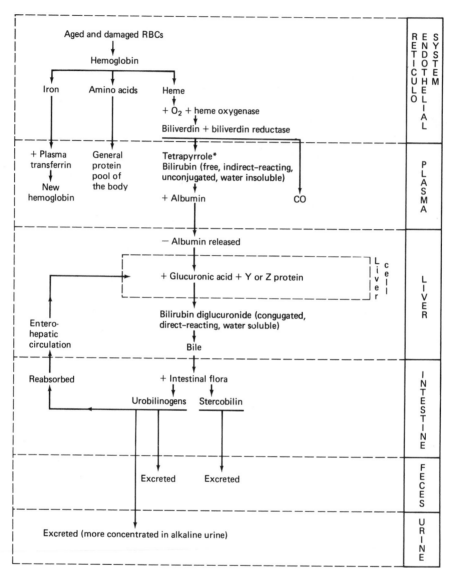

Figure 1–4. Bilirubin metabolism. (Data from Beck, 1971; Carnevali & Patrick, 1979; Sabaston, 1981; and Spencer, 1973.)
*Defined as a complex cyclic compound, an important component of myoglobin, cytochrone, catalase, as well as hemoglobin. (Levinsky, 1993.)

Pathophysiology. Jaundice is the major, overt indicator of a pathological state in bilirubin metabolism. It occurs when bilirubin is not removed or excreted or is formed in excessive amounts. At any point in the bilirubin metabolism mechanism, a congenital abnormality (an inborn error in metabolism) or an acquired abnormality can occur. Congenital abnormalities are often called constitutional hyperbilirubinemia. An example of such an abnormality would be Gilbert's disease. An increase in direct (conjugated, water-soluble) bilirubin levels is often seen in septic infants, especially with gram-negative infections. The increase may be the first clue to the presence of sepsis. Decreased levels of bilirubin occur rarely and are of little clinical significance.

Increases in total bilirubin are categorized into three mechanisms of jaundice production (see Fig. 1–5):

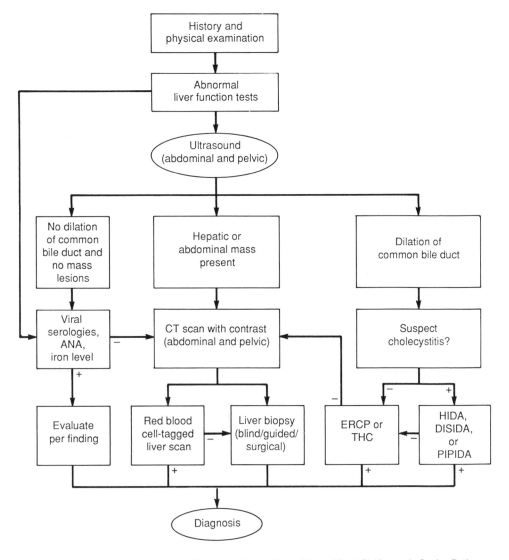

Figure 1–5. Diagnostic assessment of the jaundiced patient. (*From Albert B. Knapp, in* Senior Patient, *September 1990, p. 36, © McGraw-Hill, by permission.*)

1. Prehepatic (retention, hemolytic) jaundice, caused by overproduction of bilirubin or ineffective red cell formation
2. Hepatic (also included in the retention class) jaundice, caused by liver cell damage or inadequate albumin availability
3. Posthepatic (regurgitation, obstructive) jaundice, caused by mechanical obstruction of extrahepatic bile passages, which results in decreased excretion

Hepatic and posthepatic jaundice often occur together because a degree of obstruction usually occurs with liver cell damage that blocks the bile canaliculi. When there is liver cell damage, the cells lose their ability to conjugate bilirubin, a function normally found only in those cells. The cell damage allows the bilirubin, which has been conjugated by healthy cells, to pass freely into all liquids of the body when under normal conditions it is confined to the liver cell, the liver canaliculi, and the bile. Its distribution is determined by the protein (particularly albumin) content of the fluid. The invaded tissue is stained, and jaundice becomes apparent when the serum bilirubin concentration exceeds 2 mg/dl in the adult or child or 5 mg/dl in the premature infant.

Unconjugated (free, indirect-reacting, water-insoluble) bilirubin accumulates in adipose tissue, can be best seen in the subcutaneous fat of the abdomen and extremities, and will be excreted in the feces in increasing amounts in the adult. Also in the adult, severe hemolysis will cause serum bilirubin elevations rarely exceeding 5 mg/dl. The jaundice will be a mild pale yellow, and the urine will be free of bilirubin (recall, the elevation is of the water-insoluble, unconjugated fraction). If urine becomes darker, it will be due to an increased conjugation and excretion of direct-reacting bilirubin by the liver because of the increased loads of unconjugated bilirubin presented to it.

For the adult, chronic overproduction of bilirubin with mild serum increases, and although it may lead to the production of gallstones—which are made up primarily of bilirubin—it causes little harm. But in the full-term infant, levels of unconjugated bilirubin over 20 mg/dl may lead to kernicterus, a condition in which the unconjugated, unbound, and lipid-soluble bilirubin is able to cross the blood–brain barrier and be deposited in the basal ganglia of the brain, sometimes causing severe damage or death. The exact mechanism is not known, but the pathogenesis is seen to be almost identical with that observed in hypoxia (Whaley & Wong, 1991). Several factors affect the occurrence of kernicterus besides the initial elevation of the serum bilirubin level:

1. Conditions that decrease the binding capacity of the serum, for example, metabolic acidosis, decreased albumin levels in the serum, drugs that compete for albumin binding sites (e.g., salicylates, sulfonamides, vitamin K), or other chemicals with similar competitive binding properties (e.g., increased free fatty acid FFA levels)
2. Any condition that increases the oxygen demand (e.g., fetal distress)
3. Any condition that increases glucose demand (hypoxia). All of these factors serve to increase the amount of unbound, unconjugated bilirubin, thus increasing the risk of kernicterus occurring

Physiological jaundice that is due to immaturity of hepatic functions or increased RBC destruction is more severe and prolonged in the premature infant. The infant is also more susceptible to the aforementioned disorders that contribute to increased, unconjugated serum bilirubin levels. Because of this, the premature infant is at greater risk for the occurrence of kernicterus.

TOTAL SERUM BILIRUBIN LEVELS INCREASED IN:

1. Conditions causing overproduction of bilirubin as in
   a. Hemolytic disease causing the saturation of available albumin binding sites because of the massive amounts of bilirubin presented to the liver, for example, erythroblastosis fetalis, abnormal hemoglobins (e.g., hemoglobin S in sickle cell anemia), and abnormal RBCs (e.g., hereditary spherocytosis)
   b. Ineffective red cell formation (sometimes called shunt hyperbilirubinemia), for example, thalassemia (Cooley's anemia), pernicious anemia, porphyria
   c. Physiological jaundice of the newborn, particularly in the premature infant, that is due in part to the reduced life span of RBCs in the newborn, the lack of intestinal flora for conversion of conjugated bilirubin to urobilinogen, the inability of the liver to conjugate bilirubin, and possibly adaptation of the infant's liver to the postnatal hypoxic state after the closing of the ductus venosus at birth (Whaley & Wong, 1991)
   d. Infants of Oriental or Asian descent, which in this instance include American Indians, who tend to have bilirubin levels almost twice those seen in the black or white races (the cause is unknown). Hyperbilirubinemia is also seen in newborns of eastern Mediterranean heritage (e.g., Greek). Whether these increases are due to overproduction or excretion defects is also unknown, but the condition has been placed in this category for convenience
   e. Gilbert's disease, a retention type of constitutional (inborn error of metabolism) dysfunction with the true cause unknown. A high concentration of serum indirect (unconjugated, water-insoluble) bilirubin may be produced. This condition is occasionally associated with a hemolytic anemia as well (Henry, 1991)
   f. Escape of blood from the circulation into tissues, which may cause large hematomas or infarcts
2. Conditions causing hepatic intracellular conjugation defects as in
   a. The specific marked decrease of glucuronyl transferase activity that occurs in all newborns, or Crigler–Najjar syndrome
   b. Inhibition of glucuronyl transferase in some breast-fed infants because of chemicals excreted by their mothers into their milk. This dysfunction can occur before birth in some infants when the chemical reaches a high level in the mothers and disappears after the birth to produce a transient, familial, neonatal hyperbilirubinemia (Lucey–Driscoll syndrome)
   c. Administration of certain drugs to the near-term, pregnant mother or to the newborn (e.g., sulfonamides, vitamin K)
   d. Decreased production and stores of albumin because of the immaturity of the liver
   e. Administration of drugs that inhibit glucuronyl transferase (e.g., novobiocin [Albamycin])
   f. Viral hepatitis, which affects not only the cellular activity of the liver in bilirubin metabolism but also will quickly lead to intrahepatic cholestasis so that concentration of both the direct and indirect fractions increase in serum
   g. Laennec's cirrhosis (portal cirrhosis) in advanced stages, because of degeneration and fibrosis of the liver structure
3. Conditions causing obstruction of intrahepatic or extrahepatic biliary passages as in
   a. lCholediocholithiasis (gallstones in the common bile duct), which causes increases in direct bilirubin levels in both blood and urine, produces the characteristic dark, "Coca-

Cola" color. Clay-colored stools also occur because of the decrease in fecal urobilino-gen and stercobilin concentrations

b. Cancer of the head of the pancreas, which causes an increase in direct bilirubin levels in much the same manner as given for choledocholithiasis

c. Certain women evidencing a jaundice in the third trimester of pregnancy. These same women often develop jaundice after the use of contraceptive agents. The mechanism of jaundice is not clear

d. Biliary duct atresia in the neonate

e. The Dubin–Johnson syndrome in which the reduced capacity to excrete bilirubin is due to an inborn error of metabolism

f. The presence of renal failure, the mechanism of which is unclear

---

IMPLICATIONS FOR NURSING: TOTAL SERUM BILIRUBIN

1. Preparation for the test includes abstention from intake of anything other than water for 8 to 12 hours before blood is drawn to prevent lipemia, which interferes with the test. Hemolysis of the sample should be avoided to prevent falsely low results in some testing methods (Diazo) (Tietz, 1990)
2. Implications related to the appearance of jaundice
   a. Relieve pruritis, if present, as this symptom can be physically exhausting and emotionally demoralizing. It also tends to lead to tissue breakdown, especially when damage is done by scratching
      (1) Prevention of scratching is impossible; the person will scratch, at least in his or her sleep, unless totally restrained, and the outcomes of such restraint are usually more difficult to deal with than the outcomes of scratching
      (2) Suggest alternatives to scratching
         (a) Use a soft cloth instead of fingernails
         (b) Use counterstimulation by tickling with a feather or long-napped material such as fake fur or by small, sharp slaps. (The last should be used sparingly. Not only can the slaps become painful in themselves, but pruritis will be aggravated by the resultant capillary dilation)
      (3) Keep the environment cool and clothing and bedding light and nonrestrictive. Woolen blankets or clothing should not be used because wool fibers often cause itching and many people react strongly to wool
      (4) Do not allow perspiration to remain on the skin or in the clothing. Salt crystals can aggravate itching
      (5) Provide tub soaks with *tepid* water (to prevent capillary dilation secondary to temperature extremes or secondary to the physical stimulation of a shower spray)
      (6) Add soothing substances such as cornstarch or oatmeal to the tub soak or apply calamine lotion to affected areas, which should be considered independent nursing but may require a physician's order
      (7) Provide diversion in whatever form is acceptable to the individual and not contraindicated by his or her status; however, ensure that the activity does not unduly increase the body's metabolic rate because this would increase the body temperature and aggravate the pruritis
      (8) Administer medications ordered for pruritis (tranquilizers, sedatives, antihistamines) after first ensuring they are not principally metabolized by the liver or, if so metabolized, that the dosage has been adjusted accordingly. Careful observation for signs and symptoms of overdosage must be maintained as well as measures for the safety of the individual (decreased level of consciousness [LOC] is a common side effect) and observation for drug effectiveness
   b. Prevent skin breakdown by
      (1) Keeping fingernails clean and clipped short

(2) Suggesting the use of clean, white, cotton gloves, especially during sleep

(3) Keeping bedding smooth and well secured. (Wrinkles lead to excess localized venous stasis, which also aggravates itching)

(4) Advising frequent changes of position and instructing the individual in the need for this to prevent venous stasis, increased body heat in localized areas, and capillary dilation

c. Assess for the extent and change in jaundice or the existence of latent jaundice if the serum bilirubin level is above 2 mg/dl (adult/child) or 5 mg/dl (premature infant)

(1) Inspect the skin in daylight rather than in artificial light. Normally olive skin or a fading suntan may appear to be jaundiced in artificial light

(2) Jaundice is best seen in people with dark skin by examining the sclera, mucous membrane of the mouth, palms of the hands, or soles of the feet for color change. Also check for darkening of the urine

(3) Note the color distribution. If sclera, mucous membranes, palms of the hands, or soles of the feet are not involved, the color change is probably normal. A color change only in areas usually tanned is probably not jaundice

(4) Note the quality of color. A somewhat bronze color rather than golden or bright yellow indicates hepatic or posthepatic jaundice. A light lemon yellow tone is more indicative of prehepatic jaundice

(5) Jaundice is not seen well in edematous areas because of the increased fluid and decreased protein levels—especially albumin—in such areas

(6) Latent jaundice may be validated by

(a) Looking for scratch marks

(b) Applying pressure over bony prominences (sternum, tip of the nose) to blanch the skin, which makes the jaundice more apparent

(c) Shaking the urine sample. If an increased amount of bilirubin is present, the urine will foam, which assists in differentiating between very concentrated urine or urine with a color alteration secondary to medical treatment (e.g., phenazopyridine [Pyridium] and an actual increase in bilirubin levels in the urine)

(7) Monitor the urine and feces for color change

(a) In early hemolytic jaundice, the urine color should be normal

(b) Tea-colored urine that will stain clothing indicates the presence of increased urobilinogen found in posthepatic jaundice

(c) In hepatitis, bilirubin may appear in the urine before jaundice is evident. The urine will be dark brown and frothy ("Coca-Cola") when the concentration is high

d. Compare the serum total bilirubin concentration with related laboratory test standards to measure the effectiveness of treatment or progress of the disease process

(1) The reader is referred to Wallach's *Interpretation of Diagnostic Tests* (1991) for a rapid retrieval of information on specific tests in given diagnoses. Any thorough medical-surgical nursing text should also provide such information

(2) In all cases of jaundice the fractions of serum total bilirubin can be particularly useful in following the course of the disease or response to treatment

(3) In prehepatic, or hemolytic, jaundice, tests frequently used include red cell fragility, reticulocyte count, peripheral blood smear, red cell survival test, Coombs' test, hemoglobin, hematocrit, serum haptoglobins, WBC count, and Sickledex

(4) In hepatic or posthepatic jaundice, tests frequently used include serum transaminases (particularly gamma glutamyl transpeptidase [GGT], alamine transaminase [ALT]), hepatitis B surface antigen (HB_sAg), serum total protein, serum albumin, protein electrophoresis or immunophoresis, plasma prothrombin time, urobilinogen, and urine bilirubin

e. Monitor the adult with chronic elevated serum bilirubin levels for the occurrence of gallstones, and when appropriate, provide dietary instruction related to fat intake

f. There is no indication in the literature of the use of phototherapy to reduce jaundice in the adult, probably because the disease effects in the adult are so much less severe than in the neonate. If, however, pruritis is a major problem and the possibility exists that reduction of the jaundice may also relieve the pruritis, further investigation of this modality could be undertaken by the nurse in collaboration with the physician

3. Implications related to care of the neonate with hyperbilirubinemia. (This is only a brief synopsis of the material so well covered by Whaley & Wong [1991] with some expansion of laboratory data. The reader is referred to that text for in-depth nursing care)

   a. Prevent neonatal hyperbilirubinemia
      (1) Early introduction of feeding, even if only water, will help prevent neonatal jaundice by increasing peristalsis to remove sterile meconium and by introducing normal intestinal flora to convert conjugated bilirubin to urobilinogen and stercobilin
      (2) Encourage prenatal medical supervision and prenatal identification of Rh-type blood groups
      (3) Follow Rh-negative women during pregnancy for increased serum bilirubin levels and the presence of antibodies in the mother by amniocentesis, and the indirect Coombs' test
      (4) Administer Rh_o(D) immune globulin (RhoGAM) as ordered to Rh-negative women at delivery or at time of abortion. If there is no order for RhoGAM, follow up vigorously to attain the order. Many hospitals require mothers to sign a release if they refuse the medication

   b. Identify risk population of infants
      (1) Amniotic fluid may be dark because of the infant's increased urobilinogen or bilirubin levels
      (2) Assess the infant for jaundice at birth
      (3) Check the infant's hemoglobin and hematocrit values for possible anemia resulting from an excessive RBC lysis
      (4) Check for variations from normal central nervous system (CNS) activity: irritability (tremors, twitching, high-pitched cry, convulsions, opisthotonos) and depression (absent Moro or sucking reflexes, diminished deep tendon reflex, hypotonia, lethargy) as indicators of the onset of kernicterus

   c. Prevent the onset or minimize the effect of kernicterus
      (1) Assess for and prevent, if possible, metabolic acidosis (decreased venous CO_2, blood gases)
      (2) Check serum protein electrophoresis (or serum albumin) for a decreased albumin concentration. Report if low so that albumin may be given if indicated
      (3) Discourage the use of drugs that compete with bilirubin for binding sites on albumin molecule (e.g., salicylates, vitamin K, sulfonamides)
      (4) Decrease metabolic demands for oxygen or glucose by
          (a) Placing the infant in position for optimal respiratory exchange. Check that oxygen is delivered at the concentration ordered. If the patient is not receiving oxygen, request an order for oxygen if indications suggest a need. Use suction as indicated
          (b) Preventing hypothermia by appropriate measures
      (5) Check the serum bilirubin response if phenobarbital is given. The purpose of phenobarbital administration is to increase protein synthesis/albumin production. The desired outcome is decreased concentrations of bilirubin

   d. Assist with care of complications
      (1) Phototherapy (see Whaley & Wong, 1991), which is usually instituted when bilirubin levels reach 10 mg/dl. Provide 25 percent additional fluid to make up for increased insensible losses. The outcome criterion is a decrease in serum bilirubin levels by 3 to 4mg/dl after 8 to 12 hours of therapy
      (2) Exchange transfusion (see Section 13.5)

   e. Provide parental support to alleviate feelings of responsibility for the infant's illness, to allow mother–child bonding to occur, and to provide a realistic, positive awareness of the progress of the infant. The mortality rate in kernicterus is almost 50 percent during the first month

   f. Do follow-up care and teaching for the family of any full-term infant whose serum bilirubin levels approached 20 mg/dl at birth
      (1) Parents need to keep other members of the health team informed of the child's history of hyperbilirubinemia at birth
      (2) An early developmental and hearing assessment should be planned to determine any possible deficits resulting from CNS damage

(3) The infant's blood should be checked during the first 2 months for possible anemia and the need for supplemental iron. Hemolysis may continue in mild erythroblastosis fetalis, even though the bilirubin levels are controlled

1.11 SERUM CHOLESTEROL

Synonyms: Plasma cholesterol; total cholesterol; HDL and LDL cholesterol

Normal Ranges: mg/dl

AGE	Total CHOLESTEROL (mg/dL)		HDL-c CHOLESTEROL	LDL CHOLESTEROL
Cord blood	M	44-103	6-53	20-56
	F	50-108	13-56	21-58
0–4 years	M	114-203		
	F	112-200		
5–9 years	M	121-203	35-75	63-129
	F	126-205	36-73	68-140
10–14 years	M	119-202	37-74	64-133
	F	124-201	37-70	68-136
15–19 years	M	113-197	30-63	62-130
	F	119-200	35-74	59-137
20–24 years	M	124-218	30-63	66-147
	F	122-216	33-79	57-159
25–29 years	M	133-244	31-63	70-165
	F	128-223	37-83	71-164
30–34 years	M	138-254	26-63	78-185
	F	130-230	36-77	70-156
35–39 years	M	146-270	29-62	81-189
	F	140-242	34-82	75-172
40–44 years	M	——	27-67	87-186
	F	——	34-88	74-174
45–49 years	M	——	—	97-202
	F	——	—	79-186
50–54 years	M	——	—	89-197
	F	——	—	88-201
55–59 years	M	——	—	88-203
	F	——	—	89-210
60–64 years	M	——	—	83-210
	F	——	—	100-224
65–69 years	M	——	—	98-210
	F	——	—	92-221
70 years	M	——	—	88-186
	F	——	—	96-206

Adult risk levels: Recommended: <130 mg/dL
High risk: >160 mg/dL

Definition. Cholesterol is a fat-related chemical, a complex alcohol that can be synthesized by all body cells except the brain and ingested in the diet through animal protein. As an alcohol it can form esters (compounds "formed from an alcohol and an acid by removal of water"

[Dorland, 1989]) with fatty acid, which are the storage form of cholesterol. Cholesterol esters make up about two thirds of the cholesterol in plasma. Free cholesterol is also found in the plasma as a lipoprotein. Cholesterol itself is insoluble in plasma, but when bound as a lipoprotein it becomes soluble and can be transported. Although these two forms of cholesterol are different, for the purpose of this discussion they can be considered together because of their closely allied role in the body.

Cholesterol is a primary constituent of the low-density lipoproteins (LDL) but can be found in the high-density lipoproteins (HDL) as well as in the very-low-density lipoproteins (VLDL). "Cholesterol is the most important sterol ('a solid alcohol of animal or vegetable origin with properties like fat' [Miller & Keane, 1983]) in animal metabolism" (Sodeman & Sodeman, 1982). It is found only in foods of animal origin.

Although cholesterol is considered a body lipid, it does not, as do other lipids, serve as a source of energy for metabolism. The body is unable to disintegrate the sterol ring. It is the only lipid that is excreted in appreciable amounts. The others are metabolized, stored, or used in body anabolism. Cholesterol probably acts as a framework in the body cells for the essential metabolic changes of the other constituents of the protoplasm. It is important in maintaining the permeability of cell membranes and in the synthesis of steroid hormones as a precursor of steroids of the adrenal cortex and ovary (Henry, 1991). It is a major constituent of bile and bile acids.

Serum cholesterol determinations alone are of limited value. However, when considered together with high-density lipoprotein cholesterol (HDL-c) measurements, determination of risk of coronary heart disease (CHD) is possible. That risk is increased 25 percent with every 5mg/dl decrease in HDL-c below the mean. Risk can be calculated by using the ratio of HDL-c to either LDL-c or total cholesterol. There is an inverse association between HDL-c and incidence/prevalence of coronary heart disease. Other risk calculation can be done by calculating the ratio of HDL-c to either LDL-c or total cholesterol. The use of either LDL-c alone, or the ratio alone gives misleading information. They should always be considered in conjunction with the total cholesterol concentration. (Tietz (1990), pp. 304–305, 368–369)

Physiology. The serum level of cholesterol remains remarkably constant from day to day in a healthy person but does tend to increase with age and change with populations, and there is wide variation among individuals.

The greater part of body cholesterol is produced by synthesis, about 1 g/day. Only about one third of that amount is provided by the diet. Although an inverse ratio of synthesis to oral intake does occur, endogenous production is not completely suppressed by dietary intake, as only the hepatic synthesis is depressed. No specific serum cholesterol level has been determined as being the critical abnormal level. For individuals over 30 years of age, however, an elevated cholesterol level remains one of the better indicators of risk populations for the development of ischemic heart disease (Harvey et al., 1991).

Cholesterol is synthesized by the body from small molecules in a long and complex series of condensations, transformations, and ring closures. Of these, one vastly important reaction is that with acetyl coenzyme A (CoA) and acetoacetyl CoA because this pathway is shared with both carbohydrate and fatty metabolism. Carbohydrates, amino acids, and other fats can be converted to cholesterol by this route, which makes the reduction of serum cholesterol by dietary means a complex and frustrating effort. The major sites of cholesterol synthesis are the liver and the intestines in humans. Synthesis is depressed not only with dietary intake of cholesterol but also with increases in insulin or thyroid hormone, and increased estrogen levels shorten the half-life of cholesterol, thereby lowering its plasma level (Sodeman & Sodeman, 1982).

Cholesterol is readily absorbable from the diet. Plants do not contain cholesterol but have other sterols, poorly absorbed by the body, that inhibit cholesterol absorption when given in large quantities—one basis for increased nonsaturated fat dietary regimens in the treatment of elevated serum cholesterol levels (Howard & Herbold, 1982).

Cholesterol and all lipids are digested in the duodenum. After bile emulsification, cholesterol diffuses into the blood or lymph.

Cholesterol is removed from the circulation only by the liver. It is directly secreted into bile and has a slight secretion to bile acids. Most of the cholesterol in bile is reabsorbed from the intestine, but a small amount is excreted with feces. This small amount is approximately half of all cholesterol excreted from the body. Neutral sterols, also excreted in the feces, make up most of the rest of the total cholesterol excreted. Waste products from steroid hormone synthesis are eliminated in the urine, which makes it a minor cholesterol excretory pathway (Henry, 1991).

Cholesterol is discharged from the liver into both blood and bile, including bile acids, and the first step in the formation of steroid synthesis from cholesterol takes place within the liver. Approximately three fourths of the cholesterol esterified by the liver is transported to the body tissues where it is ingested and used. In the adrenal cortex cholesterol acts as a precursor for pregnenolone, which itself is a precursor for progesterone, testosterone, estrogen, aldosterone, and cortisol. In the skin, cholesterol is a precursor of vitamin D that is activated with the application of ultraviolet light. It also helps give the skin its water-resistant quality (Harvey et al., 1991).

SERUM CHOLESTEROL LEVELS DECREASED IN:

1. Malnutrition because of an insufficient intake of dietary protein to provide liver synthesis of lipoproteins but *only* when the caloric intake is adequate to prevent mobilization of lipid stores
2. Idiopathic steatorrhea because of a lack of intestinal absorption of amino acids, which causes decreased hepatic synthesis of lipoprotein. Blocks in carbohydrate and lipid absorption contribute but are not the major problem
3. Hepatocellular liver disease such as hepatitis. There can be marked depression with severe hepatitis, or in portal cirrhosis the damaged liver cell may not be able to convert protein and carbohydrate to fat. Determination of serum cholesterol levels is a frequently used tool in the diagnosis of hepatic disease. With liver disease there is a relatively larger decrease in esterified cholesterol than in free cholesterol
4. Hyperthyroidism, although the depression is variable and is therefore of little use in patient evaluation. Serum cholesterol is the oldest in vitro measurement of thyroid function. Although it is known that the thyroid stimulates removal of cholesterol by direct secretion into bile and bile acids, the thyroid gland also stimulates cholesterol synthesis by its control of the level of hepatic cellular function where 90 percent of endogenous cholesterol is formed (Guyton, 1982), which may account for the variability of the serum level changes in both hyper- and hypothyroidism

5. Decreased levels have been seen in cases of acute infection and anemia, possibly because of decreased protein availability

6. Cancer. "Low levels have been found to be inversely related to cancer mortality. It may be that cancer causes low cholesterol concentrations many years before it is diagnosed" (Salmond et al., 1985)

7. Cholesterol below 150 mg/dl may be a marker for disease, such as malabsorption, anorexia nervosa, short bowel syndrome, and requires further gastrointestinal evaluation (Phillips & Weiss, 1992, p. 24)

SERUM CHOLESTEROL LEVELS INCREASED IN:

1. Hyperlipoproteinemia, with the direct cause-and-effect sequence unknown. Atherosclerosis and a risk of coronary disease have been correlated with elevated lipoprotein levels and, more specifically, with elevated cholesterol levels. Persons with increased cholesterol levels tend to have myocardial infarctions at an earlier age than do those with elevated triglyceride levels alone. Although the causes of hyperlipidemia are generally unknown, Harvey and colleagues believe that it must "result from either increased synthesis or diminished removal of serum lipoproteins and their constituent lipids" (Harvey et al., 1991)

2. Cancer of the head of the pancreas resulting from blockage of excretion by biliary obstruction or interference with the circulation of cholesterol in the form of bile salts or neutral sterols. Elevations occur in obstructive jaundice as well and for the same reasons. Levels can increase to 250 to 500 mg/dl. Greater elevations should be considered a result of intrahepatic cholestasis rather than posthepatic obstruction (Henry, 1991). Increased levels are sometimes found in pancreatitis because of secondary biliary obstruction

3. Moderate amounts in uncontrolled or inadequately managed diabetes mellitus because of a decrease in carbohydrate metabolism, which causes an increased utilization of lipids and increases their serum levels as they travel to the liver. Hyperlipoproteinemia may be a contributory factor in the development of the diabetic complications of the peripheral vascular system

4. Hypothyroidism, which may reflect the overall metabolic depression. The serum level is increased in spite of a decrease in cholesterol synthesis. The increased blood levels probably reflect the decrease in tissue use, storage, and excretion of cholesterol

5. Nephrotic syndrome, a consistent feature of this disorder, because of a compensatory increase in hepatic synthesis to make up for the loss of protein through the kidney. Most plasma protein levels are decreased, but the lipid-binding proteins are not thought to pass into the urine; hence their levels, including those of cholesterol, increase in the serum. Persons with the lowest serum albumin levels in this disorder often have the highest lipid levels. This does not apply in lipoid nephrosis of children

6. The third trimester of pregnancy; the elevation remains until well after the delivery. The reason for this increase is not known

7. Individuals on diets high in saturated fats. Exogenous cholesterol will increase serum cholesterol levels in variable degrees. Factors that influence the amount of cholesterol absorbed include the total amount in each feeding, how frequently the feedings occur, the

other types of dietary fats fed with the cholesterol, past dietary intake, and the age of the person (Howard & Herbold, 1982). The liver tends to compensate by synthesizing less cholesterol with the additional intake. Ingestion of *saturated* fats, however, increases the synthesis of cholesterol

8. Early starvation, probably because of mobilization of peripheral deposits
9. Individuals who have had a hypophysectomy; this is possibly linked to the loss of adrenocorticotropic hormone, or corticotropin (ACTH), which tends to decrease serum cholesterol levels, as well as possible decreased amounts of other hormones that tend to decrease synthesis (Faulkner et al., 1968)
10. Genetic predisposition (All factors listed predispose to coronary heart disease)
    Individuals who have inherited a tendency to produce
    (1) Low levels of high density lipoproteins (HDL-cholesterol), also known as familial hypercholesterolemia and first noted in the middle years of life
    (2) Low-serum polipoprotein A-1 (a protein that attaches to low-density cholesterol)
    (3) High-serum apolipoprotein B level (a protein that attaches to LDL cholesterol)
    Individuals with
    (1) Congenital variations in coronary arterial structure
    (2) Susceptibility to adverse effects of cigarette smoke
    (3) Familial indicators, that is, high blood pressure; parents and or siblings with CHD at an early age; personal or family history of peripheral vascular diasese, diabetes and/or stroke
    (4) Increased serum lipids and lipoprotein levels (Considered to have a 50-percent inheritability factor)
    (5) Low levels of HDL cholesterol (under 35 mg), also known as familial hypercholesterolemia
    (6) Males have been found to have a risk factor 3 to 4 times greater than women. Onset usually occurs during the middle decades of life
    (7) Obesity, about 30 percent of CHD patients are overweight

(Berkow, 1990, p. 849; McCance and Heuther, 1990, p. 176)

IMPLICATIONS FOR NURSING: SERUM CHOLESTEROL

1. To provide the most accurate data possible, a serum lipid analysis should be done when the individual is at a stable weight, on his or her usual diet, and consuming the same amount of alcoholic beverages as usual. No food or drink other than water should be given for 12 hours before blood is drawn for this test
2. Prevention of secondary problems, or limitation of the severity of the initial disorder associated with increased cholesterol and other lipid levels, is a major responsibility of nursing through the nursing role of health maintenance and nursing management of populations at risk. The cornerstone for nursing intervention is the precise identification of risk factors operant and adequate explanation of these factors to the individuals involved
   a. In children who have a family history of premature cardiovascular disease (e.g., a myocardial infarction (MI) before the age of 50), encourage and facilitate screening tests for triglycerides and cholesterol by the age of 5

    b. All siblings of hyperlipoproteinemic persons should also be tested regardless of age

    c. High-risk individuals, especially children, should be receiving a low-saturated-fat diet (saturated fats in the diet being primarily coconut oil, butter fat, and animal fats). The nurse can counsel and assist in dietary planning. Preventative measures should be instituted by the late teens or early adulthood to be effective (McCance & Heuther, 1990, p. 1974–76)

    d. The nurse should also supply assistance to high-risk individuals and their home caretakers in dietary planning to include the increased use of polyunsaturated fats (corn, cottonseed, soy, and safflower oils, as well as margarine)

    e. Dietary planning should also aim to reduce the total fat content in the diet to approximately 35 percent of the dietary intake. The average diet in the United States consists of 40 to 50 percent fat intake. To reduce the total absorption of cholesterol, its intake in the diet needs to be reduced from the usual 600 to 1200 mg/day to 100 to 300 mg/day (Howard & Herbold, 1982)

    f. Water intake should be increased, unless contraindicated, to help eliminate waste products and to decrease the viscosity of the blood. A high-fat meal causes an increase in the coagulability of the blood for several hours after ingestion

    g. One of the major precipitating factors in the occurrence of hypertension is obesity. Weight loss to within one's own normal range for body build should be encouraged with dietary counseling. This should include the rationale and assistance in long-term planning for a change in eating habits. Such counseling is most effective if the counselor is seen personally to follow the precautions suggested. The use of community resources (e.g., the American Heart Association) and referral to them can help the individual comply with the diet by providing additional support and assistance

    h. Yet another risk factor is that of smoking. The individual needs to be informed as to the cause-and-effect relationship and its hazards. Again, teaching is most effective when what is taught is seen to be valued by the teacher

3. Assess all persons in your care, those over the age of 30 especially, for evidence of the presence of risk factors for coronary artery disease

    a. Presence of xanthomas (cholesterol deposits in the skin or tendons), frequently found in the achilles tendons, on the knuckles, and along the arm tendons

    b. Family history of hyperlipidemia

    c. Personal history of alcohol abuse. Ingestion of large amounts of alcohol is felt to predispose to coronary artery disease in some types of hyperlipidemia (Howard & Herbold, 1982). Alcohol has been shown to depress ventricular performance, which causes less uptake of fatty acids and leads to myocardial cell injury (Jones et al., 1982). The important factor is the amount ingested

    d. Personal smoking history, of particular importance in the occurrence of angina because of its vasoconstrictive effect

    e. Evidence of atherosclerotic arterial disease; for example, intermittent claudication; change in skin color, temperature, sensation; pain at rest; history of slow healing; easy infection and edema in the peripheral extremities, particularly the legs; faint or absent peripheral pulses (check bilaterally for comparison); bruits in peripheral arteries; trophic changes in the skin on the extremities

    f. Premature arcus senilis. When it occurs with xanthomas, it is almost always indicative of familial hypercholesterolemia (Harvey et al., 1991)

    g. Increased blood pressure. For persons over 50 a blood pressure of 160/95 indicates the need for further screening. Elevation of the diastolic pressure is more significant than elevation of the systolic pressure

    h. Significant glycosuria, or a fasting serum glucose greater than 120 mg/dl, indicates a twofold risk of CHD

    i. Increases in uric acid levels greater than 7.5 mg/dl also contribute to coronary artery disease risk

    j. Increased serum sodium levels can indicate a potential for increased blood pressure and may need further examination as a risk factor

4. If any of the foregoing indicators are positive, collaborate with the physician—or suggest that the individual confer with his or her physician—to obtain both serum cholesterol and triglyceride, specifically LDL and HDL, determinations if no recent test results are available. Any increase in normal levels, of HDL should be followed seriously. If serum cholesterol and triglyceride levels are within normal limits, a primary lipid metabolic disorder is usually ruled out (Henry, 1991)

5. Increased cholesterol levels found in women around the menopausal age should be investigated further because of the possibility of the existence of hypothyroidism. An onset at this age is frequent in women and is easily mistaken for part of the menopausal syndrome. Rather typical of hypothyroidism is an asymptomatic and concurrent increase of cholesterol, uric acid, and serum aspartate aminotransferase (AST) levels with normal liver function. Given the occurrence of increased cholesterol levels in women as described, the thyroid function should be checked

6. Gallstones should be suspected in the individual with elevated cholesterol levels accompanied by a history of gastrointestinal symptoms or fatty intolerance. With increased synthesis of cholesterol, the cholesterol contents of bile become supersaturated in relation to the other two components of bile, which leads to cholesterol precipitation and stone formation

7. Persons being treated for primary biliary cirrhosis with an elevation of cholesterol levels because of the retention of bile may show a drop toward normal in the cholesterol level, which can be secondary to liver failure. This decrease in the cholesterol concentration could easily be misinterpreted as a positive response to treatment. Locate available liver function test results, and examine the person for signs and symptoms of liver failure when cholesterol levels have reduced but the evidence of biliary cirrhosis has not. Bear in mind that symptoms and signs of liver failure occur only when there is diffuse parenchymal damage. Look for jaundice, bleeding tendencies, ascites, generalized edema, portal hypertension, hepatomegaly, and skin changes

8. Knowledge of the action and uses of medication to decrease serum cholesterol levels is basic in giving adequate nursing care

   a. A trial of diet therapy or weight reduction is usually performed before medications are started because of the possible side effects of medication and, in some cases, because the medication is very distasteful when given orally

   b. Drug therapy should be accompanied by an initial determination of serum cholesterol and triglyceride levels and the tests repeated at least at monthly intervals during treatment

   c. The effectiveness of therapy—diet or medication—should be assessed by noting any changes in the size of xanthomas, the return of pertinent laboratory values to normal range (see the previous material), a change in weight, or a reduction in blood pressure

   d. Dextrothyroxine sodium (Choloxin), an isomer of thyroxine, cannot be given to persons with known heart disease or those with a familial increase in cholesterol levels. It tends to increase the body's metabolic rate, and signs and symptoms of coronary artery disease are known side effects. The purpose in giving the drug is to prevent an extension of atherosclerosis as well as decrease cholesterol levels

      (1) Determination of protein-bound iodine is useful in validating the effectiveness of the drug. Increased levels indicate drug absorption and transport

      (2) Choloxin can cause iodism and signs and symptoms (e.g., acneiform rash, itching, runny nose, brassy taste in mouth) should be reported immediately so that treatment with the drug can be discontinued

   e. Cholestyramine resin (Questran) is used as an adjunct to diet. It combines with bile salts to form a nonabsorbable and insoluble compound that is excreted in the feces. It has many side effects. Prevent or alleviate them by

      (1) Providing a high-bulk diet and adequate fluids to prevent constipation

      (2) Reporting the occurrence of constipation and adjusting the dosage as ordered

      (3) Observing for signs and symptoms of fat-soluble vitamin deficiency with long-term use, for example, observe for bleeding tendencies

(4) Scheduling other oral medications and meals (e.g., 1 hour before giving Questran) so that their absorption is interfered with as little as possible. Questran can be given concurrently with Choloxin

9. Persons with nephrotic syndrome are sometimes placed on usual or even high-protein diets, which is not usual in other persons with increased cholesterol levels. Their need for replacement of plasma proteins can supersede their need for decreased cholesterol levels (Rakel, 1987)

10. Allow the patient 20 minutes of rest or relaxation seated or lying down prior to serum cholesterol testing. Serum cholestrol rises with mental stress and standing posture

11. If not contraindicated, suggest the inclusion of oat bran foods in diet (e.g., cereal, bread, rolls), especially to women over 50, as it has been found most effective in decreasing cholesterol levels in that age and gender group ("National Cholesterol Education Program," 1992, pp. 17–18)

12. Identify children and adolescents at risk, and provide early information and support to prevent atherosclerosis. They have been defined as those with:
    a. Family history of coronary atherosclerosis and/or coronary arteriography
    b. Family history of MI, angina, peripheral vascular disease, and/or sudden cardiac death by age 56
    c. Parent with blood cholesterol levels over 240 mg/dl ("National Cholesterol Education Program," 1992, pp. 2317–18)

13. When teaching an individual about the need to watch dietary intake, some items to include are
    a. To provide positive reinforcement for all efforts and gains. For example, a difference as small as 5 mg/dl in HDL cholesterol levels will have a significant impact on the rate and severity of any heart failure that has occurred (McCance & Huether, 1990, p. 174)
    b. The addition of oat bran to the diet of women over 50 can reduce total cholesterol and LDL cholesterol levels significantly (American Family Physician, May 1992, pp. 17–18)

14. A home test kit has been approved for cholesterol monitoring. The process is as follows:
    a. A plastic container holding a test strip is used to collect a few drops of blood on the test strip from a fingerstick
    b. The test strip changes color depending on the amount of cholesterol present in the blood
    c. The test strip color is compared to a conversion chart for a cholesterol reading. Results take up to 15 minutes. Results of the test have been found to be as accurate as those currently in use in laboratories and doctors' offices. (Female Patient "Home Cholesterol Kit Cleared for Use," May 1993, p. 81)

1.12 SERUM ENZYMES

Enzymes are special chemical catalysts of biologic origin, invariably protein. All living organisms synthesize enzymes. They are rapidly degraded and replenished. Enzymes are essential to life and enable the many biochemical reactions in the body cells to occur. There is no test to measure the intracellular enzyme concentration directly. The serum measurements done are assumed to parallel enzyme concentrations and changes within the cells, much as serum potassium levels are believed to reflect those of intracellular potassium.

Over 700 enzymes have been isolated, and because of the increasing number and the increasing application to clinical laboratory work, a standard classification system was produced for general use. Of importance to nursing is an awareness that this system provides for more than one term to be used in dealing with an enzyme. For example, the test frequently referred to as serum LDH is also known as (1) L-lactate: NAP oxidoreductose, systemic name; (2) 1.1.1.27, International Union of Biologists code designation; and (3) lactate dehydrogenase, practical name. Enzymes named in recent years have suffix endings of "ase." Those named years ago may have names that do not now fit into the classification system but are retained as trivial or common names because of their familiarity (e.g., ptyalin for amylase). The classification system assists the clinical chemist in communication with other health team members and vice versa.

Intracellular enzymes have no known physiological function in the plasma and appear in much lower concentrations there than within the cell. Serum increases occur, their cause dependent on the physiological mechanism of the enzyme involved. If an enzyme is present in fairly large concentrations in only one organ, a serum increase would help determine the affected organ. Such enzymes are called *tissue-* or *organ-specific* enzymes, examples being acid phosphatase of the prostate gland or acetylcholinesterase of RBCs. *Nontissue-* or *nonorgan-specific* enzymes, when increased in serum levels, can be compared with levels of other such enzymes for information as to the affected organ because the several enzymes are present in different tissues in different ratios. For example, damage to the liver cells will usually cause an increase in serum aspartate aminotransferase (AST), but many other cell injuries could cause the same rise. In comparing the AST level to another enzyme such as serum alanine transaminase (ALT), more specific information can be obtained. If the ALT level is increased, liver damage can be fairly safely assumed because ALT is more specific to liver cells and serum AST ($_c$SAST) is more sensitive to changes in the status of the cardiac cell. If the ALT concentration were within normal limits, liver damage could almost be ruled out (Tietz, 1990). Therefore, a single test for a serum enzyme of a nontissue- or nonorgan-specific type is of limited diagnostic value in itself. Such a test can be most useful in following the course of a disease process once diagnosed or following the response of the body to treatment. Isoenzyme fractionation of nontissue- or nonorgan-specific enzymes seems to be tissue-specific and can be used to follow up screening tests.

Decreased serum enzyme levels happen infrequently and may or may not be of clinical importance; however, the absence in the serum of an expected enzyme is usually related to a single gene abnormality—an inborn error of metabolism—that results in the loss of services of the enzyme (e.g., albinism, storage diseases [such as Gaucher's], Tay-Sachs disease, or phenylketonuria [PKU]).

Units of measurement for serum enzymes can be a great source of confusion. International units (IU) of measurement are being adopted, but in the United States at least, other units of measurement are still in use. Thus Bodansky, King-Armstrong (KA), or Bessey-Lowrey units will be given in many lists of normal ranges. Conversion from one type of unit to another can produce results that are grossly in error even when international units are used unless it is known that the exact methodologies were followed for the tests used and that ambient conditions were identical in all laboratories. Therefore, the units given in this text (in international units, whenever available) do not reflect other measuring system units, and the practitioner is strongly urged to work with the unit system given in the facility that has determined that client's serum levels. Efforts should not be made to translate results from one system of measurement to another.

In this section we deal with only three of the myriad of possible serum enzyme tests. These are used fairly consistently as screening tests. They provide a fairly broad, nontissue- or nonorgan-specific survey and offer information about several organs or systems within the body (e.g., cardiac, liver, skeletal, lung). This broad view makes them good screening tests.

1.12.1 Serum Alkaline Phosphatase

Synonyms: Phosphatase, alkaline, ALP, alkaline phosphatase, SAP

Normal Ranges (IU/L)

Adult	
Male	19–74
Female	12–63
Senior adult	
Male	19.0–74
Female	12.0–64
Pediatric	
Newborn	50–275
Infant	100–330
Child	90–230
Adolescent	100–250

Physiology. Serum alkaline phosphatase (SAP) is found in almost all body tissues. It is manufactured by bone (40 to 75 percent), liver, intestine, and placenta. It is called an enzyme of secretion. In the healthy person it is secreted constantly and rapidly from the cell into the interstitial area and thence into the serum. Alkaline phosphatase is necessary for hydrolysis of organic phosphates and is, therefore, important to digestion and absorption through the mucous membrane of the gastrointestinal tract. The component produced by the liver is in greatest concentration in the serum of adults. It is rapidly and constantly excreted into urine, bile, and the gastrointestinal tract. There is some question as to the enzyme's actual pathway and a possibility that the enzyme found in the urine is that from kidney tissue only and does not represent serum enzyme cleared by the kidney. In any case, the constant secretion and excretion produce a relatively constant and low serum level. Should one of the excretory routes be blocked, the rate of production increased, or the rate of release from the cell increased, plasma levels will rise.

Pathophysiology. The activity of SAP gives important information about bone formation (osteoblastic activity) and is clinically useful as a test of liver function, being the most sensitive test of common bile duct obstruction. It is a more sensitive index of bile stasis than is the serum bilirubin level.

SAP is frequently the first enzyme to be studied in hepatic disease and is used extensively in the differential diagnosis of jaundice. An increased serum level is said to reflect acute liver cell disease (given validation that it is the liver component that is elevated) or bile duct obstruction but is not specific to any one liver disease. The mechanism of increased SAP levels with hepatobiliary disease is not clear. It is thought to be related to both impaired excretion with regurgitation of bile alkaline phosphatase and increased formation by or release from hepatic cells. The mechanism for increase with bone formation is more straightforward in that the enzyme is formed by the osteoblast so that increased numbers of osteoblastic cells will result in increased SAP concentrations.

SAP of bone origin can be differentiated from SAP of liver origin in a rough estimation by its response to heat: SAP of bone origin is heat stable, whereas that of liver origin is not. As usually analyzed in most clinical laboratories, however, the activities of osseous alkaline phosphatase and hepatic activity are indistinguishable. There is often a significant overlap in the heat test, and it has been found to be most useful in separating bone–liver SAP as a group from tumor–placenta SAP as a group. Isoenzymes are tissue-specific but seldom used. Low levels of SAP are rarely encountered.

SAP LEVELS INCREASED IN:

1. Bone disease because of stimulation of osteoblastic activity secondary to bone destruction and remodeling, which is found in
   a. Paget's disease (osteitis deformans), which demonstrates some of the highest known levels with localized bone destruction, absorption, and abnormal new formation
   b. Osteogenic sarcoma with increases 20 to 40 times normal. Other primary bone tumors will cause similar but lesser increases (e.g., chondrosarcoma)
   c. Osteomalacia with moderate increases because of low serum calcium stimulating parathyroid activity. Active rickets will present a similar picture for the same reason with increases two to four times normal
   d. Metastatic bone tumors from any primary site but most commonly prostatic and breast cancer
   e. Healing fractures, frequently but not always
2. Liver or hepatobiliary disease such as
   a. Biliary cirrhosis or Laennec's cirrhosis because of hepatic cellular damage and the release of alkaline phosphatase, which causes marked increases but less than those in biliary obstruction
   b. Biliary obstruction, found secondary to a number of obstructive processes (e.g., gallstones, biliary atresia). Increases occur secondary to stimulation of or injury to epithelial cells of the liver or biliary tree
   c. Toxic hepatitis (chlorpromazine hepatitis), because of a hypersensitivity response. Viral hepatitis often will not cause an increase in SAP levels
   d. Space-occupying lesions or granulomatous diseases of the liver such as amyloidosis, sarcoidosis, tuberculosis, and to a lesser degree, cancer. Primary hepatomas show no consistent elevation of SAP levels
3. Faulty calcium metabolism in kidney disease such as
   a. Renal tubular acidosis because of faulty calcium and phosphate reabsorption in the tubules, which causes increased calcium reabsorption secondary to parathyroid stimulation and a reactive increase in SAP levels in an attempt to maintain normal calcium and phosphorus serum levels
   b. Chronic nephritis because of impaired calcium absorption secondary to the kidney's inability to form the active metabolite of vitamin D, which causes decreased serum calcium levels, parathyroid stimulation, bone resorption, and an osteoblastic reaction
   c. Chronic glomerulonephritis because of a decreased serum calcium level (mechanism similar to that given in item 3b)
4. Faulty or inadequate calcium absorption from the gastrointestinal tract, which causes a decrease in serum calcium levels and stimulates parathyroid activity, ultimately increasing osteoblastic activity followed by a release of alkaline phosphatase into the serum. This condition is found in
   a. Malnutrition

   b. Malabsorption syndromes in which calcium combines with the increased fats retained in the alimentary canal to form an insoluble calcium soap and decrease absorption of fat-soluble vitamin D
   c. Hypovitaminosis D
5. Hyperparathyroidism (rationale given in item 3)
6. Physiological states such as
   a. Third trimester of pregnancy with increases two to three times normal, which is believed to be due to increased production from the placenta
   b. Periods of rapid growth and bone building
   c. Aging. Normal values in healthy adults over the age of 70 may be one to one and one-half times the standard normal values

SAP LEVELS DECREASED IN:

1. Kwashiorkor, because of protein deficiency
2. Congenital hypophosphatasia because of a lack of production
3. Dwarfism
4. General debility and anemia; exact mechanism not clear

IMPLICATIONS FOR NURSING: SERUM ALKALINE PHOSPHATASE

1. Serum for testing must be free from hemolysis because of the large concentrations of alkaline phosphatase in RBCs. No special patient preparation is necessary
2. Serial determinations of SAP levels are necessary for any conclusions as to dysfunction or response to treatment
3. An increase in SAP levels without a rise in the concentration of any other intracellular enzyme is probably due to bone enzyme serum increases. Other enzymes are not present in bone to any great extent
4. Correlation with clinical and laboratory data helps to determine the importance or impact of an increased SAP level and indicate progress and prognosis
   a. Check serum calcium and phosphorus levels
      (1) Increased SAP levels with normal serum calcium and phosphorus levels occur in osteogenic sarcoma. A dramatic rise in the SAP content in patients with Paget's disease may indicate a common complication of the disease—osteogenic sarcoma
      (2) An imbalance in serum calcium, either increased or decreased levels, can ultimately cause an increase in SAP levels. (See "SAP Levels Increased in," item 3)
   b. Check the serum bilirubin levels
      (1) Serum bilirubin and serum cholesterol concentrations can be expected to be elevated together with the SAP in toxic hepatitis. An increase in bilirubin and cholesterol levels with the clinical picture of hepatitis but without increases in the SAP content may indicate viral hepatitis
      (2) A normal serum bilirubin and increased SAP levels may be suggestive of liver metastasis, given a known primary site, or may suggest other space-occupying lesions such as sarcoidosis or amyloidosis
   c. Check x-ray films of long bones for demineralization
5. Comparison of an individual case of increased SAP levels with others of the same diagnosis is not a fruitful exercise because there is considerable variation in serum levels from patient to patient
6. Correlate with changes in jaundice
   a. A rise in SAP levels usually parallels the degree of jaundice

      b. Higher levels are more likely an indicator of posthepatic jaundice than viral hepatitis
7. Correlate with therapy
      a. Administration of vitamin D for osteomalacia should cause a slow drop in the SAP concentration
      b. SAP is the best indicator of the extent and change in bile stasis; it is more specific and sensitive than serum bilirubin
8. Prevent neonatal hepatitis (see "Immunization Recommendation for Hepatitis B")

1.12.2 Serum Aspartate Aminotransferase

Synonyms: Glutamic oxalic transaminase (GOT), SGOT

Normal Ranges

Adult*	0–41 IU/L
Senior adult	8–33 IU/ml
Pediatric	
Newborn	2–55 IU/L at 31C
Over 2 yr	10–30 IU/L at 31C

*Female values are often slightly lower than male values, *see* Physiology.

Physiology. AST, an intracellular enzyme, is an enzyme of cellular metabolism with no known function in the plasma. Serum values for females are lower than for males (e.g., at ages 20 to 29, the males' range is 0.0 to 40.6, females from 0.0 to 31.8) and increase slightly with age, becoming almost equal with male values. Very high concentrations of enzyme are found intracellularly; very low concentrations are found in serum, and the enzyme may be totally absent when all cell membranes are intact.

    The function of transaminase is to catalyze transfer of an amino group from one amino acid to a keto acid, thus forming another amino acid. AST is widely distributed in the body tissues and is found in particularly high concentrations in those tissues with high metabolic activity. In descending order of enzyme concentration, these tissues are cardiac, hepatic, renal, skeletal muscle tissue, and RBCs. The enzyme is present but in lesser concentration in the cells of the lung, brain, and pancreas.

    Because of its wide distribution, AST is considered a nontissue- or nonorgan-specific enzyme and is, therefore, most helpful when its serum level is compared with the levels of several different serum enzymes. Little is known of the production, regulation, or excretion of the transaminases. Very little AST is excreted in the bile because of the blood–bile barrier, and it is not known whether the small amount found in bile is from the blood or directly from the liver cells.

Pathophysiology. When body cells containing AST are damaged or their activity impaired or destroyed because of deficient oxygen or glucose, the cell membrane becomes permeable or may rupture. The AST together with other cell contents, finds its way to the plasma, which increases the serum concentration of AST. The greater the intracellular concentration of the enzyme, the higher and the more rapid the rise in serum levels with cell damage. For example, damage to as little as 1 percent of the liver cells can raise the serum level of AST because of the relatively high intracellular enzyme concentration as well as the large number of hepatic cells the 1 percent represents. Damage to cardiac tissue produces a rather rapid rise of the SAST concentration; the degree of elevation correlates closely with the size of the infarct. Increases of over 500 units are unusual with solely cardiac involvement. In cardiac failure (congestive heart failure) elevations of over 1000 may occur. This extreme elevation is apparently due to the secondary congestion and necrosis of the liver rather than to cardiac cell injury per se. In liver disease higher levels are produced. The release of AST from the liver cells does not reflect liver function, which may well be normal even in the face of high SAST levels. The SAST concentration reflects the cells' response to injury and greater cell membrane permeability.

Functional change of the liver occurs only after cell necrosis. Prolonged elevation of SAST levels in liver disease may be the first indication of a nonresolving or chronic active hepatitis. A rapid drop may indicate total liver failure (Harvey et al., 1986). SAST levels also increase with cellular damage to skeletal muscle, but this is the least sensitive indicator of muscle involvement. Although not specific to any one organ or system, SAST changes are thought to be more sensitive to a change in liver status than the more specific liver enzymes (e.g., SALT).

Since the normal range of SAST levels includes a complete absence of the enzyme in body serum, decreases in the serum level are of interest only insofar as the speed with which the drop occurs (liver failure) or as an indicator of disease progress and response to treatment.

SAST LEVELS INCREASED IN:

1. Conditions causing injury to cardiac muscle cells as in
   a. Myocardial infarction. Serum levels may increase to 500 IU (from a norm of 10 to 40 IU) within 24 hours and will return to normal in 4 to 7 days if further cell damage does not occur
   b. Cardiac failure (congestive heart failure). Serum levels are frequently increased, but the amount of increase varies, depending on concomitant liver involvement (see "Pathophysiology")
2. Conditions causing injury to hepatic tissue cells as in
   a. Viral hepatitis. Serum levels are often high (greater than 100 IU). The major rise occurs in the prodromal-preicteric stage
   b. Hepatitis resulting from the ingestion of toxic substances. Serum levels of 30,000 IU/ml are seen in carbon tetrachloride poisoning
   c. Obstructive jaundice. Elevations are relatively modest, usually under 300 IU/ml
   d. Cirrhosis, metastatic malignancy of the liver, and less commonly, primary hepatomas, all of which can produce hepatic necrosis and a clinical picture somewhat similar to that of hepatitis
   e. Acute pancreatitis resulting from posthepatic obstruction
   f. Morphine administration, which decreases biliary secretions and increases the tone of gastrointestinal and biliary sphincters
3. Conditions causing injury to skeletal muscle cells as in
   a. Dermatomyositis. (Included among the group of collagen diseases and can be acute, subacute, or chronic. Characterized by a constant inflammation of muscles, which leads to decomposition and atrophy.) Because AST is so widely distributed in the body,

serum elevations are highly nonspecific in muscle disease, and CPK or aldolase is a more specific and useful test

  b. Progressive muscular dystrophy because of the cellular injury caused by the replacement of muscle cells with fat and connective tissue and an inflammatory process

  c. Muscular trauma because of overuse or external injury

  d. Trichinosis, possibly due to cellular inflammation and injury resulting from the lodging of larvae in body tissues such as the heart, lung, and striated muscle

4. Any condition that causes RBC lysis, which releases AST into the serum (e.g., hemolytic anemias)

5. Later stages of pulmonary thromboembolism; see "Implications for Nursing: SAST and LDH," item 3, in Section 1.12.3

6. Infectious mononucleosis at times. Possibly because of liver involvement, which occurs in 8 to 10 percent of all cases and resembles infectious hepatitis. It may also be due, rarely, to involvement of the heart and lung

7. Hepatotoxicity secondary to the administration of many drugs (e.g., narcotics (see item 2f), analgesics, antibiotics, and steroids)

SAST LEVELS DECREASED IN:

• Not clinically significant

1.12.3 Serum Lactic Dehydrogenase—Total

Synonyms: Lactic acid dehydrogenase, LDH-L, LDH

Normal Ranges (IU/L)

Adult		60–220
Senior adult		71–207
Pediatric		
Newborn		300–500
Child	6 mo–9 yr	250–425
	10–15 yr	200–350

Physiology. As SAST, LDH is an intracellular enzyme of cellular metabolism that is present in very high concentrations within the cell, comparatively low in serum concentration—although higher than that of SAST—and always present in the serum in some amount. The enzyme has no known function in the serum. LDH is involved in the end reaction of the anaerobic phase of carbohydrate metabolism: it reduces pyruvic acid to lactic acid and, in the presence of oxygen, oxidizes lactic acid to pyruvic acid. As SAST, LDH is nontissue or nonorgan specific and is present in widely distributed body cells. It is found in substantial amounts, in decreasing order, in the following tissues: skeletal muscle, liver, heart, pancreas, spleen, and brain. It is also present in varying concentrations in lymph nodes and thyroid, adrenal, and lung tissues. Its isoenzymes are more tissue specific and, although not used as screening tests, are frequently used to validate a diagnosis. Tissue specificity in the isoenzymes by American classification adheres to the following pattern: LDH, heart; LDH_2, kidney and heart; LDH_3, adrenal and lung; LDH_4, lung; LDH_5, liver. In British classification the series is reversed in mirror image.

Pathophysiology. The mechanism for the release of LDH from the cells is the same as that described for SAST with increasing cell permeability or rupture in response to injury. The resulting increases in serum levels are proportionate to the extent of tissue damage and the degree of intracellular concentrations of the enzyme in a given tissue. The elevations of LDH levels occurring after a myocardial infarction stay increased much longer than those of other intracellular enzymes. LDH is considered highly sensitive in determining MI and is more specific than CPK.

LDH is the least specific of enzymes in liver disorders and probably the most specific for pulmonary emboli. However, some 50 percent of all pulmonary emboli shows no abnormality of serum enzymes; thus the LDH specificity is, at best, only 50 percent. Therefore, pulmonary embolism cannot be ruled out in the absence of serum enzyme elevations. LDH levels may also increase in renal disorders, neoplastic disease, and liver disease. Isoenzyme levels increase long before the total LDH.

LDH LEVELS INCREASED IN:

1. Conditions causing cardiac cell damage as in
   a. MI. The increase in the LDH level occurs 12 to 24 hours after injury and remains elevated for a prolonged period—up to 2 weeks or as long as active inflammation persists
   b. Congestive heart failure, but only when there is liver involvement as with SAST. Values will be normal in congestive heart failure alone. The isoenzyme elevated will be LDH_5
2. Acute hepatitis with a large serum concentration increase. Only LDH_5 levels rise. Most liver diseases causing increased levels have increases in LDH_5
3. Approximately 50 percent of patients with a diagnosis of carcinoma. This is a nonspecific change with no particular diagnostic value
4. Untreated pernicious anemia, especially when the hemoglobin concentration is less than 8 g/dl, because of hemolysis. A slight increase occurs in severe hemolytic anemias
5. Cardiac valve prosthesis postoperatively
6. Renal infarct occasionally, but the increase is not clinically useful
7. Pulmonary infarction with a rise in LDH_2 and LDH_3 levels, but if hemolysis occurs because of hemorrhage around the infarct, LDH_1 levels may also rise
8. Skeletal muscle disease with increases in isoenzymes 3, 4, and 5. This very lack of specificity makes the test of little value in evaluating the muscle disease
9. The period after severe exercise; there is a rapid rise and fall in LDH

LDH LEVELS DECREASED IN:

- Not clinically significant

IMPLICATIONS FOR NURSING: SAST AND LDH

1. No specific preparation is usually required for the person having these tests, except in cases of suspected hepatic disease. If possible, treatment with any hepatotoxic drugs should be withdrawn for about 12 hours before testing. The person drawing the blood should ensure that the sample is free from hemolysis. Care should be taken to avoid shaking the container, and the sample should be sent promptly to the laboratory

2. Intramuscular injections should be avoided to prevent increases in serum levels in any person being followed with enzyme determinations for indication of disease progress or response to treatment
3. Because these serum enzyme tests are nontissue or nonorgan specific, relationships among the enzymes tested should be explored. Nursing care can then be planned, based on the nurse's or physician's interpretation of those relationships, to support the organ or system threatened as well as the individual's ability to cope with the physiological and psychological changes occurring. SAST and LDH changes very generally indicate dysfunction of the heart, the lung, the liver, or skeletal muscle
   a. Indications of lung dysfunction—generally limited to pulmonary embolism—differentiated from MI. Enzyme concentrations are not totally reliable in pulmonary embolism and can often be normal, especially with smaller infarcts
      (1) SAST levels will be normal in 60 to 75 percent of all patients with pulmonary embolism or only slightly increased some time after the infarct
      (2) LDH levels usually increased (isoenzymes LDH_2 and LDH_3) on the day of the embolism
      (3) CPK levels will be normal
      (4) Other laboratory data confirming the status
         (a) WBC count increased with increased neutrophils
         (b) Erythrocyte sedimentation rate (ESR) increased
         (c) Serum bilirubin level frequently increased to greater than 5 mg/dl
         (d) Chest film or lung scan showing infarct shadow
         (e) Serum aldolase concentration slightly increased
   b. Indications of MI
      (1) SAST level increased. Not usually increased in pulmonary embolism. SAST is the least useful of enzyme tests for diagnosis or prognostic application
      (2) LDH level increased. Levels of isoenzymes LDH_1 and LDH_2 elevated—LDH_1 greater than LDH_2, which is of specific diagnostic value; see Part III
      (3) CPK level increased. It is *not* increased in lung injury or liver disease. For further information regarding CPK isoenzymes, see Section 11.3.1. Enzymes are helpful not only in the prognosis but also as a "clock" to tell when an infarct actually occurred. (See Fig. 1–5 as to the amount and duration of the increase.) Any noticeable deviation from the expected curve of enzyme activity indicates a pathological change and must be reported promptly
      (4) Other laboratory data confirming the status
         (a) Technetium pyrophosphate scan for circulatory perfusion changes of the heart
         (b) Twelve-lead ECG
         (c) Ultrasound imaging (echograms/sonograms)
         (d) Those with levels over 1000 IU should have a careful investigation of recent history to identify any possible toxic ingestants
   c. Indications of liver dysfunction
      (1) SAST
         (a) Values greater than 500 IU are more likely related to liver dysfunction than cardiac
         (b) Values usually increase before the occurrence of jaundice in hepatitis
         (c) Read or obtain if not available a medical and social history for any person whose SAST levels reach concentrations in excess of 500 IU with some signs or symptoms of liver involvement (e.g., increased SAP levels, jaundice) to determine possible contacts with viral hepatitis
      (2) CPK levels normal
      (3) Other laboratory data confirming the status
         (a) Increased serum bilirubin concentration in posthepatic and intrahepatic obstruction
         (b) Increased SAP levels
         (c) Increased SALT (SGPT) content (more specific to liver disease than LDH or SAST)
         (d) Increased gamma glutamyl transferase (GGT) concentration in hepatobiliary and pancreatic disease
         (e) Decreased serum albumin and increased serum globulin levels in long-term cirrhosis particularly. The total protein (TP) concentration may be normal or decreased, rarely increased
      (4) LDH levels are not usually increased in viral hepatitis or in posthepatic obstruction. An increase will occur with an associated malignancy

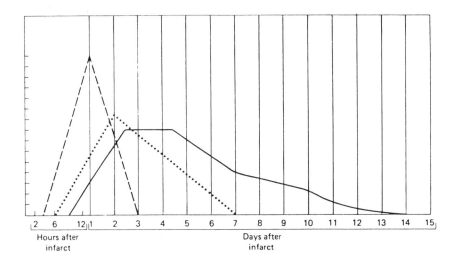

— — CPK : Increases within 2 to 5 hours; peaks during first 24 hours at 5 to 15
times normal; returns to normal by 2nd or 3rd day.

——— LDH : Increases in 6 to 12 hours after infarction; peaks in 42 to 72 hours at
2 to 8 times normal; returns to normal 5 to 6 days later, but can
persist to 10th day — or two weeks after infarct.

•••••• SAST : Increases within 6 hours after infarction; peaks in 24 to 48 hours at
2 to 15 times normal value; returns to normal after 3 to 7 days.

Figure 1–6. Elevation of enzyme levels in myocardial infarction.

       (a) Slight to moderate increase in LDH levels in cirrhosis
       (b) LDH is less useful than SAST or SALT in the diagnosis or evaluation of liver disease
       (c) Serial alterations follow a characteristic pattern; a deviation indicates a relapse or complication (see Fig. 1–6)
    d. Indications of skeletal muscle disorders
       (1) Enzyme tests should be taken at a time of maximum muscle tenderness and fever
       (2) SAST and LDH levels are usually elevated in myositis
       (3) CPK, aldolase, and SAST concentrations increase first in acute myopathies (12 to 24 hours); LDH levels increase after 48 hours
       (4) Extremely high levels of CPK and other serum enzymes occur in early and middle stages of Duchenne muscular dystrophy. CPK is minimally elevated in other forms of muscular dystrophy
       (5) Other laboratory data confirming the status
          (a) Muscle biopsy
          (b) Electromyographic studies

1.13 THYROID FUNCTION DETERMINATION AS A SCREENING TEST

Normal Ranges

FT$_4$ Free Thyroxin-Direct Dialysis	0.8–2.7 mg/dl
Thyroid-stimulating hormone (TSH)	0.3–5 uIU/ml

A. Identification of groups at risk

The Most Commonly Screened Group: Newborns. Hypothyroidism is one of the most common endocrine problems of childhood. If the diagnosis is delayed past early infancy, the chance of permanent mental retardation is great, and the neonate does not usually exhibit obvious signs of hypothyroidism. Despite the fact that congenital hypothyroidism occurs in only approximately 1 of 5000 live births, the significant risks of mental retardation and failure in physical development indicate a strong need for such screening.

Males over 50 Years of Age. This group of individuals has been found to be more likely to present with a masked form of hyperthyroidism (apathetic hyperthyroidism) in which the epinephrinelike effects are not prominent. The lack of characteristic signs and symptoms—tremor, hyperkinetic behavior, tachycardia, and heat intolerance—make the likelihood of accurate diagnosis and treatment of the thyroid imbalance difficult. Single-system predominance of hyperthyroid symptoms also occurs more frequently in this age/sex group. Hyperthyroidism should be suspected and tested for when such individuals present with unexplained congestive heart failure or arrhythmias such as atrial fibrillation or flutter, first-degree block, or multifocal premature ventricular contractions (PVC). Also suspect would be a new onset or an accentuation of previous angina pectoris or when there is a lack of response to or a requirement for unusually high doses of digitalis for control of cardiac symptoms.

Other systems can produce the major number of systemic symptoms in masked hyperthyroidism, for example, the person presenting with skeletal muscle wasting and weakness, profound weight loss without muscle wasting, unexplained severe abdominal cramps—with or without pernicious diarrhea, which, when it occurs, is unaccompanied by blood or pus—or profound depression or marked emotional lability.

Individuals with Psychiatric Problems. Masked hyperthyroidism should be screened for and ruled out in all newly diagnosed psychiatric patients. Although it has been suggested that the presence of increased thyroid levels can precipitate frank psychosis in persons with latent psychiatric problems, it is also possible that hyperthyroidism presenting only as profound depression or marked emotional lability can be misdiagnosed as a purely psychiatric problem.

Previously diagnosed psychiatric patients who suffer an unexplained decompensation in their condition should also be evaluated for thyroid imbalance.

Both hyperthyroidism and hypothyroidism can present with a single-system predominence, and signs and symptoms of the imbalance may be overlooked or treated as a totally different problem for weeks, months, and even years.

Menopausal Women. This group is less readily defined by age, but as a group, women in general have a higher incidence of almost all endocrine disorders and might benefit from closer attention to the possibility of thyroid disorders. For example, women of menopausal age, especially those showing an increase in serum cholesterol levels, should be considered with a high index of suspicion for a decrease in thyroid function.

The Elderly (over 70 Years of Age). This population was once thought to be at particular risk for hypothyroidism. More recent investigation makes the concept of routine senile hypothyroidism less easy to accept. The gland does atrophy with age, and function does decline—there is a decrease in circulating T_3—but it is more logical to assume that the decrease in normal thyroxine turnover is due to reduced peripheral need. Hypothyroidism can and does occur in the elderly, however, and should be assessed.

Individuals with a History of Low-Dose Irradiation to the Head, Neck, or Superior Mediastinum (Usually over the Age of 25). Although thyroid cancer may be associated with euthyroidism, hyperthyroidism, or hypothyroidism so that evaluation of the hormone is not specifically useful in the diagnosis of neoplastic changes, the incidence of thyroid nodule occurrence increases with each decade of life, and the probability of malignancy increases when there is a history of low-dose irradiation to the head, neck, or superior mediastinum.

Low-dose irradiation was used fairly extensively two to three decades ago to reduce the size of the thymus gland or to treat acne.

The major rationale behind the need for laboratory screening tests for thyroid dysfunction in these risk populations is that early and accurate diagnosis of thyroid imbalance cannot be made without laboratory tests.

B. Related Nursing Actions

1. The nurse needs to attain a thorough knowledge of the signs and symptoms of thyroid imbalance (increase and decrease) so that awareness of the existence of such clues is enhanced and the probability increased that such clues will be picked up and acted upon
2. Any nursing assessment should include a pertinent investigation for thyroid disorders. The skill of physical appraisal (palpation) of the thyroid should be one of the talents of the nurse, as should the ability to seek out information pertinent to the existence of thyroid disorder in history taking
3. Individuals in risk groups should be urged to request thyroid evaluation from their physicians
4. When examining the individual born and raised three or four decades ago, the nurse should inquire into the possibility of low-dose irration having been used on the thymus gland, or to treat acne

---

IMPLICATIONS FOR NURSING: THYROID FUNCTION

Newborns are frequently screened for disorders in serum chemicals other than those discussed thus far (See Chapter 15). Tests included in such screening of newborns are, among others, evaluation of the level of thyroid-stimulating hormone (TSH) and thyroxine (T_4). There exist other groups at risk for thyroid dysfunction that should be screened as carefully as are newborns, for example, the elderly. Further, any physical examination done by an health practitioner should include palpation of the thyroid and a history and physical examination that is sensitive to manifestations of thyroid disorders.

1.14 SEQUENTIAL MULTIPLE ANALYZER PROFILES

The sequential multiple analyzer (SMA) is not a test but, rather, the name of an instrument used for automatically testing a specific group of screening tests. Frequently used groupings of SMA screening tests include:

1. The *Hospital Model (SMA 12)* that tests for serum sodium, potassium, chloride, CO_2, total protein (TP), albumin, urea nitrogen (BUN), and glutamic oxalic transaminase (GOT)
2. The *Survey Model (SMA 12)* that tests for TP, albumin, calcium, inorganic phosphorus, BUN, cholesterol, glucose, uric acid, creatinine, total bilirubin, alkaline phosphatase and lactate dehydrogenase (AST)
3. The *SMA-7* that analyzes whole-blood samples for RBC count, WBC count, hemoglobin (Hg), and hematocrit (Hct) values as well as the blood indices, that is, mean corpuscular volume (MCV/MC), hemoglobin (MCH), and MCH concentration (MCHC)
4. The *SMA-6* is a short version of the hospital model that includes only six of the 12 tests: sodium, potassium, chloride, bicarbonate (or CO_2), glucose, and BUN

ADVANTAGES

- Quickly available results
- Some cost reduction (per test only; with the number of tests included in an SMA group, the overall cost is significant)
- Comprehensive chemical profiles
- Increased dependability and accuracy
- Potential for discovery and diagnosis of unsuspected disease

Recently concern has been expressed about this multiple testing approach. Little benefit is seen for the patient in terms of findings indicating problematic areas related to planned care. Outcome reviews found that 84 percent of the abnormalities discovered by the screening tests proved to be false positives. In addition, the primary reason for the use of multiple screening tests—the need to seek evidence for a disease condition that could complicate the surgical procedure—is too often superceded by the need to meet institutional requirements or the fear of medicolegal complications. It has recently been suggested that a thorough physical examination and history provides the best information on preoperative status and tests indicated. Current guidelines for routine preoperative testing have been suggested as follows ("Which Pre-surgical Tests Are Worthwhile," 1992.)

1. All testing should be first indicated as necessary by physical examination and history taking
2. Electrocardiography: all patients 50 years of age and older
3. Hematocrit and blood typing: *only* if major blood loss is expected
4. Serum electrolytes: individuals taking digitalis or diuretics or who have kidney or heart disease
5. Prothrombin/partial thromboplastin: individuals with liver disease, malnutrition, or with a history or physical signs of abnormal bleeding
6. Chest films should be done routinely for any thoracic surgery

(Data source: Which Pre-surgical Tests are Worthwhile? *Emergency Medicine,* October 15, 1992, 24.14:88–89.)

TWO

HEMATOLOGY SCREEN

Hematology is the study of blood. Hematologists are concerned with all aspects of blood such as blood volume, blood flow, and tests done on the blood for the diagnosis of disease in other organs. This chapter is limited to tests done on the major cellular components of blood, particularly tests done primarily for the diagnosis of diseases of the blood itself. Because there is a close relationship among the cellular blood components, all those components should be tested so that the relationships can be explored.

Blood consists of both fluid and solid elements. The fluid portion is called *plasma* and is made up predominantly of water. When the fibrinogen is removed from plasma, the resulting fluid is called *serum.* The cellular components consist largely of white blood cells (WBCs), platelets, and red blood cells (RBCs). RBCs normally outnumber WBCs by a ratio of at least 700:1.

COMPLETE BLOOD COUNT AND DIFFERENTIAL

The complete blood count (CBC) traditionally includes the following tests: red blood corpuscle (cell) count, hemoglobin determination, hematocrit, white cell count, and white cell differential.

Frequently included in the CBC are the Wintrobe blood indices (mean corpuscular volume [MCV], mean corpuscular hemoglobin [MCH], mean corpuscular hemoglobin concentration [MCHC]) and red cell distribution width. A platelet count, or estimation, is usually done as a part of the differential or smear evaluation. The presence of reticulocytes and nucleated RBCs are noted, and RBC morphology (determination of variance in size, shape, or pigmentation) is described. The sedimentation rate has been included in this writing, although is not usually done as a part of the CBC because of its nonspecificity. This nonspecificity makes it a screening test in the true sense of the word, and, as such, it is of interest.

The CBC is probably one of the more important laboratory tests. A great percentage of all hematologic disease can be diagnosed from the CBC findings. It is frequently part of the routine laboratory work included when a patient is admitted to a hospital and has the advantage that it can be performed on either venous or capillary blood.

2.1 TESTS RELATED TO THE RED BLOOD CELL

2.1.1 Red Blood Corpuscle Count

Synonyms: RBC count, red blood cell count, erythrocyte count

Normal Ranges ($\times 10^1/mm^3$)[a] (mil/mm^3)

Adult	
Female	4.0–5.3
Male	4.4–5.7
Senior adult	3.0–5.0
Pediatric	
Newborn	4.8–7.1
Neonate	4.1–6.4

[a]When counts are reported from automated counter, only the numerals are reported (e.g., 4.0 to 5.3). To get the total figure, multiply the reported total by 1 million (10^6).

Definition. The RBC count is simply that—a count of the RBCs in a given sample of either venous or capillary blood, venous blood being preferred. The count can be done individually "by hand" by using a counting chamber or by an automated process. The automated process is more rapid and accurate and is used more frequently.

Physiology. There are several theories on the origin of the cellular blood components including RBCs, the most commonly accepted being the monophylectic (fixed stem cell) theory, outlined in Figure 2–1. The RBC becomes progressively smaller as it matures and loses its nucleus, at which point it is more correctly called a corpuscle than a cell. Reticulocytes (young RBCs; Fig. 2–1) are found in the peripheral blood in small numbers and are grossly indistinguishable from normal RBCs. They are identified by special staining of the blood smear.

Blood cells are formed in red bone marrow (ribs, sternum, vertebrae, and pelvis of the normal adult). In infants and children through adolescence, all bone marrow produces blood cells, later some marrow is replaced with fat—yellow marrow. RBC production depends on a number of things such as an adequate intake of protein, carbohydrate, fat, minerals (especially iron), and vitamins (especially vitamin B_{12}, folic acid, vitamin B_6 [pyridoxine], and vitamin C [ascorbic acid]). Vitamin B_{12} also requires the presence of intrinsic factor to be absorbed, which is produced by the cells of the stomach lining.

Erythrocytes are carried by the blood, which is propelled by the heartbeat and somatic muscle "pumps" (peripheral muscle action that propels blood by contraction and squeezing the vasculature). RBCs function only within the vasculature, as opposed to the WBCs, which migrate into tissue when needed. The major function of the RBC is to carry hemoglobin, which in turn carries oxygen, in a weak bond, to the body tissues, and carbon monoxide, in a strong bond, from the tissues to the lungs (Henry, 1991). It also has a function in acid-base balance (see Section 1.2 on the chloride shift).

RBCs survive about 120 days. This fairly long survival is due in great part to their unique shape, being thin in the center and thick at the edges once the nucleus is lost—a biconcave disk (Frohlich, 1980). They are flexible and elastic, so they can slip through the smallest vessels by deforming and then returning to functional shape. As they speed through the blood vessels, they take on the shape of

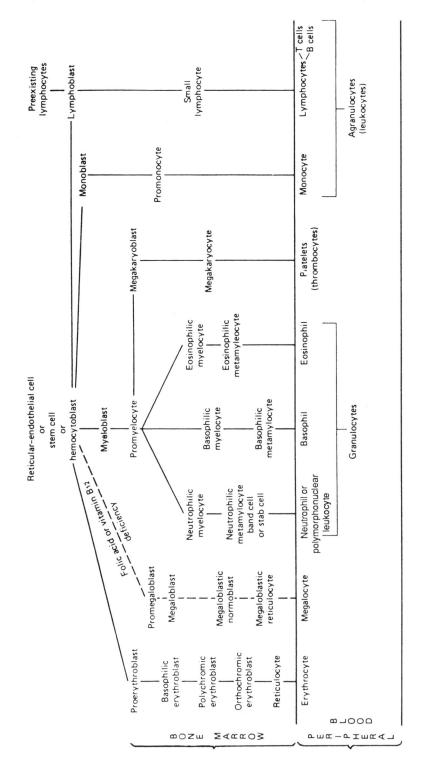

Figure 2–1. Formation of blood cells. (Adapted from Whaley, L. F. & Wong, D. L. [1979]. *Nursing Care of Infants and Children.* St. Louis: C.V. Mosby, 1979, p. 1367, with permission.)

tiny parachutes, with their central portion well in advance of a thicker edge (Greisheimer & Wiedeman, 1972). As the RBC ages, it becomes more fragile and ultimately will rupture. If the cell does not disintegrate spontaneously, it will be broken down by the spleen or other parts of the reticuloendothelial system, which also picks up the debris and degrades it to bilirubin (see Fig. 1–1).

Regulation of RBC production is very complex and depends on several factors. The primary factor for production and termination of production seems to be the level of tissue oxygenation, tissue hypoxia causing increased production. Tissue hypoxia is believed to stimulate the kidney to release the hormone erythropoietin, which increases both RBC mitosis and the rate of RBC release from the bone marrow. When tissue oxygen reaches normal levels, erythropoietin production ceases (Henry, 1991, p. 609).

A significant percentage of RBCs is in the spleen at any one time, not in storage but rather in a dynamic equilibrium with the circulation (Nordin, 1980). Epinephrine released into the system, usually secondary to stress, will alter that equilibrium and increase the number of circulating RBCs as a physiological compensatory measure.

Physiological Variations. In the elderly, ranges of normal are wider than the adult norm, not only for RBCs but for hemoglobin and hematocrit as well. In general, values are lower. At one time the so-called anemia of the aged was considered a function of aging. It is now thought to be due to the generally poor nutritional state among the elderly, which is due to a variety of factors (Carnevali & Patrick, 1979).

Blood volume and, consequently, the RBC count in the neonate depends on the amount of blood transfer from the placenta at the time of birth. Also, few new RBCs are produced for the first 8 to 10 weeks of life, which causes a physiological anemia.

Pathophysiology. When the balance of RBC production and destruction is lost, blood disorders occur. Production can be decreased if the mechanisms of control are lost such as in deficits of erythropoietin because of kidney disease. Disease can occur as well through endocrine system relationships with cell production, which may account for anemias accompanying thyroid or adrenal disorders (hypothyroidism, Addison's disease). Blood disorders can occur because of defects anywhere along the process of cell production (i.e., differentiation, proliferation, and maturation). Such defects are most commonly due to deficiency states, which are frequently congenital in origin or secondary to drug administration.

An increased rate of destruction occurs in some hereditary diseases (e.g., spherocytosis), some acquired diseases (e.g., liver failure), or with an abnormal environment for the RBC (e.g., transfusion reactions).

Increased production of RBCs occurs as a compensatory response seen in adaptation to high altitude or in pathology causing tissue hypoxia (respiratory or cardiac disease). It can also be secondary to pathological states in which there is an increase in the erythropoietin concentration without tissue hypoxia as a stimulus such as in tumors of the kidney or polycythemia vera (Frohlich, 1980) (see Table 2–3 for definition of abnormal cells).

RBC COUNT DECREASED IN:

1. Conditions related to defects in regulatory mechanisms such as a loss of adequate erythropoietin in

    a. Chronic renal disease because of decreased secretion of erythropoietin and possibly depression of the bone marrow itself by the uremia. This causes a normocytic (cell normal in size and shape), normochromic (cells normal in hemoglobin content) anemia. Anemia is roughly proportional to uremia; the hemoglobin level rarely falls below 6 g/dl (Harrington & Brenner, 1973). Recall that with an increase in the blood urea nitrogen (BUN) level greater than 200 mg/dl, the RBC life span is shortened to about half of normal (see "Implications for Nursing: Serum Urea Nitrogen" in Section 1.6)

    b. Addison's disease by a mechanism that is unclear. A normocytic, normochromic anemia results

    c. Hypothyroidism because of multiple factors. Most frequently a normocytic, normochromic anemia results. Achlorhydria is present in some cases, which increases the problem of poor intestinal absorption often present with hypothyroidism and causes a macrocytic (cells larger than normal) anemia*

    d. Chronic inflammatory disease. A normocytic, normochromic anemia with shortened RBC life results

2. Conditions related to defects in cell differentiation, proliferation, or maturation such as

    a. Defects in stem cells that lead to aplastic anemia. True aplastic anemia demonstrates suppression of all myeloid (bone marrow) elements, red cell aplasia or hypoplastic anemia (which usually refers to a depression of the RBC level only), Fanconi's syndrome (a familial hypoplastic anemia or pancytopenia [depression of all cellular production]), or Diamond-Blackfan syndrome (a congenital purely red cell anemia). Besides familial or hereditary defects, there are defects secondary to the accidental or therapeutic exposure to irradiation; administration of toxic drugs (chemotherapy); or to an autoimmune or allergic process

    b. Defects in nuclear development (DNA-RNA) because of deficiencies in folic acid or vitamin B_{12}, two critical coenzymes of nuclear development. This causes macrocytic anemia (see Fig. 2–1). This anemia can be secondary to an inadequate intake (malnutrition) or inadequate absorption (idiopathic steatorrhea, the lack of intrinsic factor from an inherent defect, or pernicious anemia, the lack of intrinsic factor after gastrectomy), the use of certain drugs (phenytoin [Dilantin], methotrexate [a folate antagonist]), or in greatly increased requirements for RBC production (hemolytic anemias, pregnancy)

3. Conditions causing increased erythrocyte destruction, such as

    a. Abnormalities of the corpuscle because of membrane defects found in

        (1) Hereditary spherocytosis, which causes rapid hemolysis of the RBCs

        (2) Acquired paroxysmal nocturnal hemoglobinuria (PNH), which has many of the characteristics of an inherited disease and causes repetitive intravascular hemolysis with morning hemoglobinuria and potential thrombotic problems (Harvey et al., 1991)

        (3) Hereditary nonspherocytic hemolytic anemias caused by enzyme defects

    b. Ingestion of and intoxication by heavy metals (e.g., lead, copper)

    c. Abnormalities in the erythrocyte's environment as found in

        (1) Microangiopathic hemolytic anemia (anemia believed to be caused by the mechanical and perhaps chemical effects of vascular lesions on RBCs that result in red cell abnormalities [e.g., schistocytes and irregularly contracted cells such as burr cells]

---

*Hypothyroidism and pernicious anemia appear together more frequently than could be due to chance. This link between the two is believed to be on the basis that both may have, at least in part, an autoimmune origin (Nordin, 1987).

and are often associated with disseminated intravascular clotting [DIC]) (Harvey et al., 1991; Henry, 1991) secondary to gas gangrene, malaria, prosthetic heart valve replacements, vasculitis, malignant hypertension, disseminated carcinoma, eclampsia, hemolylic-uremic syndrome in children, sepsis, and renal homograft rejection

(2) Intoxication with chemical agents (e.g., arsenic)

(3) Antibody responses secondary to transfusion reactions (including erythroblastosis fetalis) and certain drug reactions (e.g., quinine, quinidine, penicillin, phenacetin)

(4) Auto antibody responses in certain disease states

    (a) Malignant lymphomas

    (b) Chronic lymphocytic leukemia

    (c) Lupus erythematosus

    (d) Infectious mononucleosis

    (e) Most viral infections

RBC COUNT INCREASED IN:

1. Physiological compensatory states (see "Physiology" and "Physiological Variations") occurring in response to

    a. Blood loss resulting from hemolysis or hemorrhage. The occurrence of an actual numerical increase other than just an increase in RBC production is dependent on the severity and duration of blood loss

    b. Tissue hypoxia

       (1) Relatively long-term existence at high altitudes

       (2) Cardiorespiratory insufficiency (e.g., mild, chronic congestive heart failure, emphysema, and some forms of congenital heart disease)

2. Pathophysiological responses in

    a. Tumors (unilateral) of the kidney, liver, adrenals (Cushing's syndrome), lung, and cerebellum, which cause excessive release of erythropoietin or erythropoietinlike substances

    b. Myeloproliferative disease without a relative increase in erythropoietin activity (e.g., polycythemia vera), which increases not only the RBC count but also all cellular elements formed in the bone marrow—leukocytes (increased number of immature neutrophils) and platelets—a total increase in marrow activity.

2.1.2 Hemoglobin

Synonyms: Hgb, Hb

Normal Ranges (g/dl)

Adult	
Female	12.0–15.0
Male	13.0–17.0
Senior adult	10.0–17.0
Pediatric	
Newborn	14.0–24.0
Neonate	11.0–20.0[a]
Infant	10.0–15.0
Child	11.0–16.0

[a]During the neonatal period capillary blood values are 2 to 3 g/dl greater than venous blood values (Whaley & Wong, 1991).

Definition. Hemoglobin is the main component of the RBC, and determination of that content is one of the most frequent tests done in clinical laboratories and one of the oldest and most important tests performed (Tietz, 1990). The test has been found to be more helpful in terms of diagnosis and management of therapy in anemia than is the RBC count because it is the simplest means available for detecting anemias and their severity. It can be used as an index of the oxygen-carrying capacity of the blood.

Before automation the hemoglobin test was one of the most inaccurate of blood tests, and results were reported in terms of a percentage of a norm. There is too much variation within the normals of age and sex for that method of reporting to be accurate. Hemoglobin is more accurately reported in grams per deciliter (or in grams per 100 ml).

Physiology. Hemoglobin is produced by immature RBCs, which are nucleated. Mature cells lack the nucleus and thus cytoplasmic protein synthesizing ability. Hemoglobin is a red-pigmented protein that is found only in erythrocytes and gives them their characteristic color. Iron is essential to the formation of hemoglobin, the heme molecule being made up of a protoporphyrin globulin and iron, and is one of the few proteins whose structure is relatively well understood. Physiologically normal RBCs contain the maximum amount of hemoglobin (Tietz, 1990).

The main function of hemoglobin is the transport of oxygen to body cells from the lungs. The hemoglobin molecule contains four heme molecules, each one of which can react with and bind one molecule of oxygen—the oxygen binds directly to the iron (oxyhemoglobin). The amount of oxygen that can be carried by a hemoglobin molecule is influenced by three major factors:

1. *Oxygen partial pressure.* When that pressure is increased, the amount of oxygen combining is increased and vice versa. The changes in oxygen's ability to be bound by hemoglobin at varying oxygen tensions is frequently described graphically by the *hemoglobin dissociation curve.* This curve shows the percent saturation of hemoglobin to be expected (given the stability of factors 2 and 3 that follows) at different partial pressures of oxygen in the blood. It emphasizes the relatively high oxygen saturations with fairly low partial pressures of oxygen (e.g., 75 percent at a PO_2 of 40 mm Hgb) as well as the rapid drop in saturation below that pressure.
2. *pH (Bohr effect).* If the other factors (partial pressure and temperature) are constant, oxygen saturation is less with a low pH and greater with a high pH (Groer & Shekleton, 1983).
3. *Temperature.* Increased blood temperature causes the blood pH to fall, thus decreasing the oxygen saturation of the hemoglobin and vice versa. This phenomenon partially explains the metabolic acidosis that occurs with hyperthermia.

In muscle, myoglobin, a protein similar to hemoglobin but found only in muscle cells, conveys the oxygen from the blood and interstitial fluid to the cell. Heme can also bind with carbon monoxide (carboxyhemoglobin, reduced hemoglobin), and the binding is much stronger than with oxygen. Thus, carbon monoxide is removed from body cells by hemoglobin (Greisheimer & Wiedeman, 1972).

The hemoglobin concentration is high at birth, a carryover from fetal life when it was necessary to provide adequate oxygen in utero; it drops rapidly until well into the second year of life. Newborn hemoglobin consists of 40 to 70 percent fetal hemoglobin (hemoglobin F), which is produced by the fetus but is abnormal in the adult in amounts greater than 1 to 2 percent

(Whaley & Wong, 1991). Erythropoiesis is also decreased in the newborn, virtually ceasing for a period after birth, and the infant's RBCs are fragile and readily destroyed. Once erythropoiesis is established, however, the hemoglobin content rises slowly, with female values stabilizing at puberty and males at about the 17th year of life.

Compensatory Physiological Mechanisms

1. Intravascular hemolysis takes place all the time, yet free hemoglobin is found in the plasma in only minute amounts (less than 1 mg/dl). The levels are kept low by the binding of free hemoglobin with haptoglobin, the levels of which decrease in response to increased amounts of free hemoglobin. This mechanism works only until free hemoglobin levels reach 7 to 14 mg/dl. Above that, free hemoglobin is excreted in the urine.
2. Decreases in environmental atmospheric pressure (high altitudes) will increase the hemoglobin concentration by increasing the numbers of normal RBCs. Levels rise to 16 to 23 g/dl in the adult.

Pathophysiology. Abnormalities in hemoglobin levels most frequently involve decreases and can be due to a number of causes, for example, decreased production because of a lack of necessary materials (iron, protein), increased loss (acute or chronic bleeding—there needs to be an acute loss of 1000 ml of blood before the hemoglobin level decreases), or conditions that interfere with red cell production (see "Pathophysiology" in Section 2.1.1) because hemoglobin concentration depends mostly on the number of RBCs present, although decreased amounts of hemoglobin per cell do occur (hypochromic anemia). Abnormal forms of hemoglobin, hemoglobin variants, may prevent what appears to be a normal hemoglobin level from being effective in its major function, that of gas transport and exchange. Abnormal forms are identified by hemoglobin protein electrophoresis (Tietz, 1990).

The mechanism for synthesis of hemoglobin protein is inherited from both parents. When an abnormal characteristic is inherited from only one parent (heterozygous), the condition may be without clinical signs or symptoms except for the "trait" found on examination of the blood (e.g., sickle cell trait). A great change in hemoglobin function occurs when even a single amino acid of its four polypeptide strands is altered, and it is possible to have several abnormal hemoglobins at one time. Abnormalities in hemoglobin synthesis are usually accompanied by abnormal variations in RBC size (anisocytosis) and shape (poikilocytosis).

Acquired dysfunction of hemoglobin also occurs. An example would be the formation of methemoglobin in heavy smokers, which replaces as much as 6 to 10 percent of the total hemoglobin. Heavy-metal intoxication has the same effect (Tietz, 1990).

Compensatory Mechanisms for Pathological Change. The body is able to compensate in part for blood loss. The early response to massive changes in blood volume is hemodilution. This helps maintain the circulating blood volume but cannot replace the RBCs, so a drop in the RBC count, hemoglobin concentration, and hematocrit will occur, noticeable only after 6 to 24 hours when hemodilution is complete. Immediately after massive hemorrhage the RBC count, hemoglobin level, and hematocrit will be normal (Harvey et al., 1991). The bone marrow response is indicated by the release of an increased number of immature RBCs into the peripheral circulation (reticulocytes). If the loss is massive or the duration prolonged, the bone marrow will undergo hyperplasia. Fetal sites of red bone marrow production can revert to cell production. An increase in nucleated RBCs will be found in the peripheral circulation (Collins, 1975).

Gradual changes in blood volume can be compensated to the extent that no acute symptoms may be noted and diagnosis is unlikely unless RBC tests are undertaken (Harvey et al., 1991).

HEMOGLOBIN CONCENTRATION INCREASED IN:

1. Severe dehydration
2. The first few weeks of life

HEMOGLOBIN CONCENTRATION DECREASED IN:

1. Conditions causing a decrease in the absolute number of RBCs (see "RBC Count Decreased in" in Section 2.1.1).
2. Conditions related to impaired cytoplasmic red cell development such as
   a. Defective heme synthesis as found in
      (1) Iron deficiency anemias secondary to an inadequate intake or absorption of iron, chronic bleeding, or pregnancy with its increased need for iron
      (2) Chronic disorders causing an impaired release of iron from stores in the reticuloendothelial cells (the anemias of chronic disease)
      (3) Sideroblastic anemia, in which the pathogenic factors are not understood
      (4) Heavy-metal (lead, copper) intoxication, which also causes ineffective erythropoiesis
   b. Defective globin synthesis as found in
      (1) Thalassemia major (Cooley's anemia; β-thalassemia) secondary to a defect in total hemoglobin synthesis with the presence of fetal hemoglobin, which affects the rate of synthesis of the amino acid chains (Harper et al., 1979)
      (2) Hemoglobinopathies secondary to structural changes in the amino acid chains, which are affected by the genetic coding of their sequence (e.g., hemoglobin H, hemoglobin Bart, hemoglobin M, hemoglobin G [Gun Hill])*

2.1.3 Hematocrit

Synonyms: Hct, "crit," packed cell volume, PCV

Normal Ranges (%)

Adult		
Female	36–45	
Male	39–51	*(continued)*

---

*More recent nomenclature is the addition of the original geographic origin of the variant. Normal hemoglobin is hemoglobin A with alpha, beta, or gamma chains, and it will be found written to identify that information. That is, normal hemoglobin can also be identified as $\alpha_2 \beta_2$ (Harper et al., 1979).

Senior adult	
Female	30–54
Male	36–56
Pediatric	
0–3 days	48–70
4–8 days	42–62
9–13 days	39–59
14 days–2 mo	35–49
3 mo–5 mo	29–43
6 mo–3 yr	30.5–40.5
4 yr–10 yr	32–42
11 yr–15 yr	34–44

Laboratory of Pathology, 1991.

Definition. Traditionally, the hematocrit is defined as the percentage of RBCs per volume of whole blood. It is currently defined more as the calculated value MCV/RBC from the automated cell counter and does not include "trapped plasma." The packed cell volume (PCV) is the "spun" (centrifuged to separate the cells from plasma) hematocrit and does contain trapped plasma. PCV values average 2 to 3 percent greater. The PCV gives an indirect estimate of hemoglobin present in the blood, whereas the automated value is a calculated one. As a rule of thumb, the hematocrit is usually about three times the hemoglobin value.

The hematocrit is considered a fundamental diagnostic test in anemia as a measure of the size, capacity, and number of cells present in a person's blood. This test, together with the hemoglobin value, establishes the presence and severity of an anemia. There is close agreement between hematocrit determinations done on either venous or capillary blood; therefore, either can be used (Henry, 1991).

Physiology and Pathophysiology. In general, the physiology and pathophysiology underlying the hematocrit determination are the same as those described for the RBC count and hemoglobin concentration. Some data concerning the significance of changes in the hematocrit are worth including here.

The hematocrit is not considered a good measure of water (*not* saline) deficit because it shows relatively little change during the development of a pure water deficit, even when the loss is great enough to be life-threatening. A loss of 20 percent of body *water* would elevate a hematocrit of 42 percent *only one* percentage point, to 43 percent (Harvey et al., 1991).

Hematocrit levels are often used as a rough measure of extracellular saline excess. It will usually be low in that case, because the amount of RBCs remains unchanged while the saline component increases—a relative decrease in hematocrit.

Blood viscosity shows little variation within the hematocrit's normal range, but an increase in the hematocrit from the highest range of normal in an infant (48 to 70 percent) will double the relative viscosity and the resistance to blood flow.

Changes in hematocrit, although dependent mostly on the numbers of RBCs present, are also sensitive to changes in size, shape, and density of the RBCs. As with hemoglobin, changes do not occur in the hematocrit until several hours (6 to 24) after massive hemorrhage, and an acute drop in the hematocrit value is usually accompanied by acute symptoms of anemia (e.g., extreme fatigue, weakness, shortness of breath, dyspnea, dizziness). Also, as in changes in the RBC count and hemoglobin values, the signs and symptoms of anemia secondary to slowly advancing losses—chronic blood loss—are less evident and therefore harder to diagnose.

HEMATOCRIT INCREASES AND DECREASES IN:

- See "Hemoglobin Concentration Increases and Decreases In" in Section 2.1.2.

2.1.4 Erythrocyte Indices

Synonyms: Wintrobe red cell indices, blood indices

Definition. The word *indices* is a plural form of the word *index* and refers to something that points out, indicates, manifests, or directs attention. The erythrocyte indices point out the characteristics of size and hemoglobin content of the RBCs and the relationship of these characteristics to the number of RBCs. A rough idea of such elements can be determined by looking at a stained smear of peripheral blood and comparing results of hgb, hct, and RBC counts and size. Wintrobe introduced the indices calculation to substitute objective quantitative standards for the subjective impressions produced by such observations of stained smears. It is well to bear in mind that the complete accuracy of these indices depends on the accuracy of the values given for RBC count, hemoglobin content, and hematocrit. The process is automated in most laboratories.

The indices are useful in determining the morphological type of anemia (e.g., microcytic, macrocytic, hypochromic, hyperchromic), which in turn helps making decisions about further diagnostic or treatment needs. Knowledgeable evaluation of the results of the erythrocyte indices can prevent the need for a bone marrow examination.

The values given in the erythrocyte indices are an average, not a precise, value. Erythrocyte indices are usually reported with a CBC rather than as a separate test or separate individual tests.

A. *Mean Corpuscular Volume*

Definition. MCV can be defined as the average, or mean volume, or size of a single RBC.

Synonym: MCV

Normal Ranges (fl)[a]

Adult	81–100
Senior adult	90.5–105.5[b]
Pediatric	
Newborn	96–108
Thereafter	82–91

[a]fl = femtoliter(s) = 10^{-15} liters.
[b]Calculated from an average of normal values given ±5 fl (Henry, 1991).

Calculation of MCV

$$MCV = \frac{\text{hematocrit} \times 10}{\text{RBC millions/mm}^3}$$

Significance. Increases above 100 fl in the adult indicate a macrocytic anemia. Values above 120 fl are found in the adult with a folic acid and B_{12} deficiency (e.g., pernicious anemia). Decreases below 78 fl in the adult usually indicate a microcytic (cells smaller than normal) anemia; values below 64 fl are found with iron deficiency anemias and thalassemia. These findings should be correlated with RBC morphology (smear).

Discussion. Increases in MCH may also be found in some stages of hemolytic anemias because of an increase in immature and, therefore, macrocytic cells and large-"shift" erythrocytes (Harvey et al., 1991). (See "Pathophysiology" in Section 2.2.1 for information on "shift to the left.")

B. Mean Corpuscular Hemoglobin (MCH)

Synonym: MCH

Normal Ranges (pg)[a]

Adult	27–35
Senior adult	28–32[b]
Pediatric	
Newborn	32–34
Thereafter	27–31

[a]pg = picograms = (10^{-12} g) = micromicrograms (μμg).
[b]Calculated from an average of normal ranges given for men and women ± 2 pg (Henry, 1991).

Definition. An expression of the amount (weight) of hemoglobin per average, single RBC.

Calculation

$$\text{MCH} = \frac{\text{Hemoglobin g/l or g/dl} \times 10 \text{ or g\%} \times 10}{\text{RBC} \times 10^{-6}/\mu\text{l of blood (or millions/mm}^3)}$$

Significance. High values are found in macrocytic anemias; low values are found in microcytic anemias. Results usually parallel MCV values.

Discussion. Increases in MCH may also be found in some stages of hemolytic anemias because of an increase in immature and, therefore, macrocytic cells and large-"shift" erythrocytes (Harvey et al., 1991). (See "Pathophysiology" in Section 2.2.1 for information on "shift to the left.")

C. Mean Corpuscular Hemoglobin Concentration

Synonym: MCHC

Normal Ranges (%)

Adult	32–37
Senior adult	29–33[a]

Pediatric	
Newborn	32–33
Thereafter	32–36

[a]Calculated from an average of normal values given ± 2 percent.

Definition. MCHC is the average concentration of hemoglobin in each red cell and is expressed as a percentage of the volume of the RBC. The RBC can be called hyper-, hypo-, and normochromic.

Calculation

$$\text{MCHC} = \frac{\text{Hgb (g/dl blood)}}{\text{Hct}} \times 100$$

Significance. A higher-than-normal concentration is not possible. Values in megaloblastic (macrocytic) anemias are usually normal. A decrease will occur in iron deficiency anemias and indicate a hypochromic state (an abnormal decrease in the hemoglobin content of the RBC).

Discussion. The MCV and MCH depend on the accuracy of the RBC count. The MCHC does not. Thus, the MCHC can be reliable when automatic methods are not available to ensure the accuracy of the RBC count.

2.1.5 Red Cell Distribution Width

Synonym: RDW

Normal Range: Adult   11.5–14.5%

Definition. Red cell distribution width (RDW) is an index of the variation in red cell size, previously reported only as being present by the word *aniscocytosis* or *anis* being printed on the laboratory report. The RDW could be defined as the quantitative equivalent of aniscocytosis. Changes in RDW so far observed have been high normal or above normal. RDW is expressed as a percentage because it represents the coefficient of red cell variation.

RDW NORMAL IN:

- Hypoplastic disorders such as anemias of chronic disease, most thalassemias, and aplastic anemia.

RDW INCREASED IN:

1. Nutritional anemias (iron, folate, or vitamin B_{12} deficiency)
2. Hemoglobin H disease
3. S-beta thalassemia
4. Leukemias
5. Immune hemolytic anemia

(*continued*)

6. Posthemorrhagic anemia
7. Any long term or chronic disease

2.1.6 Sedimentation Rate

Synonyms: Erythrocyte sedimentation rate ESR, SR, "sed" rate, Westergren's sedimentation rate

Normal Ranges (mm/hr)

Adult	
Male	0–10
Female	0–20
Senior adult	
Male	15–20
Female	20–30
Pediatric	
Newborn	0–2
Neonatal to puberty	3–13

Definition. Determination of the erythrocyte sedimentation rate (ESR) is a highly nonspecific test, performed on anticoagulated whole blood. The blood is allowed to stand in a calibrated tube. The corpuscles (cells) will settle, and the plasma will displace upward. In the healthy individual the rate of settling is constant. The sedimentation rate is determined by measuring the level of plasma layer 1 hour after the blood sample is placed in the tube. The value is more often increased as compared to the norm (i.e., the rate of settling is faster) than decreased, and the rate at which it settles can vary from person to person even with the same diagnosis. It is of merit, then, in those disease processes in which its value has been found to be elevated. Changes in the degree of increase in the sedimentation rate can be a useful guide in assessing the progress and activity of the disease, but not as a diagnostic aid.

Pathophysiology. The sedimentation rate is a rough measure of abnormal concentrations of fibrinogen and serum globulins; the cause of the increased concentrations is not clear. With elevations of the fibrinogen content and to a lesser degree elevations of the globulin content in the plasma, there is increased rouleaux formation of the RBCs (rouleaux RBCs clumped together, like rolls of coins) (Miller & Kane, 1983). Such formation tends to increase the weight of the RBCs and, thereby, the speed of sedimentation (Davidsohn & Henry, 1969).

SEDIMENTATION RATE INCREASED IN:

1. All inflammatory diseases such as:
   a. Chronic infectious disease (e.g., tuberculosis). An increase in the sedimentation rate usually parallels an increase in the disease activity
   b. Diseases of the connective tissue (e.g., rheumatic fever and rheumatoid arthritis)
   c. Acute localized infection in which the increase is seen with an accompanying increase in RBCs
2. All diseases associated with tissue degeneration or necrosis such as cancer in which the increase in ESR often parallels the extent of the malignancy

3. Multiple myeloma because of the presence of abnormal immunoglobins that increase the formation of rouleaux
4. Most anemias resulting from a change in the erythrocyte/plasma ratio that favors the rouleaux formation of erythrocytes
5. Normal pregnancy after the third or fourth month of pregnancy. The mechanism is not clear, and the ESR usually returns to normal about 1 month postpartum

SEDIMENTATION RATE DECREASED IN:

1. Conditions causing increased serum albumin levels (see "Serum Total Protein Increased In" in Section 1.8)
2. Sickle cell anemia

IMPLICATIONS FOR NURSING: RELATED TO THE RED BLOOD CELL AND HEMOGLOBIN

1. Data from related tests of importance, depending on the diagnosis or probable diagnosis should be gathered and compared with known results of tests on the RBCs
   a. Stool for occult blood to detect gastrointestinal bleeding in known history of bleeding, clinical indications of bleeding, and in anemias of unknown origin
   b. WBC count is decreased with total marrow depression, decreased in macrocytic anemias
   c. WBC differential. Neutrophils are multilobulated (hypersegmented, or extra lobes in the nucleus) in idiopathic steatorrhea and pernicious anemia—macrocytic anemias. Neutrophil numbers are increased in polycythemia vera but usually not increased in compensatory polycythemia
   d. Platelet count is decreased with total marrow depression, increased in polycythemia vera, but not increased in compensatory polycythemia
   e. Serum iron levels are decreased in nutritional anemias—it is useful to check for this decrease before doing any diet teaching so as not to overload the person with iron or unnecessary and confusing information. The test results will not be valid if done shortly after a blood transfusion or when the patient has been receiving oral iron therapy
   f. B_{12} and folate levels should be checked with any macrocytic anemia
   g. Shilling test should be performed in macrocytic anemias—a test for vitamin B_{12} absorption. It is performed when vitamin B_{12} and folate levels do not respond to dietary supplementation (Nordin, 1980, 1992)
   h. Gastric analysis, but it is rarely used now. No free acid is present in pernicious anemia
   i. Bone marrow examination is indicated when there is an increased number of immature forms of all myeloid cells in peripheral circulation
   j. Reticulocyte count to determine a positive marrow response in the face of a decreased RBC count. An absence of increased reticulocyte numbers after blood loss indicates poor marrow function
   k. Serum bilirubin or urobilinogen levels to validate the presence of intravascular hemolysis. Hemoglobin breakdown serves to increase serum bilirubin or urobilinogen level (see Fig. 1–1)
   l. Red blood cell morphology (See Section 2.3.1)
   m. Serum haptoglobin levels decrease, or an absence may indicate intravascular hemolysis
   n. Increased free hemoglobin concentration is an indication of intravascular hemolysis
   o. Urine hemosiderin concentration is an indication of intravascular hemolysis
   p. Sickledex, a screening test for potential hemoglobin S carriers (trait) or sickle cell anemia
2. Check for increased values of hemoglobin, hematocrit, and RBCs in response to treatment of anemias
3. Prevent changes in RBC test results because of technical errors in obtaining blood
   a. There is no special patient preparation for tests of RBCs other than the usual instruction in preparation for venipuncture. Capillary blood is frequently used for children

    b. For capillary samples particularly, there should be no excessive massage of the ear lobe, finger-tip, or heel to improve blood flow. Massaging can increase the total number of cells in the sample over the true number or can cause mechanical injury to the cell that results in cell destruction and dilution of the sample by tissue fluid, thereby decreasing the values. Capillary blood must also be handled more carefully than venous blood because it will coagulate more rapidly (Henry, 1991)

    c. With venous samples, the tourniquet should be removed, circulation restored, and then the tourniquet reapplied when there is difficulty locating the vein. This will prevent hemoconcentration, which would invalidate the test result

    d. The sample must be sent to the laboratory as quickly as possible. Standing causes changes in the character of the blood and the distribution of the cells in the plasma (sedimentation)

    e. Timing of sample taking should be observed by the nurse. Unless specifically ordered for that time, samples should not be drawn after a transfusion or shortly after the person has acted as a blood donor. If the sample must be taken in spite of such invalidating circumstances, the nurse should note the circumstances on the request slip and in the nursing records. The presence of intravenous infusions or evident dehydration, especially in children and the elderly, should also be noted on the request slip and nursing record

4. Identify risk groups for anemia

    a. Persons having had gastric resections (loss of intrinsic factor) or intestinal resections or bypasses, especially with the loss of the terminal ilium (where vitamin B_{12} is absorbed)

    b. Persons with problems with alcohol (liver disease impairs synthesis and storage of RBC materials)

    c. The elderly, mentally retarded, or poor, especially those who are living alone (inadequate diet)

    d. Persons with long-term or chronic gastrointestinal disease (decreased absorption of necessary material for RBC production)

5. Identify high-risk groups for secondary polycythemia

    a. Persons with chronic respiratory or cardiac disease

    b. Persons who have been living in areas of high altitude

6. Identify persons at risk for inadequate oxygen transport to body cells

    a. The symptomatic polycythemia vera patient, because of slowed circulation secondary to an increased cell mass in the blood, and despite above-normal hemoglobin levels and RBC count

    b. The anemic patient because of decreased oxygen carrying power of the blood secondary to decreased blood hemoglobin levels and RBC count

    c. The major goal of the nursing plan of care in these cases is to equalize oxygen demand and available oxygen at the cellular level

7. Common nursing problems related to abnormal laboratory findings in tests of RBCs and suggested nursing actions are listed in Table 2–1.

TABLE 2–1. ABNORMAL RED BLOOD CELL TEST RESULTS AND CORRESPONDING NURSING ACTIONS

Test Result	Problem(s) to Observe for	Nursing Actions
Decreased RBC count	Fatigue; shortness of breath (SOB); dyspnea on exertion (DOE); dyspnea at rest; increased heart rate (HR); precordial pain (myocardial hypoxia); decreased level of consciousness (LOC)	Decrease metabolic needs by decreasing physical activity (e.g., passive rather than active range of motion [ROM]), preventing stress by preventing infection, and determining stressful situations in environment and controlling as possible
		Provide adequate environmental oxygen:

(continued)

TABLE 2–1. (Continued)

Test Result	Problem(s) to Observe for	Nursing Actions
		O$_2$ per cannula as indicated; O$_2$ should be given judiciously because (1) elimination of all hypoxia effectively eliminates erythropoiesis; (2) SOB, etc., may be due to a primary pulmonary problem (chronic obstructive pulmonary disease [COPD]) and depend on low O$_2$ for respiratory drive; should be an independent nursing judgment, but may require an order
		Open windows can decrease subjective dyspnea by psychological impact on the patient
		Position of comfort, arms and shoulders supported, for adequate lung expansion
		Change of position to permit equal lung expansion and prevent pooling of fluids
		Deep breathe, cough, turn, and instruct patient in procedure and rationale
		Provide for safety with decreased LOC:
		No smoking, or only when observed
		Accompany patient when out of bed
		Use of side rails
		Infections should be prevented even in simple anemias, especially in children because of cellular dysfunction caused by hypoxia
Decreased hemoglobin concentration	Potential oliguria (blood flow to kidney decreased by 50% when hemoglobin (Hgb) less than 7–8 g/dl); complaint of cold; cool, pale skin because of decreased peripheral perfusion; absence of cyanosis when Hgb less than 5 g/dl	Measure intake and output; report change; keep health team informed
		Monitor intraveneous (IV) line carefully, maintain access; adequate clothing and bedding, preferably several light layers to decrease weight and effort in moving

(continued)

TABLE 2–1. (Continued)

Test Result	Problem(s) to Observe for	Nursing Actions
		In patients with cyanotic cardiac respiratory disease, use other parameters than presence of or changes in degree, of cyanosis in evaluating level of oxygenation in response to activity
		In dehydrated patient, Hgb level should be above normal limits; otherwise, anemia is present
Increased RBC count	May precipitate congestive heart failure (CHF) or pulmonary edema in those with cardiac disease, especially the elderly	In the diagnosed CHF patient, especially the elderly, check for jugular venous distension (JVD) with head of bed elevated 30°
	Engorged color of face and extremities because of capillary sludging and stasis of blood; potential thrombus; precordial pain because of increased cardiac effort	Check peripheral circulation and venous return; assist venous return as practical (e.g., posture change), encourage leg exercises to increase action of "somatic pump"; provide adequate hydration (within limits of primary pathology) to decrease blood viscosity
Poikilocytosis (spherocytosis) (sickling)	Decreased capillary flow; potential thrombus; joint pain; intravascular hemolysis; potential jaundice; misdiagnosis of pain secondary to vascular occlusion at sites other than joints (symptoms do not occur in newborns up to 6 months of age—protected by presence of Hbg F)	See "Implications for Nursing: Sickledex" in Section 15.2.4.C; maintain adequate hydration to decrease blood viscosity
		Provide or refer for genetic counseling when both partners have the "trait" and plan a family
		Immobilize painful joint
		Provide analgesics and rest
		No aspirin should be given because of its effect on platelet function
		Practice and teach prevention of crisis
		Avoid chilling or contact with persons with infectious disease

(continued)

TABLE 2–1. (Continued)

Test Result	Problem(s) to Observe for	Nursing Actions
		Avoid high altitudes
		Avoid physical fatigue
		Identify and avoid stressful situations
		Ensure intake of adequate, balanced diet
		Ensure intake of adequate fluids
		Facilitate total immunization program and updates
		Institute good dental hygiene and checkups
Increased MCV and MCH	Increased numbers of immature RBCs or macrocytic cells in peripheral circulation, potentially causing hemolysis; lemon yellow jaundice; glossitis; stomatitis	Protect from bleeding of mucous membrane:
		Use soft toothbrush
		Monitor diet to eliminate caustic, spicy, or tart substances
		Avoid extremes of temperature in food
		Stress intake of protein and vitamins
		Provide and teach need for mouth care before and after meals:
		Provide cool, mildly alkaline mouthwashes
		Provide comfort measures if jaundice causes itching (see "Implications for Nusing: Total Serum Bilirubin" in Section 1.10)
Decreased MCV, MCH, MCHC	Possible iron deficiency/ nutritional anemia	Do diet history
		Teach management of adequate diet, e.g., iron-rich foods (liver, red meat, raisins, kidney beans, peas, dried apricots, fortified cereals and breads, molasses)
		Observe patients with anemia of unknown origin for ice eating (pagophagia), which has been observed in

(continued)

TABLE 2–1. (Continued)

Test Result	Problem(s) to Observe for	Nursing Actions
		some iron-deficient individuals
		Administer iron as ordered: prevent and teach prevention of possible constipation secondary to its use; inform patient of expected change of stool color to black
		Label any stool specimens with information that patient is receiving iron
		Iron given intramuscularly (iron dextran [Imferon], iron sorbitex [Jectofer] must be given by Z-track technique to prevent staining
Increased ESR	Inflammatory or degenerative process; potential signs and symptoms of acute infection, fever, chills, etc.	Provide measures to prevent further cross-infection, or infection of others
		Consistent decrease in the ESR can be used as one index for increasing activity levels after systemic or chronic inflammatory processes
Decreased haptoglobin content	Intravascular hemolysis; potential jaundice and pruritis	Monitor bone marrow effectiveness by checking reticulocyte response
		Provide comfort measures in cases with pruritis
Pancytopenia	Potential infection; potential bleeding	Protective isolation may be used
		Provide protective measures to prevent or minimize bleeding (see increased MCV, MCH), e.g.:
		Give all medications orally, if possible
		Give all injectables with smallest-gauge needle possible

Abbreviations: SOB, shortness of breath; DOE, dyspnea on exertion; HR, heart rate; LOC, level of consciousness; ROM, range of motion; COPD, chronic obstructive pulmonary disease; Hgb, hemoglobin; IV, intravenous line/infusion; CHF, conjestive heart failure; JVD, jugular venous distention.
From Frohlich, 1980; Howard & Herbold, 1982.

2.2 TESTS RELATED TO THE WHITE BLOOD CELL

2.2.1 White Blood Cell Count

Synonyms: WBC count, WBC, total white count, leukocyte count

Normal Ranges $(\times 10^3/mm^3)^a$

Adult	4.0–10.0
Senior adult	
Male	4.25–14.0
Female	3.1–12.0
Pediatric	
Newborn	9.0–30.0
4 wk	5.0–19.5
6 mo to 1 yr	6.0–17.5
2–5 yr	5.0–10.0

[a]Automated reports by single number only. Multiply by 1000 for total count.

Definition. A total white count is one of the routine tests done as a screening test for leukocyte disorders. Evaluation of the other myeloid cells (RBCs, platelets) is also routinely ordered with the white count because leukocyte disorders rarely occur alone. They are more usually associated with changes in the other myeloid cells. A white blood count is done on almost every patient admitted to the hospital regardless of disease. By itself it is of little value as an aid to diagnosis. It must be related not only to other clinical tests but also to the clinical condition of the patient.

No patient preparation is necessary for the test. It is subject to errors of random distribution of the cells, however, and is only as accurate as the laboratory worker involved. Most laboratories rely on automation for the white cell count, which increases the accuracy of the test. A larger volume of blood must be examined than that used for red cell counts because WBCs are far fewer in number in the blood. An increase in the total number of WBCs is referred to as *leukocytosis*. A decrease is termed *leukopenia*.

Physiology. WBCs are found in the bloodstream at approximately a 1:500 to 1:1000 ratio to the number of RBCs present. Less than 1 percent of the body's total WBCs are in the peripheral blood. The remainder are in the marrow as developing and mature cells, lining the capillary walls, and in extravascular areas throughout the body, especially the lungs, liver, and spleen. WBCs are nucleated cells that become smaller as they mature, the nucleus taking up a smaller portion of the cell space (Harvey et al., 1991). They are separated into two major categories: granulocytes (polymorphonuclear leukocytes, or polys) and agranulocytes. Granulocytes are further divided into neutrophils, basophils, and eosinophils on the basis of their staining properties. Agranulocytes (without granules in cytoplasm and with an unlobulated nucleus) are made up of monocytes and lymphocytes.

Production. Neutrophils, basophils, eosinophils, and monocytes are produced from the bone marrow and, it is generally accepted, originate from the same stem cells as do erythrocytes (see

Fig. 2–1). Lymphocytes are formed in the lymph nodes and lymphoid tissue found in the spleen and intestines. Evidence suggests that they originate from the same stem cell as the other formed elements of the blood. They are subdivided into two major systems (see Fig. 2–2). The *T-cell system* requires a functioning thymus for normal development and is responsible for cell-based immunity. The *B-cell system* is responsible for antibody production (humoral immunity) (Nordin, 1980, 1987).

Regulation. The human body produces a "colony-stimulating factor" from monocytes and macrophages (McCance and Huether, 1990, p. 262). This factor appears to have properties closely resembling those described for erythropoietin in RBC production, thus a granulopoietin. The substance, a glycoprotein, has been produced under laboratory conditions and is found in many body tissues and fluids (e.g., bone marrow, urine) (Lithium as a granulopoietic agent, 1979). It is thought to be produced in response to granulocyte breakdown rates and to endotoxemia. Granulocytes are produced at about the same rate as RBCs in response to an antigen process (Harvey et al., 1991).

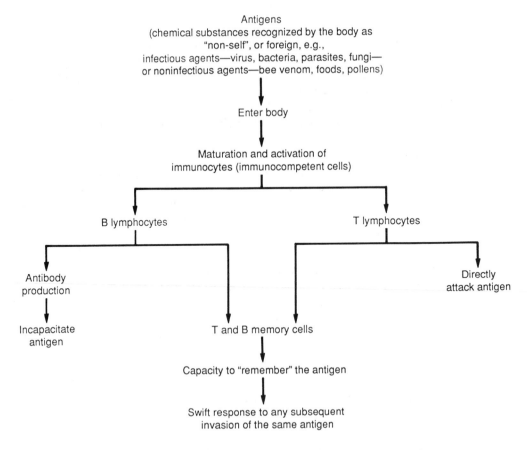

Figure 2–2. White blood cell immune response. (Data from McCance & Huether, p. 139.)

Storage. The 99 percent of WBCs not circulating are stored in bone marrow, temporarily adhered to the capillary walls, or have migrated into tissues until needed or until they die. Because WBCs do not function within the bloodstream itself but, rather, when they migrate into the tissues, those cells circulating in the bloodstream could be considered a storage pool as well.

Life Span. Granulocytes live for 10 to 14 days. They remain in the bloodstream only 6 to 10 hours and survive in the tissues for 4 to 5 days under normal conditions. Lymphocytes survive for a longer period, over 100 days. In healthy tissues the macrophage form of monocytes can survive for months.

Function. Leukocytes are considered a part of the reticuloendothelial system, and their function, as a group, is to protect the body against bacterial and protein invasion. They do this by phagocytosis (granulocytes-monocytes), antibody production (B-cell lymphocytes), and delayed hypersensitivity response (T-cell lymphocytes). Granulocytes are stimulated to migrate to areas containing necrotic tissue and bacteria where they recognize foreign objects and then phagocytize and digest them. This stimulus–response characteristic is called *chemotaxis*. Mature granulocytes enhance the migration of monocytes. Monocytes, after entering tissues, can be converted to macrophages with enhanced phagocytic and digestive ability. Plasma cells are normally not found in the blood of well persons and originate from B lymphocytes after antigenic stimulation of that tissue. Their chief function, when present, is antibody synthesis (Harvey et al., 1991).

Pathophysiology. When an infectious process occurs, neutrophils are mobilized early in the inflammatory reaction. As with RBCs, the appearance of additional immature or juvenile neutrophils (band cells) indicates that there is stimulation of neutrophil production. This state of increased numbers of juvenile neutrophils in circulation is termed a *shift to the left*. The term originated because the table of cells used for differential counting in the laboratory indicates the immature forms of neutrophils toward the left of the table. Neutrophilia (a relative increase in the percentage of neutrophils in a differential count) is usually accompanied by some degree of shift to the left in acute infections. (At times, the appearance of hypersegmented polymorphonuclear cells, as with pernicious anemia, is called a "shift to the right," but this term is much less commonly used.)

With a generalized infection the leukocytes respond in three phases:

1. *Acute, progressive.* Relative neutrophilia (increased percentage of neutrophils) may or may not have leukocytosis, a shift to the left, or the appearance of some toxic granulation in the *mature* neutrophils' cytoplasm (its presence in immature neutrophils signals marrow exhaustion). A white blood count that exceeds $100 \times 10^3/mm^3$ has a markedly increased viscosity, which can impair circulation in the small vessels of the brain, kidney, lungs, or retina.
2. *Recovery phase.* Neutrophils decrease in number, monocytes increase, and eosinophils appear.
3. *Convalescent.* Neutrophils return to a normal percentage, lymphocytes increase in number, and the shift to the left disappears.

The phagocytic activity of granulocytes is increased in anemic persons and those with a fever but is impaired in malnourished persons or those with high blood glucose concentrations such as in uncontrolled diabetes mellitus or the malnourished person receiving a prolonged concentrated glucose infusion by hyperalimentation.

WBC COUNT INCREASED IN (ABSOLUTE WBC COUNT INCREASE: LEUKOCYTOSIS)

1. Acute infections, particularly those produced by pyogenic (pus-producing) organisms (e.g., streptococci, staphylococci, pneumonococci)
2. Chronic infections (e.g., tuberculosis)
3. Administration of hydrocortisone, which decreases the rate at which neutrophils leave the blood; administration of epinephrine, which stimulates the release of WBCs in the marginal pool of the capillaries
4. Myeloproliferative disorders, defined as all disorders that involve the uncontrolled proliferation of bone marrow cells (e.g., chronic lymphatic leukemia, polycythemia vera)
5. Tissue necrosis and extreme stress as in acute myocardial infarction, burns, gangrene, convulsions, and paroxysmal tachycardia
6. Acute hemorrhage
7. Metabolic intoxications such as uremia, acidosis, and acute gout
8. Physiological states such as
   a. Physical exercise
   b. Obstetric labor
   c. Response to cold
   d. Response to pain
   e. Response to massage (states c through e are probably due to the release of cells from bone marrow)
   f. Emotional stress
   g. Menstruation (states f and g are probably due to increased release from capillary walls)
   h. Diurnal variation (increased in the afternoon)

WBC COUNT DECREASED IN (ABSOLUTE WBC COUNT DECREASE: LEUKOPENIA)

1. Response to ionizing radiation as in treatment or accidental exposure
2. Certain diseases of the blood (e.g., pernicious anemia) because of a disordered DNA synthesis
3. Response to certain infecting agents (e.g., viral infections, rickettsial infections [Rocky Mountain spotted fever, typhus] or protozoan infections [malaria])
4. Hypersplenism as in hereditary spherocytosis and idiopathic thrombocytic purpura
5. Physiological states such as prolonged rest (basal conditions decrease WBC count and production) and aging
6. Response to the administration of drugs, especially chemotherapeutic agents (e.g., cyclophosphamide [Cytoxan]) or drugs with similar action (e.g., antithyroid propylthiouracil). WBC depression has been reported as a rare and not expected response to many other drugs, perhaps as an idiosyncratic response on the part of the individual.

2.2.2 Differential WBC Count

Synonyms: Differential, blood smear, smear evaluation

Normal Ranges

	Adult (× 10³/mm)	Senior Adult (%)	Pediatric	
			Age	Percentage
Neutrophil	2.0–7.5 or 32–62% of 100 counted WBCs	As for adult with slightly wider variation in range, 43–79% (Fowler results)	Newborn 4 wk 6 mo to 1 yr 2–5 yr	61 35 32 30
Eosinophil	0.4–0.44 or 2.2%	0.0–10.0	Newborn 1 wk 2 wk and after	2.3 5 2–3
Basophil	0.0–0.3 or 6%	0.0–0.3	Not available	
Monocyte	0–1.4 or 0–4%	1.0–15.0	Newborn 2 wk 3 mo 6 mo to 1 yr 2 yr to adult	6–12 8–9 7 5 5–8
Lymphocyte	1.0–4.5 or 31% ± 5%	11–48	Newborn 4 wk 6 mo to 1 yr 2–5 yr	31 56 61 30

Definition. A differential WBC count identifies the relative proportions (percentages) of the different types of white cells that make up the total white cell count. Frequently, the differential count is reported in percentages.

Increases or decreases in the WBC count may be due to increases or decreases in one or more of the categories of leukocytes. A white cell differential gives the percentage of each category in a particular sample of blood. This differential must always be interpreted with the total white count for the blood sample being examined. An increase in the percentage of any particular category may be secondary to a true increase in the number of cells in that category or secondary to a decrease in one or more of the other categories. A true increase is termed an *absolute increase,* whereas that secondary to a decrease in other categories is termed a *relative* increase. To avoid possible misinterpretations, most laboratories report the differential count in absolute numbers for each category rather than as a percentage, thereby circumventing interpreting the percentage in light of the total count (Nordin, 1980, 1987).

Differential counts are done as chamber counts or on stained blood smears as part of the peripheral blood smear evaluation but are treated separately in Table 2–2 because of their importance as an individual test. Each leukocyte seen is identified and classified, and the percentage of each cell type observed is calculated. When "hand-counted," 200 to 1000 leukocytes should be counted for accuracy. Percentages are based on 100 cells counted, and the percent distribution of the several different types of leukocytes is given. The differential count often yields more

TABLE 2–2. DIFFERENTIAL WHITE BLOOD CELL COUNTS

White Cell	Function	Causes of Increases or States in Which Increases Are Found	Causes of Decreases or States in Which Decreases Are Found	Discussion

Neutrophil (polymorphonuclear leukocyte)	1. Phagocytosis
	2. Major phagocyte in first 12 hr of inflammatory response
	3. After death, ruptures, releases enzymes that digest tissue, to excavate the inflammed site and stimulate appearance of more phagocytes
	Major role: to dispose of invaders, foreign bodies, and debris
		Pathological
		1. Acute infections, especially in localized cocci infections (e.g., tonsilitis, otitis media); in some general infections (e.g., rheumatic fever, diphtheria)
		2. Intoxicants:
		  a. Metabolic: diabetic acidosis, uremia, burns
		  b. Chemicals and drugs: lead, mercury (especially with nephrotoxic and hepatotoxic drugs), digitalis, epinephrine, adrenocorticotropic hormone (ACTH), hydrocortisone
		3. Acute stress (e.g., severe hemorrhage, surgery)
		4. Tissue necrosis: myocardial infarction (MI), gangrene, neoplasm
		5. Myeloproliferative disease: polycythemia vera, myelocytic leukemia
		6. Thrombosis
		7. Acute hemolysis, especially intravascular (disseminated intravascular coagulation [DIC])
		Physiological
		1. (See increased absolute WBC count Sec. 2.2.1)
		2. Newborn
		3. Neutrophilia response more rapid and intense in children
			1. Acute viral infections (e.g., rubeola, viral hepatitis, viral pneumonia)
			2. Ultimately in all grave infections of prolonged duration (because of increased rate of destruction or sequestration into tissues?)
			3. Nutritional deficiencies, especially folic acid and vitamin B_{12}
			4. With splenomegaly
			5. Marrow aplasia secondary to ionizing radiation, antimetabolites
				The splenic vasculature contains only a small portion of the body pool of granulocytes. Its role in leukopenia is not clear. It is altogether likely that the spleen's role in the disappearance of granulocytes from the circulation when it is enlarged is a very minor one

Eosinophil	1. Weak phagocytic action of foreign particles and antigen–antibody complexes 2. Not all specific functions known 3. Modulate reactions that occur when most cells and basophils degranulate 4. Destroy nelminths 5. Contains substances that inactivate factors released by MAST cells and basophils, e.g., histamine, platelet-activating factor, slow-reacting substances of anaphylaxis	1. Allergic reactions (e.g., hay fever, asthma, exfoliative dermatitis, erythema multiforme), and drug reactions 2. Parasitic infections: intestinal (hook and round worms), tissue (toxocara, trichina) 3. Skin disorders (e.g., pemphigus vulgaris, dermatitis herpetiformis) 4. Neoplasms 5. Myeloproliferative disorders (e.g., Hodgkin's disease, metastatic cancer, polycythemia vera) 6. After ionizing radiation 7. Other: pernicious anemia, polyarteritis, Addison's disease because of decreased glucocorticoid production	1. Increased circulating glucocorticoid levels 2. In pancytopenia, for whatever cause	The presence of eosinophils in sufficient numbers after a rise in the neutrophil count secondary to an infection indicates resolution and healing of inflammatory reactions
Basophil	1. Actual function is unknown 2. Contains both heparin and histamine and releases histamine on contact with antigen/allergic reactions, which increases local vascular and capillary permeability 3. Bears a close resemblance to mast cells;[a] may therefore be of some help in chronic infections in the prevention of agglutination, which is part of the chronic inflammatory response 4. Involved in some delayed hypersensitivity reactions, for example contact allergies	1. Infrequently increased 2. When elevated, most often associated with a myeloproliferative disorder (e.g., chronic myelocytic leukemia) 3. Increased during healing phase of inflammatory response and in chronic inflammation	1. Not seen except in states of pancytopenia	Because the function of the basophil is not really known, its variation with disease and infection is, as yet, of no help in the management or prognostication of disease

(continued)

TABLE 2–2. (Continued)

White Cell	Function	Causes of Increases or States in Which Increases Are Found	Causes of Decreases or States in Which Decreases Are Found	Discussion
Monocyte	1. Phagocytosis: Monocytes are released into the blood, leaving randomly (1/2 time of 8.4 hr) to the tissues where they are transformed into hystiocytes or macrophages. They make up a mononuclear phagocyte system (reticuloendothelial system), which defends against microorganism, mycobacteria, fungi, bacteria, protozoa, and viruses. 2. The cells are motile and engage in phagocytosis and are integral parts of humoral and cell-mediated immunity. 3. Process antigen; interacts with antigen–antibody complement to promote phagocytosis. 4. Its multiple functions include host defense, control of hematopoiesis, and "policing the environment" of the body.	1. Certain bacterial infections (e.g., brucellosis, tuberculosis (Tbc), subacute bacterial endocarditis) 2. Certain protozoal and rickettsial diseases (e.g., malaria, Rocky Mountain spotted fever, typhus) 3. Recovery phase of inflammatory response 4. Recovery phase after marked neutropenia 5. Other: monocytic leukemia, Hodgkin's disease	1. Not seen except in states of pancytopenia	There is a special relationship between the monocyte and the tubercle bacillus, and an increase in monocytes not otherwise explained should alert the practitioner to the possibility of an active tuberculosis process. Disseminated Tbc may be indicated by the appearance of promonocytes in the peripheral blood. The monocyte is the chief cell in the formation of the tubercle of tuberculosis
Lymphocyte	1. May be the first leukocyte to enter virally infected tissue 2. Closely involved in the body's immune response and antibody formation	1. Certain acute viral infections with early increase (e.g., pertussis, infectious mononucleosis, rubella) 2. Large numbers of chronic infections (e.g., brucellosis, syphilis)	1. Increased circulating ACTH levels cause an immediate decrease; in time, lymphocytosis may occur 2. Thyoma	A progressive increase in the lymphocyte percentage is considered a favorable prognostic sign in pulmonary tuberculosis and vice versa. Increases are

3. Collagen disease (e.g., systemic levels erythematosus, rheumatoid arthritis, scleroderma, dermatomyositis, polyarteritis nodosa)
4. Other: chronic granulomatous disorders, chronic lymphatic leukemia, lymphosarcoma, Addison's disease (because of a glucocorticoid production)
5. Relative increases occur with hyperthyroidism and with neutropenia, for whatever cause
6. Physiological increases:
   a. Relative increase at expense of neutrophils at high altitudes
   b. Relative increase closely related to degree of tanning of the skin, thus seen more often in warm-weather areas
   c. Relative and absolute increase in infants and children

3. Congenital immuno-deficiency in children
4. Hypogammaglobulinemia
5. Stress, psychological and physiological
6. Prolonged depression

usually not of diagnostic significance unless at 40 percent or more, unless a baseline level is available. Percentage can vary from 14 to 45 in apparently healthy persons

Abbreviations: ACTH, adrenocorticotropic hormone; MI, myocardial infarction; DIC, disseminated intravascular coagulation; Tbc, tuberculosis.
[a] A mast cell is defined as a connective tissue cell containing heparin and believed to be instrumental in immune reactions, anaphylactic and atopic.
Data from Collins, 1975; Davidsohn & Henry, 1969; Faulkner et al., 1968; Greisheimer & Wiedeman, 1972; Groer & Shekleton, 1983; Harvey et al., 1991; Henry, 1991; Jones et al., 1982; Kintzel, 1977; The Lab, Drugs and Nursing Implications, 1978; Whaley & Wong, 1991.

helpful information than any other single procedure used to examine the blood. As with the WBC count, the differential must be related to the clinical condition of the patient and to other hematologic tests for correct and useful interpretation. (See Section 2.2.1 for related physiology and pathophysiology.)

IMPLICATIONS FOR NURSING: TESTS RELATED TO THE WBC

1. No special patient preparation is necessary. Because the major function of the WBCs as a group is to protect the body from bacterial and foreign protein invasion, the major nursing goal in caring for a person with abnormalities of any or all of the WBCs would be to provide protection from such invasions. This goal can be reached by the following steps

   a. Assess for risk populations

      (1) Primary immunodeficiency resulting from genetic defects or unknown causes, is rare and presents in many different ways—identification is a primary responsibility of the physician

      (2) Secondary immunodeficiency is very common, particularly in the hospitalized patient or the person being treated for a chronic disease

         (a) Review available data for possible immunosuppressive factors
            - Presence of severe infections
            - Presence of severe trauma (e.g., burns) or emotional stress
            - Presence of malnutrition
            - Presence of malignancy
            - Presence of a collagen disease
            - Presence of an enlarged spleen or history of splenectomy (check for surgical scar)
            - Presence of any myeloproliferative disorder
            - Lack of breast-feeding in newborn
            - Administration of immunosuppressive drugs (see "WBC Count Decreased in," item 6, in Section 2.2.1 for a partial list)
            - Treatment of malignancy with radiation or chemotherapy
            - Presence of an inheritance pattern of immunodeficiency in the family history (e.g., death of young child because of unknown cause)
            - Uncontrolled diabetes mellitus with high serum glucose level (phagocytic activity is impaired in such states)

         (b) Assess the person at risk for a pattern of immunodeficient response
            - Presence of unexpectedly severe infection
            - Presence of infection secondary to ordinarily benign organisms (see Appendix G)
            - History of recurrent infections
            - Presence of eczema or candidiasis
            - Impairment of growth and development
            - Absence of palpable lymph nodes or visible tonsils in children over 6 months of age. The presence of local lymphadenopathy (palpable enlargement of lymph glands) is a reassuring sign of an adequate body immune response to an infecting agent (Groer & Shekleton, 1983)
            - Lymphocyte count (not just a relative percentage) under 2000/mm^3 in a child or under 1500/mm^3 in an adult. If the count is this low, look for (request if necessary) a repeat count. Assess the patient with a low lymphocyte count for possible stressors that would decrease the count temporarily (e.g., viral infection, severe emotional stress, even in an immunologically healthy person)
            - Absence of pus in sites infected by pus-forming organisms
            - Absence or decreased numbers of granulocytes in biopsy specimen of pyogenic infection site

- History of frequent upper respiratory infection (URI) without evidence of pneumonia or purulent otitis media in children over 12 months of age
- Failure to thrive in infants and very young children
- Recurrent staphylococci skin infections
- Presence of chronic diarrhea, especially in children

b. Assume that any individual who is malnourished, has uncontrolled diabetes mellitus, is receiving hyperalimentation with a high concentration of glucose, is elderly, or has any change in the absolute WBC count to be a person at risk for immunodeficiency

2. Provide protective, anticipatory care to risk populations

a. Because WBC production decreases at rest, activity that is carefully graded to the capacity of the individual should be an integral part of the nursing care plan, as should education of both patient and family as to the purpose of each nursing measure instituted and the rationale behind the measure

b. Review "Implications for Nursing: Serum Globulin" in Section 1.9.2 with regard to serum globulin disorders. All are also applicable for persons with disorders of the WBC

c. Isolation of any type should be instituted only with an adequate knowledge of the individual's resistance, potential for infection, and mode of transmission of potential pathogens. Strict isolation or protective (reverse) isolation can produce emotional stress, further decreasing the individual's immunoresponse, and tends to decrease the patient's activity, which can decrease WBC production and decrease the immunoresponse. Further, improper isolation is often worse than no isolation because it can breed false confidence and important assessments for evidence of infection may not be done

d. The use of universal precautions (see Appendix I) provides for consistent safety for the immunocompromised individual

3. Assess for and prevent, as possible, specific complications in persons with disorders of the WBCs

a. White counts of 100,000 and greater (as in leukemias) increase the risk of circulatory sludging and thrombosis resulting from increased blood viscosity

(1) Provide adequate fluids within the limits of the primary pathology. Fluids are of particular importance in acute lymphocytic leukemia (ALL) because of the tendency in that disease to high uric acid levels and urate nephropathy

(2) Provide measures to prevent peripheral stasis (e.g., range of motion [ROM], frequent position change, frequent inspection of skin color and temperature)

(3) Be alert for indication of thrombus formation of vital structures (e.g., flank pain, alteration in urine output, which may indicate kidney occlusion; complaints of blurring of vision, visual cuts (e.g., right or left hemianopia [hemianopsia]), which indicate possible retinal occlusion; possible pulmonary emboli) (see "Implications for Nursing: Thrombin Time," in Section 3.10; "Implications for Nursing: Platelet Count" in Section 3.11; and "General Implications for Nursing Related to Problems in Coagulation" Section 3.12)

b. Persons with relative or absolute decreases in granulocyte number are at risk for the development of septicemia. Localized infections will not form abscesses because pus does not form. The infection is thus less likely to remain walled off locally, and septicemia results. The occurrence of fever may be the first indication of the problem

(1) Inspect the body daily for indications of infection, especially in those areas most susceptible to infection (e.g., mucous membranes, skin folds with high moisture levels—axilla, perineum, etc.)

c. Children frequently tend to develop URI even when not immunodeficient

(1) Provide excellent mouth care and pulmonary toilet

(2) Auscultate the chest for diminished breath sounds or evidence of rales

d. Inspect frequently for evidence of fungal infections (e.g., white patches on mucous membrane); report and obtain a treatment order as rapidly as possible

4. Monitor repeated white blood counts and differentials for response to therapy or changes in status

a. Changes in absolute white blood count

(1) Increases can signal the occurrence of superimposed infection or other severe stress

(2) Increases almost always accompany hereditary anemias

(3) Increases in patients with subacute bacterial endocarditis could signal an embolic complication (Sodeman & Sodeman, 1982)

(4) Decreases can indicate either a positive response to treatment or bone marrow exhaustion. Check the differential for more useful information as to what is occurring

(5) Decreases below the normal range can indicate the possibility of bone marrow exhaustion or suppression

b. Changes in differential counts

(1) The presence of some band cells or even metamyelocytes (immature WBCs), coupled with an increase in neutrophil number and the total white count (leukocytosis) indicates a healthy bone marrow response to infection (shift to the left)

(2) A shift to the left without the accompanying leukocytosis indicates an overworked and potentially exhausted bone marrow

(3) The appearance of "blast" cells in the lymphocyte or monocyte series (see Fig. 2–1) also indicates a stressed bone marrow

(4) The presence of toxic granules (large, deeply stained granules thought to consist of enzymes rather than phagocytized material) in immature neutrophils, an increasing number of juvenile forms in the circulation, and a fall in the total white count indicates inadequate marrow response—marrow exhaustion

(5) The appearance of significant numbers of immature forms of WBCs, especially metamyelocytes and myelocytes, coupled with a decrease in the total WBC count, indicates probable bone marrow exhaustion. This occurrence must be reported to the health care team, and the individual must be carefully protected from infection and injury

(6) Eosinophil increases indicate healing or recovery in inflammatory states

(7) Lymphocyte and eosinophil numbers will be decreased in acute stress responses

(8) Monocyte levels should be expected to increase relative to the decrease in neutrophils in the recovery phase of inflammatory diseases

(9) Increases in monocyte numbers alone, independent of acute infection, may indicate the onset or reactivation of tuberculosis

2.3 PERIPHERAL SMEAR

Synonyms: Smear evaluation, blood smear, stained blood film

Definition. This test is an examination of the cellular contents of the blood under a microscope by using a variety of stains. Basic dyes (blue) and acid dyes (red) are used. Certain structures take up only the acid dyes and are therefore called *acidophilic* (or oxyphilic or eosinophilic). Others take up only the basic dyes and are called *basophilic*. Those that take up both dyes are referred to as *neutrophilic*. Modern hematology began with the recognition and use of these staining properties.

Much information of great importance is available from this test. It allows for the determination of blood cell morphology (form and arrangement of structure), which can identify cell origin and maturity as well as the ratio of various cell types to each other. These data, sometimes alone, more often combined with information from the history, physical, and other laboratory tests, provide the medical diagnosis, much as would a histological tissue section. The information can also be used as a guide to treatment or as an indicator of the harmful effects of chemotherapy or radiotherapy. The differential can be a part of this examination or a totally separate count.

2.3.1 RBC Morphology

To an experienced laboratory worker the peripheral smear can give a fair indication of the amount of hemoglobin present as well as the number of red cells (see Table 2–3). Hemoglobin can be roughly estimated by the depth of staining present. This quantitative analysis is of help in characterizing a number of conditions such as microangiopathic hemolytic anemia, iron deficiency anemia, pernicious anemia, sickle cell anemia, and hereditary spherocytosis.

No special patient preparation is necessary. Either venous or capillary blood can be used, but if a platelet count is to be done, venous blood should be used (Henry, 1991). (For related physiology and pathophysiology, see Section 2.1.1.)

IMPLICATIONS FOR NURSING: PERIPHERAL SMEAR

See "Nursing Implications: Tests of RBCs and Hemoglobin," Section 2.1.

TABLE 2–3. ANALYSIS OF RED BLOOD CELL ABNORMALITIES

Morphology Abnormality	Definition	Possible Causes
Anisocytosis	Variations in size	Nutritional iron deficiency anemias
Microcytes	5 μm or less in diameter	
Macrocytes	10–20 μm in diameter	Presence of increased number of reticulocytes; pernicious anemia; folic acid or vitamin B_{12} deficiency; pernicious anemia rarely found in other conditions
Megalocytes	12–25 μm in diameter	
Poikilocytosis	Variations in shape; can be oval, pear shaped, saddle shaped, club shaped, irregularly shaped	Common occurrence, multiple causes
Burr cells	Irregular projections from RBC; also called acanthocytes or spur cells	Liver disease: albumin deficiency; kidney disease
Fragmented cells	Small fragments of RBC debris	Metastatic malignancy; angiopathic disease
Sickle cells	RBC bent in crescent or sickle shape	Sickle cell anemia
Spherocytes	Globular rather than usual biconcave cell without central pallor of normal RBC; slightly smaller in diameter than normal	Hereditary spherocytosis; some types of hemolytic anemia
Ovalocytes	Elliptic cell	Found in normal healthy persons as an inherited trait or associated with many anemias

(continued)

TABLE 2–3. (Continued)

Morphology Abnormality	Definition	Possible Causes
Target cells	RBCs with a dark peripheral rim of hemoglobin and dark central ring that are separated by an unstained ring; abnormally thin cell	Chronic anemias: hemoglobinopathies (sickle cell anemia; HbC): thalassemia; lead intoxication; severe iron deficiency; liver disease; absence of spleen
Variations in staining Polychromatophilia	Residual RNA picks up blue stain, which is mixed with usual red stain of hemoglobin	Further staining will reveal reticular structure of the reticulocyte; 1% occurrence normal in peripheral blood; increased in hemophiliac anemias and in response to blood loss; hemolytic anemias
Basophilic stippling	Variable-sized granules staining blue, found in the RBC because of degenerative changes in cytoplasmic RNA of young cells	Present after exposure to lead, no direct relationship between degree of stippling and degree of toxicity; present in some serious blood diseases (e.g., severe pernicious anemia, leukemia)
Malarial stippling	Fine granular appearance of RBC (Schüffner's granules), staining purplish red; cells larger than normal	Found in RBCs that harbor the malarial parasite in tertian malaria
Variations in structure (see Fig. 2–1) Megaloblast	Markedly larger RBC; does not divide normally	Vitamin B_{12} or folic acid deficiency, pernicious anemia; megaloblastic anemia in liver disease
Megaloblastic normoblast	Juvenile form of megalocyte	Occurs in same series as megaloblast, when coupled with presence of a shift to the left (immature neutrophils in peripheral circulation), may indicate space-occupying lesion of marrow (e.g., metastatic cancer, leukemia, multiple myeloma, Gaucher's disease)
Howell-Jolly bodies	Nucleus broken up into segments; may be singular or multiple	*Singular:* megaloblastic anemias; hemolytic anemias; postsplenectomy; leukemia; *Multiple:* indicative of megaloblastic anemia (multilobulated nucleus)
Cabot's ring	Ring, figure of 8, or loop-shaped structure in RBC	Occurs rarely; found at times with pernicious anemia or lead poisoning
Variations in degree of color Hypochromia	Enlargement of central pale area of the RBC; area is also paler than normal	Nutritional and iron deficiency anemias
Hyperchromia	Deep staining of outer ring of RBC; usually lack the pale center entirely	Pernicious anemia

Data from Davidsohn & Henry, 1991.

2.3.2 Platelet Estimation (See also platelet count 3.11)

Synonym: Thrombocyte estimation

Normal Range: On smear estimation, usually reported as adequate, increased, or decreased; normal or abnormal (for actual platelet count normals, see Section 3.11)

Definition. When a peripheral smear is examined, a comment regarding the platelets is considered a necessary part of the report. This comment usually simply describes the general impression obtained by the person doing the test. For instance, the platelets can be described as "adequate" and "normal," when found so, which refers to their numbers and morphology, or "decreased" and "abnormal." Some laboratories will routinely provide an indirect count when the numbers do not appear normal with the gross examination. This semiquantitative assessment of platelets is an effective screening test for changes in the numbers of platelets present.

The indirect method of counting is a somewhat easier technique than the direct count (see Section 3.11). The results obtained tend to be higher than are those from direct methods of counting. Roughly, the procedure involves the platelets being counted simultaneously with the red cells. The number of platelets is then calculated on the basis of the RBC count.

Physiology and Pathophysiology. See Section 3.11, "Platelet Count."

IMPLICATIONS FOR NURSING

See Section 3.11, "Platelet Count."

THREE

COAGULATION SCREEN

The coagulation screen is not usually used unless there is reason to believe that a bleeding disorder exists, and it is therefore not a true multisystem screen. Portions of the screen, including at least a prothrombin time (PT), a partial thromboplastin time (PTT), and a platelet estimation (discussed in Section 2.3), are, however, used for almost all preoperative patients. The coagulation screen does look at more than just the bleeding problem in that blood vessel integrity, blood component integrity, and by implication, the integrity of the functions of other organs such as the liver are all involved in the pathogenesis of bleeding problems. The coagulation screen can determine, quickly and efficiently, the presence of a bleeding problem, the pathway involved, and to a lesser extent, the component(s) that are defective. Each laboratory selects a few procedures from the many available that will best serve the needs of its community. They are often chosen on the basis of relative simplicity (Henry, 1991).

All coagulation tests, with the exception of the whole-blood clotting time, are done on plasma. Calcium, removed when the blood is anticoagulated, must be replaced at the time of testing.

3.1 PHYSIOLOGY OF COAGULATION

Coagulation is the process of changing the fluid plasma of the blood to a solid gel by the ultimate conversion of fibrinogen to fibrin. Its central process is that of thrombin generation. Coagulation involves the participation of at least 12 identified factors (Table 3–1) as well as many cellular blood components. The factors are thought to circulate in an inactive form. When stimulated, they become active in a sequential, not necessarily strictly numerical, order that is often called the *coagulation cascade*. The three mechanisms of hemostasis are clot formation, rapid constriction of the injured vessel, and aggregation of platelets to form a plug on the injured surface of the blood vessel. There are two introductory pathways that can initiate the process. The site of the stimulus determines the pathway (Fig. 3–1). The extrinsic pathway is the most rapid because of the presence of tissue thromboplastin (factor III), whereas the intrinsic pathway must produce thromboplastin from the activation of platelets. Coagulation is most rapid in the child and adolescent because of the superb elasticity of their blood vessels.

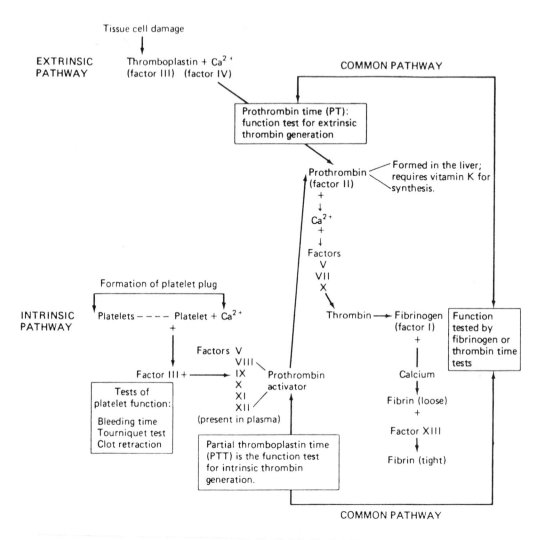

Figure 3–1. Blood clotting mechanism.

3.1.1 Formation of the Platelet Plug: Intrinsic Pathway

Damage to a blood vessel causes it to contract, an important hemostatic mechanism of the extrinsic pathway, but of lesser value in the intrinsic system. The platelet plug bridges the gap between vascular contraction and clotting. It is the self-sealing attribute for local vessel repair. It is a different process from clotting because blood can clot without the presence of platelets, but the plug cannot form without them. A platelet plug can occur in the absence of clotting but requires some thrombin for the process. The steps of the process are as follows:

1. Disruption of vessel wall because of multiple causes (e.g., antigen-antibody complexes, foreign contaminants, or products released from neutrophils)
2. Exposure of endothelial collagen fiber. The endothelium of blood vessels usually provides a nonwettable surface that is not stimulating to platelets
3. Once platelets are activated by contact with collagen (can also be stimulated by mechanical disruption of blood flow), a change in their characteristics occurs (they become sticky and adhere to collagen), and they spread out (pseudopods) to cover the maximal surface
    (a) Adenosine diphosphate (ADP) and calcium (Ca^{2+}) are released
    (b) Platelets in circulation begin to stick to platelets adhering to the wall in the presence of Ca (platelet aggregation)
    (c) Serotonin and epinephrine, which stimulate local vessel contraction and allow the platelets to anchor, are released
    (d) Phospholipid (platelet factor III, thromboplastin), which triggers prothrombin (thrombin generation, see Fig. 3–1) is released
4. The presence of thrombin continues platelet activation and aggregation
5. Ultimately, if coagulation occurs, fibrin strands produced by the activation of prothrombin-thrombin are deposited in the platelet plug
6. Platelet plugs form less readily when the blood flow is rapid (e.g., arterial vessels) and require sufficient blood loss to decrease the flow pressure before the plug will occur. Pressure exerted on the exterior of the vessel wall will thus decrease local blood flow and enhance clotting

TABLE 3–1. PLASMA COAGULATION FACTORS

Coagulation Factor Number[a]	Common Synonyms
I	Fibrinogen
II	Prothrombin
III	Tissue thromboplastin, platelet factor III
IV	Calcium
V	Labile factor, plasma accelerator (A) globulin
VII	Stable factor, serum prothrombin conversion accelerator (SPCA)
VIII	Antihemophilic factor
IX	Christmas factor, plasma thromboplastin component (PTC)
X	Stuart-Prower factor
XI	Rosenthal's factor, plasma thromboplastin antecedent (PTA)
XII[b]	Hageman factor
XIII	Fibrin-stabilizing factor; Laki-Locano factor (LLF)

[a]There is no factor VI. Although it has been described, it is not currently believed to be a separate factor and has been deleted from the list (Harper et al., 1979).
[b]Deficiency of this factor is evident only in laboratory studies. The person with a deficiency will present with no bleeding tendency (Harper, 1979).
Data from Caprini, 1976; and Whaley, & Wong, 1991.

3.2 PATHOPHYSIOLOGY OF THE COAGULATION PROCESS*

1. Problems related to small vessels (vascular phase of hemostasis)
   a. Telangiectasia
   b. Purpura
2. Problems related to the platelet plug
   a. Thrombocytopenia–decreased number of platelets
      (1) Idiopathic thrombocytopenic purpura
      (2) Systemic lupus erythematosus
      (3) Drugs
      (4) Tumors
      (5) Consumptive coagulopathy (disseminated intravascular coagulation [DIC])
   b. Thrombasthenia—decreased platelet function, thrombopathia
      (1) Glanzmann's thrombasthenia
      (2) Congenital and acquired
         (a) Combined defect (von Willebrand's disease)
         (b) Drugs: primarily dextran and aspirin
         (c) Uremia
3. Problems related to thrombin generation
   a. Factor VIII, IX, and XI depression (All clinically indistinguishable except by laboratory test)
      (1) Hemophilia A (VIII)
      (2) Hemophilia B (IX): Christmas disease
      (3) Hemophilia C (XI)
   b. Factor II, VII, IX, and X depression (vitamin K-dependent factors)
      (1) Coumarin therapy (vitamin K antagonist)
      (2) Liver disease (factor VII first to decrease) (liver synthesizes vitamin K)
      (3) Vitamin K deficiency (dietary malabsorption)
   c. Factor depression is a common pathway
      (1) Parahemophilia (V)
      (2) Stuart-Prower (X)
      (3) Calcium (IV) (very rare; unlikely as a cause of clinical bleeding except rarely in instances of transfusion of acid-citrate-dextrose (ACD) anticoagulated blood; coagulation process can take place with less CA than that necessary for usual physiological function)
   d. Antithrombin
      (1) Heparin
      (2) Endogenous–secondary to other disease processes
   e. Fibrin network
      (1) Fibrin-stabilizing factor
      (2) Congenital hypofibrinogenemia
      (3) Acquired hypofibrinogenemia

(*continued*)

---

*Data taken from Caprini, 1976, and Sodeman & Sodeman, 1982.

(a) DIC
(b) Primary fibrinolysis

Defects in platelets and clotting factors are the most common causes of bleeding in children.

3.3 BLEEDING TIME

Synonyms: Ivy bleeding time, Duke bleeding time

Normal Ranges (min)

Adult	
Ivy method	2.0–8 (reported to the nearest $1/_2$ min)
Duke method	< 3
Senior adult	As for the adult
Pediatric (Ivy method)	
Premature	1–8
Newborn	1–5
Thereafter	1–6

Definition. Bleeding time is a simple and inexpensive test that is thought to reflect the platelet function of aggregation and the vasoconstriction of the vessel. The platelet function measured is independent of the blood clotting mechanism; however, severe impairment of clotting might prolong the bleeding time (see Section 3.1.1). The time measurement reflects the time interval needed for bleeding from a small superficial wound (standardized to 1-mm-deep skin wound) to cease.

Of the two methods usually used, the Duke and the Ivy, the Ivy method is more popular and is considered the more sensitive of the two tests. It is performed by applying pressure to the forearm with a blood pressure cuff at 40 mm Hg and making a small standardized cut in the forearm. The blood is then blotted at 30-second intervals, care being taken not to touch the cut itself until the bleeding stops. The Duke method involves a standardized cut on the earlobe with the same timed blotting until bleeding ceases.

BLEEDING TIME PROLONGED IN:

1. Thrombocytopenia, thrombopathies (see Section 3.2). Aspirin is a major offender. It is thought to affect platelet adhesiveness and can increase the bleeding time up to 21 minutes if given within 1 week preceding the test (SHMC, 1991)
2. Parahemophilia
3. Von Willebrand's disease
4. Fibrinolytic states
5. Senile purpura because of the loss of elasticity and turgor of the vascular wall. It is clinically benign, the most serious consequence being cosmetic
6. Scurvy
7. Congenital afibrinogenemia
8. Fibrolytic states
9. Patients who have ingested aspirin within a week preceding the test

IMPLICATIONS FOR NURSING: BLEEDING TIME

1. Persons having the test should be informed of the possibility of slight scarring (Ivy method) from the small incision. They should also be informed if the usual practice consists of taking at least two if not more samples. Most laboratories now use a disposable device that makes two simultaneous standard cuts. In some facilities the test is repeated until two bleeding time values are not more than a minute apart when the Ivy test is used. Because the normal range is broad and the test is quite variable, such repetition is recommended

2. A relevant history should be taken for drugs affecting platelet function (see "Implications for Nursing: Platelet Count" in Section 3.11)

3. Note the administration of thrombocytopenic drugs on the laboratory request slip for a bleeding time test. This is particularly important when aspirin is being administered. Note the date and time of the last dose

4. If the patient's platelet count is less than 25,000/mm^3, a special, informed order for a bleeding test usually must be obtained from the physician or pathologist

5. If the patient is receiving therapeutic heparin, the test should not be done for approximately 4 hours after a dose is given. This precaution does not usually apply to heparin used in a heparin lock to keep the vein patent

6. Observe the skin of the arms carefully after routine blood pressure taking for petechiae in any person with a prolonged bleeding time as well as after venipuncture or the Ivy method of performing the bleeding test. A test sometimes used, which the nurse can use as a nursing observation with the aforementioned activities, is the *tourniquet test*. When the blood pressure cuff is inflated halfway between the systolic and diastolic pressures (about 40 mm Hg) for 5 minutes, petechiae will appear distally to the cuff. The normal person can form up to five petechiae. In the person with platelet or vascular defects, petechiae formation is markedly increased

7. All nursing actions relevant to platelet estimation also apply for the patient requiring a bleeding time test (see "Implications for Nursing: Platelet Count" in Section 3.11 as well as "General Implications for Nursing Related to Problems in Coagulation" in Section 3.12)

BLEEDING TIME NORMAL IN:

- Hemophilia A and B. Hemophilia A is a disorder of factor VIII, as is von Willebrand's disease, but von Willebrand's has a defect in platelet adhesion that hemophilia A does not

BLEEDING TIME DECREASED IN:

- Not clinically significant

3.4 PROTHROMBIN TIME

Synonyms: Protime, PT, quick prothrombin time, quick test, INR

Normal Ranges (one stage; sec)[a]

International normalized ratio (INR)[b]	
Medical and surgical thromboembolic states	2.0–3.0
Artificial heart valves and recurrent embolism	3.0–4.5
Adult	11.2–13.8
Senior adult	No change from adult value

Pediatric	
Premature	12–21
Newborn/neonatal	12–20
Thereafter	12–14

[a]Normal ranges are usually measured against a control. Therefore, there is variation in normal ranges between laboratories. In many instances results are expressed as a percentage of activity rather than elapsed time in seconds.

[b]The INR is usually used as a single coagulation test. The INR ranges are recommended after the patient has been stabilized on oral anticoagulants (vitamin K-dependent factors approximately 20 to 30 percent of normal), usually 5 to 7 days after start of therapy (Laboratory of Pathology, 1991).

Definition. The PT test indicates the rapidity of blood clotting and is a good test of the extrinsic thrombin generation pathway. It does not measure the amount of prothrombin generated, rather the activity. The extrinsic PT is so short that any contribution to clotting from the intrinsic pathway is usually negligible.

In the past the PT test was thought to measure prothrombin activity only. It is now known that a normal test result depends on adequate levels of factors V, VII, and X as well as all factors of the extrinsic pathway (see Fig. 3–1). It is the *only* test that measures factor VII activity (Caprini, 1976).

The protime test is widely used for differential diagnosis in jaundice. Vitamin K administered parenterally usually restores a prolonged PT to normal in a patient with obstructive jaundice and will fail to do so in patients with intrinsic hepatic (parenchymal) disease (Henry, 1991; see also Section 1.10). Probably its greatest uses are as a guide for anticoagulant dosage in the administration of warfarin (coumadin), phenindione (Hedulin), or dicumarol; as a diagnostic test in bleeding disorders; and a measure of vitamin K deficiency (Wheelis, 1979).

Physiology. Prothrombin (factor II) is synthesized in the liver and is dependent on the presence of vitamin K. There are other precoagulation factors also dependent on vitamin K for synthesis: factors X, VII, and IX (Christmas factor). Vitamin K is synthesized primarily by intestinal bacteria and, being lipid soluble, is absorbed only if bile salts are present.

Pathophysiology. Deficiencies in either of these substances, bile salts or fat, lead to deficiencies in vitamin K and thus in the precoagulation factors noted, prothrombin among them. Prothrombin deficiency is almost always associated with other factor deficiencies.

In the absence of vitamin K, the protein normally activated by the vitamin may enter the bloodstream where it acts as a competitive inhibitor of the vitamin K–dependent factors and enhances their deficiency (Frohlich, 1988).

The amount of prothrombin in the blood is actually less critical in clotting than is the availability of the other factors necessary for its conversion to thrombin (i.e., factor deficiency). The amount of prothrombin usually available provides a wide margin of safety against its being deficient. Therefore, the two-stage prothrombin test, which actually measures the prothrombin, is not frequently used. The one-step method measures deficiencies in factors V, VII, X, and II (Henry, 1991).

The stimulus for prothrombin generation through the extrinsic pathway is tissue damage, which releases tissue thromboplastin. Because fewer reactions are required to complete this pathway, the protime is about one third that of the PTT.

PT PROLONGED IN:

1. Inadequate intake of vitamin K as in
   a. Hemorrhagic disease of the newborn because of an inadequate supply of milk. Milk is the only source of vitamin K for the newborn because he or she lacks bacteria in the bowel for vitamin K synthesis (see Section 1.10)
   b. n.p.o. states before surgery in persons who have had antibiotic bowel sterilization
2. Impaired intestinal absorption of vitamin K as in
   a. Sprue
   b. Ulcerative colitis or Crohn's disease
   c. Obstructive jaundice
3. Parenchymal hepatic disease as in
   a. Cirrhosis
   b. Hepatitis
4. Persons being given certain drugs such as
   a. Cholestyramine (Questran) because of binding of bile salts
   b. Aspirin in large doses
   c. Long-term antibiotic therapy because of decreased vitamin K synthesis (or gut sterilization before surgery)
   d. Large amounts of laxative because of a decreased absorption of vitamin K
   e. Warfarin or dicumarol because of decreased vitamin K synthesis. The therapeutic level of prothrombin with these drugs is usually 1 to 2 times the normal range
5. Disease states producing decreased fibrinogen values, below 100 mg/dl (see Section 3.6)
6. Disease states producing coagulation inhibitors such as lupus erythematosus, alcoholism, renal insufficiency, malnutrition, and scurvy

PT SHORTENED IN:

1. Response to treatment with certain drugs (e.g., vitamin K, anabolic steroids)
2. Persons consuming an excessively high-fat diet or one with an excessive intake of vitamin K-rich foods

---

IMPLICATIONS FOR NURSING: PROTHROMBIN TIME

1. No special patient preparation is necessary
2. Small amounts of vitamin K are frequently given to a mother before childbirth or given to the newborn if necessary. The nurse needs to supply not only the drug but also the reason for the injection and reassurance as to its effectiveness in preventing hemorrhagic disease of the newborn
3. Any person who receives prolonged antibiotic therapy for more than 2 days or intensive therapy for gut sterilization should be supplied with foods to replace the intestinal flora as a regular part of the diet or when feeding is resumed. Foods helpful in the repopulation of intestinal flora include yogurt, acidophilus milk, buttermilk, and soft natural cheeses. These individuals also need to be carefully observed for superimposed infections from nonsusceptible organisms. Candidiasis of the mucous membrane of the mouth or, in women, of the mucous membrane of the vagina is a frequent complication
4. Plasma taken for PT determination must be tested promptly (within 6 hours of collection) or frozen for longer storage. Factor V activity is rapidly lost at temperatures of 37°C or higher
5. See Section 3.12 for general nursing implications that also apply

3.5 PARTIAL THROMBOPLASTIN TIME, ACTIVATED

Synonyms: aPTT, APTT, partial thromboplastin time, PTT

Normal Ranges[a] (sec)

	Activated Method	Traditional Method
Adult	35–45	60–85
Mean	40	70
Senior adult	No change from adult values (method not described in the literature; apparently activated)	
Pediatric		
Premature	<120	
Newborn	<90	
Thereafter	<60	
Range	39–53	

[a]The only difference between PTT and the activated thromboplastin times is that the activated method uses the addition of a silica compound to standardize the initial, or activation phase of the test, thus decreasing the length of time between the addition of calcium and visible clotting. It is felt to be the more reproducible test and almost as sensitive as the standard test (Sodeman & Sodeman, 1982). Reference ranges or "normals" for both PT and PTT depend on the commercial reagents used and vary from laboratory to laboratory (Nordin, 1980).

Definition. The PTT test is used as a screening test for deficiencies of coagulation factors in the intrinsic and common systems (see Fig. 3–1) of thrombin generation. Single deficiencies can be further isolated, especially if the deficiencies are severe. Such isolation is less useful in mild deficiencies or where combined deficiencies exist as in intravascular clotting. Factor inhibitors can also prolong the PTT. There is a further simple test (1:1 mix with normal plasma) to differentiate inhibitors from factor deficiency, and it is usually done with a prolonged value (Wheelis, 1979). The PTT is sensitive to all factors except VII (stable factor or serum prothrombin converter accelerator).

The PT and PTT tests form the basis of screening tests for coagulation factor deficiencies.

The name "partial" thromboplastin is derived from the use of a thromboplastin that lacks the ability to compensate totally for the plasma defect of hemophilia, hence, a *partial* thromboplastin.

Physiology. The intrinsic pathway of coagulation is stimulated by the release of factor III (platelet thromboplastin) and involves a longer period of time to reach its end point—the production of fibrin—than does the extrinsic pathway. It also requires a greater number of coagulation factors to complete its process. The PTT responds with prolongation primarily in persons with factor IX and VIII deficiencies: hemophilia (Harvey et al., 1991).

Pathophysiology. See Section 3.4.

PTT PROLONGED IN:

1. Hemophilia because of factor VIII or IX deficiency
2. von Willebrand's disease (pseudohemophilia), although the increase may be slight

3. Persons receiving coumarin or dicumarol therapy, although not consistently prolonged, and the increase is usually slight. The increase is due to the failure of the liver to synthesize factor IX

4. Heparin therapy, because of inhibition of the formation of thrombin from prothrombin. Heparin probably also prevents plasma thromboplastin activity. The PTT is commonly used to monitor heparin therapy. The dosage is adjusted to keep the PTT at 1 to 2 times normal

5. DIC, levels due to consumption of platelets and a decrease in factor VIII

6. Conditions requiring multiple doses of naloxone (Narcan), process unclear

PTT DECREASED IN:

- Extensive cancer, except hepatic cancer, because of the increasing amount of thromboplastin from the tumor content

---

IMPLICATIONS FOR NURSING: PARTIAL THROMBOPLASTIN TIME, ACTIVATED

1. No special patient preparation is necessary
2. Related to patients on heparin therapy:
   a. A PTT test is usually done before each heparin dose when therapy is being started; therefore, the nurse must check that the blood sample has been collected before giving the medication
   b. A PTT determination is done 4 hours postdose if heparin is being given subcutaneously or intramuscularly. Intramuscularly is the most dangerous method and should be avoided if possible. The risk of hemorrhage or hematoma at the site is great. Preferably, therapeutic heparin is given intravenously by continuous infusion (Nordin, 1980, 1987).
   c. Give any other intramuscular (IM) injections just before giving heparin to decrease the chance of bleeding. All drugs should be given orally as well, if possible (see "General Implications for Nursing Related to Problems in Coagulation" in Section 3.12). All precautions taken for any patient with a bleeding disorder should be taken with persons receiving heparin
3. Related to patients with hemophilia:
   a. Check any site of bleeding for rebleeding after the first clot has formed. Primary hemostasis is unstable in hemophilia.
   b. Prevention of crippling effects because of bleeding into joint spaces or secondary to pain on movement is a major nursing responsibility
      (1) In the acute stage, elevate the affected joint and immobilize it to encourage clotting
      (2) Assist with factor replacement (factor VIII, Hemofil, Humafac, Factorate; factor IX, Konyne, Proplex (rarely used). Most frequently used is cryoprecipitate, or antihemophilia globulin [AHG]; and AHF—antihemophilia factor [AHF]) in hemophilia A. The use of these materials is the major medical approach to both controlling bleeding and preventing further bleeding, which would prevent crippling by eliminating the cause
      (3) Institute passive range of motion (ROM) as soon as the bleeding stops and the acute phase is over
      (4) Minor pain control should be maintained with acetaminophen (Tylenol) rather than aspirin to prevent further bleeding effects, yet provide for maximum activity
      (5) Provide pain medication as ordered before activity

(6) Consult with the physician and physical therapy department in setting up activity programs. Get input from the patient and family as to preferred activities and work them into the program to increase compliance

(7) Teach patient, family, home caretaker when appropriate about the long-range effects of joint involvement to increase compliance with the activity regimen.

c. Assist patient, family, home caretaker in developing maximum independence. Refer to a home care program if available. If none available, consult with the health care team to set up the most appropriate teaching system possible

(1) Delay teaching until the major bleeding emergency is over. Teaching, except that related to prevention of bleeding should also be delayed until the process of adjustment to a new diagnosis of hemophilia has occurred for both patient and family or home caretaker. Content areas and some general guidelines on which to base a teaching plan are as follows:

(a) Bleeding control: direct pressure, immobilization and elevation, packing with Gelfoam or fibrin foam, application of topical hemostatic preparations such as thrombin, application of cold, and compression with woven elastic (Ace) bandages

(b) Self-administration of scheduled or an emergency infusion of factor replacements with emphasis on prevention of further trauma (e.g., the use of small-gauge needle, intravenous technique, minimal venous obstruction with venipuncture)

(c) Signs and symptoms of transfusion reaction (e.g., chills, temperature spike, dyspnea, rash, back pain, edema). (Reactions occur because of the presence of anti-A or -B isohemagglutinins in solution. Cryoprecipitate must be cross-matched with the recipient's blood type)

(d) Care of stored factor. Cryoprecipitate is stored frozen

(e) Use of over-the-counter drugs (e.g., no aspirin); teach patients and families to read labels

(f) Need to advise others of diagnosis (e.g., dentist); use of ID card, bracelet, or tag with name, doctor's name, and diagnosis

(2) Refer to National Hemophilia Foundation for literature, films, counseling, special children's camps, and newsletter

d. All precautions and teaching areas listed for other bleeding problems apply to the individual with hemophilia (see "General Implications for Nursing Related to Problems in Coagulation" in section 3.12)

4. Monitor related laboratory findings with bleeding problems of the intrinsic pathway

a. Whole-blood clotting time is usually prolonged

b. Prothrombin consumption time is usually decreased

c. Bleeding time is usually normal (there is no platelet deficiency in hemophilia A and B, but there is with von Willebrand's disease)

d. The PT is usually normal

3.6 PLASMA FIBRINOGEN

Synonym: Claus fibrinogen

Normal Ranges (mg/dl)

Adult	160–300
Senior adult	470–485
Pediatric	
Newborn	150–300
Thereafter	200–400

Definition. The plasma fibrinogen test is similar to the TT test in that both measure conversion of fibrinogen to fibrin by thrombin. They differ only in the method of procedure. The fibrinogen test does minimize the effects of any inhibitors of coagulation (antithrombin, heparin), whereas the thrombin test is sensitive to the presence of inhibitors. The fibrinogen test is helpful in differentiation between bleeding due to liver disease and bleeding resulting from DIC because its level is rarely decreased below 100 mg/dl in liver disease but can be much lower in DIC.

There are several different methods of measuring fibrinogen. Methods such as used for this test, which involve some form of clottable protein determination, are done rapidly; thus they make good screening tests. A chemical assay of fibrin is the most accurate method but is more time-consuming.

Physiology. Fibrinogen (factor I) is one of the major plasma proteins (see Section 1.8, Serum total protein—Physiology) and makes up about 5 percent of those proteins. Once clotting has occurred, virtually all of the fibrinogen will have been removed from the plasma. Fibrinogen is produced in the liver by what must be an extremely efficient process because it is uncommon to see decreases except in the most severe forms of liver disease and decreases that do occur are rarely below 100 mg/dl (Ravel, 1989). This soluble plasma protein is converted by the action of thrombin, in the presence of calcium and factor XIII (fibrin-stabilizing factor), to the insoluble protein molecule fibrin (see Fig. 3–1).

The peptides (A and B) that are split from the fibrinogen molecule in this process are acute-phase reactants that respond to inflammation, which makes fibrinogen's role in the body a dual one—that of clotting and inflammatory repair (Groer & Shekleton, 1983). The fibrin molecule then forms long fibrin threads that interweave and form the clot, thereby trapping blood cells. The normal presence of heparin and antithrombin in the plasma inhibits the formation and action of thrombin, thus preventing spontaneous activation of fibrinogen and generation of the fibrin clot, assuming relatively small amounts of thrombin being formed. In the face of increased tissue or platelet destruction, however, greater concentrations of thrombin occur, and clotting takes place. Blood clotting at an inflamed site helps wall off the area and potentiate other chemical responses to speed repair.

Pathophysiology. Deficiencies of fibrinogen can be congenital or acquired and can result in (1) afibrinogenemia, no measurable fibrinogen; (2) hypofibrinogenemia, fibrinogen present but in amounts less than 100 mg/dl; and (3) dysfibrinogenemia, fibrinogen decreased in function (as measured in its reaction to thrombin) but present in normal amounts (measured immunologically). Acquired deficiencies occur as a result of liver disorders, active fibrinolysis, or intravascular clotting disorders.

Clinical signs and symptoms of patients deficient in fibrinogen only, but with normal procoagulants otherwise, are less severe than the symptoms of patients with deficiencies of one of the other procoagulants. Therefore, the bleeding that occurs with many congenital forms of fibrinogen deficiencies is not usually life-threatening because the congenital form is usually an isolated fibrinogen deficiency; however, isolated fibrinogen deficiencies are uncommon in acquired bleeding disorders (Henry, 1991).

FIBRINOGEN LEVELS INCREASED IN:

1. The elderly—a physiological response, the purpose of which is not clear
2. Response to nonspecific stimuli (e.g., trauma, infections, neoplasm, hemorrhage)

FIBRINOGEN LEVELS DECREASED IN:

1. Intravascular clotting disorders with consumption in excess of production, most commonly disseminated intravascular coagulation DIC, which occurs secondarily to complications of pregnancy such as
   a. Missed abortion (long-standing intrauterine death of the fetus)
   b. Premature separation of the placenta
   c. Amniotic fluid embolism after the administration of oxytocin. (All are felt to be due to the release of thromboplastin-like substances from the placenta and amniotic fluid into the circulation)
2. DIC secondary to other conditions such as (these occur more commonly than pregnancy-related DIC)
   a. Prostatic cancer with metastasis, believed to produce a fibrolysin (plasminogen) activator (see Fig. 3–2 in Section 3.9)
   b. Septicemia
   c. Surgical and postoperative shock
   d. Postcardiac bypass surgery
   e. Massive thrombosis
3. Liver disease (cirrhosis, hepatitis) because of decreased production, which is not usually clinically evident unless accompanied by other factor deficiencies that may cause clinical signs and symptoms
4. Conditions causing increased levels of fibrinolysins (enzymes that destroy fibrinogen) and active fibrinolysis such as
   a. Cancer of the prostate with metastasis
   b. After thoracic surgery
5. Congenital deficiencies, all other coagulation factors being normal

FIBRINOGEN NORMAL IN QUANTITY BUT ABNORMAL IN FUNCTION IN:

1. Congenital dysfibrinogenemia
2. Multiple myeloma because of the presence of paraproteins that act as inhibitors of fibrin strand and clot activity

---

IMPLICATIONS FOR NURSING: PLASMA FIBRINOGEN

1. No special patient preparation is necessary. The fibrinogen test must be performed within 24 hours of blood sample collection. If the nurse obtains the blood sample, the laboratory request slip should be clearly labeled as to the time the specimen was taken, and it should arrive in the laboratory as soon as possible
2. For persons with congenital fibrinogen deficiencies:
   a. Treatment is the administration of fibrinogen by plasma transfusions. Since this factor is lost from the body by normal decay in 12 to 21 days when not used for clot formation, replacement is done routinely every 10 to 14 days. The nurse should monitor fibrinogen levels for such a person when under nursing care between infusions. Fibrinogen levels should be maintained at 50 mg/dl or higher

> b. True fibrinogen levels for diagnostic purposes can be determined only when there is no active bleeding and there has been no recent (3 to 4 weeks) transfusion of blood or plasma
>
> 3. A fibrinogen level below 100 mg/dl is rare in liver disease and can therefore be helpful in ruling that condition out as the cause of low fibrinogen concentrations. Since the alternative possibilities of cause are somewhat limited, a careful nursing history (see "General Implications for Nursing Related to Problems in Coagulation" in Section 3.12) can assist the physician in targeting the problem area
>
> 4. The test sample should not be drawn within 6 hours of a heparin dose because heparin interferes with thrombin and hence fibrin generation

3.7 WHOLE-BLOOD CLOT RETRACTION

Synonyms: None

Normal Ranges

Adult	Complete retraction with 24 hr
Senior adult	As for adult
Pediatric	Retraction may be complete within 4 hr but normal values are generally as for adult

Definition. Clot retraction is done as a part of the test for clotting time. Because it is nonspecific and unreliable, it is not presently used a great deal. Test tubes filled with blood are placed in a warm bath (37°C) to be observed for clot retraction every 30 to 60 minutes. The test is open to error because of the differences in the size of the clot formed. Approximately one half of the total blood volume in the tube should be made up of clot, the other half made up of serum for a "normal-"size clot.

Clot retraction is a rough indicator of platelet adequacy but is reliable only when packed red cell volume (hematocrit) and fibrinogen concentrations are within normal limits.

Physiology. When the coagulation cascade, or process, is complete, a clot has been formed. The fibrin of that clot is acted on by factor XIII, which causes the strands to shrink. The clot's ability to shrink depends on an adequate number of platelets being present and on the action of thrombin. It is thought that platelets may provide the necessary energy, adenosine triphosphate [ATP], for the shortening process. The fibrin strands of the clot attach to the edges of the injured blood vessel. The process of shrinking serves to pull the edges closer together, which helps to decrease blood loss and begin repair. The retraction process is therefore essential to the process of hemostasis (Watson, 1979).

The clot usually decreases to half of its original size in 1 hour, the fibrinogen free serum being extruded and a definite margin being visible between clot, serum, and test tube wall. The resulting clot, if normal, is much firmer than the original.

Pathophysiology. The absence of fibrinogen, an increase in fibrinolytic activity, or an increase in packed cell volume will cause RBCs to be released from the clot into the serum. Smaller clots than normal occur with decreased packed cell volumes or fibrinogen concentrations (Henry, 1991).

POOR WHOLE-BLOOD CLOT RETRACTION OCCURS IN:

1. Thrombocytopenia
2. Thrombasthenia
3. Fibrinogenopenia. Because of the small clot size, clot retraction is inadequate, although it may be misinterpreted as normal

WHOLE-BLOOD CLOT DISSOLUTION OCCURS IN:

- Conditions with increased fibrinolytic activity (see Section 3.9)

IMPLICATIONS FOR NURSING: WHOLE-BLOOD CLOT RETRACTION

The time span necessary for initial retraction to half-size (1 hour) and total clot retraction (24 hours) provides a rationale for the need to immediately immobilize a bleeding part and then to restrict vigorous activity of the part for 24 hours. Immobility promotes clot formation; decreased activity enhances clot stability.

3.8 WHOLE-BLOOD CLOTTING TIME, ACTIVATED

Synonyms: Activated coagulation time, ACT[a]

Normal Range: 75–105 sec

Therapeutic Ranges:
150–210 sec (general heparin therapy) (Nordin, 1980,1987)
300–600 sec (extracorporeal heparin therapy) (Widman, 1983)

---

[a]Another similar test used to monitor heparin therapy besides the ACT and the APTT is the blood activated recalcification time (BART), or recal time. The therapeutic range of the BART test is 1.5 to 2.0 times the normal clotting time, i.e., with the normal range of the activated whole-blood clotting time given previously, the BART therapeutic normal would be 113 to 210 seconds.

Definition. The activated whole-blood clotting time measures the overall activity of the intrinsic clotting mechanism, the time it takes whole blood to clot firmly. The predecessor test, nonactivated whole-blood clotting test, widely known as the Lee-White clotting test, was time-consuming and the least accurate of coagulation tests. Blood takes 4 to 8 minutes to clot firmly, and heparinized blood, the kind most often being tested, extends that time to about 20 minutes. The activated test speeds up that process and can be reproduced more accurately.

Physiology and Pathophysiology. See "Physiology" and "Pathophysiology" in Sections 3.4 and 3.5.

ACT PROLONGED IN:

- Conditions as for the PTT test (Section 3.5)

ACT DECREASED IN:

- Conditions as for the PTT test (Section 3.5)

3.9 FIBRINOLYSIN

Synonyms: Whole-blood clot lysis, clot lysis

Normal Range

Adult   Negative (no lysis of clot) in 48 hr
                             No available data for indication of any difference from adult normals
                             for other age groups

Definition. The principle underlying this test is that an increased activity of fibrolysins (plasmins [a protelytic plasma enzyme]) in the blood will cause a clot, formed from whole blood, to dissolve over a specified period of time, from 1 to 24 hours. A normal clot will remain intact for at least 24 hours. This type of evaluation of the fibrinolytic system is the more common approach used in screening tests or in emergency conditions. Other tests look at the activity of components for fibrinolysis, which components rapidly disappear from the circulation and are, therefore, of limited usefulness in emergency conditions (Caprini, 1976).

Physiology. (See Fig. 3–2 for a diagrammatic representation of the fibrinolytic system.) The fibrinolytic system is by intent a protective mechanism to rid the body of clots that are no longer needed and exists in addition to the clotting inhibitors such as heparin and antithrombin. Preactivators circulate in the blood until they are themselves activated to profibrolysin (plasminogen) by the presence of certain tissue enzymes (plasminogen), and then they are converted through further enzyme activation (fibrokinases) to fibrolysin (plasmin). Fibrolysin acts on the blood clot and on fibrinogen as well by breaking them down into products that inhibit the coagulation process (Price & Wilson, 1992). This fibrinolytic sequence is a slow process as compared with coagulation; it is as complex as the coagulation process, and it is even less well understood.

Pathophysiology. At this point in research, it is difficult to determine what level of fibrinolytic activity will result in hemorrhage. Some experts feel the fibrinolytic mechanism is of major significance, and others feel that there is little clinical significance in its role in the cause of bleeding (Henry, 1991).

IMPLICATIONS FOR NURSING

- The test should not be done (blood drawn) within 6 hours of a heparin dose.

3.10 THROMBIN TIME

Synonyms: None

Normal Ranges

Within 3 sec of control (control usually approximately 9 to 13 sec)
No data available for an indication of variations from this norm in other age groups

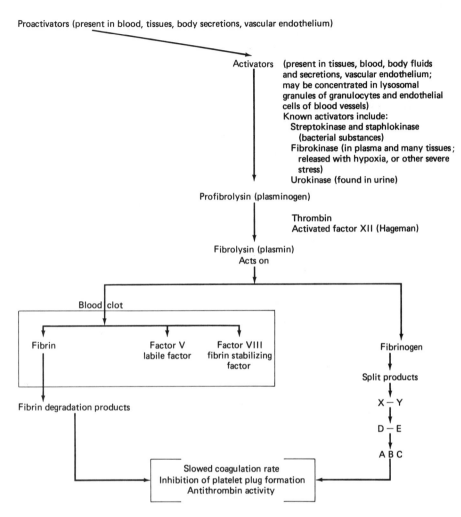

Proactivators (present in blood, tissues, body secretions, vascular endothelium)

Activators (present in tissues, blood, body fluids
and secretions, vascular endothelium;
may be concentrated in lysosomal
granules of granulocytes and endothelial
cells of blood vessels)
Known activators include:
Streptokinase and staphlokinase
(bacterial substances)
Fibrokinase (in plasma and many tissues;
released with hypoxia, or other severe
stress)
Urokinase (found in urine)

Profibrolysin (plasminogen)

Thrombin
Activated factor XII (Hageman)

Fibrolysin (plasmin)
Acts on

Blood clot

Fibrin

Factor V
labile factor

Factor VIII
fibrin stabilizing
factor

Fibrinogen

Split products

X — Y

D — E

A B C

Fibrin degradation products

Slowed coagulation rate
Inhibition of platelet plug formation
Antithrombin activity

Figure 3–2. Fibrinolysis. (Data from Caprini, 1976; Davidsohn & Henry, 1969; Frolich, 1976; Ganong, 1979; Harper, Rodwell, & Mayes, 1979; and MacBryde & Blacklow, 1970.)

Definition. As noted with the plasma fibrinogen test, the thrombin time and fibrinogen test evaluate the thrombin-fibrinogen reaction. The thrombin time detects defects in the rate of fibrin formation. The test is done by adding thrombin to plasma and timing the resulting formation of a fibrin clot. This is then compared with a control (or normal). A result plus or minus seconds of that control indicates the presence of adequate and functional thrombin. The test is sensitive to the presence of inhibitors of thrombin formation and is more sensitive in detecting heparin inhibition than is any other test.

Physiology. Thrombin formation, already discussed in the general physiology of coagulation, is the central process of blood coagulation and can be generated by both the intrinsic and extrinsic systems. Its presence is essential to the function of platelets and also seems to be a factor in activation of the fibrinolytic system (Mountcastle, 1980; see also Fig. 3–2). It is formed through the action of calcium and factors V, VIII, and X and functions as an enzyme by stimulating fibrinogen in the presence of calcium to form fibrin (see Fig. 3–1). Prothrombin circulating in the blood is not converted to thrombin at any appreciable rate, if at all. Thrombin generation is stimulated by and appears quickly after any bleeding. The rate at which it is produced sets the rate of the speed of clotting. Very quickly after maximum thrombin production has been reached, antithrombin progressively inactivates it, and it is continuously removed from the system. Were it not removed, it would have a half-life of only 3 days. The action of antithrombin and endogenous heparin prevent continuation of the clotting process beyond need.

Thrombin appears to be formed mostly in the arteries in response to roughened endothelium or collagen exposure.

Pathophysiology. One of the major pathologies directly related to thrombin generation is that of thrombosis. Clots formed in blood vessels are called thrombi (thrombus, singular), which distinguishes them from extravascular clots. The careful balance maintained by the body between blood fluidity and necessary clotting is not yet well understood. Study in the area of intravascular clotting or thrombosis is hampered by the fact that humans are the only animals known to form venous thrombosis (Groer & Shekleton, 1983).

Although thrombin is produced primarily in the arterial circulation, the production of a venous thrombus appears to be the result of venous stasis, which causes venous concentrations of thrombin to be produced at injury sites in the arteries. The venous intimal endothelium of a thrombosed vein is usually found to be normal. Because much activated thrombin is held back (sequestered) in slowed venous circulation, it cannot be adequately destroyed by the liver; thus thrombosis occurs, spreads, and may lead to embolization. Thrombosis can occur in the arterial circulation at the site of injury or at sites of slowed circulation such as atherosclerotic narrowing of coronary arteries. The elderly are a population at risk for atherosclerosis and consequently thrombophlebitis.

A second major area of pathology is a decrease in thrombin activity because of an increase in fibrinolysis, which produces anticoagulant split products, low fibrinogen levels, or the presence of endogenous circulating anticoagulants often seen as an effect of many chronic diseases (Caprini, 1973).

THROMBIN TIME PROLONGED IN:

1. Persons with plasma fibrinogen levels under 100 mg/dl
2. Persons with systemic disease causing an increased production of coagulation inhibitors such as
   a. Systemic lupus erythematosus
   b. Uremia
   c. Hyperbilirubinemia
3. Impaired fibrinogen function (abnormal fibrinogen)
4. Inhibitors of thrombin-induced clot formation such as
   a. Exogenous administration of heparin as therapy
   b. Abnormal globulin

    c. Intravascular clotting disorders that produce increased amounts of fibrinogen split end products (see Fig. 3–2 and Section 3.6 "Fibrinogen Levels Decreased in," items 1 and 2)
5. Most cases of polycythemia vera because of a relative depletion of plasma clotting factors, particularly fibrinogen and prothrombin, and because of inadequate platelet function

THROMBIN TIME DECREASED IN:

- Not found to be clinically significant. Systemic levels are not necessarily altered when either arterial or vascular thrombosis occurs. The thrombin increase is local and quickly eliminated (see "Pathophysiology," this section).

IMPLICATIONS FOR NURSING: WHOLE-BLOOD CLOTTING TIME, ACTIVATED; FIBRINOLYSIN; THROMBIN TIME

1. No special patient preparation is necessary
2. Persons at risk of thrombus formation
    a. The elderly are at particular risk of thrombosis, especially when ill and hospitalized. As a consequence, their risk of developing DIC is increased, since massive thrombosis is one etiology for DIC. The nurse then should take a meticulous history and do a thorough, continuing physical appraisal of the elderly patient. Particular attention should be paid to persons at even higher risk within the elderly as a group. These include females taking oral replacement hormones and persons with varicose veins, a history of congestive heart disease, and conditions tending to decrease mobility (to include the loss of visual or hearing acuity, which can tend to immobilize the elderly because of fear or social embarrassment). A continuing appraisal for indicators of thrombosis or bleeding should be carried out
    b. The individual with polycythemia vera (a fairly rare disorder) is also at dual risk of thrombosis and bleeding from the increased viscosity of the blood and potential heart failure and from decreased fibrinogen and prothrombin levels and ineffective platelet function
        (1) Do not treat increased blood viscosity by the provision of increased fluids in this case because of the presence of hypervolemia. Phlebotomy (venisection) removing about 500 ml of blood every 2 or 3 days and the use of marrow suppressants are the medical approaches to decrease blood viscosity
        (2) Observe particularly for bleeding from a peptic ulcer (Hemoccult or guaiac test for all stools or vomitus) because this is a common problem with this diagnosis (Harvey et al., 1991)
3. Other pertinent tests to monitor with a prolonged thrombin time include PTT and one-stage PT. Hypofibrinogenemia will be indicated by prolonged values in one or all of these. No clotting will occur in afibrinogenemia; therefore, the prolongation of the tests will be indefinite
4. If a repeat thrombin time is reported as "corrected at 50/50" (or 90/10) control/patient mixture, a coagulation factor or element deficiency is present. If uncorrected, anticoagulant (heparin, fibrin split products) activity is indicated (Caprini, 1976)

3.11 PLATELET COUNT

Synonym: Thrombocyte count

Normal Ranges (per mm^3)

Adult   250,000–500,000

(continued)

Senior adult	
Age 50[a]	
Female	255,000–1,392,000
Male	330,000–1,430,000
Age 94[a]	70,266–175,000
Pediatric	
Premature	100,000–300,000
Newborn	140,000–300,000
Neonatal	150,000–390,000
Infant	200,000–473,000
Thereafter	150,000–450,000

[a]Dameshelk method.

Definition. The platelet count is most consistently accurate when done on an automated counter. Platelets are difficult to count because of the speed and ease with which they disintegrate. In a blood sample drawn for analysis platelets are stable only at room temperature, not refrigerated, and are stable for only 24 hours. Thus there are virtually no functional platelets in stored blood. Bank blood frequently will have the platelets removed immediately for use in platelet transfusion.

The use of venous, rather than capillary, blood is recommended for this test. The results from venous blood tend to be more reproducible. Capillary sticks tend to lower counts because of the loss of platelets adhering to the wound.

Physiology. Platelets are formed from megakaryocytes in the bone marrow (see Fig. 2–1). They are not true cells because they have no nuclei, but they are highly active metabolically when stimulated. They are stimulated by any foreign substance with a negatively charged surface, including glass, which explains blood clots forming in a test tube.

Platelet function is primarily that of hemostasis ("thrombo" means clot and "cyte" means cell, hence a clot cell), actively engaging in the formation of the platelet plug to maintain blood vessel integrity (see Section 3.1.1). They are one of two sources of thromboplastin (or factor III), the other being injured tissue; they are an essential element in the process of coagulation (see Fig. 3–1). They produce serotonin to stimulate blood vessel contraction at the site of injury. Further, they are essential to clot retraction (see Section 3.7).

Platelet regulation is not too well understood. After acute blood loss, production increases; larger platelets appear in the peripheral circulation; the platelet count rises. The body produces platelets at a constant rate (from 50,000 to 100,000/mm³/day), which maintains the normal level. Their life span is from 4 to 11 days. There is a circulating substance called thrombopoietin that stimulates increased speed in the formation and the development of platelets (McCance and Huether, 1990, p. 771). Approximately one tenth of the circulating platelets are used to maintain the blood vessels' endothelial integrity, and about one third are sequestered in the spleen in the normal person (Henry, 1991).

Pathophysiology. An increase in platelet numbers can occur. When it does, there is a tendency to thrombosis and, less frequently, a tendency to hemorrhage as well. An extremely high count apparently has an anticoagulant effect, which may be that of inhibition of thromboplastin (factor

III) generation. Increases can occur secondary to increased production or increased release. Decreases, felt to be of more clinical importance, can occur secondary to a decrease in production, an increase in pooling (sequestration) in the spleen, or increased destruction. Platelets can also be adequate in numbers but ineffective in function.

PLATELET COUNT INCREASED IN:*

1. For physiological causes of changes in platelet levels with platelet estimation, see "Implications for Nursing" in this section
2. Myeloproliferative syndrome, including the initial response in polycythemia vera, causing a thrombocythemia. Platelets are abnormal and lead to thrombosis
3. Response to acute stress (e.g., injury, surgery), with an increase in production rather than release from bone marrow. A similar increase occurs when adrenal corticosteroid hormones are used therapeutically
4. The period after a splenectomy. Increases are greater if a preexisting anemia is not corrected by the surgery and always higher than the levels reached after other surgeries
5. The period after hemorrhage (usually a physiological response)
6. Metastatic cancer, particularly that of the lung and other epithelial cancers
7. Acute infections possibly related to the stress response

PLATELET COUNT DECREASED IN (THROMBOCYTOPENIA):

1. Conditions causing decreased production such as
   a. Bone marrow failure secondary to the administration of drugs, chemotherapeutic agents, or irradiation
   b. Bone marrow replacement by primary bone marrow malignancies or metastatic malignancies
   c. Idiopathic thrombocytopenia purpura (ITP), cause unknown. ITP occurs secondarily to many things and may have an autoimmune mechanism; autoantibodies (IgG) to platelets' protein are often present. ITP is known to occur secondarily to viral infections (especially in children), the administration of quinine and quinidine, pernicious anemia, and paroxysmal nocturnal hemoglobinuria
2. Conditions causing increased destruction, such as
   a. Immune thrombocytopenia
   b. disseminated intravascular clotting (DIC)
3. Conditions causing increased pooling (e.g., splenomegaly)

PLATELET COUNT NORMAL IN NUMBER BUT ABNORMAL IN FUNCTION IN:

1. von Willebrand's disease. Platelets lack the ability to aggregate
2. Persons with high triglyceride levels. Platelets have a decreased ability to aggregate. High cholesterol levels have no effect on platelets

---

*Two terms are used, frequently interchangeably, to describe platelet increase: *thrombocythemia* and *thrombocytosis*. Thrombocytosis seems to refer to an absolute increase in circulating platelets above 500,000/ml. Thrombocythemia is used to describe conditions that involve an increase in the number of megakaryocytes in the bone marrow and an increase in circulating platelets over 1,000,000/µl (Frohlich, 1988).

3. Persons taking a high dosage of aspirin, which causes inhibition of platelet aggregation because of decreased ADP release (a 0.5-mM concentration of aspirin in the blood can be achieved by as little as four 5-g aspirin tablets and can cause a bleeding tendency [Groer & Shekleton, 1983])

4. Nitroglycerin and prostaglandin E_1, which also inhibit platelet aggregation

---

IMPLICATIONS FOR NURSING: PLATELET COUNT

1. Assess for cause of abnormal platelet count: physiological causes for normal changes in platelet levels:
   a. Newborns have fewer platelets during the first few days of life.
   b. Decreases occur for 2 weeks before menstruation. The decrease is progressive over that period and starts to rise again by the third day of menses
   c. Daily variations occur within one individual for unexplained reasons
   d. Compensatory increases are found in high altitudes
   e. Levels are generally higher in winter than in summer
   f. Levels are increased after violent exercise, possibly because of a change in distribution
   g. Platelets can be normal in number but deficient in function; a normal laboratory count does not ensure normal function
2. Determine importance of abnormal platelet count:
   a. Differences in count occur between laboratories. Always use the ranges of the laboratory doing the testing
   b. Only great variations from normal in platelet counts have clinical significance:
      (1) Decreases in count are usually considered of more clinical importance than are increases
      (2) Differences in count less than 25 percent from normal are rarely considered significant
   c. If platelet variation from the norm is greater than 25 percent of normal; if the variation is a decrease and is a major one; if bleeding tendencies are observed and/or if the person is routinely taking drugs that alter platelet function; the nurse should:
      (1) Document significant findings in writing
      (2) Check repeat platelet counts. If not available, request that one be ordered
3. Areas of assessment for cause of abnormal bleeding (thrombocytopenia):
   a. Check pertinent laboratory tests results other than the platelet count (e.g., increased bleeding time; poor clot reaction)
   b. If not available or if no abnormality present, do a comprehensive history of drugs presently in use as well as those taken over the previous week or two. The best documented and most universal offender in causing bleeding is aspirin. (Platelets affected by drugs do not "recover" and will remain ineffective until they disintegrate. Their life span is variable, in a range of 4 to 11 days)
4. Nursing actions to prevent trauma and bleeding:
   a. Provide a soft toothbrush, and instruct the client in its use and the rationale for its use
   b. Advise the use of an electric razor to minimize skin trauma during shaving
   c. Request that medication be given by mouth rather than parenterally, if possible
   d. Reduce trauma related to venipuncture and intravenous administration of medication by:
      (1) Organizing requests for blood work so that as many as possible are done with one sample
      (2) Suggesting the use of a heparin lock for repeated blood sampling if feasible. (Although heparin has an effect on platelet aggregation, this is not its main physiological function in coagulation disorders, and the amount of heparin actually present in the blood tested would be minuscule, especially if the first portion of blood drawn via a haparin lock is discarded. Testing norms could be readily adjusted for the variance, should one occur)

(3) Maintaining patent intravenous (IV) lines to prevent the need for repeated venipunctures. If the facility procedure requires automatic intravenous line restarts after a certain period of time, consult with those responsible to arrange an exception for this individual. Keep diligent watch for irritation or inflammation at the needle site in a long-term IV. Change to a central line pump that can be used over long periods might well be suggested in some instances

e. Maintain skin and mucous membrane integrity by:

    (1) Examining the skin and all mucous membrane (especially of the nose and mouth) at least daily for evidence of bleeding or changes in the amount and pattern of bleeding

    (2) Inflating the blood pressure cuff no more than the mean between previous baseline systole and diastole levels, unless a change in blood pressure is evident. Remove the cuff as soon as possible and try not to have to reinflate it

    (3) Determining any history of excessive menstrual bleeding, tarry stools, nose bleeds, and recent viral infections. (Viral infections are found to cause temporary platelet production failure. It is of special importance in children aged 2 to 6, who tend to have acute idiopathic thromboyctic purpura—postinfectious thrombocytopenia—more frequently than adults [Jones et al., 1982])

    (4) Informing the individual of the reason for the above measures and eliciting his or her cooperation in preventing trauma (e.g., no forceful nose blowing or removal of crusts from nares: use water-soluble gel for application to the nasal mucous membrane to prevent crusting; when up, the patient should wear slippers with hard soles or wear shoes; keep finger and toe nails short and smooth)

f. Be aware of problematic platelet levels to anticipate, prevent if possible, or take immediate corrective action with bleeding or hemorrhagic tendencies

    (1) Platelet counts from 100 to 50,000/mm^3 correspond to a hemorrhagic tendency

    (2) Spontaneous hemorrhage usually does not occur until the count is less than 20,000/mm^3

    (3) Platelet levels under 10,000/mm^3 may be life-threatening

        (a) A person demonstrating such low platelet levels requires intensive nursing care and may require a platelet transfusion

        (b) If a platelet transfusion is probable, the nurse should supply information and explanations about the process, the risks, and the role of donors to the patient and family as soon as possible or reinforce previously given information

        (c) Cross-matching of platelets is not strictly necessary, especially with a single transfusion, but in some cases it is done

        (d) Inquire about presence or history of excessive menstrual bleeding

5. Identify risk populations for thrombosis

    a. With metastatic malignancies, especially of the lung

    b. Over age 60 with sedentary life-style

    c. At bed rest or otherwise immobilized

    d. With atherosclerosis

    e. With diagnosed myeloproliferative syndrome, including polycythemia rubra vera

    f. In acute stress reaction (e.g., post trauma, surgery)

    g. After acute hemorrhage

    h. With severe iron-deficiency disease

    i. With various epithelial malignancies (An important cause for the tendency to venous thrombosis in malignancy is thrombocytosis and increase in fibrinogen. [Laboratory of Pathology, 1991])

6. Implement nursing measures to help prevent thrombus formation in conditions of an increased platelet count (thrombocytosis). Measures to decrease venous stasis include:

    a. Use of properly fitted, properly worn elastic hose, which are removed at least once daily and left off at night if the person sleeps in a prone position. Visually examine the legs when hose are off for evidence of venous stasis (e.g., cool extremities, varicose veins, capillary dilation). Hose should be reapplied with the leg elevated at least to the level of the rest of the body

    b. Frequent change of position, independent or assisted

    c. Sequential elevation of dependent parts of the body

    d. Elimination of any pressure in the popliteal area, (e.g., use no knee pillows)

e. When possible, body weight should be evenly distributed over the largest body area possible: no crossed legs; lying down is better than sitting; sitting is better than standing

f. *No* massage of leg muscles because of risk of embolism entering the bloodstream

g. Bed exercises should be passively instituted, then taught and actively practiced by the patient when possible. Examples of bed exercises include flexion and extension of the knees, alternating the legs; foot lifted from the back of the mattress with the back of the knee pressed to the mattress; flexion, extension, and rotation of the ankle with the heel off the bed; gluteal muscle setting (buttocks tightly contracted, then relaxed)

  (1) Exercises should be done independently by the patient, if possible. Set up mutually agreed-on environmental clues to remind the person of the exercises, such as doing a set of exercises each time a nurse enters the room, or, if that seems to predict too little exercise, each time a commercial comes on television

  (2) Passive range of motion (ROM) is still indicated in a patient at risk for thrombosis, even if that person is up and walking. Not all muscles are used equally in ambulation, and some not at all

h. When the patient is out of bed, similar isometric leg exercises while in a chair need to be taught and positively reinforced. Assessment of the usual clothing worn can be done in preparation for discharge to help eliminate the risks caused by the use of girdles or control top hose. If the patient is overweight, the benefits of weight loss should also be explored

i. Suggest and encourage swimming or wading in water as a recreational pursuit, or if a pool is available in the physical therapy department, consult with appropriate members of the health team to foster this activity while the person is hospitalized. Water exerts equal pressure about the leg, and during wading, the water pressure is exerted most strongly in the area with the most need of venous support. Muscular activity requires less effort when swimming, with an equal increase in muscle pumping of blood

3.12 GENERAL IMPLICATIONS FOR NURSING RELATED TO PROBLEMS IN COAGULATION

1. Observe persons with undiagnosed bleeding problems carefully for the origin of bleeding. Although the specific diagnosis is ultimately made by the physician primarily on the basis of laboratory data, data collected by the nurse based on the following generalizations can also be helpful. Bleeding into deep tissue spaces or joints usually indicates a coagulation disorder, whereas superficial bleeding is more often due to a vascular or platelet disorder (Caprini, 1973)

2. Principles that are helpful in understanding how diagnoses of coagulation defects are made include:

   a. Factors I, II, V, VII, IX, and X are synthesized in the liver; therefore, liver disease may affect their production

   b. Liver-synthesized factors II, VII, IX, and X depend on vitamin K; therefore, any process that interferes with vitamin K intake, absorption, or utilization may affect their production

   c. Only factors I, II, V, VIII, and XIII and platelets are consumed in the process of blood clotting. Other factors act as true enzymes. Therefore, in conditions of rapid or prolonged clotting (e.g., DIC), the listed factors may be depleted

   d. Banked blood as well as platelets will be deficient in factors V and VIII because they are unstable on storage. Replacements are possible only with fresh blood or plasma

e. Platelets, which must be used immediately, and cryoprecipitate, which can be frozen and is rich in factors I and VIII, are commonly removed from banked blood for individual administration (see Table 13–4)

3. Certain requirements should be met in obtaining blood samples for coagulation tests. Although this activity is not always the responsibility of the nurse, seeing that the requirements are met may well be in order to ensure valid test results:

a. Select a vein of adequate caliber; the use of the veins on the back of the hand is not recommended

b. Use at least a 19-gauge, thin-walled needle to help prevent hemolysis

c. A clean venipuncture (no residual bruising) will give the most accurate results

d. Before use, the first few milliliters of blood collected should be discarded to remove tissue thromboplastin generated by the tissue trauma of venipuncture

e. The tourniquet should not be left in place for over 1 minute because stasis facilitates blood clotting and changes the normal distribution of blood cells

f. Use only a very light pressure to immobilize the vein without compressing it. This avoids mobilizing vessel wall enzymes that can falsely elevate fibrinolytic levels (Caprini, 1976)

g. Usually, blood should not be taken from a patient who was given heparin within 6 hours before the time of sample taking, and blood is best taken from the arm without a heparin lock

4. Complete an accurate history taking and physical appraisal are of great importance in the determination of the cause and thus the treatment of bleeding disorders. In addition to those observations suggested with the nursing implications for platelet estimation (Section 2.3.2) and those given with individual tests in this chapter, the nurse can assist the physician in the assessment process by observation or inquiry into the following areas:

a. Duration of bleeding tendency—lifelong or of only recent origin

b. Presence of chronic disease originating before or concurrent with the bleeding problem, especially hepatic or renal disease

c. Diet history, with special emphasis on deficiencies in protein, fat, and vitamins K or C intake

d. In the newborn, bleeding from the umbilicus that is prolonged or occurring after normal clotting time (24 to 48 hours). This may indicate a defect of the extrinsic pathway or a fibrin defect. Inquire into the family history about bleeding or a consanguineous union (such bleeding is a hallmark of a rare autosomal recessive trait)

5. Active observation should be done for bleeding or thrombosis in all risk populations (e.g., at the time of delivery [bleeding], the elderly [thrombophlebitis], patients with a medical history of bleeding problems in themselves or their families). With these persons it would be sensible to perform guaiac or Hemoccult tests on all urine, stools, or vomitus

6. Institute nursing actions to reduce trauma and prevent bleeding. Review "Implications for Nursing" in Section 2.3.2. In addition:

a. Teach and help the person to practice good dental hygiene to prevent extractions and probable severe hemorrhage

b. Avoid taking rectal temperatures because of the possibility of damage to the fragile mucous membrane, particularly if the platelet count is less than $20,000/mm^3$

    c. Persons taking oral anticoagulants may be advised by their physicians to carry vitamin K at all times. This individual may need instruction as to the purpose and effect of vitamin K and how to use it in self-treatment of spontaneous hemorrhage

7. Despite the need for calcium in almost all the steps of the coagulation process, a low serum calcium level is not considered a cause of abnormal bleeding. A deficiency of calcium low enough to cause bleeding is incompatible with life (Sodeman & Sodeman, 1982)

F O U R

URINALYSIS SCREEN: URINALYSIS ROUTINE

The routine urinalysis is one of the first tests used in identification of pathology of the urinary tract and is an indispensable part of clinical pathology. It can provide an estimate of renal function, give information as to possible causes for dysfunction, and can even indicate systemic disease. Urinalysis is a careful, systematic study of the physical, chemical, and microscopic properties of urine. Data thus obtained help provide only a tentative diagnosis at times, but at the same time guide the selection of more specific tests for more definitive diagnosis.

Tests commonly included in a routine urinalysis are gross examination, specific gravity, pH, glucose, protein, ketone bodies, occult blood, bilirubin, and a microscopic examination of the urinary sediment if indicated or ordered. To understand the implications of abnormalities in results to these tests, it is necessary to understand how urine is formed.

4.1 PHYSIOLOGY OF URINE PRODUCTION

Urine is formed by the filtering of plasma through the glomeruli, the selective reabsorption and secretion activity of the tubules, and the excretion of the formed urine by the urinary tract. All blood circulating through the body eventually passes through the kidney. The blood enters the nephron(s) of the kidney at the glomerulus. Glomerular filtration occurs in almost exactly the same manner that fluid is filtered out of any high-pressure capillary. The filtrate leaves most of its protein content in the capillaries. If the glomerulus is healthy, the resulting plasma, which contains most of the organic and inorganic chemicals of the blood (e.g., glucose, amino acids, urea, uric acid, sodium, potassium, chloride, and bicarbonate) goes into the tubule system of the nephron (Fig. 4–1). The tubules selectively secrete waste products not useful to the body and reabsorb those needed by the body (Table 4–1). The waste products, together with at least enough water to keep them in solution, are excreted into the kidney pelvis, ureter, and bladder to be removed from the body when sufficient amounts of this waste solution, now called urine, stretch and stimulate the bladder muscles to contract (see also "Physiology" in Section 4.6, urine specific gravity).

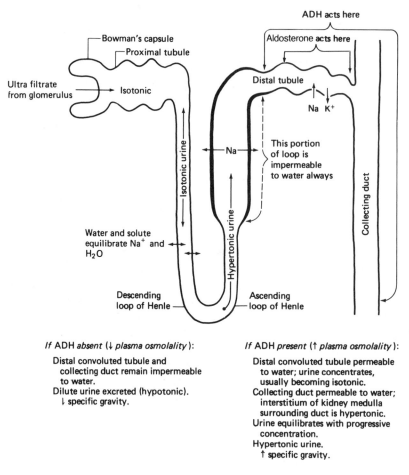

Figure 4–1. Dilution and concentration of urine. (Adapted by Tami Bruce from Harvey, A. M., Johns, R. J., McKosick, V. A., et al. [1968]. *Principles and Practice of Medicine* (19th ed.). New York: Appleton-Century-Crofts, with permission.)

Some 180 L of fluid are filtered daily in the healthy adult. The filtrate forms approximately 1 to 1½ L of urine. About 25,000 mEq of sodium and 25 g of urea, the major inorganic and organic solutes, are processed with the water, and of that amount, about 150 mEq of sodium and 15 g of urea are excreted.

There are some age-related physiological changes in kidney function. Urine osmolality decreases slowly from a high at age 30 to a low at age 80, and other slight tubular function changes occur as a result of a loss of tubular cell mass with age progression. In infancy all renal functions are less efficient because of immaturity; however, these changes are not felt to be clinically important in the healthy infant or older person. They do pose a threat in illness or in an imbalance of fluid, electrolytes, or acid-base levels because of their influence on the body's ability to adapt.

TABLE 4–1. SEGMENTAL FUNCTIONS OF THE RENAL TUBULES

Segment	Functions
Proximal tubule	Reabsorption 　70% filtered H_2O and NaCl 　Glucose 　Urea 　Uric acid 　Amino acids 　K^+, Mg^+, Ca^{2+}, HPO^- 　HCO_3 (reabsorbed and regenerated; accomplished through secretion of H^-) Secretion 　Organic acids and bases 　H^+ and NH_3
Henle's loop	Reabsorption through countercurrent multiplier NaCl in excess of H_2O
Distal tubule	Reabsorption 　Filtered H_2O and NaCl (small fraction only) Secretion 　H^+, NH_3, K^+ (depends on aldosterone concentration)
Collecting ducts	Reabsorption 　NaCl 　H_2O (depends on ADH concentration) 　Urea Secretion 　H^+, NH_3 (pH of urine may be reduced to 4.5–5.0) 　K^+ (depends on aldosterone concentration)

Abbreviations: ADH, antidiuretic hormone; HPO^-, phosphate.

From Maureen E. Groer, & Shekleton, M. E. (1983). *Basic Pathophysiology: A Conceptual Approach* (2nd ed). St. Louis: C. V. Mosby, p. 342, with permission.

Individual renal thresholds vary, sometimes widely, and nursing assessment should include the possibility.

4.2 PATHOPHYSIOLOGY OF URINE PRODUCTION

Dysfunction of urine formation and excretion has a profound effect on the body's homeostasis. The kidney is primarily a volume organ. Although one of its major functions is to excrete waste, that process depends on an adequate circulatory volume that is composed of a specific balance of certain chemicals and water. Should fluid volume decrease, more waste will be retained; if there is a proportional increase of solute to water, additional water is required to remove additional solute. The kidney strives to maintain the body's extracellular fluid (ECF) osmolality at a norm, usually 285 mOsm. The person with renal insufficiency loses this flexibility. The lack of or a decrease in the functional ability of either antidiuretic hormone (ADH) or aldosterone can alter the kidney's flexibility as well because kidney function is controlled mostly by these hormones.

When circulatory volume decreases, the glomerular filtration rate (GFR) will also decrease. Any alteration in the GFR will alter urine production. This can be due to changes in arterial blood pressure for any reason, an increase or decrease in oncotic pressure (pressure of plasma proteins), an increase in glomerular permeability (e.g., nephrotic syndrome), or a decrease in the filtration area of the glomeruli.

The next priority for kidney function, after volume, is that of acid-base balance. The kidney works to excrete fixed acids in the free state as well as in combination as titratable acids and ammonium; it also reabsorbs bicarbonate (HCO_3) as needed. When the extracellular volume (ECV) is threatened, however, that threat takes precedence, and the kidney is stimulated to increase sodium reabsorption in exchange for hydrogen (H^+) or potassium ions (K^+) by means of the distal tubule's cation pump to maintain the ECV despite any effect on the acid-base balance. This is the basis for persistent metabolic alkalosis resulting from a K^+ or chloride (Cl^-) deficit.

4.3 RISK POPULATIONS

Senior adults, especially females, are more prone to urinary tract infections (UTI) that are due in part to the shortness of the urethra, a decreased immunologic response, a delayed and prolonged kidney response in acid-base regulation, and decreased tubular cell mass. Glucose reabsorption is also decreased. Glucose absorption is also increased in the elderly, which can enhance nutritional problems.

Newborns have a less efficient buffer system, both in the blood and in the kidney, and acidosis is more likely to develop in newborns. The kidney's ability to adapt to changes in serum Na^+ levels is reduced, which leads to fluid volume problems, and as in the elderly, the infant's kidney reabsorbs glucose less efficiently (Whaley & Wong, 1991).

Pregnancy also predisposes females to UTI because of the occurrence of dilation of the urethra and urinary stasis.

4.4 GROSS EXAMINATION OF URINE

Synonym: Visual examination of urine

Normal Ranges

Color	Pale to dark yellow
Transparency	Clear or slightly cloudy
Odor	Mild, faintly pungent, or aromatic

The appearance and odor of a urine specimen are often reported only when they are abnormal. Newborns and the aged tend to have less ability to concentrate urine; therefore, the urine is more likely to be pale when normal. When less precise laboratory measurements were available, much unwarranted importance was given to the gross characteristics of urine. Presently, such examination does not, perhaps, receive enough attention. Active awareness of changes in the characteristics of a patient's urine is highly recommended as an independent nursing action of no small value (Table 4–2).

TABLE 4–2. CHANGES IN URINE AND CORRESPONDING NURSING ACTION

Change in Urine	Cause	Related Nursing Action
Color and transparency Colorless	Very dilute because of inability to concentrate (infant, diabetes insipidus, inappropriate ADH in some diuretics), increased fluid intake	Check history; monitor intake and output (temporary increased output = diuresis; prolonged = polyuria); observe for change
Cloudy	Most often due to phosphate precipitation in alkaline urine	Report; manipulate diet to provide acid ash foods, restrict alkaline ash
	Presence of phosphates, carbonates, urates, uric acid (precipitate in acid urine)	Report; manipulate diet to provide alkaline ash foods, restrict acid ash (see "Implications for Nursing," Section 1.7)
	Presence of leukocytes, bacteria, yeasts, clumps of pus, calculi, gravel	Depends on how specimen is obtained; may be normal; observe urine and patient for signs/symptoms of UTI
Smoky	Microscopic hematuria, minimal red cells, prostatic fluid, spermatozoa; mucin, mucous threads	Usually normal urine, possible menses
Milky	Many polymorphonuclear (PMN) leukocytes (pyuria)	Obtain culture; institute infection control measures
	Chyluria (filariasis)	Check for lymph enlargement, especially of lower extremities
Opalescent	Fat from nephrosis; crush injuries, especially of long bones	Check for concentrated urine, signs and symptoms of renal insufficiency; monitor for potential fat embolism
	Bacteria	Check for characteristic unpleasant ammonia odor; obtain culture
Bright yellow	Many drugs (e.g., acriflavine, quinacrine [Atabrine], nitrofurantoin [Furadantin], riboflavin—large doses)	Instruct patient/family that this color change is an expected effect; instruction best if done before medication started
Yellow-orange	Concentrated urine because of increased metabolic rate (fever, thyroid increase), lack of water intake, or excessive losses (dehydration)	Increase water intake if appropriate; place on intake; determine cause of losses and correct if possible or refer
	Urobilin in excess because of liver or gallbladder disorders (colorless until exposed to light)	Will cause a white or colorless persistent foam when shaken

(continued)

TABLE 4–2. (Continued)

Change in Urine	Cause	Related Nursing Action
	Bilirubinuria because of liver or gallbladder disorder	Will cause a yellow persistent foam when shaken
		Both indicate a bilirubin disorder (see "Implications for Nursing," Section 1.10)
	Phenazopyridine (Pyridium) (urinary disinfectant)	Instruct patient/family that this is an expected effect
Yellow-green	Bilirubin—biliverdin due to bilirubin dysfunction, possible hemolysis; some drugs: senna, cascara; some foods: rhubarb	Causes a yellow persistent foam when shaken (see "Implications for Nursing," Section 1.10); assess bowel management; assess diet
Red	Hemoglobin (Hbg) (bright red when fresh) resulting from intravascular hemolysis greater than haptoglobin can bind	Seek source, report (possible transfusion reaction) (see Table 13.6); check RBC count, Hgb, and hematocrit (Hct)
	Red blood cells (RBCs) because of trauma of urinary tract/kidney or may be menstrual contamination	Seek source; if not menstrual, blood in urine always significant; report and follow up with routine urine specimens
	Myoglobin	Look for muscle damage; report
	Porphyrin because of genetic disease (colorless until exposed to light)	Check medical history; report
	Phenindione (Hedulin) (anticoagulant similar to coumarin)	Causes benign color change in alkaline urine, inform patient and family to expect this; the drug can also cause urinary bleeding with similar color changes that can be differentiated by acidifying urine; benign color change will disappear
	Some foods: beets, candy, and some other foods containing fuscin dye	Response to beets is genetic; check diet history for possibly dyed foods
	Menses	Look for accompanying clots and mucus
Red-pink	Phenophthalein (found in many laxatives, e.g., Ex-Lax, Feen-a-mint); senna, cascara, rhubarb	Usually occurs in response to the drugs and/or food listed when urine is alkaline; check medications being taken and inform patient and family of cause-and-effect relationship when found
	Sulfobromophthelein and phenolsulfonphthalein used in certain gallbladder tests	Inform patient of possible color change of urine after test and that it is temporary

TABLE 4–2. (Continued)

Change in Urine	Cause	Related Nursing Action
Red-purple	Phenolphthalein	As above
	Porphyrin	As above
Red-brown	RBC, older cells	As above
	Hemoglobin on standing	As above
	Methemoglobin (an abnormal hemoglobin associated with excessive smoking or heavy-metal poisoning)	Assess smoking history and record; check complete blood count (CBC) for report of basophilic stipling of white blood cells (WBCs) (lead intoxication); record findings, report if positive
	Myoglobin	As above
Brown-black	Methemoglobin	As above
	Homogentisic acid resulting from a rare genetic disorder—alkaptonuria	Color change occurs in alkaline urine on standing
	Phenols; melanin resulting from Addison's disease, but a rare occurrence	As above
Blue-green	Dyes used in diagnostic tests and/or in medications (e.g., Evans blue, methylene blue, indigo carmine, indicans) such as Urised	Inform patient and family about to have such tests or recieve medication containing dyes of the probability of urine color change
	Pseudomonas infection	Check for characteristic odor (rather pleasant, fruity, but somewhat cloying); obtain culture if necessary to establish diagnosis; requires antibiotic susceptibility test before treatment because of resistance to many antibiotics[a]
Odor—physiological changes		
Strong, sharp, vitamin B, penicillin-like	Multivitamin ingestion	If client or family is upset by urine odor, it is sometimes helpful to explain the cause
Pungent, grasslike	Asparagus	Foods can be avoided
Penetrating, ammoniacal	Decomposing urine	Urine should be disposed of as soon as possible
Odor—pathological changes		
Sweet, heavy, thick (at times described as pleasant/fruity)	*Pseudomonas* infection	See "Blue-green" above
Stale urine, ammoniacal	Uremic acidosis	See "Implications in Nursing," Section 1.5
Acetone odor, heavy, sickening, sweet	Ketonuria with diabetic acidosis; lighter or no odor, usually with	Ketonuria associated with glucosuria places the patient

(continued)

TABLE 4–2. (Continued)

Change in Urine	Cause	Related Nursing Action
	appearance of ketones in urine in starvation	at special risk for infection and overgrowth of monilial infection, especially in women; frequent and meticulous perineal care needed
Sharp, acid, "fishy," unpleasant even fresh; as it becomes older, more markedly ammoniacal	UTI—bacterial	Culture and sensitivity tests should be run and followed by treatment; depending on medication used, the urine pH may need manipulation, so frequent pH checks should be made; maintain urine at most advantageous pH; increase fluid intake as appropriate
"Mousy," "horsey," musty odor—in infant	Phenylketonuria	Report notice of odor; routine testing usually done for this condition on newborns (see Section 15.2.4.C)
Asparagus odor	Hepatic failure	Less noticeable odor in urine than in other body secretions such as breath vapor
Fecal odor	Usually due to a rectal fistula	Report; institute infection control measures (see Section 5 Nursing Implications Specimen Collection)

Abbreviations: PMN, polymorphonuclear (leukocytes); Hgb, hemoglobin; RBC, red blood cell; Hct, hematocrit; CBC, complete blood count; WBC, white blood cell.
[a]This section from Beck, 1971; Davidsohn & Henry, 1969; Govoni & Hayes, 1985; Harrington & Brenner, 1973; Price & Wilson, 1992; Ravel, 1989; Watson, 1979.
Other data from Beck, 1983; Sorensen & Luckmann, 1979; Whaley & Wong, 1991.

4.5 pH OF URINE

Synonyms: None

Normal Ranges

Adult	5–7 pH units[a]
Senior adult	No age-specific difference
Pediatric	
Newborn/Neonatal	5–7
Thereafter	4.5–8

[a]This normal range is for a group of hospitalized persons, a group that might be expected to have a more alkaline urine than the general population because of the combination of the effects of immobility and posttraumatic tendency to extracellular alkalosis (Sabiston, 1981).

Definition. The urine pH is a fairly simple test to perform. It reflects the kidneys' ability to maintain the hydrogen ion (H^+) concentration of the body's plasma and ECF.

Physiology. Ultimately it is the kidneys' function to correct acid-base disturbances. Its action is more thorough and selective than that of body buffers and respiratory control. The urine can sustain an H^+ concentration 1000 times greater than that of the blood. The maximum urine acidity is pH 4.5; that of blood is 7.35. The kidney can eliminate hydrogen in three ways:

1. Formation of ammonia (NH_3) in the distal tubular cells (60 to 75 percent of all H^+ is excreted from the body by this mechanism)
2. Excretion as a titratable acid (e.g., sulfuric, phosphoric, hydrochloric, pyruvic, lactic, citric) and some ketones from the glomerulus and the proximal tubule (25 to 40 percent of all H^+ is excreted by this method)
3. Excretion as free H^+ in exchange for Na^+, which usually returns a bicarbonate ion with it

The process has the net result of conserving sodium and bicarbonate and excreting the acid products of metabolism. More acid than alkali is formed by the body in its metabolic process, yet the normal ratio of bicarbonate to acid is 20:1 in the body. This results in an acid urine in health.

Physiological Alterations in Urine pH

1. Alkaline urine occurs in (increased pH)
   a. Infancy. Hydrogen excretion is reduced—less acid is secreted—in the first year of life. In the first few days of life the infant has a diminished capacity to produce ammonium ions as well
   b. Urine that has been left standing because of the loss of carbon dioxide or the action of some bacteria on urine
   c. Individuals receiving a primarily vegetarian diet
2. Urine pH increases after a meal because of the increased secretion of HCl into the stomach for digestion (alkaline tide, reducing blood pH)
3. Urine pH decreases (increased acidity) in
   a. Early morning urine samples or after any fairly prolonged period of sleep because of the mild respiratory acidosis occurring with sleep and the renal compensation to that acidosis
   b. Individuals receiving a diet high in meat protein and some fruits (e.g., cranberries [acid ash])

Pathophysiological Alterations in Urine pH

1. Alkaline urine occurs in (increased pH)
   a. Renal disease such as
      (1) Chronic glomerulonephritis because of decreased glomerular filtration, which causes a diminished excretion of phosphate, sulfate, and other acid buffers
      (2) Renal tubular acidosis because of impaired distal tubular function, which causes a decreased ability to exchange H^+ (secretion) and a decreased formation of ammonia

     b. Metabolic or respiratory alkalosis from any cause as a result of the kidneys' compensatory action in retaining H^+ and eliminating excess base. Ammonia production is also decreased

     c. Hypoaldosteronism (Addison's disease) at times because of H^+ retention secondary to sodium loss. Potassium often is retained, even preferentially, which allows H^+ to be excreted. In that case the urine pH would be within normal limits

     d. The presence of some bacterial infections (e.g., *Pseudomonas, Proteus*)

     e. Individuals who are immobilized

  2. Increases in urine acidity occur in (decreased pH)

     a. Metabolic acidosis and respiratory acidosis from any cause as a compensatory response to retain bicarbonate and eliminate excess acid. Titratable acid production is increased, as in ammonia production

     b. Hypokalemic, hypochloremic alkalosis (such as occurs in hyperaldosteronism or with prolonged vomiting). This is a paradoxical aciduria that occurs despite the presence of metabolic alkalosis. Both K^+ and H^+ are excreted in response to the elevated aldosterone levels, which obligates Na^+ reabsorption. In the absence of chloride, bicarbonate is reabsorbed with the Na^+, thereby prolonging the alkalotic state and increasing urine acidity

Pharmacological Alteration in Urine pH. Although alkalinity may occur only as a side effect of the administraton of drugs, drugs can be given specifically for that purpose. Usually this is done to facilitate the action of other drugs that are most effective in an alkaline medium (e.g., neomycin, kanamycin, streptomycin, sulfadiazine, and sulfamerazine).

Acidic urine suppresses the growth of both gram-negative and gram-positive organisms, including *Escherichia coli, Staphylococcus aureus, staphylococcus albus,* and some streptococci. Gram-negative organisms are one of the most frequent urinary tract contaminants. *E. coli* accounts for roughly 80 percent of cultured infections.

  1. Alkaline urine occurs with the administration of

     a. Excess amounts of sodium bicarbonate and other antacids that are absorbable (e.g., calcium carbonate [Tums], magnesium hydroxide)

     b. Potassium citrate, sometimes used as an expectorant with other drugs or as potassium replacement as in K-Lyte

     c. Acetazolamide (Diamox) or other carbonic anhydrase inhibitors (e.g., methazolamide [Neptazane])

     d. Chlorothiazide (Diuril), a diuretic that promotes K^+ loss and bicarbonate excretion

  2. Acidic urine occurs with the administration of:

     a. Ammonium chloride, sometimes used as a mild expectorant, a diuretic, or systemic acidifier. It is only effective in creating acidic urine for short periods of 1 to 2 days because of the renal compensatory mechanisms it stimulates.

     b. Methenamine mandelate (Mandelamine). However, the use of this drug or other methenamine compounds such as methenamine hippurate (Hip-Rex) contributes to urine acidification only when the urine pH is at 5.5 or less at the time of administration

     c. Methionine, which is useful over prolonged periods

     d. Ascorbic acid

IMPLICATIONS FOR NURSING: pH OF URINE

See "General Implications for Nursing, Urine Screen" at the end of this chapter.

4.6 SPECIFIC GRAVITY OF URINE

Synonyms: None

Normal Ranges[a]

Adult	1.003–1.030
Senior adult	1.016–1.022
Pediatric	
Newborn	1.001–1.020
Thereafter	1.001–1.030

[a]1 unit specific gravity = 40 mOsm.

Definition. The urine specific gravity test can be defined as a comparison of the weight of urine with the weight of an equal volume of distilled water. It can also be defined as a measurement of density, which depends not only on weight but also on the number of solute particles in solution. This definition is probably a more accurate reflection of the kidney function being measured. The kidneys' capacity to concentrate is related to the concentration of particles in a solution (osmolality), not to their weight. The correlation between specific gravity and osmolality is close enough to use specific gravity as a clinical guide to urine osmolality, even though methods for measuring specific gravity are not as precise as those for measuring osmolality.

It is a relatively simple, inexpensive, and convenient method for evaluation of the kidneys' ability to dilute and concentrate urine. The test gives some information about renal tubular function.

Physiology. The cells of the kidney tubules in each nephron function to modify the glomerular filtrate presented to them by removing some of the substance from the filtrate (tubular reabsorption) or by adding more of a substance to the filtrate (tubular secretion). Most of the reabsorption occurs in the proximal tubule. In a healthy kidney with a "normal" filtrate, about 98 percent of the filtrate is reabsorbed. It is through this process of tubular absorption and secretion that the final composition of urine is determined. Part of the process is the ability of the tubules to respond to the osmolality of the filtrate and keep it constant. This serves to either concentrate or dilute the urine. Figure 4–1 describes the fairly specific process of tubular function by nephron segments.

The function of concentration of urine is directly under the control of ADH. Na^+ and water diffuse passively in or out of the descending limb of Henle's loop as the interstitial and intravascular fluids equilibrate with the glomerular filtrate; however, in the ascending loop, the membrane is impermeable to water, and Na^+ must be actively transported out of that section of the loop. Beyond this point, at the beginning of the distal convoluted tubule, ADH, if present, acts on the membrane to allow water to flow out. If ADH is absent, the entire distal tubule is impermeable to water, and the hypotonic urine produced in the ascending portion of Henle's loop is excreted unchanged. The collecting ducts, under the influence of ADH, progressively concentrate the urine (see Fig. 4–1) (Harvey et al., 1991).

Pathophysiology. In renal disease and in many conditions causing renal dysfunction, the mechanism most commonly lost is the ability to concentrate urine, which can threaten or cause severe water loss. A specific example of this occurrence is found in pyelonephritis. The kidney no longer responds to the presence of ADH. The actual loss of the hormone, as in diabetes insipidus, will obviously cause the inability to concentrate urine. Yet, there is otherwise a relatively normal tubular function.

Concentration of urine depends in part on the amount of water available for excretion, assuming adequate ADH secretion and the kidneys' ability to respond to it. The amount of water available for excretion, then, in turn depends on the amount of water taken in, the amount lost through the lungs or skin, and the amount of blood perfusing the kidney. In conditions of reduced blood perfusion of the kidney, renin is secreted, and angiotensin and aldosterone are produced, all of which enhance the production of a highly concentrated urine almost without sodium.

Although there is a general, moderate decrease in specific gravity with aging, the decrease is not thought to influence findings in any clinically important way, being a reflection of the loss of cell mass rather than a loss of function of the existing tubules.

During the neonatal period an infant's GFR is very low and remains low for several months. In addition, an infant's ability to concentrate urine is very limited. The infant then has the potential for difficulty in both concentration and dilution of urine.

SPECIFIC GRAVITY INCREASED IN:

1. Inaccurate reading because of the use of too small an amount of urine for testing or too narrow a vessel in proportion to the size of the urinometer
2. Inaccurate reading because of the use of refrigerated urine or urine that is colder or warmer than room temperature (20°C). A correction by adding 0.001 for each 3°C the sample is above or by subtracting 0.001 for each 3°C the sample is below 20°C should be made (Henry, 1991). Normal room temperatures may be calculated differently in different places. Check the local laboratory for the proper calculation
3. Individuals who have had an intravenous pyelogram for a day or two after injection of the dye
4. States of dehydration or water deprivation because of a lack of available water to be excreted. This can occur in many situations and conditions (e.g., diarrhea; vomiting; excessive sweating; inability to respond to thirst, as with decreased levels of consciousness)
5. Excessive ingestion of sodium chloride, which causes true hypernatremia
6. Urine with glucose or protein in excessive amounts (e.g., uncontrolled diabetes mellitus, nephrotic syndrome)
7. States causing a decreased GFR such as shock or heart failure

SPECIFIC GRAVITY DECREASED IN:

1. Conditions that increase the GFR such as severe hyperthyroidism or fever
2. Conditions causing decreased tubular absorption such as
   a. Diabetes insipidus because of the loss of hormonal influence of ADH
   b. Early pyelonephritis

   c. Occasionally sickle cell anemia

   d. Acute renal failure. The specific gravity is fixed at 1.00 to 1.012

3. Individuals on diets severely restricted in salt or protein because of an inadequate intake of solute

4. Individuals taking potent diuretics that decrease the tubular reabsorption of salt and water

5. Individuals having a marked increase in water intake. This can occur because of the oral intake or parenteral administration of electrolyte-free solutions such as 5% glucose in water

6. Severe K^+ deficiency or calcium excess because of a possible inhibition of tubular reabsorption

7. Inaccurately measured samples because of the use of warm urine. Urine measured when it is at 35°C will measure 0.005 too low (see the correction formula given in "Specific Gravity Increased in" earlier in this section)

8. Urine containing large amounts of urea

IMPLICATIONS FOR NURSING: SPECIFIC GRAVITY OF URINE

The nurse can perform specific gravity tests totally independently and without increasing the patient's cost for care. Because the procedure can be so helpful in determining the state of hydration of a patient and can also indicate acute renal failure, the nurse should not only become adept at the technique but also should become as knowledgeable as possible about the implications of the changes in specific gravity values.

1. Test procedure (urinometer)*
   a. The urine sample should be fresh and at room temperature. It should also be well mixed, that is, it should be a representative sampling of the urine. Urine taken from the bottom of a catheter bag, for example, would not yield accurate results
   b. Check that the urinometer to be used is the correct size for the container. There are varying sizes available, and the urinometer from one set, used with the container of another, will produce inaccurate readings
   c. Test the urinometer if unsure of container size or accuracy of the calibration by filling the container at least three-fourths full of distilled water. (In many areas tap water contains many solutes and should not be used.) Insert the urinometer (process given in f). The reading should be 1.000. If the reading is incorrect, be sure to correct your urine sample reading by the same variation. Have the urinometer recalibrated as soon as possible
   d. Dry the urinometer thoroughly before using for the test
   e. Fill the container with urine—three fourths at least or to the marked level. There must be sufficient fluid to "float" the urinometer
   f. Insert the urinometer gently without allowing it to touch the sides or bottom of the container. Before releasing the urinometer, twist it between the finger and thumb to cause it to spin. It should then float freely without touching the sides or bottom of the container
   g. Read with the meniscus of the fluid at eye level
   h. The urinometer is calibrated with lines similar to those of a thermometer. The denser the solution, the higher the meter will float in it. Therefore, the greater numbers are toward the base, the smaller ones toward the top. The numbers usually range from 1.060 to 1.000
2. Correlation with other tests

---

* Electronic measurement (refractometers), a much simpler and more accurate procedure, available in many health settings.

   a. Specific gravity should correlate fairly closely with osmolality. A minimum specific gravity of urine is 1.001, which corresponds with about 40 mOsm. The maximum specific gravity of urine is about 1.040 or 41.6 mOsm (1 unit of specific gravity = 40 mOsm)
   b. Specific gravity can be expected to be increased in the presence of glucosuria or proteinuria. It will be decreased in the presence of increased urea excretion
   c. Specific gravity exerts effects on other tests. The patient demonstrating proteinuria will appear to have a greater amount of protein in the urine in the face of an increased specific gravity. The amount of protein excreted remains the same, but its concentration in solution changes, depending on whether the urine is dilute, normal, or concentrated

3. General guidelines for evaluating specific gravity findings
   a. The specific gravity of an individual kept n.p.o. overnight should be at least 1.022 to be considered normal (Henry, 1991)
   b. If the urine does not concentrate overnight, this may be an early sign of renal disease
   c. Expect a decreased urine specific gravity in persons on diets severely restricted in sodium or protein because of the decrease in available solute
   d. A first morning urine specimen tested for specific gravity might be considered adequate if it reaches 1.016, given that it is negative for glucose or protein
   e. The oliguria of acute renal failure can be differentiated from that of a water deficit by the presence of a fixed specific gravity of 1.010 to 1.012 in acute renal failure

4. Special concerns in caring for infants:
   a. Because of their limited ability to concentrate urine, infants require feedings rich in protein, which help increase the urine concentration
   b. Urea excretion is hampered in the infant because of the difficulty in urine concentration. To ensure excretion of urea, the protein-rich feedings must contain adequate amounts of water—an excellent rationale for breast-feeding
   c. At times it is difficult to acquire enough urine (approximately 15 ml with small urinometer sets) for a specific gravity test for the infant. There are available on the market so-called specific gravity beads, supplied in a series of different weights, that will sink in urine of equal or matching specific gravity. The weight is inscribed on the bead; however, even this method requires 10 ml of urine

4.7 URINE GLUCOSE

Synonym: Urine sugar[a]

Normal Range: Random test: negative for all age groups
                   24-hr urine test: 0–0.25 g/24-hr specimen

[a]The term *urine fractional* may still be heard as a synonym for a urine glucose test, particularly those tests done outside the laboratory. The so-called fractional was once the gold standard for urine testing. It has been supplanted by the methods described in this section. The urine fractional was the testing of a certain group of urine voidings, excreted in a given time frame. The purpose was to determine when the most glucose was excreted and plan insulin dosage accordingly. An example of timing and procedure is as follows. All urine voided during the period between breakfast and lunch (e.g., 7:00 A.M. to 12:00 noon) is collected in a container. The collection is mixed, and a sample (an aliquot) is tested for glucose and acetone. A second collection is then started from 12:00 noon to 5:00 P.M., a third from 5:00 to 10:00 P.M. and a final collection made from 10:00 P.M. to 6:00 A.M., each collection being tested when complete (Phipps et al, 1983).

Definition. The random urine glucose test is a qualitative test, that is, one that simply determines the presence or absence of a substance. Although it is sometimes used in the laboratory as part of a routine urinalysis, it is probably more often used by other health care workers and the clients themselves to monitor diabetic control. Over time the pattern of control can be estimated by using Clinitest tablets or various dipstick and tape methods. Urine testing has never been a *pre-*

cise measure of diabetic control, and blood glucose testing has become the method of choice ever since simple and accurate means have been available for use. However, urine testing is still a very useful alternative for the person to whom cost or the discomfort of blood glucose monitoring is a concern. The elderly with noninsulin-dependent diabetes mellitus (NIDDM) are probably as well if not better served by urine glucose monitoring.

Urine testing is done by using a dipstick dipped into the urine sample, a test strip or tape on which drops of urine are placed, or a Clinitest tablet. The Clinitest is a reduction test. Certain metal ions are included in the tablet and are reduced (heat reaction, forming a precipitate) when glucose is present in the urine. The reaction changes the color of the urine; however, the Clinitest reaction is not specific for glucose alone. The presence of other sugars (fructose, galactose, lactose, maltose, and xylose) or substances such as ascorbic acid can trigger the same reaction. Because of this, test strips, tapes, or dipsticks are more frequently used. The chemical response for these agents is an enzymatic one. The testing material is impregnated with glucose oxidase, which is very sensitive to the presence of glucose and changes color at very low concentrations (0.1 g/dl). The Clinitest is sometimes used as a confirmatory test after a positive strip or dipstick test result.

Physiology. When the blood sugar level, specifically glucose, rises, the glomerular filtrate may contain more glucose than can be reabsorbed. Tubular reabsorption of glucose is limited by the concentration of an enzyme necessary to the process in the tubule cell. The rate limit is approximately 350 mg/min. When this rate is exceeded, the excess glucose is excreted into the urine. The result is glucosuria. The blood level at which this spillover occurs is approximately 170 mg/dl and is called the *renal threshold* for glucose. The concentration thus spilled into the urine is sufficient to be detected by the usual screening methods. Variations from this threshold norm can and do appear on an individual basis.

Pathophysiology. The most frequent cause of glucosuria, at least in the adult, is diabetes mellitus in which the lack of insulin or the presence of ineffective insulin causes increased blood glucose levels; however, nine other precipitants of increased glucose levels and subsequent glucosuria have been listed previously (see "Serum Glucose Levels Increased in" in Section 1.4).

Glucosuria can occur without increased blood glucose levels, although it occurs much less frequently. Renal diabetes, also known as renal glucosuria or nondiabetic glucosuria, is so named because of the source of the defect, a renal tubular deficiency in the reabsorption of glucose. This defect, coupled with two other renal defects (vitamin D–resistant rickets in children or idiopathic osteomalacia [milkman's syndrome] in adults and excessive excretion of amino acids) is usually referred to as Fanconi's syndrome or more recently as de Toni-Fanconi's syndrome.

Another glycosuria occurring without increased blood levels of glucose has been found in a small percentage of pregnant women. Their renal threshold becomes lower, and they spill glucose. The condition is usually temporary, and the cause has not been defined.

POSITIVE URINE GLUCOSE TEST RESULTS OCCUR IN:

1. Conditions causing an increased blood glucose concentration beyond renal threshold maximums (see "Serum Glucose Levels Increased in" in Section 1.4)
2. Renal tubular defects resulting from genetic inheritance
3. Rare instances during pregnancy because of a decreased renal threshold
4. Conditions causing false-positive reactions such as   *(continued)*

a. Individuals tested with Clinitest tablets who may be taking one of a number of different drugs and excreting specific metabolites in their urine that test positive when using this method. The following is a partial list of such substances:
   (1) Salicylates, paraaminobenzoic acid (PABA)
   (2) Cephalosporin antibiotics of all generations with the exception of one third-generation preparation—moxalactam
   (3) Some sedative hypnotics such as chloral hydrate or paraldehyde
   (4) Ascorbic acid, high doses
b. Individuals tested soon after ingestion of a large amount of carbohydrate
c. Postgastrectomy in some persons

FALSE-NEGATIVE URINE GLUCOSE RESULTS OCCUR IN:

1. Some older diabetic patients with arteriosclerosis because of an increased renal threshold
2. Individuals taking large quantities of ascorbic acid (vitamin C) when using reduction-type (dipstick, test strip or tape) testing methods for urine testing

---

IMPLICATIONS FOR NURSING: URINE GLUCOSE

1. See "Implications for Nursing: Serum Glucose" in Section 1.4
2. Collection of urine specimens
   a. Single void, or random urine sample
      (1) To measure *current* blood glucose levels, a second or even third voided specimen is still considered best. *Double-voided* specimens are collected as follows: the individual being tested urinates, and that specimen is discarded. She or he then drinks a full 8-oz glass of water and one-half hour later voids into a clean container. This second-void specimen is then tested. Some practitioners suggest testing the first voided specimen as well until a personal normal pattern has been defined
      (2) For information about *control over time*, several days or weekly, the more concentrated first void of the morning can provide a useful sampling of urine "over time"
      (3) The urine should be collected midstream as a "clean catch," (see Section 4.12–General Implications for Nursing), and there should be adequate cleansing of the area before the void
      (4) Catheterization for the purpose of specimen collection to monitor urine glucose levels is to be avoided if at all possible because of the high risk of infection for the glycosuric person
   b. 24-hour urine collection (applicable to *all* 24-hour urine tests)
      (1) While explaining the client's role in the collection process, stress the importance of collecting *all* urine over the 24 hours. The test will not be valid, and will therefore be useless, if even one void is not included. Repetition of the test is also costly
      (2) At a set time, the client begins the process by voiding and *discarding* that first specimen
      (3) All urine thereafter is to be collected and placed in a selected container for the next 24 hours
      (4) Urine is best collected using a "hat" (a round, plastic basin with a wide lip on 2/3 of the basin and an indented pouring spout on the one flat side) placed on the front portion of the toilet (under the seat for females)
      (5) Each void should be poured into a large collecting bottle
      (6) The collection ends in exactly 24 hours from the time of the *first collected voiding*. The final void should be as near as possible to exactly 24 hours
      (7) Preservatives are placed in the collecting bottle for some of the tests and vary with the test to be done. Preservation of urine stability can also be accomplished by refrigerating the

urine collection throughout the process. The use of refrigeration and/or preservatives varies from laboratory to laboratory. Check with the laboratory doing the test. For examples, see Table 4–3

TABLE 4–3. PRESERVATION OF URINE STABILITY

Example 1.		
Samples Refrigerated	*HCL Added for (ml)*	*Na Carbonate Added for (5 g)*
Aldosterone[a]	Calcium (10 ml)[a,b]	Coproporphyrine (a.k.a. Uroporphyrin)[b]
Pregnanetriol[a]	Catecholamines[a] (10 ml)	
Prednanediol[a]	5-HIAA (10 ml)[b] (hydroxyindole acetic acid; serontonin) Phosphate/Phosphorus (10 ml)[b] Vanillylmandelic acid (VMA)[b]	

Example 2.		
	33% Acetic Acid Aldosterone Pregnanetriol Catecholamine Phosphorus	

[a]Same in both labs.
[b]Process differs (see Example 2).
Data from Corbett, 1992, and Laboratory of Pathology, 1991.

3. Because the accuracy of urine glucose testing depends on the technique of the person doing the test, the nurse should learn, teach, and practice meticulous technique:
   a. There are a number of different types of dipstick or test strip materials available for use (e.g., Combistix, Tes-Tape, Clinistix, Diastix). They vary in color response, the time required for the reagent to be exposed to the urine, and the number of urine tests that can be done on the same strip or stick. For these reasons as well as acceptance of the concept as a sound one in almost any case, the nurse is cautioned to read directions with care and to carry them out precisely
   b. Some generalizations concerning urine tests done with glucose oxidase reagent strips or sticks include
      (1) Protect the materials from moisture or excessive heat. Reagents tend to lose sensitivity when so exposed. Store in a cool dry area but not a refrigerator
      (2) If the strip or stick is brownish in color, do not use it. Such a color indicates a significant loss of sensitivity
      (3) Do not take more out of the container than will be immediately used. Recover the container immediately
      (4) Do not touch test areas or allow them to touch other areas. Lay the stick or strip on a clean piece of paper if it must be put down
      (5) Be sure that the urine to be tested is well mixed
      (6) Completely wet the reagent area so as to completely cover it
      (7) Avoid prolonged dipping, which can leach reagent from the strip
      (8) Read at the time indicated, exactly. Time with a secondhand
      (9) Hold the strip immediately alongside the appropriate color chart to compare the color. Do not use one company's chart for another company's product, even if the colors seem identical

    (10) Reading is best done in direct daylight. In any case, lighting conditions should be the best possible
    (11) Comparison of urine glucose levels to appropriate serum glucose levels helps clarify the client's true body glucose status
  c. If the test material used does not include a testing area for ketones (acetone), that test should usually be done in addition to the glucose test. The presence of ketone bodies indicates the seriousness of the diabetic's condition. The absence of a positive ketone test result in the presence of a glucose strongly positive urine also demands prompt attention. In an older (50 or above), known diabetic in a state of dehydration and with a decreased level of consciousness, the possibility of a nonketotic, hyperosmolar, hyperglycemic coma should be suspected and checked out
4. Measurement of urine glucose response: Most urine glucose testing is now conducted and reported in terms of grams per decaliter rather than in terms of scores of 1 through 4 +, even when done with the relatively imprecise methods of dipsticks, strips, tapes, or tablets. Table 4–4 may be useful as a guide should the materials in use *not* provide such a readout (Table 4–4 is a Clinitest scale)

TABLE 4–4. CONVERSION FROM NUMERICAL SCALE TO g/dl SCALE FOR CLINITEST

Concentration (g/dl)	Numerical Scale
0.25	Trace
0.5	1 +
0.79	2 +
1.0	3 +
2.0	4 +

5. General instructions for the individual with insulin-dependent diabetes mellitus (IDDM)
  a. It is important to keep a record of both the time and the results of all urine testing done. The information should be kept all in one place
  b. The results of each urine test should be used to adjust the insulin dosage on a scale prepared by the physician; this scale should take into account dietary intake and exercise as well
  c. The testing and insulin administration record should be shared with the physician at each visit
  d. Usually for IDDM the urine is checked four times daily. It may be a good idea to increase the frequency of the checks if any of the following occurs
    (1) Urine test results show an increase in glucose levels to 1.0 g/dl or higher
    (2) Signs and symptoms of hyperglycemia occur (e.g., polyuria, polydipsia)
    (3) There is evidence of increased physiological stress (e.g., an infection)
6. General instructions for the individual with NIDDM:
  a. Urine glucose levels should be tested daily. A good time for testing is about 2 hours after the largest meal of the day
  b. Increased testing is indicated with positive findings, with signs and symptoms of hyperglycemia (see the previous discussion of hyperglycemia), or in the presence of fairly prolonged stress
7. If there is no glucose found in a 2-hour postprandial (after meals, or p.p.; also sometimes called p.c. [postcibum, after eating]) urinary glucose test, it is unlikely that untreated diabetes mellitus is present
8. Related tests
  a. Elevated 2-hour p.p. blood glucose level (greater than 160 mg/dl) in repeated tests, with or without positive urinary glucose results, confirms the diagnosis of diabetes mellitus (Henry, 1991)
  b. Glucose tolerance test (GTT) is done when the aforementioned finding is doubtful
  c. A 24-hour urine specimen for glucose determination is performed when the aforementioned finding is doubtful or instead of a GTT
  d. Serum sodium (Na^+) test is performed to determine possible fluid loss with osmotic diuresis secondary to glucosuria
  e. Serum potassium (K^+) test is done in cases of possible or diagnosed ketoacidosis to determine the need for replacement

4.8 URINE PROTEIN

Synonyms: None

Normal Range: 0.0–0.15 gm/24 hr specimen[a]

[a]Newborns have higher levels of protein in the urine the first few days of life, but no specific value alterations are available (Henry, 1991). No normals established for random specimen (Laboratory of Pathology, 1991).

Definition. Measurement of urinary protein levels is an important evaluation of glomerular function. As with the screening test for urinary glucose, the screening test for urinary protein is most frequently performed by using a reagent-impregnated strip or stick—a qualitative test. Also, as in the urinary glucose test, the quantity of protein present can be roughly estimated on a scale of increasing concentration. The scale can be roughly quantified as shown in Table 4–5.

The reagent test (dipstick test such as Albustix, Combistix, or a strip test such as Albutest) is most sensitive for albumin and least sensitive, if sensitive at all, for globulin. It does have the advantage of avoiding many of the false positives that plague globulin-sensitive proteinuria tests. It is important, then, to confirm a positive reaction to the reagent test with another qualitative or quantitative test, particularly if there is any question as to the significance of the proteinuria. To do this, frequently a 24-hour urine sample will be analyzed for confirmation; the method for this provides a fairly accurate evaluation of urine protein concentration. It also avoids the problems of variation in dilution or concentration found in random-sample testing.

Physiology. Not all urine protein is pathological, and not all pathological proteinuria is persistent. But measurable, significant, persistent proteinuria almost always indicates renal disease (Price & Wilson, 1992).

The healthy glomerular membrane prevents most of the protein constituents of blood from entering the tubular ultrafiltrate (see Fig. 4–1). The small amount of the smaller molecular proteins that do get through may be reabsorbed by the tubules. Less than 0.1 g/24 hr is normally excreted. This amount usually cannot be detected by routine screening tests but may be detected in 24-hour samples. An increase in the GFR can increase normal protein excretion slightly.

Pathophysiology. According to Price & Wilson (1992), "the direct cause of proteinuria is always an increase in glomerular permeability." As with most generalizations, that is not quite true. Protein can appear in the urine because of postrenal problems, in which case glomerular permeability is not a factor.

TABLE 4–5. CONVERSION FROM NUMERICAL SCALE TO mg/dl FOR PROTEIN CONCENTRATION

Protein Concentration (mg/dl)	Numerical Scale
Less than 5	Negative
5–10	Trace
10–30	1 +
40–100	2 +
200–500	3 +
500 or more	4 +

Data from SHMC, 1984.

Proteinuria can be classified in at least two ways:

1. Extent (Henry, 1991)
   a. Heavy proteinuria (more than 4 g/day; nephrotic syndrome)
   b. Moderate proteinuria (0.5 to 4 g/day; most renal diseases in some phase and most systemic diseases with nephropathy [e.g., diabetes mellitus, multiple myeloma, preeclampsia])
   c. Minimal proteinuria (less than 0.5 to 1.0 g/day; chronic glomerulonephritis, postural proteinurias)
2. Relationship of the proteinuria's etiology to the kidney and the mechanism involved (Ravel, 1989)
   a. Functional. Not obviously associated with pathology, renal or systemic
   b. Organic. Associated with pathology, renal or systemic
      (1) Prerenal—not resulting from kidney disease primarily
      (2) Renal—resulting from primary kidney disease
      (3) Postrenal—resulting from the release of protein into the urine at a point below the kidney parenchyma (e.g., renal pelvis, ureters, bladder, urethra, or contamination from vaginal, prostatic, or seminal secretions)

POSITIVE REACTION IN URINARY PROTEIN SCREENING TESTS FOUND IN:

1. False positives because of the presence of hemoglobin or contamination of urine with chemicals such as phosphates and urates secondary to drug metabolites (i.e., sulfonamides or high doses of penicillin) or such as the ammonium compounds
2. Functional, nonpathological conditions such as
   a. Severe muscular exertion. Proteinuria is seen quite frequently in pregnant women at the time of labor
   b. Severe dehydration because of the increased concentration of solute in solution
   c. Orthostatic proteinuria, which occurs only when the person is standing erect, and may be due to renal congestion or ischemia secondary to an exaggerated lordotic position
   d. Response to temperature change (e.g., internal temperature: fever; external temperature: exposure to cold)
   e. Severe emotional stress
   f. Contamination with vaginal secretions
3. Prerenal pathology such as
   a. Conditions leading to a hypoxic renal state (e.g., shock, severe acidosis, acute cardiac decompensation, severe anemia, preeclampsia of pregnancy)
   b. Multiple myeloma (Bence Jones protein—primarily globulin excreted, so a false negative is possible)
   c. Hypertension
4. Renal pathology such as
   a. Glomerulonephritis, poststreptococcal infection; less commonly, postcollagen disease, or very rarely after sickle cell disease. It can also be idiopathic
   b. Nephrotic syndrome
   c. de Toni–Fanconi's syndrome or renal tubular acidosis
   d. Tumors or infarcts causing destruction of the parenchyma of the kidney
5. Postrenal conditions such as

a. Infection of kidney pelvis or ureter
b. Cystitis
c. Urethritis or prostatitis

FALSE-NEGATIVE RESPONSES TO URINARY PROTEIN SCREENING TESTS OCCUR IN:

1. See item 3 in "Positive Reaction"
2. Dilute, random urine samples, or the reaction may be falsely low
3. Highly buffered alkaline urine

4.8.1 Protein Electrophoresis, Urine

Synonym: Albumin and globulin fractionation, Urine

Normal Range: Individual interpretation usually done

Definition. Considered a more accurate evaluation of urine proteins than the A/G ratio calculation. *Electrophoresis* is the term applied to the movement of charged particles suspended in a liquid on various media (Miller & Keane, 1983, p. 363). Urine proteins consist of a minimal trace of albumin and globulins alpha 1 and 2.

Pathophysiology. In renal disease states urine protein distribution can assist in differentiating glomerular and tubular disease. Testing identifies the presence and amount of low-molecular-weight proteins (albumin, alpha-1-globulin or beta globulin fractions) not usually seen in normal urine (Laboratory of Pathology, 1991).

Findings

1. A predominance of globulin fractions with minimal albumin occurs in renal tubular proteinuria (Laboratory of Pathology, 1991)
2. Low-molecular-weight proteins (albumin, alpha-1-globulin, or beta globulin fractions) usually occur with glomerular disease (Laboratory of Pathology, 1991)
3. Urine protein fractions are the method of choice for diagnosis of Bence Jones proteinuria. However, the reaction is doubtful when only a small amount of Bence Jones protein is present (Laboratory of Pathology, 1991)
4. False-positive reaction can occur
   a. When other globulins are precipitated by acetic acid in the heat preparation method
   b. With high concentrations of Bence Jones protein (Henry, 1991)

IMPLICATIONS FOR NURSING: URINE PROTEIN

1. Some renal disease can be prevented or its severity modified by consistent preventative measures. Nursing measures to help prevent infection are given at the end of this chapter. Awareness of these measures will help the nurse to include appropriate prevention in the care of all patients

2. Encourage the culturing of all sore throats, especially in school-age children, a high-risk group. Although costly, this method is considerably less costly than the treatment of glomerular nephritis, even including treatment of the sore throat, should it be indicated

3. In taking a history of a patient with proteinuria, inquire into recent acute infections, even those seemingly far removed from the present problem, some 10 days or 2 weeks previously
   a. Check voiding history for changes. Decreased or increased volume? Increased frequency? Change in color? Change in odor?
   b. Check for the presence of edema (periorbital in morning?) or undue fatigue

4. Assess related laboratory test results
   a. Urine. The presence of pyuria (pus cells found in the urine) in the absence of proteinuria tentatively indicates a postrenal infection. Pursue questions concerning pain or discomfort related to urination with the occurrence of pyuria
   b. Urine: specific gravity. Values will increase in uremia and will increase markedly in the nephrotic syndrome until the late stages
   c. Blood: RBC count, Hct, Hgb. Anemia accompanies almost all renal disease and is roughly proportional to the severity of the uremia. The blood urea nitrogen level (BUN) increases in uremia. The RBC life span is reduced to about one half normal when the BUN level exceeds 200 mg/dl
      (1) Serum sodium—markedly increased in nephrotic syndrome
      (2) Serum potassium—may decrease because of urinary washout. May increase with urinary obstruction
      (3) Serum total protein—albumin, decreased with severe to moderate prolonged proteinuria

5. Teach the patient, family, home caretaker the purpose of any prescribed regimens and/or medications
   a. Severe anemia secondary to renal disease may be treated with androgens, which act directly on the bone marrow to increase renal secretion of erythropoietin. One happy side effect for males may be the return of libido, which kidney disease can suppress. Side effects for women are masculinizing changes, for which they should be prepared. The changes are reversible, but not immediately, on cessation of treatment with the drug. (Children may be given corticosteroids)
   b. Transfusions are rarely used because of the depressive effect on erythropoietin and bone marrow
   c. Increased blood pressure may not be treated medically. Explain the rationale to the patient/family if a lack of therapy is questioned. A decreased blood pressure causes a decreased GFR, decreased renal perfusion, and further renal damage. When there is reason to believe that treatment of the original pathology will effectively decrease the blood pressure, given time, the risk of prematurely decreasing it is not taken
   d. Edema resulting from decreased protein levels in the circulating volume (decreased serum protein causes decreased oncotic pressure intravascularly, causing movement of fluid out of the capillaries) is treated frequently with sodium restriction and diuretics to remove the excess sodium (e.g., nephrotic syndrome). Plasma expanders can be used when the circulating volume is very low, particularly when potent diuretics are given. Most, however, contain sodium. A high-protein, high-carbohydrate diet is usually prescribed to attempt replacement of renal losses of protein and to provide a ready form of energy in the proteinuria of the nephrotic syndrome. This may be given as a tube feeding because such a diet is found unpalatable by most people. Antibiotics are frequently given because of the renal patient's increased susceptibility to infection as well as to treat renal disease resulting from infection. The nurse should see that he or she is personally informed as to the expected effects, desired effects, side effects, and untoward effects; the dosage and how it should be adapted to this patient's renal condition; and the desired outcomes of its use

6. For nutritional needs, see "Implications for Nursing: Serum Total Protein," items 4b, 5b, and 6, and 8 in Section 1.8

7. For nursing measures related to anemia, see Section 2.1.6, item 1f

8. For nursing care in renal disease, see "Implications for Nursing: Serum Creatinine," items 1 to 8, 12, and 13 in Section 1.5

9. For nursing care in azotemia, see "Implications for Nursing: Serum Urea Nitrogen" items 2, 3, and 9 in Section 1.6

4.9 URINE BILIRUBIN

Synonym: Urine bile

Normal Range: Negative for all age groups

Definition. Bilirubin is normally not found in the urine. When present it is an indicator of an increase in the serum levels of conjugated (direct-reacting, water-soluble) bilirubin, which may be due to liver disease or biliary obstruction. When present in great amounts in urine, the color changes to very dark amber or a deep yellow-orange and produces a persistent yellow foam when agitated (see Section 4.4).

Physiology. See "Physiology" in Section 1.10.

Pathophysiology. (See also "Pathophysiology" in Section 1.10.) Bilirubin, conjugated by the liver, may be unable to be excreted into the bile because of obstruction of bile canaliculi from many causes. With the blockage of its normal excretory route, the conjugated bilirubin is ultimately excreted into the urine (see Fig. 1–1). Its appearance in the urine can even precede the appearance of jaundice.

Indirect-reacting, or unconjugated, bilirubin apparently cannot pass the glomerular filter and does not appear in the urine. Increased serum levels of this substance will ultimately cause an increased production of direct-reacting, or conjugated, bilirubin, which eventually enters the urine.

At the same time that urinary bilirubin excretion increases, the production of urobilinogen is increased, and there is an increased excretion of that substance into the urine. Thus, when a serum bilirubin test result indicates an increase in the unconjugated (indirect-reacting) bilirubin concentration, one would expect to see a rise in urine urobilinogen levels and, later, frequently increased urine bilirubin levels (Sodeman & Sodeman, 1982).

When increased red cell destruction alone causes the serum bilirubin concentration to rise, only the unconjugated (indirect-reacting) fraction is increased, and consequently, bilirubinuria will not occur.

Despite a physiological jaundice, little or no conjugated bilirubin is found in the neonate's serum or urine during the first few days of life (1 to 4) because of the immaturity of the liver, which cannot form conjugated bilirubin.

POSITIVE REACTIONS TO URINE BILIRUBIN FOUND IN:

1. Liver disease resulting from
   a. Obstructive jaundice because of gallstones or other mechanical obstructions, such as cancer of the head of the pancreas
   b. Inflammation because of infectious processes in the liver such as hepatitis
   c. Fibrosis of the biliary canaliculi in conditions such as cirrhosis
   d. Exposure to toxins or ingestion of certain drugs that are hepatotoxic
2. See also "Total Serum Bilirubin Levels Increased in," items 2 and 3 in Section 1.10

NEGATIVE REACTIONS TO URINE BILIRUBIN:

- Not clinically significant

IMPLICATIONS FOR NURSING: URINE BILIRUBIN

See "Implications for Nursing: Total Serum Bilirubin," item 2 in Section 1.10.

4.10 URINARY HEMOGLOBIN

Synonym: Occult blood

Normal Range: Negative for all age groups

Definition. The test for urinary hemoglobin, or occult blood, indicates the presence of microscopic (occult, hidden) blood, macroscopic blood (visible indications of blood can be changes in urine color), intact RBCs, or lysed cells with free hemoglobin present. An abnormal number of RBCs in urine is called "hematuria." The presence of free hemoglobin in the urine is called "hemoglobinuria." Normal urine may contain about 1000 RBC/ml. Some 66,000 RBC/ml are usually required to be clearly detected in a microscopic examination of urine (Henry, 1991).

The test can be done with a reagent strip or a tablet or as a wet chemical test. The reactive substance is usually orthotolidine, which is sensitive to a hemoglobin level equivalent to 10 million RBCs/L (10,000 RBC/ml) of urine, and reacts positively to myoglobin and the intermediate hemoglobin chemical derivatives as well as to hemoglobin. It is more sensitive to hemoglobin than to RBCs, but free hemoglobin occurs in at least 90 percent of all urine specimens containing RBCs.

Physiology. Ordinarily, proteins of large molecular structure such as the RBC do not pass the glomerular membrane in any significant number. (Significant is defined by Ravel [1989] as over six RBCs per high-power field (HPF) on microscopic examination.)

Pathophysiology. In hemolytic anemias or other types of intravascular lysis of RBCs, free hemoglobin is produced in excess of the available haptoglobin for binding. The excess is excreted by the kidney (see "Compensatory Physiological Mechanisms:" in Section 2.1.2). Free hemoglobin also occurs in the urine in response to severe, unaccustomed exercise; in a deficiency of glucose-6-phosphate dehydrogenase as a result of the ingestion of certain drugs or fava beans; in autoimmune hemolytic anemias; and in several abnormal hemoglobinopathies (Henry, 1991).

Hematuria occurs with damage to the endothelial lining of the small glomerular arterioles. This damage can occur secondarily to a number of different precipitants (e.g., trauma, hypertension, systemic disease). Hematuria also occurs secondary to problems of the lower part of the urinary tract (e.g., infections, tumors, or mechanical trauma resulting from renal stones).

Causes of hematuria or hemoglobinuria can be organized as follows (Harvey et al., 1991):

1. Local disorders of the kidney and genitourinary tract
   a. May have slight (rarely more than a few hundred milligrams per day) proteinuria
   b. Are often associated with some discomfort or pain (e.g., suprapubic discomfort, dysuria, renal colic)

    c. May cause blood to appear only at the beginning or end of micturation

    d. Do not cause casts in the urine

2. Diffuse renal disease

    a. Is usually associated with proteinuria

    b. Usually produces painless hematuria or hemoglobinuria

    c. Produces a uniform distribution of RBCs or hemoglobin in the urine

    d. Characteristically produces RBC casts, which unmistakably identify the nephron as the source of bleeding

POSITIVE URINARY HEMOGLOBIN TEST RESPONSES OCCUR IN:

1. As a false-positive reaction in urine contaminated with a high bacterial content because of the presence of bacterial peroxidases

2. In some physiological conditions such as

    a. After vigorous exercise undergone immediately before the test, which produces a microscopic hematuria

    b. In benign recurrent hematuria, which is found in children and frequently precipitated by a viral respiratory infection or other mild febrile illness. There is no loss of renal function (Whaley & Wong, 1991)

3. Consistently after renal trauma. The severity of the bleeding into the urine is not a reliable indicator of the seriousness of the injury

4. In infections of the lower part of the urinary tract, particularly in acute cystitis

5. In genitourinary tumors. Hematuria is the most frequent sign of urinary tract cancer and often may be the only sign. Tumors are unlikely to occur in children (Ravel, 1989)

6. In the presence of renal calculi. It may also be an isolated finding with painless renal calculi

7. In inherited disorders such as

    a. Hemoglobinopathies where hemoglobinuria is usually grossly visible without other signs or symptoms

    b. Polycystic kidney disease, which may be rapidly fatal in infants but consistent with a normal life span in adults

8. In thrombocytopenia purpura. In small children aged 6 months to 3 years, a similar condition known as hemolytic-uremic syndrome occurs. It is an uncommon disease but of importance in that it is one of the most frequent causes of acute renal failure in children

9. In diffuse renal lesions resulting from glomerulonephritis (acute and chronic); autoimmune hemolytic anemia seen with systemic lupus erthematosus, lymphomas, polyarteritis, viral pneumonias, Goodpasture's syndrome (lung purpura with nephritis), and allergic nephropathies (Henoch-Schönlein syndrome); malignant hypertension (severe); or focal embolic glomerulitis (usually secondary to bacterial endocarditis)

10. In conditions resulting from the ingestion of such drugs as sulfonamides, phenacetin, quinine, arsenic, carbon tetrachloride, or those that inhibit glucose-6-phosphate dehydrogenase activity such as primaquine, nitrofurantoin, and phenothiazine

11. In systemic infections such as blackwater fever *(Plasmodium falciparum)* or clostridial infections

12. Secondary to incompatible blood transfusions causing intravascular lysis, an immunohemolytic process. RBCs or hemoglobin can occur in the urine both as a result of direct hemolysis and secondarily to renal damage occurring because of hemoglobin obstruction in the renal tubules
13. In paroxysmal nocturnal hemoglobinuria

FALSE-NEGATIVE URINARY HEMOGLOBIN REACTIONS OCCUR IN:

- The presence of large amounts of ascorbic acid in the urine. Large amounts of ascorbic acid are present in many parenteral antibiotics as a preservative (e.g., tetracycline)

IMPLICATIONS FOR NURSING: URINARY HEMOGLOBIN

1. In risk populations
   a. Check the microscopic examination of the urine for the presence of red cells as well as a positive reaction to blood. If the specimen examined was not fresh, total hemolysis may have occurred. Conversely, the absence of a positive reaction for blood does not necessarily rule out the presence of RBCs in the sediment
   b. If the urinalysis is positive for hemoglobin but the urinary sediment is normal, suggest that a fresh urine specimen be examined. The presence of both RBCs and hemoglobin is expected; the absence of RBCs suggests urine that has been standing for a prolonged period
   c. Check each voiding for a change in color. A smoky color indicates small amounts of blood; red or brown indicates gross hematuria
   d. Get a complete voiding history: changes in the amount of urine, change in color, pattern of occurrence with color change (e.g., only after unusual exercise, just at the start and completion of the urinary stream [may indicate the urethra or bladder as the source of bleeding])
2. With the presence of massive amounts of hemoglobin in the urine and the absence of other indicators of kidney disease
   a. Observe for bleeding tendencies
   b. Check coagulation screening tests if available. Request such tests if evidence of bleeding tendencies is found
   c. Look for report of RBC casts. Their presence indicates kidney disease and their absence, a disorder of the lower portion of the urinary tract
3. Hematuria accompanying UTI usually disappears as the acute infection subsides. If this does not occur, the possibility of relapse or reinfection with another organism should be explored. Consult with the physician regarding the need for further cultures
4. Hematuria or hemoglobinuria accompanying or after transfusions
   a. Reactions usually appear during the infusion, but hematuria or hemoglobinuria may not be evident for several hours, even after all other signs have been allayed
   b. Specially diligent monitoring should be instituted with those individuals who are felt to be at risk for a transfusion reaction (e.g., known history of a previous transfusion or a prior pregnancy)

4.11 URINE KETONES

Synonym: Ketone bodies

Normal Range: Negative for all age groups

Definition. Testing for ketone bodies in the urine is another fairly simple, straightforward test. Ketonuria of sufficient concentration to produce a positive response in testing reflects an alteration in carbohydrate metabolism with secondary disturbances in lipid metabolism.

Diabetes mellitus is the only disease in which ketonuria has a true diagnostic importance. Ketonuria in slight to moderate amounts is fairly common. But in most cases it is only incidental to the variety of conditions in which it can occur. The presence of ketonuria in diabetes mellitus is a major indicator of impending or established ketoacidosis. Its absence or a less-than-strong testing response does not rule out diabetes mellitus, however, if other signs or symptoms of the condition are present.

With the advent of the laboratory use of reagent strips, especially the combined strips, testing for urine ketones has become a more frequent part of a routine urinalysis. In the past it was often routinely done only on young children. The reagent strip is the simplest form of testing. There is also a tablet form of the same testing material (nitroprusside and alkali) that is similar in sensitivity. The strip test is most sensitive to acetoacetic acid (also referred to at times as diacetic acid) and less sensitive to acetone. It does not react at all with the third ketone body—ß-hydroxybutyric acid. It is felt, however, that there is little need to distinguish between acetone and acetoacetic acid, as both have essentially the same significance.

Table 4–6 presents a comparison of testing responses and provides a rough quantification of urine ketone test results.

Physiology. (See also "Physiology" in Section 1.4.1.) When fat is used as a body fuel, as in dieting for weight loss, one of the first steps in processing it for use involves lipolysis, that is hydrolysis of triglycerides to glycerol and free fatty acids (FFA). Thus FFA formation is increased. The glycerol fraction is broken down for glucose by the liver as it reverts from glucose utilization to glucose production. The remainder of the fat molecule, approximately 90 percent, becomes waste products such as ketone bodies and must be eliminated. Usually the body metabolizes all ketones produced, but in the face of markedly increased ketone production, not all ketones can be metabolized, and the excess must be excreted in the urine (ketonuria). For the dieter this process is a compensatory one, at least for a while (Howard & Herbold, 1982; Tietz, 1990).

Pathophysiology. When ketone bodies are produced in excess, as occurs when fat is mobilized for fuel, their levels may rise from 1 mEq/dl to as high as 30 mEq/dl. They circulate in the bloodstream (ketonemia) and are subsequently excreted in the urine. The body is in a state of ke-

TABLE 4–6. URINE KETONE TESTING

Sodium Nitroprusside Tests		Approximate Level of Total Ketone Bodies (mg/dl)	
Reagent Strip Scale	*Tablet Test Scale*	*Concentration of Acetoacetic Acid*	*Concentration of Acetone*
—	Trace	5	20–40
Small	1 +	10	100
Moderate	2 +	20–100	250–500
Large	4 +	100–300	800–4000

From Davidsohn & Henry, 1969.

tosis. In the absence of glucose (e.g., starvation) or the inability of the body to use it because of a lack of insulin (e.g., diabetes mellitus), the body can to some extent use ketones in lieu of glucose. In diabetes mellitus with the absence of insulin to transport the liver-produced glucose into the cells, however, the body soon reaches a state of cellular starvation. The unused ketones are excreted rapidly because of a low renal threshold. Ketone bodies are organic acids, but few of them can be excreted as acid. Instead, they require sodium for their excretion, which causes sodium loss. They are also fairly large molecules and tend to add to the osmotic diuresis, rapidly depleting the ECV.

Because ketone bodies are organic acids, they produce excessive amounts of free hydrogen, thereby causing metabolic acidosis. Slight to moderate degrees of ketonuria are fairly common conditions that are secondary to a number of causes. Ketoacidosis is not as frequent an occurrence as ketonuria, but it can and does occur in uncontrolled diabetes mellitus. The amount of ketones present in the urine in such states is in fact a good indication of the severity of the ketoacidosis and may provide warning of impending coma.

POSITIVE URINE KETONE TEST RESPONSES OCCUR IN:

1. Physiological conditions, treatments, or other illnesses causing nondiabetic positive responses as in:
   a. Individuals ingesting high-fat, low-carbohydrate diets for weight loss or for control of certain types of seizure activity
   b. Persons receiving L-dopa (Parkinson's disease) or who had liver function tests or medications using phthalein compounds (bromsulfalein), which may cause low-grade false positives
   c. Infants with untreated phenylketonuria, although high enough levels are seldom present in the disease state to cause positive reactions to general screening tests for ketonuria
   d. Individuals occasionally after exposure to cold or severe exercise
2. Pathological conditions such as
   a. Diabetes mellitus in which the presence of ketones is an indicator of metabolic acidosis
   b. The first trimester of pregnancy in latent or otherwise controlled diabetic women. The stress of fetal growth can cause a hypoglycemic state that, when coupled with nausea, vomiting, and decreased food intake, actually produces a starvation ketosis with ketonuria and decreased serum glucose levels. This state can have an effect on the fetus's mental development (Metheny & Snively, 1983). Ketoacidosis is more common in the second half of pregnancy of diabetic women as a result of an increase in placental hormone levels, which are antagonistic to insulin. Ketoacidosis can be fatal to the fetus, particularly during the second trimester (Howard & Herbold, 1982)
   c. Starvation because of the lack of available food or an inability to digest or absorb food adequately or as a result of an increased and excessive body demand for nutrients (e.g., cancer, thyrotoxicosis, and increased tissue catabolism). A type of starvation occurs in postanesthesia patients. Because of tissue destruction during the surgery, the stress response increasing tissue catabolism, and the lack of nutritional intake, perhaps before and certainly after the surgery, such patients are prime candidates for nondiabetic ketonuria

d. Febrile diseases and toxic states, usually or especially in children, accompanied by vomiting or diarrhea

e. Glyocogen storage disease (e.g., Gierke's), in which ketonuria is accompanied by hypoglycemia

IMPLICATIONS FOR NURSING: URINE KETONES

1. Diabetic patients who evaluate the effectiveness of their treatment by urine tests do not necessarily have to do the test daily. After the initial learning period when the process should be practiced several times daily, the diabetic with a stable blood sugar level who has never had evidence of hypoglycemia or ketonuria during his or her stabilization period on a treatment regimen usually may test for acetone only when glycosuria is increased beyond his or her "norm." Many diabetics routinely show a trace or more of sugar

2. The diabetic person must become capable of examining his or her own urine for ketones, or a family member or home caretaker must have this skill if the patient is to live outside a hospital setting. Because the process varies slightly or greatly, depending on the product used, the process per se will not be discussed here. Generally, the dipstick or reagent strip is more convenient for home use. Care of these products and general instructions in the use of testing material are given with nursing implications for urine glucose. The procedure to be followed at home should be the same as that taught in the hospitals, and any adaptation to the home environment should be worked out before discharge

   One of the more important points to clarify in the teaching process is the knowledge and understanding of the patient, family, home caretaker as to what to do should he or she get a positive result. There are several options available: repeat the test, increase the insulin dosage, note any accompanying signs or symptoms of ketoacidosis, assess for possible precipitants of ketoacidosis, increase the frequency of testing, call the doctor, or inform a clinic or visiting nurse. Usually, the doctor likes to be notified *whenever* ketonuria occurs, but this needs to be validated with the doctor as well as other steps to be taken

3. The use of the combined Keto-Diastix (acetone and glucose) has the disadvantage of giving a falsely low glucose reading when there are moderate or large amounts of ketones present. The patient, family, home caretaker needs to be aware of this possibility if using this product. Further, he or she needs to know how to retest the urine with Clinitest tablets and to understand the rationale

4. Further, subjects to be covered in preparing the diabetic patient to go home include understanding the need for and the process of evaluating the testing material for deterioration. (Measures to prevent deterioration are included under urine glucose, this chapter.) Any strips produced by the Ames Company can be tested for effectiveness of the acetone reagent by placing the strip in a solution composed of one-quarter teaspoon of *freshly* opened Cutex or Revlon nail polish remover (or any remover that is known to contain primarily acetone) and mixing with two thirds of a cup of water. Any result showing less than "small," or one that produces a color response that does not match those of the color chart indicates deterioration, and the testing material should be discarded

5. Identification of risk groups for ketonuria in a hospital population, or in any situation in which patients contact nurses is of importance for provision of complete preventive care. Risk populations include

   a. Any pregnant women, particularly those with a history of diabetes in the family or "prediabetes" themselves and certainly those diagnosed as diabetic
      (1) Check the urine for ketonuria on each visit, whether glucosuria is present or not
      (2) Teach the procedure and rationale to the women, and set up a regimen for preventive testing
      (3) Be especially alert during the first two trimesters. Women should be impressed with the need for daily testing during that time

   b. Postoperative patients
      (1) Particularly those who had extensive periods without food before surgery
      (2) Those who face prolonged periods receiving parenteral nutrition only (not to include those undergoing hyperalimentation)

(3) Those who had extensive preparation of the gut before surgery (gut sterilization)
    (a) If possible, check the urine daily for ketones
    (b) If (a) is not possible, monitor any routine urinalyses that are done for the presence of ketones
    (c) If at all appropriate to the case at hand, discuss with the physician the possibility of increased nutritional intake for the patient as soon postoperatively as possible. Elemental diets through nasogastric tubes have been given immediately postoperatively in at least one study with totally beneficial rather than detrimental results (Moss 1977, pp. 73 to 82). The better the nutritional state, the more rapid the recovery, and a person demonstrating ketonuria is also demonstrating starvation
6. For related nursing implications, see also "Implications for Nursing: Serum Glucose" in Section1.4 and "Implications for Nursing: Urine Glucose" in Section 4.7

4.12 MICROSCOPIC EXAMINATION OF URINE

Synonyms: None

Normal Ranges

Cell count
  RBC 2–3/HPF
  WBC 4–5/HPF
Casts
  Occasional hyaline casts
No age variation in the healthy infant, child, or senior adult

Definition. Examination of urinary sediment can indicate or confirm evidence of renal disease. It provides information about the kidneys and urinary tract not found elsewhere when correlated with the clinical status of the patient. Because there is no widely accepted standardized procedure for this examination and inasmuch as urinary sediment is concentrated by centrifuging to greater or lesser degrees, depending on many variables, strict interpretation of quantitative reports is difficult.

The urinary sediment is routinely examined for cells, casts, crystals, and oval fat bodies. The cells and casts are often called *formed elements* and are usually of the most importance. Any other materials found in the urine are reported and discussed. Further testing is done as indicated to confirm the findings (e.g., urine culture for a finding of urinary bacteria) (Henry, 1991).

As in all tests included in the routine urinalysis, proper collection and handling of the urine are vital in obtaining valid results. For example, urine sediment will lyse rapidly. Some 50 percent of the WBCs present can be lost in 2 to 3 hours at room temperature. Therefore, examination of urinary sediment should be prompt.

Physiology

Cells. Cells are normally found in urine and come from either normal desquamation of the lining of the urinary tract (epithelial cells) or from the blood (WBCs and RBCs). Epithelial cells appear in very small numbers as a result of normal cell aging and sloughing. Certain epithelial cells cannot be easily identified as to source and at times may not be distinguished from WBCs. In some counting procedures (Addis counts) WBCs and epithelial cells are counted together. An increased number of epithelial cells will be found after prostatic massage in males.

Just how WBCs and RBCs enter the urine when there is no pathology present is not known, but in proportion there are a greater number of WBCs to RBCs in the urine than in the blood. The excretion rate of WBCs by way of the urine varies from hour to hour in the same individual. Excretion rates also increase with strenuous exercise or fever. Females tend to have a greater concentration of WBCs in urine than do men.

Casts. Normally, the number of cells present in urine is too small to form casts, so very few casts are seen in normal urine. An occasional hyaline cast may be seen, often after exercise or in the person with postural proteinuria (see Section 4.8), because cast formation is closely tied to the presence of renal protein and hyaline casts are almost entirely protein. Hyaline casts are hard to see on microscopic examination, and when they are seen, if they are the only type of casts present, they have little significance (Ravel, 1989).

Crystals. The importance of crystal formation in urine is questionable. Except when an unusually large number of one type is seen or when the crystals are abnormal, they are not routinely reported. They may have been somewhat overemphasized in the past. Crystals can, however, contain clues to calculus (stone) formation or certain metabolic diseases. Crystal formation is pH dependent. Crystals that normally appear in acid urine include calcium oxalate, uric acid, and urate. Alkaline urine produces phosphate and carbonate crystals. Neutral urine can also produce crystals such as calcium oxalate and calcium phosphate. A generalization can be made. If the urine is alkaline, phosphates crystalize; if the urine is acid, urates crystalize (Henry, 1991).

Pathophysiology

Cells. Epithelial cells increase in number in relationship to the amount of tissue deterioration present. Fatty degeneration of the epithelial cells occurs in some conditions. The epithelial cell includes fatty droplets with inflammatory changes in the tubule cells. In the presence of marked proteinuria, the cell degrades to the point of becoming only a fatty droplet found floating free in the urine. This is called an oval fat body and occurs in conditions such as the nephrotic syndrome. The source of the fat is thought to be the lipoproteins that can pass the damaged glomerulus in this condition. Oval fat bodies are also found in many other diseases (e.g., lupus erythematosus, subacute glomerulonephritis, the nephrotic stage of glomerulonephritis, with certain tubular poisons [mercury], and in rare hypersensitive states). Active degeneration of the tubules with increased epithelial cell excretion occurs in acute tubular necrosis or necrotizing papillitis (Ravel, 1989).

RBCs. A significant increase in microscopic hematuria occurs in substantially the same disorders given previously in this chapter for urinary occult blood, or hemoglobinuria. Some conditions related to only occasional gross bleeding in the urine but with significant microscopic hematuria include bleeding and clotting disorders (e.g., purpura, effects of anticoagulants); blood dyscrasias (e.g., sickle cell anemia, leukemia); renal infarction; malignant hypertension; subacute bacterial endocarditis; collagen disorders (e.g., lupus erythematosus, periarteritis nodosa); and various bladder, urethral, or prostatic conditions. Extrarenal sources can also contribute to microscopic hematuria (e.g., acute appendicitis; salpingitis; diverticulitis; tumors of the colon, rectum, and pelvis) (Henry, 1991).

WBCs. Increased numbers of leukocytes, particularly neutrophils, are seen in almost *all* renal disease or disease of the urinary tract. They can come from any point in the urinary tract and are generally accompanied by significant proteinuria if of renal origin. Bacteriuria usually accompanies lower UTI with only slight proteinuria (Ravel, 1989).

Casts. Casts are formed protein gel conglomerations outlining the shape of the renal tubules in which they are formed. They are produced in two ways: (1) by the precipitation and gelling of protein from a high-solute concentration of tubular fluid or (2) by clumping of the cells in the tubules into a matrix of protein (Henry, 1991); see Figure 4–2.

Some factors that influence the formation of casts include:

1. pH. Protein casts tend to dissolve in alkaline medium, so an acid pH favors formation
2. Concentrated solutions. High-solute solutions favor cast formation, whereas very dilute media tend to disolve casts
3. Proteinuria. Because protein is the basic matrix for cast formation, proteinuria from a renal or prerenal source is a necessity for cast formation

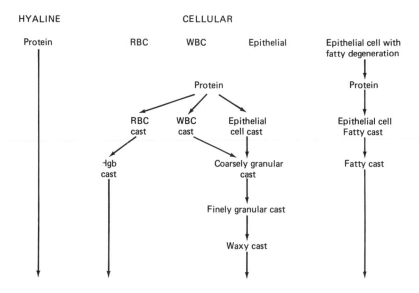

Figure 4–2. Formation of casts. (From Ravel, R. [1984]. *Clinical Laboratory Medicine: Application of Laboratory Data [5th ed.].*

4. Stasis. To provide the time for protein precipitation in the tubules, a slowing of the urine flow through the tubules is necessary. This usually occurs with a protein obstruction intratubularly. Ordinarily, the distal, or collecting, tubules are where casts are formed. This may be due to the fact that urine acidification takes place there as well as the fact that urine concentration is the greatest at this point

There are three main types of casts formed (see Fig. 4–2). The cellular cast may be made up of one or all of the cells present in the urine. As the cellular cast is excreted, disintegration may take place and leave only coarse or fine granules, or the full cast may be expelled. *Broad casts,* which are casts of the larger collecting tubules where large ducts drain several small ones, indicate a more widespread and severe stasis and are often found in kidneys close to total renal shutdown; hence, another name for broad casts is *renal failure casts* (Ravel, 1989).

An increase in the number of casts appearing in the urine is called *cylinduria,* and an increased number is diagnostic of renal rather than lower urinary tract disease, since they are formed in the nephron (Henry, 1991).

IMPLICATIONS FOR NURSING: CASTS, CRYSTALS, AND CELLS IN URINE

Microscopic Findings	Cause and Significance	Assessment and Nursing Care
Casts		
RBC	Localizes source of bleeding as the kidney; presence of any casts indicates presence of proteinuria, increased urine concentration, and renal stasis	1. Any urine specimens must arrive at lab immediately 2. Mark any urine sample with time of collection 3. Report the presence of increased numbers of casts; bring to the attention of the physician
WBC	Localizes source of infection as the kidney	
Fatty	Indicates renal tubular damage; frequently present because of nephrotic syndrome	4. Increase fluid intake if appropriate—especially important in the aged 5. Manipulate diet for alkaline ash if appropriate (see Section 4.5); again of particular importance in caring for the aged 6. See "Implications for Nursing: Urine Protein," Section 4.8.1
Broad	Indicates severe stasis, potential renal shutdown	Report immediately to physician
Hyaline	If persistent and increasing in the face of therapy, can suggest serious intrarenal problem; further diagnostic workup indicated Individual occurrence or only occasionally found, usually benign but does indicate that conditions necessary for formation were present	Bring persistency to attention of physician; assess for change in urinary output

(continued)

Microscopic Findings	Cause and Significance	Assessment and Nursing Care

Crystals
  Cystine, tyrosine
  leucine, sulfonamide
	All abnormal in urine; indicate loss of amino acids through urine; may be due to an inherited metabolic disease	Report; usually a recheck will be done; presence and identity confirmed; cystinuria in itself benign, easily overlooked; can cause massive renal calculi

Cells WBC in clumps	Strongly indicates renal infection, but not conclusive	Urine specimen should go to lab immediately or be kept cool; WBCs lyse on standing and in alkaline urine
With WBC or mixed epithelial and WBC casts	Definitely shows kidney origin of infection	
Many	Usually with acute infection	Obtain a culture; with repeated sterile cultures, continued WBCs may indicate tuberculosis or a lupus nephritis
Gross amount	May indicate rupture of renal or urinary tract abscess	Look for changes in vital signs (decreasing temperature, for example) or complaint of pain
Slight increase	Usually indicates urethral calculi, renal calculi, or acute or chronic cystitis, urethritis, prostatitis	To determine presence of urethritis over renal or bladder infection, a two-container specimen may be ordered: initial voiding in container 1, rest in container 2; in urethritis, most leukocytes will be in container 1
Epithelial clumps	Seen in acute tubular necrosis	
RBCs	Poorly preserved in dilute or alkaline urine; specific gravity; 1.006–1.010	If RBCs expected and not reported by lab, consult with physician for second order; might be well to check specific gravity before requesting second order Report should have been positive for hemoglobin or occult blood because of hemolysis; if not, no RBCs present, hemolyzed or intact. Prevent contamination of urine specimen, especially in females; bacteria from vagina or rectum may be cause of alkalinity in urine
Bacteria	Could be due to UTI or contamination of specimen	Prevent contamination by proper technique (see "General

Microscopic Findings	Cause and Significance	Assessment and Nursing Care
		Implications for Nursing" at the end of this chapter); suspect contamination when numerous bacteria and squamous epithelial cells are reported
Trichomonas	Almost always a contaminant	Report; may indicate need for WBCs

From Harper et al., 1979; Henry, 1991; and Saxon & Etten, 1987.

GENERAL IMPLICATIONS FOR NURSING: URINE SCREEN

1. Identify risk groups for UTI (e.g., females, because of the short urethra, extremes in age, the debilitated in health, adult diabetics)
    a. Assess risk groups for signs and symptoms of UTI. They may be easily missed because the signs or symptoms are often vague. A high index of suspicion should be applied in a general assessment of any member of a risk group
        (1) Check for UTI any time an elderly person presents signs or symptoms of an altered state of health
        (2) Check for lethargy or a change in mental status as possible symptoms of uremia
        (3) Anorexia, vomiting, and restlessness can also relate to a UTI
        (4) Any change in voiding habits (nocturia, dribbling, incontinence) as well as the more specific signs of UTI (e.g., frequency and dysuria) should be noted and monitored
    b. Keep careful intake and output records on all risk patients, particularly when urinary problems are suspected. Such records kept routinely on all risk individuals are of great value. Such a record is *the* most effective nursing assessment tool
    c. Urinary dipstick or strip screening can be used independently by nursing personnel to help determine increased UTI risks (e.g., alkaline urine)
    d. Individuals with a history of bacteriuria should have
        (1) A careful inquiry into the history of the frequency of previous occurrences and possible causes
        (2) A history taken of the type(s) of treatment used in the past and their response to the treatment(s)
        (3) A history taken of the type of follow-up care done in the past to help prevent further occurrences and enhance its effectiveness
        (4) A flow sheet kept that documents daily voiding patterns, general health status, intake and output, and dipstick findings (if done)
        (5) Instruction in maintaining the individual's own flow sheet after discharge in order to detect early signs and symptoms of UTI, which should then be shared with the physician
    e. Preventative measures should be instituted for *all* patients, but such measures are imperative for the groups at risk
        (1) Fluid intake should be increased with any signs or symptoms of UTI unless contraindicated by other disorder(s)
        (2) Teach and assist the individual to carry out measures to prevent urinary stasis or infections such as:

    (a) Providing easy and safe access to bathroom, day and night (night light, bedside com-mode)

    (b) Preplanned waking to use the toilet during night if sleep patterns are not unduly disturbed

    (c) Maximizing physicial mobility during the day

    (d) Appropriate positioning to urinate: females seated upright, no slouching or crouching, elevating the fatty "apron" with the palms of both hands, bending forward at the hips to help empty the bladder; males standing with back in alignment, bending forward at hips to help empty bladder

    (e) Preventing urinary tract contamination because of poor hygiene
- Provide for or remind the individual to change underwear, keeping it clean and dry
- If diapers are used at night, change them as soon as possible after they have been wet
- Discourage elderly women from using a sanitary napkin throughout the day, or make sure that it is changed as soon as it becomes wet. A wet napkin provides a good environment for bacterial growth and will tend to irritate and inflame the perineal area
- Provide and teach the need for excellent perineal care daily. Show women the technique of cleansing with a cloth by stroking toward the rectum only, never from the rectum forward. The same technique is to be practiced with the use of toilet paper after voiding
- For patients on bedrest, use disposable bedpans or urinals, or establish routines of *thorough* cleansing and routine disinfection and culturing of nondisposable items. Provide cleansing, disinfection, and culturing of bathtubs

    (f) Providing sexually active older women with special instruction as needed (e.g., voiding immediately after intercourse to flush the urethra; bathing just before or after intercourse; change of position for the sexual act if the male superior position is usual, as it can cause extraurethral stress and irritation).

  (3) When a UTI does not respond to the administration of an antimicrobial agent (cultures remain positive; signs and symptoms remain active)

    (a) Request a Gram stain, culture, and sensitivity test

    (b) Consult with the physician for a change in treatment

  (4) At times dietary manipulation to foster acid urine is indicated (e.g., in the presence of a *Proteus* infection or in the care of a sedentary person with urinalysis findings of phosphate crystals [which tend to precipitate in alkaline urine and may form calculi])

    (a) Provide acid ash foods (cranberries, plums, prunes, eggs, meat, fish)

    (b) Consider the need to restrict the use of alkaline ash foods (whole milk, nuts, other fruits*)

2. With systemic diseases that predispose to acid-base imbalances, the individuals at extremes in age must be closely monitored and protected against such imbalances because they have little reserve for adapting in acid-base disorders

  a. Testing urine for pH is one way to monitor acid-base balance

    (1) Only fresh urine should be used

    (2) The testing strip or stick should be left in the urine for just a few seconds; excessive fluid can wash away the reactive chemicals

    (3) Observe for changes in color in a good light by using the proper scale for the test agent being used

---

* A rather thorough study was done on the effect of cranberry juice in decreasing the urinary pH. It was found that in young subjects given 450 to 720 ml of 80% cranberry juice per day (not a commercially available preparation) there was a significant decrease in the urinary pH. Little or no effect was noted in other age groups or at lower concentrations of cranberry juice. There were also side effects of frequency of voiding—increased body weight and diarrhea in the successful group (Kinney & Blout, 1979).

(4) When accuracy is imperative, use a fresh urine sample taken between meals and when the patient has been awake for several hours. (Recall, sleep causes a slight respiratory acidosis, which leads to a more alkaline urine, and food intake will alter the acid-base response, depending on what has been eaten and on the "alkaline tide"[†] after meals because of hydrochloric acid utilization)

b. Individuals receiving intensive or prolonged antacid therapy, particularly those among the elderly with diminished renal adaptation to correct acid-base disorders, should be taught to

   (1) Observe themselves or have a family member assess for symptoms of milk-alkali syndrome (nausea, vomiting, confusion, polydipsia, polyuria, and a profound distaste for milk). The potential for this problem is greatest in those taking readily absorbed base products, such as Tums

   (2) In caring for the hospitalized patient receiving antacids, the nurse should monitor laboratory values for urinary pH and venous CO_2 levels, which are indicators of the base content of the blood

3. Proper urine collection is absolutely essential in getting accurate test results in cases of pyuria (presence of WBCs in urine) and is important in almost all tests on urine. Contamination from the periurethral area and the vagina is a significant factor in causing inaccurate visualization of WBCs in the urinary sediment

   a. Procedure (female: clean catch, or midstream)

      (1) Wash hands and rinse well. If the patient is collecting his or her own specimen, this must be stressed

      (2) Spread the labia

         (a) Using three separate cleansing wipes (prepackaged wipes, soft clean cloths saturated with cleansing detergent or povidone-iodine [Betadine], or (last choice) cotton balls, also saturated), wash downward from just above the inner labia on one side, and stop before reaching the rectum. Discard the wipe

         (b) Repeat on opposite side

         (c) With third wipe, cleanse between the inner labia

      (3) Rinse well with water pouring from front to back

      (4) Continue to hold the labia apart, and when rinse water has dripped off, the individual should begin voiding

      (5) As soon as some urine has cleansed the urethral opening, place the collecting container in position with your free hand, not touching the inner surface or edge about the opening with fingers or the body

      (6) When the specimen is in the container, cap it as soon as possible to prevent bacterial contamination from the air. Do not touch the inner surface of the cap. The container and cap *must* be clean, preferably sterile. The fuller the specimen container, the less the chance of bacterial contamination

      (7) Take immediately to the laboratory, or if it *must* wait more than 1 hour, refrigerate the specimen

      (8) If the individual has been having difficulty with either concentration or dilution of the urine, for whatever reason, that fact should be indicated on the laboratory request slip or on the specimen label

   b. Procedure (male: clean catch, or midstream)

      (1) Retract the foreskin of the uncircumsized penis

      (2) Cleanse the glans by using a circular motion from the tip of the penis to the foreskin, and discard the wipe. Do not retrace with the same cleansing wipe. Repeat with remaining wipes. Often two are sufficient

      (3) Follow steps (5) through (8) in 3a. The tip of the penis should not touch any part of the collecting container at any time

---

[†]The *alkaline tide* is thus called because of the change in pH from acidic to alkaline in the digestive tract after meals when most if not all of the available hydrochloric acid has been used and alkaline pancreatic enzymes are at a high level of secretion.

Part

II

Diagnosis of Infectious Disease

DEFINITION OF TERMS

There is a difference between infection and infectious disease. Many terms used to describe infection tend to be used interchangeably and are confusing for that reason. The following defines frequently used terms for the purpose of this book

- **Colonization.** The presence in the body of a bacterium, virus, yeast, fungus, protozoa, or rickettsia that may or may not be capable of producing disease. The interactions between bacteria and humans are more often than not equally beneficial (mutualism). The presence of such an organism in the body is most commonly trivial and unapparent or helpful (e.g., normal flora of the intestinal tract digest protein for absorption by the body). The person is indeed colonized, but he or she is *not sick*.

  For an insight into the microorganisms normally present (normal flora), the common contaminating microorganisms, and the unusual—or abnormal—microorganisms most likely to cause an infectious process in a given body site, see Appendix G
- **Infectious process.** The state occurring when the invasion of organisms or their toxins is in sufficient numbers and virulence to stimulate an inflammatory response in the part of the body overwhelmed so that notable signs and symptoms occur (e.g., fever [local or systemic], redness, pain, discomfort)
- **Infectious disease.** A condition occurring in much the same manner as an infectious process but capable of being transmitted from one person to another by transfer of the organism. The term is used interchangeably with *communicable disease*. An infectious disease *is* an infectious process, but an infectious process is localized and not considered a disease in the truest sense of the word. As a person can be colonized and not "sick," so may a person have an infectious process but not be considered "diseased"
- **Local infection.** An infectious process confined to one area of the body (e.g., an abscess, a furuncle)

- **Focal infection.** A local infectious process with systemic symptoms (e.g., increase in body temperature with a postoperative wound infection)
- **Systemic or generalized infection.** Organisms spread throughout the body—may be a septicemia or pyemia (see under organism)
- **Opportunistic infection.** Infectious process caused by organisms of low pathogenicity, often endogenous to the host, because some factor or set of factors has compromised the intrinsic defense mechanisms of the host or has in some way altered the ecology of the normal resident microbes (see the next section)
- **Secondary or superimposed infection.** An opportunistic infection that occurs during the course of another infection, the *primary infection*
- **Nosocomial infection.** The term applied to hospital-acquired infections as opposed to community-acquired infections. They are usually but not necessarily opportunistic in type
- **Iatrogenic infection.** An infection induced by the effects of medical treatment by a physician or surgeon, or by exposure to the health care environment, and implying that the effects could have been avoided by proper care or history taking
- **Acute infection.** An infectious process characterized by a rapid onset, usually severe symptoms, and a fairly rapid course
- **Chronic infection.** An infectious process characterized by a slow, probably insidious onset, although it can be a residual state after an acute infection. Symptoms are insidious and often nonspecific. The course is protracted. Chronic disease may have periods of remission and exacerbation
- **Bacteremia.** Presence of bacteria in the blood; may be transient or constant; may be a sign of an infectious process or a momentary happening before bacterial destruction
- **Septicemia.** Presence of bacteria or their toxins in the blood that is usually associated with a severe infectious process and involves active multiplication of the microorganism in the bloodstream and production of toxin. It is known in lay terms as *blood poisoning*
- **Pyemia.** A type of septicemia with the presence of pyogenic (pus-forming) microorganisms in the bloodstream (e.g., streptococci, staphylococci). Secondary abscesses can form wherever the microorganisms lodge. Organisms causing pyemia kill the neutrophils that phagocytize them. The resulting cellular debris is called pus. (Nonpyogenic organisms [e.g., *Salmonella, Brucella, Mycobacterium*] persist within the macrophages that attack them rather than kill them and cause chronic, low-grade infections)
- **Toxemia.** A term used to imply a concentration of bacterial toxins in the blood when applied to infectious diseases. It may also refer to metabolic toxins (e.g., toxemia of pregnancy)

GENERAL INFORMATION ABOUT INFECTIOUS DISEASE AND ITS CONTROL

It is no longer possible to classify microorganisms as pathogens and nonpathogens in humans. Many organisms, supposedly part of the "normal flora," are now found to cause disease. There are multiple causes for this change. Drugs have been discovered to eliminate certain pathogenic organisms. In their absence the usual ecological balance is upset, which allows a previous nonpathogenic organism to emerge and grow out of all proportion and cause a disease state. Further, some therapies developed since the 1960s depress the normal immune mechanism.

Most interactions between humans and bacteria are unaccompanied by disease. Many body parts are always colonized with normal flora, and most infectious diseases in humans are mild (see Appendix G). The acute, fulminating, and highly contagious bacterial diseases of the past are less frequently seen because of environmental sanitation and preventive medicine. When they do occur, such acute infectious diseases are relatively simple to diagnose, and there is specific and effective therapy for most. More difficult in the present is the interpretation of a culture to determine the primary infective agent, because the likelihood of secondary contributors to the infectious process is greatly increased.

Control of infectious disease is a great deal broader than are the identification and treatment of a given infectious disease. The diagnosis is only the beginning of the control process, and that process is most frequently contained in the scope of nursing practice. Control consists of prevention based on known methods of microorganism transmission and identification of the population at risk; surveillance through identification of outbreaks, extensive data collection, organization, and reporting; and preparation, implementation, and updating of infection control techniques specific to the locale and infestive agent.

PHYSIOLOGY

(See also "Physiology" in Sections 1.9.2 and 2.2.1, and Table 2–3.) The body has a great number of natural barriers to infection as well as a variable number of acquired defenses. The natural, or innate, barriers include the intact skin and endothelial linings of body organs, the limited ability of the skin and endothelial linings to decontaminate themselves by the "washing" action of area fluids (e.g., sweat, urine flow, mucus, and through the presence of antibacterial substances on those surfaces [e.g., lysozymes, hydrochloric acid, digestive enzymes, sebaceous secretion]), cilia and ciliary movement in the respiratory passages, phagocytosis, and antibody response. Many microorganisms cannot survive in the environment of a healthy body because of the ambient temperature or the oxygen tension.

Acquired defenses include active immunity secondary to immunization, usually including diphtheria, tetanus, pertussis, poliomyelitis, measles, and at times mumps, rubella, and smallpox; active immunity occurring secondarily to certain infectious diseases (e.g., mumps, chickenpox); and passive immunity resulting from the administration of immune serum or gamma globulin.

PATHOPHYSIOLOGY

Infections occur secondary to invasion and colonization of a susceptible body by microorganisms that infect humans. The process occurs only if each step, or link is present and can occur only in specific sequence:

1. Presence of sufficiently virulent and numerous causative agents or of one capable of destroying normal tissue
2. Presence of reservoirs in which the organism can thrive
3. Presence of a portal through which the agent can leave the host
4. Presence of a mode of transfer

These microorganisms include:

- **Bacteria.** Unicellular forms of plant life classified as to shape and visible only under a microscope
- **Viruses.** Chunks of genetic material (DNA, RNA) that are obligate intracellular parasites, that is, they cannot live apart from animal cells and can insert themselves into host cells. They tend to remain there in a dormant state in many cases. Individual organisms are visible only with electron microscopy
- **Fungi.** Multicellular moldlike organisms. These are often "opportunistic" infectors because they are not usually particularly pathogenic unless they enter an already compromised host. Many forms tend to occur in rather typical geographic distribution (e.g., histoplasmosis in the midwestern and eastern parts of the United States)
- **Protozoa.** Single-cell animal organisms that are motile and much more structurally complicated than are bacteria
- **Rickettsia.** Biochemically resembling bacteria and spread by vermin (e.g., ticks, fleas, and lice) and, like viruses, cannot live apart from animal cells

FIVE

IDENTIFICATION OF CAUSATIVE ORGANISMS AND FOREIGN HARMFUL AGENTS

5.1 METHODS FOR DIRECT EVIDENCE OF INFECTIOUS ORGANISMS

5.1.1 Examination of Direct Smears

A. Gram's Stain

Synonyms: None

Reported Results

Negative	Expected result from a specimen taken from a normally sterile site, indicates no visualization of microorganisms
Presence of mixed flora	Indicates the identification of expected resident flora (normal flora) from the site
Positive for shape and Gram result	Indicates the identification of the probable causative organism by virtue of the number seen or its presence in a normally sterile site
Presence of an increased number of polymorphonuclear neutrophils (PMN)	Increases the index of suspicion for infection

Definition. In most laboratories the examination of specimens received involves examining direct smears, unstained and stained, and culture on appropriate media. There are many staining procedures, the most common and useful being the Gram's stain. It is the one most likely to provide valuable information about the greatest number of organisms and is, therefore, usually indicated whenever staining is indicated. It is routinely used to examine cultures to identify organisms and determine purity of the colonies (i.e., single microorganism's growth).

The Gram's stain provides a method of distinguishing between the many bacteria that have similar morphology. It artificially groups bacteria into gram-positive (stain purple) and gram-negative (stain red) categories and makes the bacteria more visible on the slide so that form, size, and other structural details can be identified. There is a correlation between the Gram's stain and many other morphological properties of related forms. The microbiologist can accurately predict by expert reading of the Gram's stain some forms of anaerobic infection, which can result in early specific therapy.

Portions of gram-negative bacteria cell walls have endotoxins (toxins retained in the bacteria) that can produce lethal shock states, yet some gram-negative bacteria form part of the normal flora of the intestinal tract of humans and animals. Their endotoxins are not released into the host in the disease-free state.

Certain gram-positive rods are spore formers that tend to contaminate soil (e.g., *Bacillus anthracis, Clostridium botulinum*). Many gram-positive cocci produce exotoxins (toxin released from the body of the organism, e.g., staphylococci, streptococci, and/or enterotoxins [toxins specific for the cells of the intestinal mucosa], which cause food poisoning).

When a smear is stained and examined, the presence and type of inflammatory cells are noted as well as the staining characteristics of the microorganisms present. If there are no accompanying inflammatory cells, it may indicate the presence of colonies of the organisms unable to elicit an inflammatory response, although they can cause an invasive infection—the infected but *not* sick individual discussed in the definition of terms previously—or may indicate an immunodeficient host.

IMPLICATIONS FOR NURSING: GRAM'S STAIN

See Chapter 6, "In Home Management" 6.2.3.B.

B. Acid-Fast Stain

Synonyms: Ziehl-Neelsen method, acid-fast bacilli stain, AFB; Kinyoun carbolfuchsin acid-fast stain

Reported Results: No AFB (acid-fast bacilli), negative, positive for acid-fast bacilli (false positives possible with occurrence of saprophytic [nonpathogenic contaminants] acid-fast bacilli, differentiation made by correlation with the clinical picture)

Definition. Acid-fast organisms cannot be stained readily by Gram's stain. Therefore, in cases of a suspected acid-fast bacterial infection (e.g., tuberculosis or leprosy, the most common conditions caused by acid-fast bacilli), special staining methods must be used. (Leprosy is caused by *Mycobacterium leprae.*) *Mycobacterium tuberculosis, Mycobacterium kansasii,* and *Mycobacterium bovis* (almost never isolated in humans) cause most tuberculosis in humans, but a tuberculosis-like disease is caused by other *Mycobacterium* organisms, known as atypical, group III, or Battey strains of *Mycobacterium*. There are still other forms (e.g., group II) that cause cutaneous lesions and lymph node infections and are seen more frequently in children. It is important that atypical strains be identified, as treatment will differ. Atypical strains tend to be resistant to currently available drugs.

The term *acid-fast* is derived from the staining characteristics of the bacteria. The organisms have such an affinity for certain stains (e.g., carbolfuchsin) that they retain the dye when washed with strong acids, a procedure that decolorizes most other types of bacteria. They are also quite resistant to strong alkaline solutions; thus both acid and alkaline solutions can be used to cut down on the presence of other organisms in the specimen. Such decontamination is necessary to culture the acid-fast organism because it is much slower growing than most bacteria—it needs 2 to 6 weeks for culture growth. Left with other organisms in the specimen, the culture would soon be overgrown.

Because the culture takes so long to yield results, treatment for disease caused by acid-fast bacilli is usually begun on the strength of the smear/stain identification. In suspected tuberculosis, sputum for smear evaluation is usually gathered in a series of not less than three first-morning-cough specimens collected on three separate days to catch the sporadic discharge of the bacilli from the tubercle.

IMPLICATIONS FOR NURSING: ACID-FAST STAIN

1. The acid-fast stain can be done on any body fluid or exudate
2. Gastric washing may be done for AFB that have been coughed up and swallowed. No food or drink other than water may be ingested for 8 hours before the test. The specimen must be taken to the lab immediately (properly labeled in a sterile container with a top), before the concentrated stomach acid can kill the bacteria
3. Sputum staining requires three to six early morning specimens collected in sterile, capped containers
4. Urine staining requires three to six early morning clean voided specimens in sterile urine bottles

---

5.1.2 Specimen Culture

Synonyms: None

Reported Results

No growth	Expected in cultures from normally sterile sites
Mixed flora	Reported with the identification of expected resident microorganisms from the site; any organisms found that are not normally present in the area or "normal" organisms that are present in increased numbers are specifically noted by the microbiologist, and an antibiotic sensitivity test is often done and reported as soon as possible thereafter

Definition. A culture involves the collection of the suspected material in an aseptic manner, or sterile collection from normally sterile body sites if possible, and introduction of that material to an environment in which the organisms present can grow—an appropriate culture media, gel, broth, or living cells. The cultures are then incubated and observed for growth for a specified length of time under specific conditions of ambient temperature and the presence or absence of certain gases (e.g., CO_2). Different types of nutrients can be added to the agar or broth culture to be inoculated to meet specific microorganism's needs; and growth or the lack of it on the different media help to identify the organism.

Specimens for culture can be collected from blood, sputum, urine, feces, the discharge or scrapings from wounds, spinal fluid, and throat secretions. Droplets can be collected on a "cough plate" for the detection of pertussis, although it is not often done at present.

Culturing an organism is done for three purposes:

1. Isolation of an organism—accomplished by streaking on an agar plate to ensure the appearance of isolated and, it is hoped, pure colonies when incubated
2. Identification of the organisms present by the characteristics of colony growth such as color and morphology of the colony, growth requirements (e.g., specific nutrient media, anaerobic conditions), effect on media nutrients (e.g., fermentation of carbohydrates), and response patterns to the addition of certain antimicrobials or serological tests
3. Maintenance, or preservation, of the live organism for further study. Staining kills the bacteria

Identification of organisms from culture characteristics is validated by the use of a direct smear or stain evaluation.

The decision whether to interpret the laboratory findings as normal, an infection, an infectious process, or an infectious disease is made by the physician or pathologist on the basis of symptoms, clinical history, clinical findings, antimicrobial findings, and any other relevant data.

IMPLICATIONS FOR NURSING RELATED TO SPECIMEN COLLECTION: REQUIREMENTS AND PRECAUTIONS

1. Universal precautions *must* be used when collecting any specimens. (See Appendix I.)
2. Usually the laboratory does not collect culture specimens, except perhaps blood cultures. Most are collected by the nurse or other unit personnel. Some general requirements and precautions related to collection of any specimens include:
   a. The quantity of the specimen collected should be as large as necessary for laboratory processing: 5 to 10 ml of sputum for routine AFB or fungus culture, 2 to 3 ml of urine for routine urine testing, and 100 to 200 ml of first-morning-voided urine for AFB culture. Check with the lab personnel
   b. All specimens should be collected as early in the disease as possible, preferably before antibiotic therapy or other therapy has begun
   c. Note the time of collection on the test request form and specimen label. The lab usually records the time the specimen is received and inoculated but needs to know the collection time to ensure adequate recovery of all significant organisms. Immediate processing must be done to recover certain ones (cocci such as gonococci, meningococci, pneumococci), and knowledge of the collection time will provide information as to the possibility of recovery
   d. Labels/request forms should include the following information:
      (1) Give *complete* information as to type and source of the specimen (e.g., "throat swab from posterior pharynx through mouth," which helps identify contaminant organisms)
      (2) If a full routine culture is not necessary (e.g., the physician wants only to rule out the presence of a specific organism), order the culture accordingly: "For beta strep only"
      (3) Note any antimicrobial therapy being administered before the specimen collection and specify it by name and dosage so that proper techniques can be used to identify or grow the organism

    e. Deliver culture specimens, particularly those collected on swabs, as soon as possible to the lab to prevent drying of the organisms. (Check with the lab regarding the availability and use of "transport media")

    f. Specimens should be collected where the suspected organism is most likely to be found with as little external contamination as possible (e.g., well within a draining wound rather than from the surrounding skin)

    g. If possible, collect specimens at a stage of the disease when the organisms are present in greatest numbers (e.g., the diarrheal stage of intestinal infections, the first 3 to 5 days of viral infections)

    h. If the patient is to be involved in the collection of a specimen, he or she will need precise and full instructions in the process as well as the reasons for the requirements. Further, he or she will need to be encouraged in the process by reminders and positive reinforcement

    i. The container for the specimen must be sterile for collection from a sterile site. Clean, disposable plastic containers with tightly fitted lids (preferably screw caps) may be used for such specimens as expectorated sputum, clean voided urine, and the like. The specimen should be introduced into the container so that the outer surfaces are not contaminated. This will prevent contamination of the specimen with outside organisms as well as contamination of health care personnel handling the container

    j. Frequently advance notice to the lab about the type of organism to be cultured is necessary so that special media or handling can be prepared. Check with the lab servicing the facility in which you work for a list of such organisms. Organisms such as *Chlamydia*, viruses, legionnaires' disease bacillus, or botulism bacillus, for example, require materials or transport media that may not be immediately available

3. Specific requirements and precautions for specimen collection are needed for:

    a. Abscesses, wounds, exudates (to include genital area—vagina, urethra, Bartholin's cyst, Skene's glands, etc.):

      (1) Specimen should be collected by sterile swab (many labs have special swabs that do not shed lint) or aspirated with a sterile needle and syringe from the most moist area. Bacteria from the absolute center may be nonviable. Therefore, the near periphery should be cultured where organisms are most viable and active

      (2) Carefully expel air from syringe after collection. Cap, properly label, and send stat to the lab

      (3) Genital area cultures (cervical, urethral, vaginal) should be clearly marked as to origin because they are usually cultured for gonococci as well as other pathogens

    b. Catheter tips (intravascular):*

      (1) Cut the tip with *sterile* scissor 4 to 5 inches from the skin by holding it directly over a sterile specimen cup or wide-mouthed bottle. (The cup is better because it allows the broadest opening for collecting the tip and also allows the tip to be cultured in the lab without removing it from the container)

      (2) Sterile technique is *essential* because catheter infections are usually due to common skin organisms, which will also be the contaminating organisms if a sterile technique is not used

      (3) Deliver as soon as possible to prevent drying of the organisms

    c. Catheter sites:

      (1) Culture at the time of catheter removal or at the puncture site if culturing a venous catheter

      (2) Veins may be carefully "milked" or pressure placed on nearby tissue to express fluid

      (3) Send a sample from a catheter site to the lab with the catheter tip, both properly labeled

    d. Nasopharyngeal and throat:

      (1) Nares: Insert swab and culture as far back as possible without bending the swab. Rotate the swab gently but use some pressure against the side

      (2) Pharyngeal: Use a swab through the mouth and explore any obvious lesions or visible crypts. Rotate the swab and get it below the surface. In the absence of lesions, vigorously

---

*Culture of urinary catheter tips is not advised because they tend to grow a plethora of bacteria whose significance is not well determined in disease.

rotate the swab over the tonsillar or any inflamed area. Avoid touching the tongue or teeth, because many contaminating microorganisms from these areas can overgrow cultured pathogens from the posterior part of the pharynx

(3) Nasopharyngeal: Use a swab attached to a narrow flexible wire. Clear the nares, insert the swab, and take a mucus sample from above and behind the uvula. If only a small quantity of the specimen is available for collection, some labs suggest moistening the swab with sterile saline beforehand

(4) Throat: Swab the posterior wall of the throat below the level of the uvula. Depress the tongue with a tongue blade, and do not touch the tongue with the swab

e. Rectal:

(1) Wearing a clean (not sterile) glove, insert the swab approximately 1 inch into the rectum, which has been cleared of feces if possible. If the swab does enter the stool, discard it and start over, except when culturing *Shigella*. In that case the swab should be totally covered and saturated with stool. This may require deeper insertion of the swab—3 inches—and help of the patient in bearing down

(2) Move the swab from side to side to sample crypts. Allow 10 to 30 seconds for organisms to be absorbed into the swab

f. Spinal fluid (collected by the physician in most cases):

(1) Keep container tightly capped

(2) Keep the fluid warm in the tube during transport. You can use body heat from a warm hand or place the tube in a glass of tepid water. A common pathogen sought from spinal fluid is *Neisseria meningitidis*, which is very sensitive to cold (anything less than 35°C).

g. Sputum:

(1) Have the patient rinse his or her mouth well with water without swallowing before trying to raise material by coughing. This decreases the amount of saliva present. Do *not* use mouthwash because this will kill the bacteria

(2) Demonstrate the technique of effective coughing for the patient and assist him or her in learning the process (e.g., need for several deep breaths to help mobilize secretion, hands on diaphragm to coordinate the expulsion of air with upward hand pressure, preparation by intake of adequate fluids to thin secretions if needed). Explain the need for sputum and not saliva and the difference between them

(3) If sputum is difficult to raise, have the patient lie with head and shoulders below chest level for a few minutes if not contraindicated by his or her condition

(4) If the specimen does not contain mucoid or mucopurulent material, consult with the physician if necessary for alternate procedures (e.g., induced sputum or nasotracheal aspiration)

(5) Early morning is often the best time for sputum collection because it takes advantage of the overnight collection of pooled bronchial secretions

(6) With nonproductive coughs, the use of cold steam or nebulized vapor may help raise sputum. The use of propylene glycol in the nebulizer should be avoided if the specimen is to be tested for *Mycobacterium tuberculi* because it will inhibit growth or could even kill the bacteria

(7) If the sputum cup is left with the patient, he or she will need careful instruction in its use—the need to keep the inner surfaces untouched and to keep it closed when not in use

h. Stool:

(1) Stool specimens must be delivered to the lab while still warm, usually within 30 minutes or less. If allowed to stand longer, normal resident organisms may overgrow the less adaptive pathogens

(2) Keep the lid and outside of the container clear of stool. The container should not be completely filled

(3) Presence of barium in the stool does not usually interfere with most cultures if adequate feces is obtained. Barium will, however, interfere with parasitic studies

(4) If the stool is to be tested for occult blood, a meat-free diet *might* be ordered for 3 days before the test. This precaution is unnecessary if the guaiac method is used for testing but important if the HemeQuant test is used. The guaiac method is probably the least sensitive

test, with a minimum of false positives, therefore useful for screening purposes. HemeQuant testing is a more sensitive measure of gastrointestinal bleeding and felt to be more likely to detect lesions of the right (proximal) part of the colon (Ahlquist, et al., 1985, p. 1427)

(5) Excessive amounts of vitamin C (greater than 500 mg/day) can cause a false negative for occult blood. Other drugs that interfere with the guaiac test are iodine (sometimes given in the treatment of respiratory disorders to liquefy secretions), inorganic iron, bromides, boric acid, cimetidine, and colchicine (for gout)

(6) If there is a suspicion of gastrointestinal bleeding, a history of aspirin ingestion should be suspected and checked. (See also Section 9.6 "Stool Examination")

i. Tissue, biopsy samples: (Usually obtained by the physician)

(1) Place in a sterile tube or sputum cup with a small volume of sterile *nonbacteriostatic* saline or a sterile moist gauze

(2) Do *not* place the sample in a preservative solution such as formalin or alcohol

j. Urine:

(1) See collection procedures in Section 4.7, Urine Glucose–24hr Urine Glucose Test

(2) Endeavor to see that urine cultures are taken before antimicrobial therapy is started, especially in the case of an elderly patient or a patient recently rehospitalized and suspected of urinary tract infection (UTI). The pathogen is likely to be more resistant to antimicrobials in these instances

5.1.3 Living-Tissue Culture

As discussed previously, two forms of microorganisms, virus and rickettsia, are obligate intracellular parasites and require animal cells to live. Thus the ordinary means of culture growth is not feasible for these microorganisms. Also, at times all usual means of isolation of a bacterium can fail. Another approach is necessary, and living-tissue culture can be used.

A. Animal Inoculation

The only available source of living cells in the past was the living, intact, experimental animal. Animals used included mice, hamsters, rats, guinea pigs, rabbits, and monkeys. The animal used depended on the microorganism to be grown. Animals were inoculated intracerebrally, intranasally, or intradermally, again depending on the microorganism. The animal was then observed for a set time, usually a matter of weeks rather than days, sacrificed, and carefully autopsied. If successful, the organism was isolated in the living host and could then be identified by indirect (immunologic, biochemical, pathological) methods.

Animal inoculation is still used on rare occasions as an aid in the final identification of acid-fast bacteria or for recovery of fastidious microorganisms when there are doubtful outcomes from stain or culture processes. The guinea pig (negative Mantoux reaction) is the animal of choice in human or bovine tuberculosis.

B. Chick Embryo

Since its introduction, chick embryo inoculation has been used more frequently than has animal inoculation. The process is less expensive than animal inoculation, better accepted by the general public, and in most cases, equally effective in isolating some microorganisms such as viruses. Lesions are produced on the membrane of the egg yolk sac and are examined by a number of techniques to identify the organism.

C. Dispersed Cells in Culture

Dispersed cells in culture is the more recent living-tissue culture method. Microorganisms, especially viruses, grow and multiply when introduced into the culture. As viruses grow in the tissue culture, they produce biologic effects on the cells present in the culture, which permits identification of the agent. The presence of the virus is confirmed by the use of a type-specific antiserum (see Section 5.2.1). The cell or tissue culture is the most widely used method for isolating viruses from clinical specimens.

5.1.4 Colony Count

A colony is a discrete group of organisms on a culture. At times such as in UTI, it is important to count the numbers of discrete colonies of a specific organism found on a given culture; 100,000 colonies/mm^3 of urine from a voided specimen; 10,000 colonies/mm³ from a catheterized specimen is felt to be significant. Lesser counts are usually attributed to contamination with urethral flora and in the absence of prior therapy largely rule out bacteriuria.

5.1.5 Biopsy

A biopsy is an examination of tissues taken from a living body. At times, a biopsy can be a useful diagnostic aid in infectious disease. For example, in many cases of prolonged fever of unknown origin (FUO), all the routine tests—culture, smear, and so on—fail to isolate and identify the causative organism of the fever. Surgical exploration of the suspect area may be done, and a biopsy with histological examination of the tissue cells may produce the identification of the microorganism and the diagnosis.

In miliary (disseminated) tuberculosis, clinical and culture investigations may fail to confirm the presence of the mycobacterium. Without evidence of the organism the diagnosis is not absolutely certain, and biopsy of the bone marrow, or less frequently the liver, may be done, successfully demonstrating the microorganism through culture and acid-fast stain.

The use of biopsy and examination of the biopsy specimens are important in the diagnosis of some types of systemic fungi and in legionnaires' disease.

5.1.6 Antibiotic Sensitivity

Most organisms are either sensitive (susceptible) or resistant to a specific group of antimicrobials. Although this reaction can help identify microorganisms, that is not the purpose for which a test is usually performed. The decisive factor in the physician's choice of antibiotic in the treatment of infectious disease is the relative susceptibility of the invading microorganism to the antibiotic.

Each antibiotic tested is listed, and its effect on bacterial growth is indicated as:

- Resistant   Bacterial growth not inhibited
- Sensitive   Bacterial growth inhibited (see the discussion of minimum inhibitory concentration [MIC] in the next section)
- Intermediate   Some inhibition (usually considered resistant)

Antibiotic susceptibility (sensitivity) testing, when available, helps the physician select the most effective agent for treatment of the organism in question. The narrower the spectrum of action of the antimicrobial, the more preferred its use when the specific organism is known. Broad-spectrum antibiotics have value when treating an as-yet-unknown infection.

A. *The Kirby-Bauer Agar Disk Diffusion Test*

The Kirby-Bauer test and its modifications are indirect approaches to describing the MIC of certain antimicrobials. The MIC is defined as the "lowest concentration of an antimicrobial at which no bacterial growth occurs for a given bacterial strain" (Henry, 1991). The test is performed after isolation of the suspected bacteria. The bacteria are placed on an agar plate, completely covering it. Specially prepared disks of a variety of antibiotics thought to be effective against the suspected microorganism are then placed at intervals on the agar plate surface. The plate is incubated and examined for clear areas (inhibition of bacterial growth) around the antibiotic-impregnated disks. The clear areas are measured and compared with a predetermined norm for MIC. Commercially prepared dilution sets are available as a modification of this method. Automated methods are rapidly replacing the Kirby-Bauer test and will give the MIC directly.

B. *Microbroth Dilution Tests*

A form of MIC test, the microbroth dilution test is a modification of the Kirby-Bauer test and is still in frequent use. It uses a standard suspension of antibiotics and a single concentration of bacteria derived from the patient's infection. If a low dilution does not inhibit growth, the therapy is thought to be ineffective.

The information gained tells the physician the inherent susceptibility of the infecting organism to the antibiotics tested. The most appropriate agent can then be selected for treatment.

Other considerations in the selection of an antibiotic include:

1. The clinical pharmacological properties of the antibiotic: What concentrations will be achieved in the blood at the recommended dosage, whether it can reach the site of infection (cross the blood–brain barrier, for example), or the route of administration and excretion (a drug not excreted by the kidney would be of little value in a UTI)
2. Previous clinical experience with the antibiotic and the organism (e.g., difficulty in maintaining a therapeutic blood level without the danger of toxicity or ineffective levels—narrow therapeutic antibiotic concentration)
3. The nature of the underlying pathological process (e.g., infectious disease in some body areas with some microorganisms makes it difficult to get adequate blood concentrations to the site as with multiple abscesses or the tubercle of tuberculosis)
4. The immune status of the patient. Individuals with little or no immunologic defense will require greater concentrations of the antibiotic and run a greater risk of secondary or opportunistic infections

Susceptibility tests are considered unnecessary by some authorities in the treatment of certain organisms that have shown little or no tendency to change in resistance (e.g., *Streptococcus pyogenes, Streptococcus pneumoniae, Neisseria gonorrhoeae)* (Henry, 1991).

There is no total agreement on this approach.

C. *Other Tests Related to Sensitivity Testing*

Antimicrobial assay—determination of the concentration of an antimicrobial present in serum and other body fluid—is used to help predict the likelihood of success in the use of a given antimicrobial and to prevent potential toxicity and is of particular concern in the patient with compromised renal or liver function. Types include

1. Radioimmunoassay (RIA)—a direct and absolute measurement
2. Bioassay
3. Enzymologic assay. Both bioassay and enzymologic assay give individualized information about each drug and do not base data on general norms
4. Bactericidal assays (-cidal assays or Schlichter tests) measure effective levels of antibiotics in the blood. They look at the combined effect of an isolated culture of the patient's infected body fluid and the antibiotic he or she is receiving. Bactericidal activity is anticipated at a given dilution. Such an indirect test can also predict success in the use of the drug as well as monitor the appropriateness of the treatment

Susceptibility tests usually reflect organism growth inhibition levels (MIC). However, certain categories of infections (e.g., bacterial endocarditis or subacute bacterial endocarditis) may require knowledge of minimal bacterial concentrations (MBC) or minimal lethal concentrations (MLC) of the drug in use (Henry, 1991).

5.1.7 Nucleic Acid Probe (DNA Probe)

Definition. The DNA probe is a complex identification system that has as its basis the unique ability of strands of nucleic acid, such as DNA, to bind specifically to fragments of nucleic acid of a complementary sequence. Under proper conditions of hybridization (i.e., nucleic acid strand combination, see definitions in Appendix K), strands of nucleic acid will bind to one another only if they are perfectly complementary one to the other (or nearly so). This enables one to be quite certain that a DNA or RNA sequence specific for a particular microorganism is present in the sample to be tested. The process involves construction of a nucleic acid sequence (called a "probe") that will match (i.e., complementarily bind to) a sequence in the DNA or RNA of the target tissue sample to be examined. Because the most frequent target molecule, DNA, exists as a double strand in the body, the DNA strands in the target sample must first be separated to permit binding of the probe; this is usually accomplished by heat denaturation (separation) of the native double-stranded DNA. The probe is then allowed to attempt to bind to the target nucleic acid molecule, a process know as *hybridization*. If the probe sequence does match a sequence in the target, the probe will complementarily combine (hybridize) with the target single strand, again forming a double-stranded helix.

The probe nucleic acid sequence is usually "labeled" with (i.e., covalently bound to) a radioisotope or chromogenic enzyme prior to use, so that its bound presence in the target DNA can be detected following the test. Nonattached (nonhybridized) probe single strands are washed away, and an indicator system (e.g., gamma counter or chromogenic substrate) then demonstrates if any of the probe remains attached to (i.e., hybridized with) the target molecule.

This system is potentially more sensitive than present antibody assays. By varying conditions of hybridization, it can also be made specific to either the genus, species, or even specific serotype of an organism. For example, using different hybridization conditions, one may ask whether a biopsy of the uterine cervix contains evidence of infection by *any* human papilloma virus (HPV) or only HPV subtypes associated with the development of cervical malignancies (e.g., HPV serotypes 16 and 18). DNA probes have the potential for use with any organism or clinical specimen and offer the additional advantage of rapid results. The cost is, however, very high, especially when used on a single-specimen basis (Ravel, 1989, pp. 188–189).

The discussion applies principally to nonamplicative methods of DNA detection. The reader should be aware of the existence of methods by which DNA sequences in target samples may be "amplified" (i.e., duplicated in millions, billions, or trillions of copies) prior to their detection by labeled nucleic acid probes. The principal amplicative method used to date is termed *polymerase chain reaction* (PCR) (Conn, 1991, p. 546). Details of these methods are beyond the scope of this text. However, the amplification step adds the potential to dramatically increase sensitivity, so that, in theory, such tests can detect a single malarial parasite in a tube of blood or positively identify a rapist on the basis of a single spermatozoid. To date, however, these tests have been plagued by difficulties due to false positives that may result from DNA "contamination" of target samples, or unexpected cross-reactivities of target sequences (witness the recent controversy about admissibility of so-called "DNA fingerprinting" in forensic and criminal cases). With improvements in these techniques, one may expect to see an ever-increasing role for like tests in the diagnostic laboratory (P.A. Treseler, MD, PhD. Personal communication).

New approaches with recombinant DNA testing also contribute to the rapidity and accuracy with which testing of *Mycobacterium tuberculosis* cell viability to an array of antibiotics can be done. Cloned luciferase (firefly) genes are delivered to the mycobacteria and luciferin is added. This produces an impressive glow within minutes. If the glow goes out after several hours, the medication has worked. If the strain is resistant to the drug, "the light stays on" (Boschert, 1993; See also Appendix K: "Terminology and Definitions Related to Recent Testing Methods").

5.1.8 Immunologic Testing

Definition. Immunoassays are based on a variety of techniques to quantify antigens or antibodies. "Labeled" reagent assays have greater sensitivity (Henry, 1991, p. 852). (See also Section 5.2.1 and Appendix K, "Terminology and Definitions Related to Recent Testing Methods.")

5.2 METHODS FOR INDIRECT EVIDENCE OF INFECTIOUS DISEASE

5.2.1 Serological Tests (Immunologic)

Serological tests are those based on observation of antibody–antigen reactions. They are of diagnostic value only late in the course of an infection. Their use in short-term illnesses is primarily for epidemiological purposes, that is, identifying a disease in retrospect so as to prevent from or treat the disease occurring in others. In some cases, as in very mild infections or those treated with antibiotics before a specific diagnosis, serology may be the only way a diagnosis can be made.

Serology is used to collect evidence of past infections. Antibodies formed in response to the infection are identified and their concentration (titer) measured at different stages of the disease process. This provides a tool for following the course of an active infection and monitoring therapy. A single test seldom provides adequate information (e.g., whether a disease is active or whether a negative response rules out a given disease). Usually, at least two tests are necessary, one during the active process and one during the convalescent stage. Paired testing such as this provides comparative data. A fourfold or greater rise in titer to a specific microorganism is usually considered diagnostic.

Blood serum is the only body fluid that gives adequately high antibody titers to be useful. No other body fluid is usually tested. The five categories of serological tests generally used to identify infectious disease are given and defined and some examples shown in the following sections.

A. Agglutination Tests

Agglutination is the result of an antibody attacking an antigen (defined as a protein that may be an organism, tissue cell [leukocytes], or other large protein molecule) that causes clumping of the antibody, antigen, and the microorganism. Agglutinins are specific antibodies developed in response to an antigenic agent (in infectious disease, the infective microorganism). They are protein—gamma globulins—and are part of the immune mechanism of the body. Agglutination tests (Table 5–1) can be done in test tubes or directly on slides by mixing the patient's serum with a specific antigen.

B. Complement Fixation Tests

Serum complement is a globulin and makes up an important serum enzyme system. There are nine major components of the complement system that are identified by letter–number designations, C1 through C9. The numbers assigned are *not* in the order of their sequence in activating the system and are, therefore, confusing. The total system, total complement, is also referred to as C. Most pathological conditions tend to decrease total complement levels.

Complement fixation tests (Table 5–2) are based on the activity of complement in the serum. During an antigen-antibody reaction, all available complement is bound, or "fixed." If complement is activated, which indicates that an antigen-antibody reaction did *not* take place, complement will hemolyze the red blood cells (RBCs). Therefore, the presence of hemolysis in a complement fixation test is interpreted as a negative response; the absence of hemolysis, as a positive reaction.

C. Precipitin Tests

Precipitin tests are used primarily in the identification of antibodies produced in response to certain fungi and bacterial exotoxins. They are also helpful in typing various bacteria and in identifying unknown protein. When properly done, they are very sensitive and highly specific. The tests are done by producing antisera, usually in rabbits, by immunization with a known protein antigen. The antisera taken from the rabbits contain precipitins (antibodies produced by the reaction of soluble antigens with antibodies). These precipitins, when placed in solution with the protein used for immunization, will form a distinct white cloud—a visible precipitate.

Two examples of the use of precipitin tests are the typing and grouping of Beta streptococci (Lancefield method) and the test done to identify schistosomiasis (a disease caused by fluke infestation, which is rare in the United States).

D. Neutralization Tests

Neutralization tests are used to detect viruses and rickettsiae. They are the most common method used to confirm and serotype viral or rickettsial microorganisms. Neutralization signifies the process on which the tests are based. The unknown virus (patient's serum) is mixed with

TABLE 5–1. AGGLUTINATION TESTS

Name (Synonyms)	Reaction Results: Reference Range	Purpose	Comments
Antistreptolysin O (ASO, ASL)	Normal: 12–100 Todd units Significant: 100–2500 Todd units	Diagnosis of acute glomerulonephritis (AGN) and rheumatic fever	Until recently the ASO was felt to be the most helpful of the many antistreptococcal antibody measurements
Brucella agglutination test (brucellosis test, undulant fever test)	Normal: 1:40 or less Significant: 1:80 or greater	Diagnosis of brucellosis	Because of many cross-reactions (false positives), results confirm but do not diagnose brucellosis; history (e.g., drinking raw milk or working with large domestic animals: cattle, pigs, goats) helpful in increasing certainty
Cold agglutinins	Normal: less than 1:32 to 1:65	Diagnosis of primary atypical pneumonia (PAP)	Called "cold" because agglutination occurs only at 37°C or lower; formed in response to a number of diseases other than PAP at lower titers; high titers in vivo can cause hemolysis; a Coombs' (indirect) test also usually ordered to check for this
Febrile agglutination group (febrile agglutinins, febrile screen)	Can include any or all of the following tests: Salmonella-typhoid (paratyphoid and enteric, rickettsial disease (those included depend to a great extent on which ones are endemic in an area; see *Proteus* OX19) (see the Widal test for typhoid), brucellosis, tularemia; see specific tests for further information		
Heterophile screen (monospot, test for infectious mononucleosis, heterophile glutination)	Normal: negative (no agglutination)	Diagnosis of infectious mononucleosis	Heterophile refers to having an affinity to more than one antibody; there are close similarities between a normally appearing antibody in all human serum (Forssman) and the specific antibody found 2–3 weeks from the onset of infectious mononucleosis

(continued)

TABLE 5-1. (Continued)

Name (Synonyms)	Reaction Results: Reference Range	Purpose	Comments
Proteus OX19 (Rocky fever test, test for Rocky Mountain Spotted Fever [RMSF])	Negative: 1:60 or less Significant: 1:80 or greater	Diagnosis of Rocky Mountain Spotted Fever (RMSF)	A high percentage of people have a normal low titer because *Proteus* organisms are common infective agents not necessarily causing disease; important that more than one titer be done with at least a fourfold rise between acute and convalescent sera for diagnosis confirmation
Streptozyme	Negative: less than 1:100 (correlates with less than 166 Todd units)	Diagnosis of AGN and rheumatic fever	Similar to the ASO but thought to be more sensitive, detecting 95% of streptococcal infections (ASO 80–85%); also thought to be quite specific—90% chance to detect recent streptococcus infection; good correlation between the tests
Tularemia	Negative: no agglutination Significant: 1:40–1:80 or higher	Diagnosis of tularemia	Titers of 1:80 are diagnostic of actual infection; elevations may persist for years, but at less than 1:80; history of visits in endemic areas or work or leisure activity causing exposure (game warden or hunting)
Widal	Negative: 1:40 or less Significant: 1:80 or greater	Diagnosis of typhoid H and O, paratyphoid A and B	Two serotypes of *Salmonella* organisms, somatic (0) and flagellar (H), cause typhoid and paratyphoid fever; other serotypes of *Salmonella* cause a well-known type of food poisoning (salmonellosis); many variables affect results: titers increase in

| | | disease course; agglutination not due to disease found in elderly, drug addicts, previous vaccination, effect of antibiotics early in the disease |
| Venereal Disease Research Laboratory test (VDRL, RPR) | Negative: no agglutination of antigen (reagin) or less than 2+
 Positive: more than 2+ agglutination of antigen | Diagnosis of syphilis | The rapid plasma reagin (RPR), a modification of the VDRL, is the most commonly used *screening* test for syphilis (reagin) |

Abbreviations: ASO, ASL, antistreptolysin O; AGN, acute glomerulonephritis; PAP, primary atypical pneumonia; RMSF, Rocky Mountain spotted fever; RPR, rapid plasma reagin; VDRL, Venereal Disease Research Laboratory.

TABLE 5–2. COMPLEMENT FIXATION AND PRECIPITIN TESTS

Name (Synonyms)	Reaction Results: Reference Range	Purpose	Comments
Influenza serology (influenza A and B, flu test)	Negative: hemolysis Positive: no hemolysis	Diagnosis of influenza A or B	Titer increase of fourfold or greater indicative of recent infection; confirmed by viral isolation
Rickettsial serology	(Usually a group of rickettsial diseases are tested and reported as a group, including rickettsial pox, Q fever, RMSF [New World spotted fever or tick-borne typhus fever], epidemic louse-borne typhus fever) Negative: hemolysis Positive: no hemolysis		A fourfold difference between acute and convalescent titers probably significant for all the aforementioned diseases
Serological test for syphilis (standard test for syphilis; STS; Wasserman)	Negative: hemolysis Positive: no hemolysis	Diagnosis of syphilis	Rarely used now, but of historical interest as the first practical serological test; antibody produced is not specific to the syphilis causative organism and thus called a "reagin" rather than antibody; the most used test to confirm syphilis at present is the fluorescent treponenal antibody absorption test, or FTA-ABS (see the appropriate section)
Precipitin tests Beta streptococci	Typing and grouping Lancefield method	Identification and typing of bacteria	Replaced by blood culture in most laboratories
Schistosomiasis test	Visible precipitate	Identification of infestation by flukes	Rare in the United States. Increased numbers with immigration from Third World countires

a type-specific antiserum (an antiserum developed against the suspected infective microorganism). At the same time a control with known virus, antigen to the type-specific antisera, and the antisera are also mixed. After a short incubation both are inoculated into appropriate tissue cultures. The two are compared for neutralization effect on viral growth.

E. Fluorescent-Antibody Tests

Synonyms: FA; immunofluorescence tests

FA tests of this type (Table 5–3) are meant to identify suspected, specific organisms and cannot be used to identify unknown organisms. Fluorescent testing is based on tagging either a specific antibody or an antiimmunoglobulin (an antiantibody) with fluorescein labeling. If the specific microorganism is present in the patient's sample, the fluorescent antibody, or antiantibody, attaches, and the organism will be visible under a fluorescent microscope. Two methods are available for the test, the direct and the indirect. The indirect method is simpler and is used more frequently.

5.2.2 Allergy/Sensitivity Testing: Skin Tests

Skin tests are generally used to determine hypersensitivity or immunity. Hypersensitivity refers to an alteration in the strength of the reactivity of the body to a foreign or harmful agent. Allergy is a form of hypersensitivity. Immunity is the resistance of the body to the effects of harmful agents.

Many agents can, without causing obvious illness (subclinical disease states), trigger cell-mediated immunity. A fairly simple way to test cell-mediated immune function is by doing skin tests with commonly encountered antigens. The absence of any skin reaction to these antigens indicates a probably impaired immune function in the person tested.

In infectious disease, hypersensitivity, or "infectious allergy," is demonstrated by a positive, delayed inflammatory response at the site of an intracutaneous (intradermal) injection of the antigenic agent. The positive or inflammatory response indicates two things: (1) the individual being tested has an intact cell-mediated immune function, and (2) it indicates either a present or a past experience with the specific antigen used—evidenced by the "sensitized" response. A negative response indicates two possible causes: (1) no prior exposure to the infective agent, or (2) active infection with temporary loss of reactivity, a state known as *anergy*. A good example of this hypersensitive response to infectious disease is the Mantoux test to detect tuberculosis.

Anergy, as defined, occurs not only in the far-advanced stages of many infectious diseases but also accompanies some chronic diseases (e.g., Hodgkin's disease and sarcoidosis). It accompanies some of the exanthems of childhood (e.g., measles) and is found in individuals receiving immunosuppressant drugs such as the corticosteroids and anticancer or antithyroid drugs.

There are three types of biologic or diagnostic skin tests:

1. Tests to determine possible susceptibility or resistance to an infection (see Schick or Dick tests in Table 5–4)
2. Tests for "infectious allergy," described earlier

TABLE 5-3. FLUORESCENT ANTIBODY TESTS

Name (Synonyms)	Reaction Results: Reference Range	Purpose	Comments
Fluorescent treponemal antibody (FTA); treponemal antibody test; syphilis confirmation test	Negative: nonreactive Positive: 1+ to 4+ (weak to strong reaction)	Confirmation test for positive or weakly positive VDRL, STS tests	The VDRL test, a flocculation test, is rarely used as it has many cross-reactions; the FTA helps confirm a positive diagnosis but has many cross-reactions as well
Fluorescent treponemal antibody absorption test (FTA-ABS)	As for FTA	As for FTA	Also rarely used, this test is a modification of the FTA to eliminate many of the cross-reactions; it causes cross-reacting antibodies to be absorbed and increases test specificity (see Section 6.3.2.D, Tests for Syphilis)
Immunofluorescent study, urine (antibody coating, urine)	As for FTA but without indication of strength of positive reaction	Differentiation between cystitis and pyelonephritis	If bacteriuria is due to cystitis, the test response will be negative; if due to pyelonephritis, it will be positive; false positives occur with auto-fluorescence of staphylococci and *Pseudomonas* organisms
Legionnaires' serology (indirect fluorescent antibody; legionnaires' indirect antibody test)	Normal is negative or nonreactive; if positive, a titer is reported	Diagnosis of legionnaires' disease	Several different tests can be done to identify this disease (culture, direct immunofluorscent [IF] stain, tissue stain—Warthin—Starry); this test was included because it is simple and can be reported rapidly; diagnosis is by fourfold increase in titer or, in an "outbreak," a single positive, plus clinical signs and symptoms; very high titers have been reported in nonaffected individuals

| Direct fluorescent antibody tests: FA (fluorescent antibody) for specific microorganisms (Group A beta-hemolytic streptococci, *Neisseria gonorrheae*, legionnaires' bacillus, *Bordetella pertussis*) | Negative: no fluorescence
Positive: fluorescent staining of suspected microorganisms | Demonstration of suspected etiologic agents of disease in patient exudate or secretions | The simplest of fluorescent tests; diagnosis of etiologic agents is more rapid than by traditional culture methods (Harris, 1980) |

TABLE 5–4. SKIN TESTS

Test Name	Disease	Antigen	Reaction Time	Criteria for Positive Reaction/Discussion
Skin tests to determine susceptibility or resistance to infectious disease				
Dick	Scarlet fever	Erythrogenic toxin	18–24 hr	Induration 3–5 mm, very red erythema, marked by swollen sharply raised edges; indicates insufficient circulating antigen and susceptibility to scarlet fever
Maloney	Diphtheria	Plain toxin	12–24 hr	12-mm or greater erythema; used to detect hypersensitivity before immunization; with a positive reaction toxoid may be given only in very small doses and carefully monitored to prevent anaphylaxis
Schick	Diphtheria	Diphtheria toxin	24–48 hr	Induration 25–50 mm in diameter; erythema not measured; fading leaves brownish pigmented area; positive reaction indicates lack of antitoxin and need for immunization
	Control	Heated toxin	12–24 hr	Used to indicate immediate inflammatory response resulting from an allergic reaction to the protein; control compared with delayed response to eliminate false positives
Skin tests used primarily to test immune competence[a]				
Candidin	*Candida albicans*	Candidal cell wall	48–72 hr	10-mm or greater induration plus erythema; most persons with active immunocompetence systems will show a positive reaction; negative response, no reaction: anergy of T-lymphocyte response
Streptokinase-streptodornase (SK-SD)	Streptococci infections	Streptokinase-streptodornase (Varidase) streptococci enzymes	48 hr	Induration of 10-mm or greater; used to assess cellular immune response (immunocompetence); also used to evaluate anergy
Trichophyton	Ringworm	Extract of *Trichophyton*	48–72 hr	Induration of 5 mm or more; used to assess cellular immune response; most persons react positively; positive response increases with age
Diagnostic skin tests				
Brucellin	Brucellosis	Killed bacteria or protein nucleate	24–48 hr	Over 5-mm induration; not well standardized; serological test may be more helpful
Coccidioidin	Coccidioidomycosis	Culture filtrate of *Coccidioides immitis*	24–72 hr	Over 5-mm induration

Foshay	Tularemia	Killed bacteria	48 hr	Over 5-mm induration
Herpes simplex	Herpes simplex	Killed virus	18–24 hr	Induration of 15 mm or more; positive reaction indicates a primary infection and nonsusceptibility to systemic spread (i.e., encephalitis); local recurrence possible
Histoplasmin	Histoplasmosis (systemic fungal infection)	Killed fungi	48–72 hr	Induration of 5 mm or more; negative reaction, no response or erythema less than 5 mm; doubtful, induration less than 5 mm; positive, erythema more than 5 mm
Kveim	Sarcoidosis	Sarcoid tissue extract	4–8 weeks	Papule develops; biopsy and examine histologically for typical sarcoid pattern; positives less likely in chronic states of the disease
Frei	Lymphogranuloma venereum	Killed chlamydial agent	48–72 hr	8–20-mm induration indicates past or present infection with any of the psittacosis group
Mantoux	Tuberculosis	Purified protein derivative (PPD) or old tuberculin (OT) tests	24–72 hr	Induration of 10 mm or larger; National Tuberculosis Association criteria on 0 to 4+ scale: Doubtful (+/–1) Erythema, edema 5 mm or less; 1+ (+) Erythema, edema 5–10 mm; 2+ (++) Erythema, edema 10–20 mm; 3+ (+++) Marked erythema, edema exceeds 20 mm; 4+ (++++) Erythema, edema, and central necrosis (Davidsohn & Henry, 1969)
Mumps	Mumps	Inactivated vaccine		Erythema of 15 mm or more, with or without induration, indicates some protection against mumps; in a case of active mumps and no previous exposure, the skin test will not become + for several days; + reactions at onset of mumps-like disease may rule out mumps
Schultz-Charlton	Scarlet fever	Antitoxin or convalescent scarlet fever serum	18–24 hr	Injected into area of bright rash suspected to be scarlet fever; + reaction, a blanched area 2–8 mm surrounding needle puncture in cases of scarlet fever; differentiates rash from that of measles, rubella, drug allergies; response increased with allergy to horse serum

(continued)

TABLE 5–4. (Continued)

Test Name	Disease	Antigen	Reaction Time	Criteria for Positive Reaction/Discussion
Tine	Tuberculosis	PPD or OT	48–72 hr	2-mm or more palpable induration around one or more of the four puncture sites; useful screening test; doubtful reactions should be rechecked with a Mantoux test
Trichinin	Trichinosis	Killed larvae	15 min	Wheal and erythematous reaction; delayed reaction occurring after 24 hr is less specific; test remains + for many years, thus possible false positives; many commercial antigens too insensitive, thus causing false negatives

Abbreviations: SK-SD, Streptokinase-Streptodornase; PPD, purified protein derivative; OT, old tuberculin.
[a]Often done at the same time as other skin tests.

3. Skin tests to determine sensitivity to environmental materials that induce an exaggerated reaction in the sensitized host (e.g., hay fever, asthma, food allergies)

The first two categories are discussed in this section (see Table 5–4). The reader is referred to a general medical or surgical nursing text for information about the last category because it is beyond the scope of this section.

In the first two categories no attempt has been made to include all possible skin tests. Instead, a fair sample of the more commonly used tests are presented, which should provide an understanding of the process.

IMPLICATIONS FOR NURSING: SKIN TESTS

1. Skin tests by injection are done by using an intradermal (intracutaneous) approach. Because the reliability of the test response depends in great measure on the injection procedure's being faultless and because these injections are often the nurse's responsibility, the procedure is reviewed briefly here
   a. Explanation of the process. Because there are almost always side effects of some kind from skin tests, the patient and family need to be fully informed as to what to expect; thus the nurse needs to be fully informed before beginning the procedure. The patient and family also need reassurance that the benefit of the skin test outweighs the risks involved. The nurse can only undertake such assurance if indeed the benefit *does* outweigh the risk. Therefore, the nurse needs not only to know the expected benefit for *this* individual but also to have at hand or undertake a thorough history and physical of the individual so that specific risks peculiar to this one individual are also known (e.g., history of hypersensitivity of any kind, presence of rash of unknown etiology)
   b. Selection of site. The area selected should be free of any edema, chronic skin disease (e.g., eczema), infectious process, scarring, or potential for irritation from clothing or from use of the body part. The inner aspect of the forearm is frequently used
   c. Selection of materials:
      (1) Needle: Short bevel, 3/8 to 5/8 inches in length, 25 to 27 gauge
      (2) Syringe: Tuberculin or other calibrated in 0.01-ml units, 1-ml capacity
      (3) Antigen: Usually kept refrigerated (some exceptions, such as for the tine test)
   d. Check antigen with that ordered. Measurement of the antigen in the syringe *must* be precise. Overdosage could cause anaphylactic shock. Underdosage would fail to stimulate an antibody response, the purpose of the skin test
      (1) Be sure that the dilution of the antigen is correct. Antigens for skin testing can be provided in many strengths. The most commonly used dilution is 1:100, but not all tests are done with that dilution. Check the physician's order. Usually, the *smallest* concentrations of any given series of dilutions is given first. The use of more concentrated antigens can result in serious side effects in hyperimmune individuals
      (2) Do not use an air lock in the syringe and needle after drawing up the antigen. (An air lock is 0.2 to 0.3 ml of air in syringe to prevent trailing of an irritating substance intradermally when giving a subcutaneous or intramuscular injection.) The skin test injection is intradermal and is supposed to irritate the tissues
   e. Check the five Rs of medication administration. Right patient, right medication, right dosage, right time, and right route. Use the recommended skin preparation of the facility. It is most important that *any* substance used to disinfect the skin be allowed to dry thoroughly before injection. Materials on the skin will trail the needle if wet and can cause a false skin reaction
   f. Injection. With the skin held tautly, the needle is inserted bevel up, just under the top layer of skin at about a 10° to 15° angle, almost flat with the skin. The needle should be inserted only

enough to cover the bevel, the outline of which should be almost visible under the skin. If injected too deeply, a false-negative reaction may occur.

Inject antigen slowly, making a small bleb, or wheal, under the skin. In some places and some instances, the wheal is outlined with indelible ink when the needle has been withdrawn to facilitate location of the injection site at the time of reading the reaction

g. Observe the patient carefully for 20 to 30 minutes after the injection for any systemic response to the antigen (hypersensitivity). Epinephrine in a 1:1000 solution for parenteral administration should be on hand. At times, standing orders suggest that it be injected directly into the skin at the needle mark of the test site upon appearance of untoward effects.

Systemic signs and symptoms to observe for include decreased blood pressure; a general feeling of apprehension or doom; weakness; pruritis; signs of perspiration, angioedema, urticaria, dyspnea or shortness of breath (SOB), wheezing, or changes in pulse (fast, irregular, weak, absent); and signs of changes in level of consciousness

2. Reading skin test reactions is frequently a nursing responsibility, or it may be the responsibility of the nurse to instruct the patient and family in the process

a. To quantify skin reactions accurately, a metric ruler should be used to measure the diameter of the indurated or erythematous area. Erythema is not usually included in the positive response, but will be in certain selected tests such as mumps (see Table 5–4, "Diagnostic Skin Tests")

b. Reading of reactions should be done in optimum light, preferably daylight

c. A rough grading system that does measure erythema can be made of the +/- approach using a target wheel guide (Brunner & Suddarth, 1988)

–	No reaction
+	Erythema smaller than a nickel in diameter
++	Erythema larger than a nickel (21 mm)
+++	Erythema and wheal (induration) without pseudopod formation (foot-like protrusions out from the wheal)
++++	Erythema and wheal with pseudopod formation

d. Erythema measurement is felt to be of no diagnostic value by some and induration (hardness) of the injection site is thought to be a better measurement (Luckmann & Sorensen, 1987)

5.3 TESTS FOR SPECIFIC DISEASES

5.3.1 Lyme Disease

Definition. Lyme disease is a multisystem inflammatory disorder caused by a deer tick-borne spirochete (*Borrelia burgdorferi*). Different ticks are carriers.* Lyme disease is of particular interest at this time because of a marked increase in incidence since 1991. It is difficult to diagnose by current methods, particularly early in the infectious process. The vector is not seen on direct examination of blood.

Signs and Symptoms. Generally early symptoms are vague and vary from person to person. A latent period, also extremely variable, of a few months to more than a year occurs in many cases. This is often followed by recurring or chronic arthritis. Some individuals complain only of lethargy and aches and pains similar to a flu syndrome.

---

*In the United States the following ticks have been identified as bearers of the disease: *Ixodes damnini* in the Northeast; *Ixodes pacificus* in the Northwest; and *Ixodes scapularis* and *Amblyomme americanum* in the Southeast.

Wallach (1992) has described stages of the disease process that are useful, if not applicable in all cases:

- *Stage 1*. Nonspecific febrile and viral-like symptoms 3 to 33 days after tick bite occurrence; characteristic erythema chronicum migrans (a small red bump at the site with a surrounding rash). Diagnostic tests during this period are seldom useful as they lack sensitivity and the diagnosis cannot be ruled out by a negative test.
- *Stage 2*. Approximately 4 weeks after the tick bite, appearance of other signs or symptoms (no standard occurrence or frequence). Ten percent of affected individuals have cardiac involvement (carditis), which is the most frequent cause of death in this disease. Fifteen percent present with neurologic symptoms (aseptic meningitis; Bell's palsy; peripheral neuropathy). Testing in this period may be inaccurate because of the use of early antibiotics in stage 1, which prevents antibody response.
- *Stage 3*. Six weeks to several years after tick bite, approximately 60 percent of untreated cases experience a recurrence of symptoms with arthritis the most common disorder. In young people this is often mistaken as juvenile rheumatoid arthritis. Diagnostic tests are primarily serological at this time, although many types of testing are being developed as present serological tests tend to lack sensitivity and specificity. Therefore, clinical observation and judgment are still of major importance in determining patient status.

Tests

STAGE 1: Western Blot. (See test details in section 6.3.2.E.) This test is more sensitive and specific than the enzyme-linked immunoabsorbent assay (ELISA) and therefore of greater value during the first month of Lyme disease infection. It is, however, technically difficult, not available in many areas, and not standardized at this time.*

STAGE 2. ELISA Test. (See test detail in Section 6.3.2.E.) This test measures antibody produced by the body in response to infection, specifically IgM (increased in the first 3 to 6 weeks) and IgG that increases more slowly. It is positive for IgG in almost all patients with complications in stages 2 and 3 on the first specimen. In most cases that single positive specimen, along with physical signs and symptoms, is considered adequate for confirmation of diagnosis.

However false positives can occur with high titers when other spirochetal diseases are present (e.g., syphilis, yaw, pinta; and low titers in the presence of hepatitis B; infectious mononucleosis; and some autoimmune diseases [e.g., conditions causing the presence of rheumatoid factor]).

Early treatment with any antibiotic can prevent *any* antibody response.

---

*It has been noted that the Western Blot test commercially available is often designed to detect *outer surface proteins* unique to the spirochete, which may not appear for months after acute infection, in which case serum can test positive by ELISA, but negative or indeterminant by Western Blot. It is suggested that the most appropriate use of the immunoblot (Western Blot) test is for low clinical suspicion for Lyme disease and multiple positive ELISA tests (Yost, 1992, p. 1218).

IMPLICATIONS FOR NURSING

1. Prevention: Information to be included in teaching:
   a. For individuals who expect to be at risk for infection, use of protective clothing, which in turn is treated with a protectant and skin repellent, is required
   b. DEET is a strongly recommended skin repellent in concentrations of 50 to 75 percent (higher concentrations can cause toxic reactions). Application should cover exposed skin (except near the eyes, mouth, on open cuts, irritated skin, or on the hands of children), as well as on clothing. It should be applied as infrequently as possible and washed off the skin on return indoors (Recommend Commercial Insect Repellents to Help Ward Off Lyme Disease, August, 1992, *Modern Medicine*, Vol. 60 #8, p. 23)
   c. Clothing for outside: Long pants, tucked into high-top shoes, long-sleeved shirt (light-colored clothes display the presence of ticks best, which can be as small as a pinhead)
   d. Inspection: Check self, children, and pets daily or more frequently, using thin-tipped tweezers for removal of ticks (which are smaller than dog ticks; immature ticks (nymphs) are smaller than a pinhead). Use a slow, steady pull without twisting which can break off the mouth parts leading to infection at the site. Place ticks in a covered jar of alcohol that can be taken to a health department, clinic, or physician for identification
2. Precautions with children: DEET can cause allergic reactions in some children. A repellent designed especially for children (Skedaddle) that contains only 10% DEET in an oil-based medium is available. The oil base allows slow release of the compound and limits its absorption through the skin. It can be used by adults with sensitivity to DEET as well (provided in individual application pouches) ("Lyme Disease Update," 1992, pp. 1–2.)

5.3.2 Epstein-Barr Test Battery

Tests Included: Epstein-Barr antibody; Epstein-Barr virus by immunofluorescent assay (EBV-IFA); viral capised antigen (VCA-IgG/IgM); early antibody (EA); Epstein-Barr associated nuclear antigen (EBNA)

Definition. The Epstein-Barr virus (EBV) is perhaps best known as the causative agent of fairly rare and exotic disorders such as lymphoma or lymphoproliferative disease or immunodeficiency (Chediak-Higashi's syndrome). Knowledge of its role as the etiologic agent in mononucleosis is fairly recent.

Serological testing

1. Determines susceptibility, immunity, or primary EBV infection
2. Helps determine the significance of presence of heterophile antibody or antibody negative mononucleosis syndrome, as well as to show association of EBV with other syndromes

Common Serological Patterns*

	IgM	IgG	EA	EBNA
Newborn (maternal)	–	+	–	–
Susceptible	–	–	–	–

*Laboratory of Pathology, 1991.

	IgM	IgG	EA	EBNA
Recent primary infection	+	+	+/–	–
Immune (latent quiescent)	–	+	–	+
Reactivation	–/++	++	+	+
Chronic	–/+	++	++	+
Heterotypic (findings not focused on EB—nonspecific)	++	+	–/+	+

Findings: High Titers

1. *Viral capised antigen-IgG (VCA-IgG).* IgM rises early in the primary infection. Once elevated, it persists for life. IgG and IgM peak during acute stage, decline 1 to 2 months after infection; IgG titers persist at lower levels for a few years. The VCA-IgG has been the most commonly used single test

2. *Antibody to EBV nuclear antigen (EBNA).* Absent in acute phase, appearing weeks to months after onset. Consists of six distinct DNA-binding nuclear proteins with the following known functions
   a. EBNA-1: essential for maintenance and replication of episomal viral DNA
   b. EBNA-2: involved in the initial phase of B-cell immortalization
   c. EBNA-3-6: Have been identified; genome coding defined; function still under study

3. *Early antibody (EA).* The *diffuse component (EA-D)* appears briefly in the acute stage of infectious mononucleosis. Antibodies to the *restricted component of EA (EA-R)* are found in pediatric primary infection, epidemic Burkitt's lymphoma (BL), and some acquired immunodeficiency states (e.g., AIDS)

4. *Elevated levels of IgG antibody to VCA and EA* usually indicate active viral replication. Antibodies to EBNA appear late in the process and may be related to T-cell immunodeficiency. (Because there is considerable overlap in the last three serological patterns, correlation of clinical findings is important in the diagnosis [Laboratory of Pathology, 1991])

5. *Related tests of significance.* Examination by culture of peripheral blood lymphocytes and lymphoid cells from lesions and throat washings can help support diagnosis. At one time saliva sampling was the most effective test available.

Physical findings of EBV include fever, pharyngitis, lymphadenopathy, and, less often, splenomegaly. Lymphocytosis with atypical lymphocytes is also present in most cases.

Pathophysiology. The EBV is a human herpes virus that infects B-lymphocytes and certain kinds of epithelial cells. The infected B cells are "immortalized," growing continuously. There are only two known patterns of its development. In the first a latent infection develops; in the second, an active infection occurs in which many copies of the genome and mature virons are produced and released.*

After an EBV infection, a variety of viral antigens appear in the infected B cells. EBNA, which is made up of six different DNA-binding proteins, is expressed first, followed by cellular

---

*A *genome* is defined as the complete set of hereditary factors contained in the haploid set of chromosomes. *Haploid* is defined as the condition of having half the number of chromosomes characteristically found in the somatic (diploid) cells of an organism. (Miller & Keane, 1983, p. 521).

DNA synthesis, the function of which is still being studied. Thereafter, the infected B cells divide, secreting immunoglobulin.

EBV FOUND IN INDIVIDUALS WITH

1. African Burketts lymphoma
2. Nasopharyngeal carcinoma
3. Infectious mononucleosis
4. AIDS, as a secondary infection

Immunity to the EBV suggests immunity to infectious mononucleosis.

5.3.3. Kawasaki's Syndrome

Synonyms: KS; Kawasaki's disease; mucocutaneous lymph node syndrome; infantile periarteritis nodosa (PAN)

(*Conn, 1991*, pp. 114–44)

Definition. KS is a fairly recently described acute febrile illness, first described in 1967 as infantile PAN. Approximately 80 percent of cases occur in children under the age of 5. The cause is unknown but appears to have some link to streptococcal erythrogenic toxins. Data suggest that it is transmitted by an anthropod vector or animal reservoir (Leung, 1991, p. 42). It primarily affects infants and children:

1. Under 5 in the United States, between 12 and 24 months of age most frequently
2. In late winter, early spring (> 80 percent)
3. Of male sex
4. Of every race (order of prevalence: Asians, blacks, whites)

If untreated, its most common sequelae are coronary artery abnormalities with chronic cardiac insufficiency, myocardial infarction, and possible sudden death secondary to aneurysm rupture. In the United States and Japan, KS has become one of the leading causes of acquired heart disease in children (Leung, 1991, p. 30).

Pathophysiology. KS is a self-limiting disease of unknown etiology but believed to be caused by an infectious agent. Therefore, diagnosis is based primarily on signs and symptoms. The disease process is characterized by immunoregulatory imbalance and lymphocyte activation, as indicated by the following laboratory findings:

1. Increased numbers of activated helper T lymphocytes and monocytes
2. Decreased CD8+ suppressor/cytotoxic T lymphocytes
3. Marked polyclonal B-cell activity

In the acute phase

1. Elevated serum-soluble interleukin (IL)-2 receptor levels
2. Circulating antibodies are cytotoxic against stimulated vascular endothelial cells appear (Leung, 1991, p. 32).

Disease phases. (Signs and symptoms are included as diagnostic criteria in the absence of specific testing.) There are three phases:

1. *Acute phase* (duration 10–14 days after onset of fever):
   a. Prolonged high fever, unresponsive to antibiotics, lasting 1 to 2 weeks. Any child with prolonged temperature increase that is unresponsive to antibiotics and not attributable to another cause is considered to have KS (Whaley & Wong, 1991)
   b. One or more oropharyngeal changes:
      (1) Injected, dry, fissured lips
      (2) Injected pharynx
      (3) "Strawberry" tongue
   c. One or more changes in extremities:
      (1) Peripheral edema
      (2) Periungual (nail bed) desquamation
      (3) General desquamation
      (4) Cervical lymphadenopathy
      (5) Hyperemic areas with desquamation of palms or soles
      (6) Diffuse macular or plaque-type blanching
      (7) Arthritis with small-joint involvement
   d. Major causes of death at this stage are acute myocarditis and cardiac arrhythmia
2. *Subacute phase* (15–25 days after onset of fever)
   a. Resolution of fever
   b. Risk greatest for:
      (1) Coronary artery aneurysm
      (2) Hypercoagability leading to thrombocytosis and coronary thrombosis
   c. Arthritis in long-boned, weight-bearing joints
   d. Periungual desquamation (shedding of skin around the nails) of hands and feet
   e. Major cause of death at this stage include ischemic heart disease, rupture of an aneurysm, and acute myocarditis associated with lesions of the conduction system
3. Convalescent phase (70 days)
   a. Resolution of all clinical signs of KS
   b. Erythrocyte sedimentation rate increased secondary to continued inflammation
   c. Arthritis in late phase due to involvement of weight-bearing joints
   d. Coronary complications due to thrombotic occlusion of coronary aneurysm and stenosis
   e. Major cause of death at this stage is myocardial infarction in children with ischemic heart disease due to residual coronary artery aneurysms and stenoses

Diagnostic tests. In the absence of specific tests for diagnosis of this disease, guidelines for diagnosis are based on clinical findings and associated laboratory test results (diagnosis of exclusion).

1. Hematology:
   a. Decreased RBC count: normocytic, normochromic anemia
   b. Persistent increased (6–8 weeks) erythrocyte sedimentation rate (ESR) suggestive of ongoing inflammation

    c. White blood cell count (WBC) increased with a shift to the left (increased immature WBCs) leading to an inflammatory response with lymphocytic predominance, which indicate immunologic responses (Cunha, 1992, p. 210)

    d. Increased platelet turnover and count (week 2 or 3) (thrombocytosis), a hallmark finding that is persistent and profound and thought to be suggestive of an inflammatory or immune response

    e. Increased liver transaminase, possibly secondary to hepatic swelling and often concurrent with increased bilirubin and alkaline phosphatase

2. Urinalysis: Increased mononuclear WBCs indicative of so-called sterile pyuria

3. Echocardiograms to monitor myocardial and coronary artery status (see also Section 17.6.1.C)

4. Ultrasound: to monitor fluid accumulation (hydrops) in the gallbladder (see also Section 17.6.1.G)

IMPLICATIONS FOR NURSING

Nursing care requires understanding of the disease process and acute as well as pertinent observation to provide individualized care and to prevent or identify the occurrence of complications

1. Medications:
    a. Aspirin is the mainstay medical treatment because of its antiinflammatory and antithrombotic actions.
        (1) Usual dosage: 80–100 mg/kg of body weight per day
        (2) Daily serum salicylate level of 20–25 mg/dL maintained during the acute phase
        (3) After fever is controlled, dosage is reduced to 3–5 mg/kg of body weight for platelet activity inhibition
        (4) Continued until platelet count, ESR, and echocardiograms become normal
        (5) If coronary artery aneurysm(s) persist, platelet inhibition is continued indefinitely
    b. Intravenous gamma globulin (IVGG) at 400 mg/kg of body weight is given for 4 consecutive days (total dose 1,600 mg) and combined with aspirin therapy. (This therapy has been tested in Japan and in the United States and has been found to be effective in reducing development of coronary artery abnormalities if given early in the course of the illness [Leung, 1991, p. 48].) It has been found to prevent the formation of the most serious complication of KS, the development of giant aneurysms. Administration of a single infusion of 2 g/kg over 10 hours may be given in preference to a 4-day infusion regime (400 mg/kg/d). The single prolonged infusion has been found to significantly lower the prevalence of coronary artery abnormalities in the children receiving it (Leung, 1991, p. 48)

2. Provision of symptomatic relief:
    a. Skin care: With temperature elevation, gentle application of soothing, nonperfumed body lotion; loose clothing; frequent position change (during "fretful" periods) can be helpful
        (1) Ensuring adequate fluid intake can help prevent skin breakdown, as will frequent position change while the child is awake
    b. Irritability of the child is a difficult problem for the caretakers, to include the family.
        (1) Maintain as quiet and peaceful an environment as possible
        (2) Provide the family with support (e.g., respite time away from the bedside without guilt; information about irritability as an integral part of the disease process)
    c. Pain and decreased range of motion (ROM) secondary to arthritis:
        (1) Provide and teach passive ROM to the affected joint as often and as much as is tolerable for the child (best accepted when the joint is warm, e.g., during a bath)

    (2) Administer aspirin as ordered, and teach the family its purposes and when to hold, rather than give, the medication, that is:

        (a) With signs or symptoms of aspirin toxicity (tinnitus, headache, dizziness, unusual confusion)

        (b) With exposure to many infectious diseases (e.g., chickenpox; influenza) because of the drug's association with Reye's syndrome

3. Ensure that the parents or caretakers are aware of, and knowledgeable about, signs and symptoms of cardiac complications to report in the future, should they occur, and are able to perform CPR.

4. Defer any live immunization (e.g., measles, mumps, rubella) until 3 months after gamma globulin treatment as appropriate antibodies will not be produced (Whaley & Wong, 1991, pp. 1586–87)

Six

Infectious and Sexually Transmitted Diseases

6.1 PREVENTION

One of the major nursing roles in communicable diseases is that of prevention.

6.1.1 General Approaches to Prevention
1. Identification of populations at risk for infectious disease secondary to decreased or absent immune response, or increased probability of exposure.
    a. Infants and young adults, particularly for those with viral and upper respiratory infections (URIs), especially in infants of low birthweight, because of ineffective or immature body defense against infection and a lack of acquired immunity
    b. Patients with chronic disease or malignancies because of decreased resistance
    c. Persons receiving immunosuppressive drugs (e.g., organ transplant patients) or cancer patients taking chemotherapeutic drugs
    d. Postoperatively in debilitated and obese patients as a result of impaired blood supply to affected tissues, particularly those persons with diabetes mellitus
2. Identification of populations at risk for complications of infectious disease
    a. The elderly, particularly progressive viral pneumonia or respiratory failure after an URI
    b. Persons with chronic obstructive pulmonary disease (COPD) and/or asthma, particularly lower respiratory infections or respiratory failure
    c. Persons with diabetes mellitus
    d. Pregnant women, particularly for lower respiratory tract infection (e.g., influenza, viral pneumonia, and urinary tract infections (UTIs) resulting from inadequate expansion with mechanical restriction)
    e. Persons with heart disease due to impaired blood supply, which decreases the numbers of white blood cells (WBCs) available to fight infection and reduces the body's ability to remove waste and debris from infection, added to the inability of the heart to cope with increased metabolic rate, further decreasing perfusion
    f. Postoperative patients, who are particularly prone to respiratory infection because of decreased ventilation secondary to pain or immobility and the irritant effect of inhalant anesthesia; also wound infections with potential for septicemia
3. Maintaining a high index of suspicion for manifestations of infectious disease, especially in high-risk populations

6.1.2 Identification of Infectious Disease

Initial identification is often done by a family member or the patient. The nurse is, however, very frequently the first member of the health team contacted for validation of his or her conclusions. To screen out innocuous complaints such as diaper rash, the nurse needs to have acquired a sound knowledge base about the major characteristics of infectious disease commonly occurring in the locality to make pertinent assessments. The base should include the order and progression of signs and symptoms in commonly occurring (e.g., the type, initial location, and progression of skin rashes), knowledge of which diseases are endemic in the geographic area, and knowledge of the method of transmission of commonly occurring or endemic diseases.

Given this knowledge base, the nurse must then be able to transfer it into clinical action by:

1. Pertinent questioning about possible contact with infectious individuals; recent changes in environment—travel in areas where certain diseases are endemic; contact with many household pets; rats in a poor environment; raw animal products such as wool, hides, and blood—or initiation of drug therapy with an immunosuppressant effect. A nursing history can only be as thorough as the knowledge base of the history taker
2. Visual inspection and careful history taking about progress and changes in signs and symptoms

6.1.3 Teaching in Prevention of Spread of Infection

The nurse can assist the person and family with an infectious disease or process in two general ways: direct care and teaching. Teaching should include the patient and any other populations contacted during care.

1. See Implications for Nursing: Urine Screen, Section 4.12 for nursing implications related to the spread of UTIs
2. Use of vaccines in the prevention of influenza (a broad term for a number of different infections)
   a. Risk groups, as defined by the Centers for Disease Control (CDC) in Atlanta, who should be immunized and given priority for immunization: critical health care workers; police; firefighters; people with COPD, heart disease, diabetes mellitus, or Addison's disease; persons taking immunosuppressive drugs or therapy (this group is rarely immunized, however, because of the risk of overwhelming infection from the vaccine); and those over 65. It is recommended that the elderly receive full vaccination yearly
   b. Vaccination is the preferred prophylactic method in influenza
3. Use of medications in the prevention of influenza
   a. Risk groups, as defined by the National Institutes of Health (NIH), for the use of amantadine (Symmetrel)
      (1) All ages with underlying serious illness
      (2) Individuals in whom shortening of a symptomatic illness by 24 hours is judged important
      (3) Unvaccinated adults performing activities essential to community function
      (4) Unvaccinated individuals in semiclosed environments, especially the elderly. (This last recommendation is modified by the fact that the benefit–risk considerations for the elderly are less clear than for other ages [Marks, 1980])
   b. Information about amantadine use for patient and family teaching

      (1) Used when vaccine is not available, is contraindicated, or in high-risk groups who have just been vaccinated. Used only until antibodies to vaccination appear. Must be started within 24 to 48 hours postexposure to be effective

      (2) Side effects: Usually dose-related (>200 mg/day). More frequent in elderly persons with congestive heart disease or impaired renal function. A divided dosage, AM and PM, helps to decrease the incidence of side effects. Central nervous system signs and symptoms (from dizziness to frank psychosis and convulsions) and cardiovascular signs and symptoms (from simple orthostatic hypotension to frank congestive heart failure) are the most common

4. Vaccines are also available for numerous diseases and should be studied as to use, type of immunity provided (active, passive), and special precautions. Some diseases for which vaccine can be provided include cholera, plague, rabies, Rocky Mountain spotted fever (RMSF), smallpox, typhoid fever, typhus, yellow fever, tuberculosis, and strains of *Streptococcus pneumoniae*

5. Immunization program for normal infants and children
    a. A dramatic decline in the incidence of the "common" childhood infectious diseases occurred over the last several decades as a result of routine immunization programs. A less desirable outcome has been the decreased reporting of infectious disease probably due to the decreased importance attached to the need for immunization by some because of a lack of experience in widespread infectious disease outbreaks or severe epidemics. The responsibility of the nurse to stress the "whys" of immunization for all infants and children is increased proportionately. A good resource to prepare for such teaching is a pamphlet available from the CDC (Atlanta, GA 30333) called "Vaccines and Immunizations"
    b. Recommended immunization schedules:
      (1) Infants and young children generally follow this pattern (Whaley & Wong, 1991, American Academy of Pediatrics, 1986, p. 9)

2 months	Diphtheria, tetanus toxoid, and pertussis vaccine (DPT); trivalent oral polio virus vaccine (TOPV) (aka-OPV); can be initiated as early as two (2) weeks in high-risk areas (epidemics)
4 months	DPT and TOPV (2-month interval recommended between the two to avoid interference from initial dose)
6 months	DPT, optional TOPV (e.g., if polio is endemic in area)
1 year	Tuberculin test (ITBC) to precede or coincide with measles vaccine now *or at 15 months*
15 months	*Haemophilus influenza* vaccine (HIB). Any HIB conjugate vaccines may be used. ITBC, measles, rubella, and mumps vaccines (MMR/MMRV) combined vaccines, e.g., MMR, preferred to individual doses. (TBC testing may be done at the same time.)
18 months	Hemophilus influenza (HBP) vaccine
4–6 years	Diphtheria, pertussis, tetanus (DPT) and trivalent oral poliovirus (TOPV) vaccines
11–12 years	Repeat HIB on entrance to middle or junior high school
14–16 years	Tetanus and diphtheria toxoid (Td), repeated every 10 years throughout life

      (2) Adults (See Table 6–1)

TABLE 6–1. RECOMMENDED IMMUNIZATION SCHEDULE FOR ADULTS

Infectious Disease Name	Immunization Recommended	Risk Populations
Tetanus/diphtheria	If immunized with DPT as a child, only booster immunization is required. Boosters are given every 10 years	All individuals are at risk as the infection does not stimulate circulating antitoxins
Hepatitis B	Series of three intramuscular (IM) (deltoid) injections, widely spaced (2nd and 3rd dose 1–6 months after first). Hemophiliacs injected subcutaneously (SC), not IM. Not given in the buttocks because of poor immune response. All three doses necessary for protection	Individuals requiring administration of blood or blood products (to include hemodialysis); health care workers; sexually active individuals with multiple partners, any person from a country or area with a high hepatitis B infection rate
Influenza	Annual vaccination for risk populations in single dose (whole virus) or divided doses (2; split virus) 4 weeks apart. Usually given before flu season (fall)	Individuals 65 or older, and/or with chronic illness (diabetes/anemia/heart/lung/ kidney disease; persistent anemia; immune system deficiency; persons living in nursing homes). Allergy possible
Measles	Frequently given with rubella; live virus given SC.	Persons born before 1957 considered immune. Contraindicated in persons with tuberculosis, immunodeficiency, or allergy to eggs/neomycin
Pnuemococcal infections	May be given IM or SC. A booster not required but at times given for high risk	Two to three times increased risk in the elderly and/or individuals with chronic disease
Rubella	Live virus given SC, often with another vaccine (mumps). Not given to pregnant women or those planning pregnancy because of possibility/risk of fetal infection	Women of childbearing age or any persons who have not had the disease or have not been previously vaccinated
Tetanus	Can be given as trivalent vaccine, DPT. Tetanus booster injection given thereafter in case of injury that allows contaminated soil contact with mucous membrane. Immunization does not follow infection: circulating antigens are not stimulated	Survival rate in adults approximately 50% with tetanus infection. Booster injections given every 10 years

Data from Burrell, 1992, Table 8–1, pp. 91–92.

6.2 NURSING MANAGEMENT

6.2.1 Necessary Knowledge Base

Once a specific infectious process is definitely suspected or diagnosed, the nurse can only provide safe and effective care when in possession of the following knowledge about the suspected or actual microorganism

1. The class of infectious agent (e.g., bacteria, virus). Check lab reports for results of culture and evaluation of smears and stains
2. The body parts or secretions infected with or harboring the infectious microorganisms and thus contagious (e.g., blood, feces, sputum, wound exudate). Assess the patient, and review the microbiology of the suspect organism
3. The method of transmission of the microorganism from host to host. Review the microbiology of the suspect organism
4. The principal portal of entry for the microorganism. Review pertinent microbiology
5. Unhealthy environments for the organism; what affects its survival in the host and in the environment. Review the microbiology
6. What, if any, immunity occurs after the infection and the duration of that immunity (permanent, temporary?). Review the microbiology
7. What, if any, induced immunity is available (vaccine? toxoid? antisera?) and the duration of that immunity. Review the microbiology. Consult with the physician, infection control officer, or microbiologist

6.2.2 Application of Knowledge Base

Given the aforementioned necessary knowledge base, nursing care to support the patient's defense against the organism, to prevent spread of the infection to others, and to prevent reinfection or secondary infection of the patient can be planned

1. The type of isolation, if any, is predicated primarily on knowledge of items 1 to 5 in Section 6.2.1. Care of items in contact with the patient is also based on that knowledge
2. The selection of health care workers to implement nursing care should be determined primarily from the knowledge of items 6 and 7
3. Medical treatment has its premise in knowledge of items 1, 2, 4, and 5. The nurse follows the response of the patient to the treatment prescribed by checking for changes in clinical signs and symptoms of the infection, the appearance of negative lab reports on cultures and slides, and decreasing titers in serological tests. Collection of specimens for laboratory examination is based on the knowledge of items 1, 2, and 5. (See also Section 5.1.2.)
4. Methods of disinfection require a knowledge of items 1 to 3 and 5

6.2.3 Maintenance of Infection Control Procedures

A. Introduction

The scope of this book does not allow coverage of the principles and methods of infection control. Probably the most consistently used approach, and most effective, is the use of the *Universal Precautions* prepared by the CDC, which focuses on control of blood-borne pathogens. (See Appendix I). The effectiveness of infection control is primarily in the hands of the nurse caring for the patient. There is also the obligation to teach the importance of the control procedures, role modeling consistent practice of them. Further, it is the obligation of the nurse to help *all* other members of the health team practice them as well. It is imperative that the nurse, by careful study and updating of information, ensure that the infection control methods used are indeed based on an accurate understanding of the infectious process present *and* are effective in control of the infection if properly followed.

B. *Precautions Related to In-Home Management*

1. *Housekeeping*. Wear *intact* gloves impermeable to liquids. Walls, floors, and other surfaces of that nature are not associated with transmission of infections to patients or health care workers. Therefore, cleanliness is to be encouraged, but sterile environments are unnecessary. Routine cleaning and soil removal are suggested whenever indicated (e.g., after spills or soiling). Any surface used should be cleaned after use. Scrubbing is at least as important as using any antimicrobial cleaning agent; both are recommended.

2. *Spills of blood or other body fluids*. Use of chemical germicides approved as hospital disinfectants is recommended. Visible material should first be removed and then the area decontaminated. If the spill is large, first decontaminate the area by flooding with a liquid germicide before cleaning.

3. *Care of clothing*. Risk of actual disease transmission through handling soiled clothing is negligible. Use common sense. Handle soiled linen as little as possible in the cleaning process. Minimal agitation (e.g., shaking) prevents gross microbial contamination of the air and persons handling the clothing/linens. Bag all soiled linen where it is used: do not sort or rinse in living areas. Articles soiled with blood or body fluids should be placed in fluid-impermeable bags. For materials that can be washed in hot water, use water at 160°F (71°C). Low-temperature laundry should be washed at l58°F (70°C). Use chemicals made for low-temperature washing (CDC, 1987a).

6.2.4 General Approaches to Nursing Management of Acute Infectious Disease Related to Common Patient Problems

1. Nursing diagnosis: Alteration in fluid volume deficit; dehydration due to fever or decreased intake
   a. Encourage fluid intake; frequent small amounts up to 2500 to 3000 ml/day minimum unless contraindicated
   b. In respiratory infections, sipping hot fluids has been found to be of greater value than drinking cold fluids. Sipping hot chicken soup was found to be the most beneficial. It provides fluid and at the same time increases nasal mucus velocity, which supports the respiratory tract's first line of defense by removing pathogens. Cold fluids have been found to suppress nasal mucus activity*
2. Nursing diagnosis: Alteration in body temperature, fever due to infectious agent's effect on the body's temperature control center and due to the inflammatory response

---

*Januszkiewics, S. A., & Sackner, M. A. (1978). Effects of drinking hot water, cold water, and chicken soup on nasal mucus velocity and nasal air-flow resistance. *Chest, 74*, 408–410; cited by Scoggin & Sahn, 1980, p. 29.

a. Of particular concern in the elderly or debilitated patient because of the accompanying tachycardia, vasodilatation, and loss of intravascular volume with perspiration

b. For adults, aspirin is best given on an around-the-clock basis, when possible, every 4 to 6 hours, and administration started with the first systemic symptom of infection, not necessarily fever. This precaution is especially important in respiratory infections. Its use should be continued even after the temperature returns to normal. Prolonged use will help to eliminate the drenching sweats that occur with rapid fever drops and will lessen the malaise, arthralgia, myalgia, or sore throat throughout use. Aspirin administration is a comfort measure only, but it should be remembered that the presence of body comfort assists in supporting the body defenses. Obviously, aspirin is not to be used when contraindicated by other conditions (e.g., ulcer, bleeding disorders), and is *absolutely contraindicated for children with acute illnesses* because of its association with the development of Reye's syndrome

c. Room temperature should depend on the needs of the patient for comfort when possible. Any rapid changes in temperature should be avoided because both shivering and sweating require energy that should be saved

3. Nursing diagnosis: Actual or potential reinfection, or secondary infection, and spread of infection to others

   a. In long-term infections check the red blood cell (RBC) count and the mean corpuscular volume (MCV) for evidence of anemia

   b. One of the simplest and most effective, yet most neglected, methods of infection control is the practice of *thorough hand washing* by the nurse *before* and *after any* patient contact

4. Evaluation of nursing plan of care

   a. Of necessity, the physician's therapeutic plan of care is also evaluated. As a general rule, expect some improvement 24 hours after antimicrobial therapy is started. Subjective improvement: verbalized sense of feeling better. Objective improvement: temperature decrease. WBC count may begin to return to normal (may have been increased totally (leukocytosis), may have had a relative increase [e.g., lymphocytosis], or may have been depressed [e.g., neutropenia]). A shift to the left may occur in any case (see Section 2.2.3); erythrocyte sedimentation rate (ESR) will decrease

   b. The elderly tend to have a smaller increase in WBC count; the temperature response may be decreased, but if present, it more often indicates infection than it might in younger adults. Signs and symptoms tend to be insidious or unusual, with sepsis, confusion, agitation, and hypotension present instead of the more typical symptoms of fever, chills, and prostration (Larson & Edwards, 1986, p. 21)

   c. Check tests of function of specifically involved areas, for example:

      (1) In UTIs: subjective: verbalized decrease in pain on urination; objective: urine less cloudy; red cell casts in urine

      (2) In hepatitis: objective: check liver enzyme function—ALT (GPT), GTT, AST (GOT); check platelet dysfunction (i.e., bleeding time), bilirubin—blood, direct and indirect, and urine

6.2.5 Antibiotic Levels: Therapeutic and Toxic

1. Indications for the use of level testing

   a. Administration of antibiotics that have a high frequency of nephrotoxic, ototoxic, or similar severe toxic side effects

TABLE 6–2. ANTIBIOTIC LEVELS: THERAPEUTIC AND TOXIC

Drug Name	Normal Range	Therapeutic Level	Toxic Level	Effective Level
Amikacin (Amikin)	0	Trough: <5 µg/ml Peak: 15–30 µg/ml	>5 µg/ml >35 µg/ml	<5 µg/ml 15–30 µg/ml
Gentamicin (Garamycin)	0	Trough: <2 µg/ml Peak: 4–10 µg/ml	>2 µg/ml >12 µg/ml	
Sulfisoxizole	0	90–100 µg/ml	>350 µg/ml	
Tobramycin (Nebcin)	0	Trough: 2 µg/ml Peak: 4–10 µg/ml	>2 µg/ml >12 µg/ml	
Vancomycin (Vancocin)	0	Trough: 5–10 µg/ml Peak: 30–40 µg/ml	Rare at <30 µg/ml May be safe as high as 90 µg/ml	

Abbreviations: t$_{1/2}$, half-life; IV, intravenous infusion or injection; IM, intramuscular injection; GI, gastrointestinal; s, second(s). *Data from Govoni & Hayes, 1985; and SHMC, 1991.*

    b. Nonresponse to the administration of an antibiotic to determine whether there is a therapeutic level of drug in the blood, especially in cases of life-threatening infection. If a therapeutic level is found in such cases, then other testing (i.e., sensitivity or susceptibility tests) may be done to monitor the appropriateness of treatment. (See Section 5.1.6, minimum inhibitory concentration [MIC], minimum bacterial concentration [MBC], Kirby-Bauer, or Schlicter tests [bacterial assays])

2. Patient preparation
    a. Blood is usually collected at times that coincide with peak and trough levels of the antibiotic in the blood. Therefore, it is usually necessary that the laboratory be told the *specific* time the blood should be drawn and that the time of collection be recorded. The patient should be informed of the time(s) for blood collection and the rationale behind the time selection
    b. No further patient preparation is usually necessary

3. Patient assessment and teaching related to antibiotic therapy. (See also "Related Nursing Implications," items 1 through 5, in Chapter 18.)
    a. Double-check for possible allergies before giving the *first* dose of any antibiotic
    b. Become familiar with the side effects of the drug being given
        (1) Which side effect usually develops first?
        (2) Which are the "expected" side effects, if any (e.g., sore mouth or tongue with more than 1 week's administration of cephalosporin)?

TABLE 6–2. (Continued)

Metabolism in the body	Comments

$t_{1/2}$: depends on rate of renal clearance: 2–3 hr
Peak: 60 s past IM
    30 s past end of 30-s IV
    Immediately at end of 60-s IV
Plateau (steady state): 10–15 hr (see $t_{1/2}$)
	Causes ototoxicity and nephrotoxicity. Sample collection time: at trough level, just before next dose, and/or at peak level (see Metabolism)

$t_{1/2}$: 2–3 hr Plateau: 10–15 hr Peak: As for amikacin	Sample collection time as for amikacin. Used primarily for gram-negative infections. Potential for oto- and nephrotoxicity. Baseline creatinine levels should be drawn before use of the drug and checked periodically
$t_{1/2}$: 3–6 hr Peak: 2–4 hr with oral and IM, 30 s with IV Plateau: Rapid excretion	Tasteless, thus useful in treating children; potential for ototoxicity and nephrotoxicity as well as agranulocytosis and other blood dyscrasias
$t_{1/2}$: 2–3 hr Peak: as for amikacin Plateau: Dose-dependent	Eliminated by the kidney, thus renal dysfunction can increase blood levels. Ototoxic and nephrotoxic. Low therapeutic index. Check creatinine levels
$t_{1/2}$: 6 hr Peak: 2 hr Plateau: 30 hr	Extravasation after IV can cause severe necrosis. Especially useful with GI infection because it is poorly absorbed from the gut. Ototoxic and nephrotoxic

(3) What nursing measures should be implemented to facilitate compliance and minimize side effects?

(4) What side effects or untoward effects indicate hypersensitivity to a given drug?

c. Observe and question the patient about the onset of side effects

d. Check for possible drug interactions between ordered antibiotics and other medications being taken concurrently. Inform the physician about any possible incompatibilities before giving the antibiotic

e. Assess the patient daily as well as relevant laboratory data, if available, for specific signs of toxicity, especially when ototoxic, neurotoxic, or nephrotoxic antibiotics are being given

f. As early as possible, identify patients at risk for toxicity (e.g., the elderly because of a decreased glomerular filtration rate [GFR] causing prolonged action of the drug and individuals with hepatic [decreased drug metabolism] or renal [decreased elimination of drug metabolites] dysfunction)

g. Serum drug levels may be drawn on a routine or a one-time-only basis with the patient at risk (see item f), when a drug has a narrow therapeutic range (i.e., the therapeutic range is very close to the toxic level) or signs and symptoms of toxicity are difficult to recognize clinically

h. If results of the drug level test indicate it is at or above the toxic level, the nurse should hold the next dose (if being administered intravenously, the infusion should be changed

to a compatible isotonic solution at a "to-keep-open rate" [TKO]) until the physician
can be contacted for a change in orders

i. Patient and family teaching

(1) Determine what the patient and family already know. Correct any misinformation.
Determine what knowledge is wanted, and start teaching with that information.
Keep it as clear and simple as possible. Use written materials to support verbal in-
formation with complex subjects

(2) As with the administration of any medication, those responsible need to be fully
informed as to its purpose in *this* case, expected effects (how will they know when
it is working?), "expected" side effects and how to cope with them, and what other
side effects to recognize and report

(3) If the patient and family are to be responsible for administering the medication, the
importance of following the dosage and time schedule exactly must be stressed by
repetition and information as to what will happen, or not happen, should compliance not occur. Help to establish a reminder system to make the process easier

(4) Share measures to prevent side effects and to alleviate any discomfort resulting
from the side effects, e.g., avoiding direct or artificial sunlight when taking tetracycline to prevent sunburn resulting from hypersensitivity, or eating yogurt, if diet
allows, to reduce candidal growth on mucous membranes in conjunction with the
administration of many antibiotics

Table 6–2 presents therapeutic and toxic levels of some representative antibiotics.

6.3 DIAGNOSIS OF COMMON SEXUALLY TRANSMITTED DISEASES

6.3.1 Introduction: AIDS Status, 1992

As of the date of the Eighth International AIDS Conference in Amsterdam, July 1992, the status
of AIDS was no vaccine, no cure, no indisputably effective treatment. The epidemic has slowed
somewhat in developed countries, such as the United States, but has shown rapid spread in poor-
er, less developed nations. The population affected in the United States has changed. An increased number of women have been infected (30 to 50 percent of all new patients in the clinics
of San Francisco and New York are related to heterosexual contact) (Gorman, 1992, p. 34). HIV
prevalence rose significantly in all age groups in the United States; in many urban areas particularly, with the greatest percentage raise among adolescents (Quinn et al., 1992, p. 252). The current worldwide adult infection status (1992) was estimated at 10 to 12 million by the World
Health Organization (WHO) (Quinn, 1992, p. 33). WHO also projected at least 30 million people infected worldwide by the year 2000. Other experts predicted a much lower number, close to
that estimated for the year 1992 by WHO (Quinn, 1992, p. 33).

Probable mutations of the HIV virus structure helps the virus elude detection (quite a few
cases of "non-HIV AIDS" have been reported) and have certainly caused many of the drugs used
to date to become ineffective over time as resistance builds. The drugs used *do* slow the AIDS infection some 2 or 3 years, but death is still the expected outcome. Infections that had been "under
control," such as tuberculosis, have become major threats to the immunodepressed AIDS victim.

Much remains to be discovered and to do about AIDS, such as:

1. Determining why AIDS remains dormant or asymptomatic, often for years, after infection
2. What triggers the infection phase
3. How the immune system is destroyed. (HIV particles are found only in one per 100 CD_4 T cells, even at the height of infection)

Some things have become known about AIDS: HIV can:

1. Alter proteins in its outer coat, disguising itself from targeted medications, such as AZT. The coat itself is laced with sugar molecules, shielding it from the human immune system
2. Only reproduce by invading a living cell, by preference the CD_4 T cell

Some things are believed to be true about AIDS:

1. By the year 2000 AIDS could become the largest epidemic of the century; worse than the 1918 influenza epidemic that killed 1 percent of the population at that time and *twice* the number killed in World War I
2. Two different strains appear to be present, caused by slightly different HIV and with predilection for slightly different host cells (Gorman, 1992, pp. 29–34; Quinn, 1992, p. 34)

The incidence of other sexually transmitted diseases (STDs) has increased dramatically in the United States. More than 12 million new STDs have occurred, caused by more than 20 different infectious processes, this despite increased public education and treatment efforts. Two major causes for the increase have been identified:

1. Unknowing disease spread by the asymptomatic patient
2. Reliance by many primary physicians on diagnosis based on past or present symptoms, plus checking for lesions as major screening methods

Very frequently more than one STD is found in the same person. Forty-five percent of gonorrhea patients and trichomona patients have been found to also have a concomitant chlamydial infection.

Groups now considered at highest risk for STD infections are those who are sexually active with multiple partners (especially prostitutes) and who are younger than 25. Further identified risk factors include those individuals who have histories of STDs or of illegal drug use (Borucki, 1992, pp. 77–78).

6.3.2 Specific Disease Testing of STDs

A. Gonorrhea

Definition. Gonorrhea (*Neisseria gonhorroeae*) is a specific, contagious, catarrhal infection of the genital mucous membrane of either sex that may affect other body structures (e.g., conjuctiva, oral mucous membrane, rectum, or body joints). Females may also have involvement of the urethra, vulva, vulvovaginal glands, vagina, endocervix, Skene's and or Bartholin's glands, or fallopian tubes. In males, prostatic involvement can occur. Dysuria and purulent urethral discharge are hallmark indicators of gonorrhea, although the discharge can be scant and watery. Females are more often asymptomatic (60–83 percent) than males (10–15 percent) (Ravel, 1989, p. 196). Symptoms manifest themselves 3 to 5 days after sexual contact with an infected individual.

Laboratory testing is essential for accurate diagnosis as the signs and symptoms are relatively nonspecific, especially in the female.

Symptomatic rectal gonorrhea is found in females and homosexual males. Oropharyngeal gonorrhea occurs, usually transmitted by fellatio, or less often cunnilingus. Adequate sexual history is imperative (Ravel, 1989, p. 196), and testing should include testing of all potential sites of infection (e.g., oropharynx, vagina, rectum) (Burrell, 1992, p. 1679). (See also Section 15.2.3.A, "Culture for Gonorrhea.")

Diagnostic Tests

Gram's Stain/Smear. (See also "Examination of Direct Smears—Gram's Stain," Section 5.1.1.A.)

1. Sample collection for testing: In a symptomatic male urethral exudates or scrapings are both sensitive and specific in establishing a gonorrhea diagnosis. The samples are usually collected with a sterile smooth platinum wire loop. Cultures should be made with negative or inconclusive smears. In testing women, gram-stained smears of either vaginal or cervical exudate lack sensitivity and specificity (Henry, 1991, pp. 1033–1034)
2. Findings of Gonorrhea and diagnosis are made on the basis of the presence of gram-negative intracellular diplococci. The Gram's stain detects fewer than 50 percent of gonorrhea infections of women, making tissue culture the test of choice
3. If a specimen is not to be examined immediately, it should be refrigerated (Henry, 1991, p. 1033)

Tissue Culture. For females it is the test of choice. It is more reliable than Gram's stain because certain *Acinetobacter* bacteria can be confused with *N. gonorrhoeae*. Bacterial samples should be obtained from several sites, including cervix and rectum. For males tissue culture is indicated if gram-stained smears are inconclusive (Pien, 1991, pp. 42–43). (For more information on cultures see Section 5.1.2, "Specimen Culture.")

FINDINGS. Gonorrhea diagnosis is made on the basis of

1. Typical colony morphology on the Agar plate
2. Gram's stain of typical colony is gram-positive. Resistant strains are identified by further testing (e.g., positive oxydase test for penicillinase producing *N. gonorrhoeae*)

Alternative Approach: Monoclonal Antibody Tests
The newest and most rapid approach to diagnosis, the enzyme immunoassay of urogenital specimens (e.g., Gonozyme Test [Abbott Laboratories]) uses three monoclonal antibodies to cover several strains of the bacteria

1. Used when doing a culture is not possible after positive findings on a Gram's stain

2. Can be used instead of a Gram's stain as a screening test but is not as accurate as the Gram's stain in testing women

FINDINGS. Sensitivity of 90 percent, specificity of 98 percent.

B. Genital Herpes

Synonyms: Herpes simplex virus types 1 and 2; HSV-1, HSV-2

Definition. Herpes simplex virus types 1 and 2 are now *reportable* STDs, but only the *initial* infection must be reported. The purpose of reporting is primarily for data gathering to determine the population involved and incidence of the diseases.

The virus is an obligate intracellular organism characterized by its ability to become latent and to produce persistent infection. In its latent period, the virus is found in regional sensory ganglia (i.e., the sacral nerve root ganglia, the trigeminal ganglia). Asymptomatic shedding of the virus occurs, especially in the first 3 months after the initial symptomatic episode ("Herpes Shedding during Remission," Emergency Medicine, July 1992, p. 77). When reactivated, the virus moves back along the sensory nerves and produces recurrent infection with blisterlike lesions, such as genital lesions, cold sores, pharyngitis, ocular keratitis, and encephalitis (McCance & Huether, 1990, pp. 739–741).

Previously, herpes simplex virus, type 1 (HSV-1) was believed to cause only cold sores and HSV-2 to be responsible for genital infection. However, both viruses have been found to cause primary and recurrent genital herpes in adults. Transmission of HSV-1 is usually nonvenereal but requires close contact (e.g., hand to mouth, kissing). HSV-2 is most often due to veneral transmission (Henry, 1991, p. 1229) and causes more than 80 percent of initial symptomatic infections (Emergency Medicine, July 1993). Although each appears to have a predilection for specific body areas (HSV-1 affecting the oral cavity [cold sores, fever blisters, skin lesions above the waist]; HSV-2 affecting the genital area [herpes labialis/neonatal/progenitalis, skin lesions below the waist]), both have been found to cause primary and recurrent genital herpes in adults. The herpes simplex viruses are probably the most common human viral pathogen, as well as the cause of one of the most common STDs. Their clinical manifestations can range from inapparent to fatal (Laboratory of Pathology, 1991).

Neonatal disease usually results from the HSV-2 and can be acquired by the infant in either the intrauterine or perinatal period, most commonly the latter (Henry, 1991, p. 1229). Delivery may require a cesarean section to prevent transmission of the infection to the neonate (Cohen et al., 1991, p. 775).

Diagnosis
A presumptive diagnosis can be based on the presence of typical genital lesions (McCance & Huether, 1990, p. 741).

Viral Tissue Culture (HSV-1/HSV-2). Must be done early in the course of the illness when viral levels are highest. Virus may be recoverable for only 2 to 3 days after onset of signs and symptoms. Specific sites are sampled, depending on the site of the infection, using aspiration or premoistened (sterile saline) swabs. Many samples require placement in a transfer media after collection; all should be kept cool or refrigerated (Lab. of Pathology, 1991). Samples may be taken from almost any affected area. Areas frequently sampled include:

1. Brain tissue (during preplanned surgical procedure)
2. Buffy coat of blood sample
3. Cerebral spinal fluid
4. Corneal ulcer
5. Saliva
6. Vesicular fluid
7. Conjunctiva of the eye
8. Rectum
9. Throat

Monoclonal Antibody Tests (with Immunofluorescence [IF] or Immunoenzyme Methods). This is the preferred test for direct detection of antigen in tissues. It can detect the virus in body fluids as well as tissues and it shows good agreement with the elaborate, time-consuming and expensive viral DNA test that is the good standard test for herpes diagnosis. It has the capacity to type the virus as well, which is important in selecting treatment and determining patient prognosis, because the recurrence rate of HSV-1 is less than that of HSV-2.

It requires neither a cultured specimen nor an "expert eye," making this test more rapidly available and less subjective.

PROCEDURE WITH TYPING. Monoclonal antibodies that react specifically with HSV-1 and -2 are labeled (mixed) with fluorescein isothiocyanate, a fluorescent tracer. The cell specimens from the culture are transferred to a slide and placed in separate wells. One well is stained with HSV-1 reagent, the other with HSV-2. The cell specimens will bind with the reagent in one or both wells if the specific virus type is present. After it is rinsed to remove unbound antibody, the specimen is viewed under a fluorescence microscope.

FINDINGS. An apple green staining of the cytoplasm indicates a positive reaction to the reagent, that is, the presence of the specific virus type. A red stain indicates a negative reaction.

PROCEDURE (DIRECT SMEAR). Monoclonal antibody testing can also be done directly from patient cell specimens. The specimen is placed on the slide with the technique appropriate to the type of specimen, incubated with the monoclonal HSV-1 or -2 antibody, and tested as before. The major asset of this approach is its speed. It is quite sensitive (70 to 90 percent), but its accuracy depends on the quality of the specimen obtained (Fife & Corey, 1984, p. 848).

ELECTRON MICROSCOPY. It is a rapid technique but one that requires specialized equipment that is not always available. It has an evident low sensitivity. It has been found to be especially useful in cases of neonatal infection or in the review of brain tissue biopsy specimens.

IMMUNOPEROXIDASE TEST. A rapid and fairly sensitive test (70 percent) used to detect viral antigens in cells directly from the patient that are resistant to the therapeutic effects of penicillin.

RESTRICTION ENDONUCLEASE ANALYSIS OF VIRAL DNA. This test is used when more specific testing is desired, one that determines the particular herpes virus involved and whether a newly developed lesion represents spread from the original infection or is the result of a new virus. It is also used in medicolegal situations and provides epidemiological tracing of a specific herpes virus. At present it is done only in reference laboratories (Noble, 1986, p. 64).

POLYMERASE CHAIN REACTION (PCR). Not yet in wide usage. Data on its use with herpes are limited, but PCR (a DNA amplification test) may prove more useful than culture in identifying asymptomatic genital herpes in pregnant women at term (Gershon, 1991, p. 109).

C. Chlamydia Trachomatis

Chlamydia trachomatis is one of a group of obligate intracellular parasites now recognized as unique, bacterialike organisms, possessing a gram-negative cell wall, unable to grow outside an animal cell, and containing both RNA and DNA (see Fig. 6–1 for life cycle). Disease states associated with *C. trachomatis* include trachoma, inclusion conjuctivitis, nongonococcal urethritis, cervicitis, salpingitis, epididimitis, pneumonia (in infants), and lymphogranuloma venereum (LVG). Asymptomatic carriers are common and more frequent than in gonorrhea (Henry, 1991, pp. 1259–60). Chlamydia was identified as an etiologic agent of STDs in the early 1980s and is a reportable disease. It is the most prevalent STD in developing countries. (Rapid Diagnostic Test, May 1992, p. 2335).

   C. trachomatis, the only chlamydia known to affect humans, causes a number of acute and chronic infections (e.g., chronic keratoconjunctivitis, acute conjunctivitis or keratitis, urethritis, cervicitis, endometritis, salpingitis, perihepatitis, epididymitis, and lymphogranuloma venereum [LVG]). It commonly has asymptomatic carriers, more so than does gonorrhea.

   It is transmitted primarily by sexual intercourse even though the organisms can be found in all body fluids, including tears. Signs of infection usually occur from 7 to 21 days after intercourse (about one-third of infected males are asymptomatic, and so are 20 to 30 percent of fe-

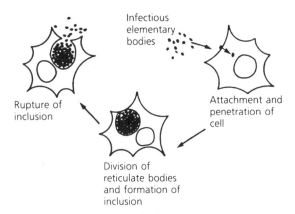

Figure 6–1. Life cycle of *C. trachomatis*. (From Emmons, J., & Courtner, p. [1985]. Towards control of chlamydial infections. *Nurse Practitioner 10*, 21, with permission.)

males) (Ravel, 1989, p. 218). It can also pass from a mother to a neonate, thereby resulting in yet another list of infections suffered by the neonate (e.g., ophthalmia neonatorum, pneumonia, otitis media, and even the possibility of an URI).

The bacterium *C. trachomatis* requires living eukaryotic cells (i.e., a highly organized cell bounded by a nuclear membrane, which is characteristic of higher organisms) for host cells, where it causes intracytoplasmic inclusions (i.e., round, oval, or irregularly shaped bodies in the cytoplasm or nuclei of cells) (see Fig. 6–1).

Symptoms of infection are usually fairly mild and may be totally absent. Males usually have a clear discharge from the penis (drip) and burning with urination; some have no symptoms. Female symptoms and signs may be an increased vaginal discharge and occasional bleeding with intercourse, but women are less likely to have overt signs than males.

Until very recently, simple, rapid diagnostic methods were not available, which has resulted in many undiagnosed carriers and in particularly harsh effects on women, who have only mild early symptoms, if any, but who have ascending infections—pelvic inflammatory disease (PID)—and a high risk of tubal scarring, ectopic pregnancy, or infertility. The risk to newborns in mothers with undiagnosed *C. trachomatis* infections is equally harsh.

Chlamydial infections often occur as coinfections with other organisms. Treatment may be effective against the other organisms without affecting the chlamydia, which leaves the woman with a persistent, occult chlamydia infection—a carrier.

Populations at Risk

1. Contacts of known *C. trachomatis*–infected individuals
2. Women with other infectious disease of the urogenital tract
3. Young women (in one survey, those less than 20 years old; in another, those less than 25 years of age) who are
   a. Unmarried
   b. From the "inner" city
   c. Taking oral contraceptives (using nonbarrier methods) or using no contraceptives
   d. Sexually active, having had three or more sexual partners in the previous year. (Emmons & Courter, 1985, p. 16)

Diagnostic Tests

Clinical signs and symptoms. Because of the low incidence of definitive signs and symptoms, cases are easily overlooked, especially in the female; mucopurulent endocervical discharge occurs in the female, whereas a mucopurulent urethral discharge is found in the male.

Tissue cell culture. Considered necessary for most standard testing of chlamydial infections as it provides an adequate sample of organisms or inclusion bodies for diagnosis. It may no longer be the gold standard test, however, if the DNA probe is available (see Section 5.1.7).

DISADVANTAGES. Very expensive, especially as a routine test; time-consuming, requires 2 to 6 days, thus delays treatment; a complex procedure; not practical as a screening test; requires centrifuge of the culture to drive the elementary bodies (EBs), the infectious form of the organism, into the monolayer.

Direct microscopy

DISADVANTAGES

1. Presence of mucus, debris, other microorganisms, or a low number of infected cells cause problems with this approach
2. Direct samples have low sensitivity
3. Reading results requires the "educated eye"

PROCESSING METHODS FOR DIRECT MICROSCOPY

1. GRAM'S STAIN A positive gram's stain but with *no* diplococci and more than five polymorphonuclear neutrophils (PMN) leukocytes is highly indicative of the infection. If the sample is from the endocervix, there should be *more* than 10 PMNs per microscopic field.
2. GIEMSA STAIN
    a. Useful in diagnosing severe conjunctivitis in infants but not accurate enough in genital specimens (Emmons & Courter, 1985, p. 21)
    b. EBs stain, purple or blue. Intracytoplasmic inclusions stain dark purple
    c. Preferred stain for use with HeLa cell culture
3. MACCHIAVELLO STAIN. EBs stain red; reticulate bodies (RB, the metabolically active replicating form, see Fig. 6–1) stain blue.
4. IODINE STAIN
    a. Intracytoplasmic inclusions stain brown
    b. The preferred stain with McCoy cell culture
5. IMMUNOFLUORESCENCE (IF)
    a. More sensitive and specific than the other staining methods; inclusion bodies appear as a sharply defined yellow-green mass not attached to the nucleus
    b. Permits earlier identification than other staining methods, often after overnight incubation
6. DARK-FIELD. Chlamydia are autofluorescent
7. SEROLOGY. Not useful because of low antibody response to chlamydial infections.
8. MONOCLONAL ANTIBODY (FLUORESCEIN LABELED) TEST*(also known as the "direct slide antigen test"). Monoclonal antibodies have been prepared against the major membrane protein present for all known serological variants (serovars) of *C. trachomatis* in both of its forms, the infectious EB and the metabolically active, replicating RB (see Fig. 6–1).
    a. Procedure: The specimen is labeled with an IF material. The suspected infected area is swabbed and, in the direct test, applied directly to the slide well, which is then stained, allowed to incubate 15 minutes in a high-humidity environment, and ultimately mounted and examined through a coverslip with a fluorescent microscope. Examination of a specimen from a culture can be done by using this technique after 48 hours of growth at 37°C.

---

*A significant number of positive monoclonal antibody direct specimen screening test results may not agree with cell culture results in populations of low prevalence, i.e., incidence of 5 percent or less of chlamydial infection. The test should be repeated or a DNA probe done on positive reactions in such populations.

The antibody conjugate combines specifically with any *C. trachomatis* present and demonstrates apple green inclusion bodies that can be read immediately after staining
  b. Advantages as a screening test
     (1) Rapid, can be read in 30 minutes
     (2) Less expensive, about half the cost of a culture
     (3) Provides information as to the accuracy of the sample being tested; helps prevent false negatives

DIRECT ANTIGEN TEST

  1. ADVANTAGES AS A SCREENING TEST
     a. Does not require a highly skilled microscopist to interpret
     b. Simple process that can be performed in a medical office having a spectrophotometer
     c. Results available in 4 hours
  2. DISADVANTAGES AS A SCREENING TEST
     a. Not as sensitive or specific as cell culture
     b. Published values vary considerably

DNA Probe Assay. (See Section 5.1.7 for information about the process of DNA probes.)

ADVANTAGES. Compared to the previous gold standard test, the tissue/cell culture, the DNA probe (assay) is a reasonable and rapid alternative. In a study comparing the two tests there was 98 percent agreement on results. Both were "essentially equivalent in terms of sensitivity, specificity, and positive and negative predictive values." The probe is much faster, approximately 2 hours for results. The DNA probe can also be used to test for *N. gonorroeae*, which is a frequent coinfection with *C. trachomatis*. Given the often "silent" onset of gonorrhea—especially in women—testing for both would seem indicated in any case (Rapid Diagnostic Tests, 1992, p. 1344; McCance & Huether, 1990, pp. 728–29).

DISADVANTAGES. At the time of this writing, the testing process is relatively new, and the factors of availability and cost must be considered.

IMPLICATIONS FOR NURSING RELATED TO CHLAMYDIA (See also Section 5.1.2, "IMPLICATIONS FOR NURSING: SPECIMEN COLLECTION.")

1. Sexually active individuals should be tested at least once a year (Sexuality Update, 1986, p. 8)
2. The patient having completed treatment for chlamydia infection should be scheduled for a return visit and test
3. Instruction at the client's level of understanding, after a review of what is known and accurately understood and beginning with what the client wants to know, should be provided to help prevent future infections. The following can apply to most STDs (Planned Parenthood of Seattle-King County. Chlamydia, 1986)
   a. Use a condom during intercourse
   b. Limit oneself to one sexual partner
   c. Ask partner(s) about any signs of infection (sores, rashes, discharge) before intercourse

d. Wash genitals before and after intercourse, gently but thoroughly
e. Urinate before and after intercourse to help cleanse the area
f. Have regular checkups for STDs
g. Women should have annual Papanicolaou (Pap) smears

D. Syphilis

Definition. Syphilis is one of the oldest documented venereal diseases, and one which is still very active. Its annual incidence in 1992 in the United States was 136,000 (Burrell, 1702), affecting primarily heterosexual men and women between the ages of 20 and 21 years (McCance & Huether, 1990, p. 729). It is a disease with both local and systemic manifestations, caused by the spirochete Treponema pallidum (an anaerobic bacterium), and is present in mucosal or cutaneous lesions of an infected individual. It is usually transmitted through macroscopically invisible abrasions caused by sexual intercourse, and can be transmitted from a pregnant woman to her fetus as early as the ninth week of gestation. (Oddly enough there is a lesser risk of gestational transmission the longer the mother had the infection. After 8 years, the mother's infection, even when untreated, is evidently not transmitted to the fetus) (McCance and Huether, 1990, p. 730).

Clinical Manifestations by stages. Syphilis develops in the following stages.

The *primary stage* (incubation period) starts approximately 3 to 6 weeks after infection. A chancre (shallow ulcer), which is easily overlooked unless it becomes secondarily infected, is present near the site of entry, usually on the genitalia. Lymph nodes in the area may become enlarged but nontender. Even untreated, the chancre heals in 2 to 8 weeks and disappears. However, the disease is readily transmitted during this stage. (Price and Wilson, 1992, pp. 923–924).

In the *secondary stage*, approximately 4 to 6 weeks (some authorities consider the time period to be 6 weeks to 6 months; some authorities say 2 to 6 weeks) after appearance of the chancre (Thompson, et al., p. 100), lesions develop on mucous membranes. Those called condylomata lata are elevated and moist. Frequently the lesions are wide spread, usually on bilateral areas of skin and almost always include the palms and soles. These lesions are quite painful and coupled with multiple signs and systemic symptoms of illness. The cutaneous lesions disappear in a few days or weeks, but relapses can occur for several years. During this stage, bacteria enter the blood stream and are carried to all major organ systems. All lesions of the secondary stage are contagious.

The *third* or *latent stage* lasts three to 5 years; it can be 1 to 40 or more years (Price & Wilson, Ibid). In rare cases it may last the lifetime of the individual. The patient is contagious throughout. Skin lesions disappear; there is no further increased evidence of infection; no clinical manifestations.

The late latent stage occurs in approximately 25% of patients. They do not progress out of the latent stage and have no recurrence of signs and symptoms. They are still contagious throughout this stage however.

Another 25% (again an approximate number) enter the final stage, called the *tertiary stage* developing neurologic, cardiovascular or ocular syphilis. (Henry, 561) During this stage the patient is no longer infectious to others. Soft tissue lesions, called *gummas* develop, as well as destructive lesions of bones. Cardiovascular destruction, such as aneurysms or valvular lesions, lead to cardiac insufficiency and central nervous system deterioration (McCance & Huether, 1990, pp. 730–32).

Congenital Syphilis. Newborns with neonatal syphilis are often premature, showing evidence of growth retardation, enlarged liver, and many other disorders (Cohen et al., 1991, p. 516). Fetal infection with stillbirth can occur. The infection is transmitted via the placenta, usually after the eighteenth week of pregnancy (Whaley & Wong, 1991, p. 522).

Tests

Rapid Plasma Reagin

Synonym: RPR

Normal Range: Nonreactive

INDICATIONS. A serological screening test for syphilis, using serum or plasma if necessary, is available. It uses cardiolipin antigen to identify syphilitic antibodies and replaces the Venereal Disease Research Laboratory (VDRL) test (see Table 5–1), except for spinal fluid examination. As it is nonspecific (positive reactions can occur with many other conditions, e.g., pinta, malaria, yaws, leprosy, lupus erythematosus, infectious mononucleosis, rheumatoid arthritis, aging), positive reactions should be further tested using the MHA-TP (see following section). It is much less sensitive in tertiary syphilis and is therefore used primarily to track success of therapy in primary or secondary stages, indicated by a reversal to negative (Laboratory of Pathology, 1991). Note that in patients with syphilis being tested by serological tests for syphilis (STS), spontaneous loss of test reactivity is well documented. In tertiary syphilis 20 to 30 percent of previously reactive STS test results revert to nonreactive status without treatment (Ravel, 1989, p. 563).

Microhemagglutination Assay-Treponema pallidum

Synonyms: MHA-TP; treponemal antibody test; syphilis confirmation test (this test replaces the fluorescent treponema antibody test—see Table 5–3)

Normal Range: Nonreactive

INDICATIONS

1. Confirmation test for any RPR
2. Suspicion of third-stage syphilis

Definition. The MHA-TP is presently the most sensitive and specific serological test for syphilis, used to confirm positive reactions in nontreponemal antigen tests (e.g., rapid plasma reagin [RPR], VDRL, see Table 5–1) and is recognized as a standard treponemal test by the CDC and U.S. Public Health Service. It can be used during the latent stage for a spinal fluid examination to confirm the presence of treponemes, indicating onset of neurosyphilis. It remains positive for life. An acute biologic false-positive (BFP) reaction can be due to many viral or bacterial infections and febrile reactions (i.e., hypersensitivity, vaccination) and generally produces low-grade or moderate (1 to 2+) serological test results for syphilis, returning to normal within a few weeks (Burrell, 1992, p. 1681; McCance & Huether, 1990, pp. 732–33; Ravel, 1989, p. 563; and Laboratory of Pathology, 1991).

E. Acquired Immunodeficiency Syndrome

Cause and process. HIV (Human immunodeficiency virus) invades many types of cells but preferentially selects one particular class that is vital to immune defense, that is, the T-lymphocyte/T-helper cells (also referred to as CD_4 cells). The virus reproduces itself very rapidly, in the process destroying most of the T-helper cells. This leaves the individual open to infection by normally nonpathogenic organisms (opportunistic infections) as well as the usual pathogens.*

The process of AIDS development is speculated upon in Figure 6–2. Because much is as yet unknown about the mechanisms of this disease, the reader will need to accept the figure as speculation, not fact. (See Table 6–3 for disease stages.)

Diagnosis of AIDS

Clinical findings. See Fig. 6–2 for a speculative progression chart.

1. There may be *no* clinical signs or symptoms except for the positive antibody reaction for HIV (and there is an indeterminate amount of time after infection before the antibody will appear). The individual with AIDS may be "perfectly healthy," again, for an indeterminate length of time but may also be able to infect others during this time
2. The CDC's criteria for a diagnosis of AIDS based on clinical signs and symptoms have been
   a. Presence of a disease that is at least moderately predictive of a defect in cell-mediated immunity, the diagnosis of which is based on strict histological and microscopic criteria. This includes such conditions as Kaposi's sarcoma (KS), primary intracranial lymphoma, or opportunistic infections (Tables 6–4 and 6–5)
   b. Absence of another probable cause for immunosuppression (e.g., corticosteroid or cytotoxic drug therapy, extremes of age [younger than 28 days, older than 60 years], or widespread lymphoreticular disease [Bender & Quinn, 1984, p. 62]) (See also "Implications for Nursing: Definitions Related to AIDS" for recent CDC criteria)
3. The AIDS incubation period is unknown. It may be as little as 5 months to as much as 15 years. In a few instances, in the very early stages, HIV infection is not detectable by serology in adults; detection in the first 15 to 18 months of life is also difficult (Henry, 1991, p. 1249). End-stage AIDS patients may lose their capacity to make antibodies as their immune systems deteriorate. Note that the virus cannot *always* be cultured from the blood of people who have the antibody (Harvard Medical School, 1984, p. 1)

---

*T cells are one of three kinds of lymphocytes:
1. T-cell lymphocytes mature in the thymus (hence the "T"). These are divided into "helper" T cells and "suppressor" T cells.
2. B-cell lymphocytes secrete antibodies (IgG, IgM, etc., also known as immunoglobins) that are specific in response to a given antibody (recognition).
3. The third kind are natural killer cells (granular lymphocytes), which go into action without prior stimulation and attack and kill other cells. (Most normal cells are resistant to killer-cell activity. Tumor cells infected with a virus are very susceptible.)

    B cells require stimulation to react, and this is provided by the T-helper cells. When antibodies are no longer needed, the T-suppressor cells "turn off" the B cells. T cells also secrete lymphokine elements (e.g., interferon) that stimulate many other cells and substances as in inflammatory response, and some can destroy corresponding antigens (Office of Research, Reporting and Public Response, 1983, pp. 3–7).

Acute Infection: AIDS positive (diagnosed HIV infection)

↓

Asymptomatic Phase: Only indicators: positive AIDS antigen test; possible signs of immune dysfunction

↓

Symptomatic Phase: Often a period of 10-12 years. Similar to stage previously called AIDS-Related Complex. Presence of opportunistic infections (e.g., thrush, tuberculosis, diarrhea); Lymphadenopathy

↓

AIDS Disease: Multisystem involvement with secondary invasive neurologic, oncologic, or infectious disease

Figure 6–2. AIDS progression.

AIDS Tests

Enzyme-Linked Immunosorbent Assay (ELISA) Test

Synonyms: Test for HIV (or Virus-1); HIV antibody; AIDS screen; antibody to human T lymphotrophic virus type III (a.k.a. HTLV III, more recently as HIV-1)

Normal Values: Negative

Henry, 1991, p. 1249.

See Definition on page 254.

TABLE 6–3. STAGING CLASSIFICATION SYSTEMS FOR HIV INFECTION

CDC Classification

Stage I	Acute HIV infection (at time of exposure)
Stage II	Asymptomatic HIV infection (may have some signs of immune dysfunction)
Stage III	Progressive generalized lymphadenopathy (PGL)
Stage IV	HIV disease:
IVa	Constitutional disease: one or more of the following symptoms: fever for >1 month; 10 percent weight loss; diarrhea lasting 1 month—no other conditions explain findings
IVb	Neurologic disease: AIDS dementia complex (ADC), myelopathy, or peripheral neuropathy—no other conditions explain findings
IVc	Secondary infectious disease
	1. Opportunistic infections (one of the following):
	Pneumocystis carinii pneumonia
	Cryptococcosis; cryptosporidiosis; toxoplasmosis; strongyloidiasis (extraintestinal); isosporiasis; candidiasis (esophageal/bronchial/pulmonary); histoplasmosis; mycobacterial disease (disseminated); cytomegalovirus; herpes simplex (disseminated); progressive multifocal leukoencephalopathy
	2. Symptomatic/invasive disease (one of the following):
	Oral hairy leukoplakia; multidermatomal herpes zoster; salmonella bacteremia (recurrent); norcardiosis; tuberculosis (extrapulmonary); oral candidiasis

TABLE 6–3. (Continued)

IVd	Cancers (one of the following): Kaposi's sarcoma; non-Hodgkin's lymphoma; primary brain lymphoma
IVe	Other conditions: Lymphoid interstitial pneumonitis; constitutional symptoms not meeting subgroup IVa; infectious disease not meeting subgroup IVc; cancers not meeting subgroup IVd

Walter Reed Staging[a]

Stage	HIV Status (antibody or virus)	Lymphadenopathy (chronic)	CD₄ count (#/mm³)	Skin Tests (delayed hypersensitivity)	Oral Thrush	Opportunistic Infections
WR0	negative	no	>400	normal	no	no
WR1	positive	no	>400	normal	no	no
WR2	positive	yes	>400	normal	no	no
WR3	positive	yes or no	<400	normal	no	no
WR4	positive	yes or no	<400	partial defect	no	no
WR5	positive	yes or no	<400	complete defect	yes	no
WR6	positive	yes or no	<400	and/or partial or complete	yes	?

[a]Uses specific immune parameters to establish patients' disease status from WR0 or HIV exposure through progressive immune dysfunction: WR6 = AIDS.
Data from Centers for Disease Control, 1990.

TABLE 6–4. FREQUENT INFECTIONS RELATED TO DEFECTS IN CELL–MEDIATED IMMUNITY

Disease	Infective Agent
Bacterial Infections	
Extrapulmonary tuberculosis, disseminated tbc	*Mycobacterium tuberculosis*
Disseminated tbc, cavitory	*Mycobacterium avium*
Pneumonia, encephalitis meningitis	*Pseudomonas aeruginosa*
Fungal Infections	
Thrush, esophagitis, fungemia, entercolitis	*Candida albicans*
Meningitis, encephalitis pneumonia, fungemia	*Crytococcus neoformans, Aspergillus fumigatus*
Protozoa Infections	
Chronic diarrhea (>1 month)	*Cryptosporidium, Isosporabelli*
Pneumonia	*Pneumocystis carinii*
Brain abcess	*Toxoplasma gondii*
Encephalitis	
Viral Infections	
Chorioretinitis, encephalitis, entercolitis	*Cytomegalovirus*
Disseminated infection	
Pneumonia	
Disseminated infection	*Epstein–Barr Virus*
Pneumonia, encephalitis, meningitis	*Herpes Simplex Virus*
Severe mucocutaneous lesions	*Herpes Zoster Virus*

Modified from Bender, B.S., & Quinn, T. C. (1984, May). What to know about AIDS detection.
Diagnosis: Medical Economics Co., p. 69, with permission. Other data form Fischi & Dickinson, 1987.

TABLE 6–5. MALIGNANT NEOPLASMS ASSOCIATED WITH HIV INFECTION

Cancer Name	Pathogenesis	Incidence	Characteristics and Area Involved
Kaposi's sarcoma (KS)	Origin of the KS cell is debated. Found to induce tumors histologically similar to KS but of mouse origin. Able to express high levels of interleukin, a basic fibroblast growth factor, and other cytokines. KS cells produce two types of cytokins; those that support their own growth and those that support growth of other cell types. Activation of the immune system may play a role in AIDS-KS pathogenesis	>24000 cases reported to date. Early in the AIDS epidemic 30 to 40 percent of reported cases of AIDS had KS. By April 1992 only 24 percent of reported cases of AIDS had KS. KS occurs in all risk groups.	*Comparison* AIDS KS Classical KS Age: Average 34 Over 50 yrs Tumor area: Widespread; Localized; often involves lower skin extremities
Non-Hodgkin's lymphoma (NHL)	Most commonly presents with systemic B-cell lymphoma symptoms, suggesting an infectious process, and/or as a rapidly enlarging mass. The B-cell lymphoma in an HIV-infected person is considered to be an AIDS-defining condition. Extra nodal sites may involve any body parts; usually CNS (26%), bone marrow (22%), gastrointestinal tract (17%), and liver (12%). Causative mechanisms are still under study; no single mechanism explains all occurrences. Association with EBV and development of B-cell lymphoma in immunodeficient individuals would seem to indicate a link. Oral hairy leukoplakia (a benign process highly predictive of AIDS development) is due to squamous cell proliferation, in turn due to EBV. EBV may play a role in tumor development or may be only a "passenger"	Data from the CDC show that 2.9 percent of AIDS cases reported in one study had high-grade NHL. This is 60 percent higher than in the general population, including all grades of NHL. Men are slightly more at relative risk than women to develop lymphoma. There appears to be no variance between risk groups (e.g., homosexual men and IV drug abusers). NHL has been found more likely to develop among those who have KS, a history of herpes simplex infection, and a low neutrophil count.	May have onset with symptoms characteristic of infectious disease. Median survival has been noted at only 5 months in one group of patients. Deaths are due to progressive lymphoma and/or opportunistic infection. Lymphocyte counts have been significantly higher in immunoblastic disease rather than small-cell disease.

TABLE 6–5. (continued)

Cancer Name	Pathogenesis	Incidence	Characteristics and Area Involved
	virus (EBV is able to "immortalize" B cells). Chromosomal alteration or rearrangements ultimately occur. No one mechanism is adequate to explain pathogenesis in all cases.		
HIV-associated-cell lymphoma	A true association between this disease and HIV infection has only been suggested, but there have been several well-documented cases of peripheral T-cell lymphoma with no single phenotype dominant. Some chronic T-cell leukemias suggest that a new form have been reported (unusual). Cutaneous T-cell lymphomas, often with unusual phenotypes, have been described. The EBV genome (see section 5.3.2) has been implicated in the pathogenesis of these disorders.		
Cervical dysplasia	Incidence of cervical dysplasia has increased in frequency in women with HIV infection. Human papillomavirus (HPV) is thought to have a key role in the malignant transformation of cervical dysplasia-neoplasia.		
Smooth muscle tumor	Given the low incidence of smooth muscle tumor in pediatric groups, the occurrence of six reportings from two separate groups of children who were HIV infected is difficult to attribute to chance. Presence of circulating transforming growth hormone would seem to have a role, similar to that in KS.		

Data from Burrell, 1992, pp. 1000–01; Henry, 1991, p. 706; and Safai et al., 1992, pp. 74–91.

DEFINITION. This test is an enzyme immunoassay screening test used to measure antibody to HIV-1 in serum or plasma for ruling out, rather than diagnosing, AIDS. Because the test does have a small potential for a positive response in persons who do not have AIDS, it cannot be considered 100 percent accurate. However, its sensitivity is 99 percent or better and has a similar specificity. When checked on persons with known AIDS, or those in a high-risk category for AIDS, there was close to 100 percent positive response.

PATHOPHYSIOLOGY. AIDS is caused by a RNA retrovirus (a virus carrying genetic information in RNA rather than DNA) transmitted in body fluids.* Transmission occurs through intimate sexual contact; exposure to blood and some blood products from infected individuals; and from an infected mother-to-be to the fetus in utero or during birth (SHMC, 1991). The HIV binds to the surface of a susceptible target cell via a receptor. The viral core consists of two strands of RNA and several proteins. (One core protein, called p_{24}, is unique to HIV. It induces antibody production in the host early in infection and is used to identify HIV infection [Hook & Fernandes, 1992, p. 486]). The virus inserts its own RNA into the cell, fusing with it. The viral RNA converts to DNA in the cell's nucleus (the genetic material), integrating into the cell's own DNA (thus, a double-stranded DNA). It could lay dormant for the life of the individual, or, more likely, be activated. The period of dormancy is thought to be related to the AIDS virus's ability to infect a cell (i.e., insert RNA into the nucleus) only when the cell is actively dividing (Davis, 1992, p. 20.) Once activated, infectious virons are produced, ultimately lysing the original host cell and spreading to other cells (Henry, 1991, p. 1249). HIV infects CD_4-positive/T-helper (T4) lymphocytes. (CD_4 is a surface antigen developed [expressed] by T-helper cells. It may infect some central nervous system [CNS] cells that also express the CD_4 antigen.) The process (infection/activation/cell lysis/cell death/viron spread) ultimately causes a marked decrease in CD_4 (T-helper) cells. The AIDS patient may be in any one of the following stages when diagnosed:

1. Positive HIV antibody only—No AIDS symptoms
2. Full blown AIDS (McCance & Huether, 1990, pp. 270–74)

POSITIVE REACTIONS IN (LABORATORY OF PATHOLOGY, 1991):

- AIDS/HIV disease (used to screen donated blood/plasma products before administration with the donor's consent; untested blood is not used)

FALSE-POSITIVE REACTIONS (RARE) IN:

1. Asymptomatic (non-AIDS) blood donors (<0.5 percent)
2. Persons with subclinical (non-AIDS) infections
   a. active carrier states
   b. cross-reactivity to other viruses (SHMC, 1991)
3. Persons (non-AIDS) with a history of:
   a. Multiple pregnancies or repeated transfusions due to the presence of antibodies to HLA antigens DR_4 and DQw_3 (usually acquired because of exposure to the antigens used in blood testing)
   b. Chronic hemodyalysis

---

*A retrovirus is characterized by a nucleic core of RNA and an enzyme that can translate RNA into DNA. It usually attacks the T4 lymphocytes but can also replicate in circulating monocytes, macrophages, deep layers of dendrite cells, and microglia of the central nervous system (Nadler, 1992, pp. 133–34).

  c. Active lymphoproliferative diseases or alcoholic hepatitis (Henry, 1991, p. 1249)

  d. Recent administration of therapeutic or prophylactic globulin (may persist for up to 6 months after administration) (Ravel, 1989, p. 149)

Retesting should be done on all positive responses.

Western Blot: Confirmatory Test

Normal Value: Negative

Purpose of the Test: A confirmatory test establishing the presence of antibody to HIV

Process of the Test: This is a more complex and time-consuming test. It uses electrophoresis to separate the killed virus antigen into its component parts on a special gel. The separated antigens (proteins) are then transferred to a special nitrocellulose sheet by an electrophoretic "blotting" technique (thus the name). The last step involves incubation of the patient's serum specimen with the antigens and comparison of the reaction, if any, with two control specimens (Damrow, 1986). It is much more expensive than the ELISA test.

DEFINITION. Because of the risk of a false positive in the ELISA screening, an HIV antibody test is not considered truly positive without the confirmation of a positive Western Blot test. The Western Blot test is more sensitive and specific than the ELISA test but also more expensive, labor-intensive, and time-consuming. Therefore, it is not used for screening purposes (Conn, 1991, p. 209).

PATHOPHYSIOLOGY. (See ELISA Test.) *Positive reactions* are defined by positive findings of specific protein bands of p_{41} or p_{24} when compared with two standard strips (Damrow, 1986) and are found in autoimmunodeficiency—AIDS. *False-positive or false-negative reactions* are estimates based on proficiency testing that indicate false-positive rate of up to 5 percent; a false-positive rate of up to 10 percent has been observed (Hook & Fernandes, 1992, p. 496). False reporting is considered to be due to:

1. Lack of standardized reagents or procedures for performance of the test
2. The fact that results of the test are based on variable reporting and interpretive data
3. Subjective interpretation of the test strip reactions (Hook & Fernandes, 1992, p. 497)

It takes from 4 to 24 hours to report findings depending on the method used for incubation. A positive ELISA and a negative Western Blot result do not rule out the possibility of antibody to HIV being present and should not be interpreted as a biologic false-positive (BFP).

There are several steps in the test process:

1. The HIV virus is cultured and grown
2. The virus is lysed (killed)
3. The lysate (the killed virus antigen) is electrophoresed, separating the proteins (killed virus antigen) into bands
4. The proteins are "blotted" on to a special nitrocellulose sheet by an electrophoretic technique
5. Desired bands of killed viral antigen/protein are cut from the nitrocellulose
6. The samples are washed, then incubated with a substrate of anti-IgG
7. The strips are washed again, and a substrate to allow visualization of the bands where antibody has attached to bound HIV proteins is applied (Calabrese & Condoluci, 1992, p. 496; Damrow, 1986)

TESTS THAT HELP DIAGNOSE AIDS

1. White blood count: Often decreased; may be normal, *rarely* increased
2. Lymphocyte count: Markedly decreased. In early disease states the lymphocyte count may be increased, but this is a rare finding. (T-helper [T4] to T-suppressor [T8] lymphocyte ratio is altered; if reversed, AIDS is severe [i.e., normal ratio of T4:T8 is greater than 1:2, e.g., T4 1.0 as to T8 3.5], with early suppression it is less than 1:0, and in the presence of opportunistic infections, the ratio is often less than 0:2.] It is important to look at total numbers, not just the ratio, however. T-helper cell numbers [T4] may remain normal or increase. Reversals of this ratio that occur with other viral infections or in response to vaccinations are rarely as severe as that seen with AIDS)
3. Platelet counts are often markedly decreased (thrombocytopenia)
4. Anergy-panel: Nonreactive (anergic) or poorly reactive
5. Quantitative immunoglobulin: IgG levels are frequently increased; IgA occasionally has increased levels
6. Lactic dehydrogenase (LDH): All fractions, LDH 1 to 5, have elevated levels, especially in the presence of *Pneumocystis carinii* pneumonia, and infiltrative disease
7. Serum albumin concentration is decreased
8. Total protein: increased levels because of increases in IgG/IgA content (see item 5)
9. Cholesterol levels are severely depressed, more so than can be expected secondary to usual malnourishment
10. Transaminase concentrations may be increased (e.g., glutamic oxalic transaminase [GOT], also known as aspartate aminotransferase (AST); glutamic pyruvic transaminase [GPT], also termed alanine aminotransferase (ALT); and gamma glutamyl transferase [GGT], also known as gamma glutamyl transpeptidase (GGT), may all have elevated levels)

CAUTIONS CONCERNING FINDINGS FROM PRESENT TESTING METHODS

1. Neither the ELISA nor the Western Blot test is infallible. False positives *are* more likely than false negatives
2. The less likely it is that someone has been exposed to HIV, the more likely it is that positive tests are in error. (Follow-up and Feedback, 1984)

FIVE MARKERS THAT MAY PREDICT DISEASE PROGRESSION

1. A dramatic decrease in the number of T4 lymphocytes (CD_4)
2. An increase in suppressor T8 lymphocyte levels (CD_8)
3. A reduction in the overall level of diagnostic antibody to HIV
4. Increased levels of antibody titer to cytomegalovirus
5. History of sex with another person in whom AIDS subsequently develops (Jenks, 1987, p. 32)

T4:T8 RATIO

Synonyms: T-cell helper:suppressor ratio; T-cell subsets; CD_4:CD_8 ratio

Normal Values: Adult 19–60

Total WBC and CBC see Chapter 2, Hematology Screen

T cells (T11)	700–2700/cmm	65–90% lymphs
Helper (T4)	400–1500/cmm	30–65% lymphs
Suppressor (T8)	200–800/cmm	12–36% lymphs
B cells (B4)	40–400/cmm	3–8% lymphs
T4:T8 ratio >0.8		

Laboratory of Pathology, 1991

TABLE 6–6. TESTS USED IN MANAGEMENT/EVALUATION OF HIV DISEASE

A. Tests to predict probability of disease progression

Test Name	*Comments*
1. CD_4 count	The most established test. Opportunistic infection risk increased with levels <200 Increased risk of death with levels <50 Not a reliable predictor of individual patient prognosis
2. CD_4 %	Indicates increased risk of pneumocystis carinii pneumonia (PCP) at 20% Use not as well established as CD_4 count May be useful as an indicator for treatment with antiretroviral therapy
3. Beta-2 Microglobulin	NON-specific marker of T-cell activation. Levels >3.5 correlated with disease progression.
4. p_{24} Antigen	In seroconversion illness, may be positive before ELISA test becomes positive

B. Tests used to measure HIV burden (infection severity)

Test Name	*Comments*
1. DNA polymerase chain reaction (PCR)	Measures HIV DNA in cells. Most useful in early disease. May be useful in diagnosis of neonatal infection.
2. RNA PCR	Method not yet standardized; most useful in advanced disease.
3. Cell Dilution/ HIV Culture	Not standardized nor available commercially. Most promising currently available test. Titrates peripheral mononuclear cells to estimate fraction carrying HIV
4. Time to HIV+ Culture	Peripheral mononuclear cells inoculated into culture of fresh cells. Time needed for culture cells to turn HIV+ noted -> estimate of HIV amount in original cells. Cumbersome process.

C. Tests used to control drug toxicity

Test Name	*Comments*
1. Complete blood count (CBC)	(See also section 2.1.1) Anemia, nutropenia are common with advanced HIV disease and many drugs used in its treatment (e.g. ganciclovir; trimethoprine, sulfamethoxazole)
2. Amylase	Used to follow patients receiving certain toxic antiretroviral drugs [Didanosine videx (ddl) & dideoxycytidme (ddc)] which can cause severe pancreatitis. Can completely suppress amylase production.[*]

[*] Most AZT resistant HIV-1 strains are susceptible to ddl and ddc. Data from Sanford, et al (1992). "Tests used in evaluation and management of HIV infection/disease." Table 12, p. 59, *The Sanford Guide to HIV/AIDS Therapy.* Antimicrobial Therapy, Inc. Dallas, Texas.

DEFINITION. The T4:T8 ratio is the primary test used to define the extent of T-helper (CD_4) and T-suppressor (CD_8) cell loss and thus the susceptibility to, or stage of, clinical disease (AIDS). (CD_4 and CD_8 are antigens expressed on the surface of the T-helper and T-suppressor lymphocytes [cells], respectively.) Measurement of the CD_4+/T-cell numbers helps establish decision points for initiating *Pneumocystis carinii* pneumocia prophylaxis and/or antiviral therapy, as well as monitoring for the efficacy of the treatment. The measurement of absolute CD_4+/T-cell levels in whole blood requires doing a WBC count; determining the percentage of WBCs that are lymphocytes (differential count) and the percentage of lymphocytes that are CD_4+ T cells (Centers for Disease Control, 1992, p. 1). Monitoring both T and B cells can be done on peripheral blood and is useful in determining both prognosis and clinical course of patients with AIDS (Laboratory of Pathology, 1991).

PATHOPHYSIOLOGY. The HIV usually infects CD_4+ T-helper lymphocytes, but it can infect some cells of the CNS that also express CD_4 antigen. (See also ELISA test.) Other antigens may be used as markers of the disease stage or progress but are not in general use as yet because of lack of long-term analysis, unproven findings, or difficulty in the testing process (Henry, 1991, p. 912).*

SPECIMEN COLLECTION

1. Anticoagulated whole blood is used
2. The specimen must be tested within 6 hours for hematology and immunophenotyping done within 30 hours, no later than 48 hours after drawing the blood
3. Usually requires two tubes of whole blood
4. Maintain specimen between 10 and 37°C (Centers for Disease Control, 1992)

IMPLICATIONS FOR NURSING: STDs

Specific Requirements for Obtaining Herpes Simplex Organism Samples

1. Cultures: HSV. (Use a sterile and protective technique)
    a. Rub a cotton-tipped swab vigorously in the ulcerated lesion
    b. Crusted lesions should not be cultured
    c. Fluid from vesicles may be used if obtained directly from vesicles and not the surrounding skin
    d. Place in transport medium immediately
    e. Send to hospital laboratory immediately
    f. If the sample is being sent to an outside laboratory, store it at 4°C until it can be sent
    g. Hold no specimen longer than 24 hours. After that time a new specimen is necessary
2. Viral stain (usually a Pap or Wright/Giemsa stain of an active lesion)
    a. Using a scalpel blade, gently unroof a vesicle and scrape the base, again gently, with the blade
    b. Transfer to a central location on the slide

Multinucleated giant cells are highly specific for herpes simplex, but only 30 to 60 percent of patients with positive cultures will have a positive stain. Therefore, stains are not highly sensitive (McKenna & Sparling, 1985, pp. 72, 75)

---

*According to Henry, protein B_2-microglobulin appears in increased concentrations in the serum of HIV-infected persons because of lymphocyte and macrophage destruction. The change predicts exacerbation of the disease. Testing of HIV p_{24} antigen and antibody to p_{24} core antigen is most specific 2 to 6+ weeks after infection. Their presence may coincide with the onset of acute symptoms related to infectious disease (e.g., mononucleosis) and disappear with seroconversion. p_{24} antigen/antibody remains nondetectable for a variable time, up to 7 years. Reappearance of antigen usually precedes AIDS symptomatology (Henry, 1991, pp. 912–13).

Precautions for Health Care Personnel Working with AIDS Patients

These precautions should be practiced with all patients, regardless of diagnosis. It protects the patient from health personnel-transmitted organisms and the health care worker from the undiagnosed infectious patient

1. Avoid needle sticks
   a. Do not recap or clip needles
   b. Use impermeable containers (heavy polyvinylchloride [PVC]) for disposal of syringes and needles in the patient's room
2. Avoid secretions
   a. Use gloves when exposed to any body secretions (i.e., doing venipuncture; an acutely bleeding, stooling, and/or incontinent patient). Gloves prevent secretions from getting under the nails where it is most difficult to remove them. Polyvinyl gloves are considered best but are also most expensive, and allergies to them are frequent.
   b. Gowns or plastic aprons are useful in keeping clothing clean, although clothing has not been shown to transmit infectious organisms
   c. In some instances double gloving may be useful, as for surgical procedures
   d. Have a disposable ventilating (Ambu) bag at the bedside for emergencies. (Few viruses are found in saliva. The risk in mouth-to-mouth resuscitation is greater if there is blood in the mouth) Special "no-contact" ventilating masks are available for use.
   e. Use goggles for procedures with a significant spray or aerosol effect (e.g., dental drilling) or with patients not in control of their secretions (e.g., many patients in intensive care units)
3. A mask is usually indicated only with a patient who has a productive, uncontrollable cough or is otherwise not in control of his or her secretions
4. Double bagging of linens is only necessary if
   a. the laundry of the facility does not treat all linens as if contaminated
   b. the bag is in danger of having fluids seep through
5. Disposable dishes are necessary only if there is free bleeding from a part of the patient that comes in contact with them
6. Pregnant women probably should be particularly careful when caring for the AIDS patient because of their increased susceptibility to infection, especially by cytomegalovirus
7. Wear bandages over wounds or abrasions. Materials such as Op-Site are best
8. Change and wash clothing soiled with blood or semen as soon as possible. Usually soap and water are sufficient to kill the organism. Disinfectant is not really necessary but can certainly be used. Household bleach is very effective
9. A private room *is not* mandatory if the patient is in control of his or her secretions (Benson, 1985; Dodge, 1985)
10. Hand washing, with particular attention to the fingers and thumbs, before and after patient care (*all* patient care) is probably the single most important precaution the nurse can take both for self-protection and protection of the patient (Lynch, et al., 1986)

Patient Teaching: Self-Care Guidelines for People with AIDS Living in the Community

1. Do not share any body secretions, particularly blood or semen. Use condoms if sexually active; dress own cuts
2. Maintain personal cleanliness with regular bathing and washing of hands frequently, especially after any contact with body fluids (semen, mucous, blood) or after using the bathroom
3. Kitchen and bathroom facilities may be shared with others. Clean surfaces regularly with a disinfectant (household bleach, freshly mixed, 1 part bleach to 10 parts water). Careful cleaning of the shower floor to prevent fungus growth is necessary as AIDS patients are at high risk for fungus infection. Soap and water are usually adequate for cleaning enclosed kitchen surfaces such as refrigerators
4. Dishes may be shared if they are washed between use with soapy water that is hot enough to require gloves or in a dishwasher. Disinfectant is unnecessary

5. People with AIDS can safely cook for others if they
   a. Wash their hands well before beginning
   b. Do not sample food by licking their fingers or tasting from a mixing spoon during preparation
6. Do not share towels or washcloths without laundering them between users. Any materials that may come in contact with blood or other body fluids should not be shared (e.g., toothbrushes, razors, enema equipment). This protects the AIDS patient as much as it does visitors and roommates
7. The AIDS patient should protect against infections transmitted from pets by
   a. Using gloves for cleaning out bird cages or kitty litter boxes
   b. Getting someone else to clean the fish tank
8. Keep living quarters well ventilated to decrease airborne disease
9. Cover mouth with tissues or handkerchiefs when coughing or sneezing (Lusby & Schietinger, 1983)

Definitions Related to AIDS

1. AIDS was originally defined clinically as
   a. A febrile prodrome of weeks to months followed by opportunistic infection
   b. Abrupt onset of opportunistic infection
   c. Presentation with Kaposi's sarcoma
2. The definition was revised by the CDC in June 1985. It is now more specifically defined and has been made a nationally reportable disease. Persistent generalized lymphadenopathy is not reportable, despite the fact that the incidence of progression to AIDS may be at least 10 percent
3. The CDC definition of AIDS now in use can be found in Appendix J. Table 6–4 lists frequent infections found with cell-mediated immunity defects. Previously called "AIDS related conditions (ARC)."

Nursing Approach to Care of STD Patients

The focus of health care team management (particularly those involved in community health) related to clients with a possible or diagnosed STD is multiple, each facet as important as the next:

1. Identification of high-risk groups
2. Identification of active infections
3. Identification of contacts of actively infected individuals
4. Identification of effective control and treatment approaches
5. Use and evaluation of the effectiveness of these approaches
6. Education of the involved individuals and the community in preventive measures

Much of the care provided by nursing involves individual counseling, and for that to be effective the health care provider needs to establish his or her "credentials" with each individual, e.g., is the provider trustworthy (will she or he "tell")? Is she or he accepting of life-styles other than his or her own? Does the health care provider have up-to-date information? Will he or she judge? Preach?

The first step in assisting the STD patient to overcome these concerns would be to deal with the realities and emotions of a given situation. Approaches that have proved helpful include:

1. Determine the meaning and context of the STD to such patients: A violation of their body? A sore? An itch?
2. Acknowledge their meaning and context and reflect your understanding in your own words (e.g., the infection feels like a violation? The sore is from an infection)
3. Determine how their words or actions may relate to how they feel about the clinician to whom they have come or been sent with the STD
   a. Embarrassment: May give little or no information
   b. Denial: "It can't be true because. . . ." Patients who use denial are unlikely to follow up on instructions

    c. Miracle worker or savior: "They'll get rid of it for me. It's not my job." These patients are also unlikely to follow instructions

    d. Anger: "You're supposed to know what to do! You're supposed to fix it! I'm not coming back here."

    e. Shame: Feels the STD is not a "normal" or acceptable medical problem, rather a sexual one. These patients are unlikely to give an adequate or accurate history

    f. Frustration: Does not expect (or perhaps does not *get*) a sense that the clinician can handle or discuss the sexual implications

    g. Fear of
       (1) loss of confidentiality, especially teens
       (2) need to "tell on" contacts
       (3) effect on spouse or partner

4. Ease the psychological discomfort (for both patient and clinician) by

    a. Acknowledging that discomfort exists ("These things can be embarrassing for both of us")

    b. Avoiding words that are frightening (incurable, hopeless) or that judge (abnormal, promiscuous, sleep around)

    c. Trying to normalize the discussion of an STD; make it a disease like others, just having particular transmissions and locations

    d. Being sensitive to and aware of differences in sexual preferences and practices (e.g., do not assume a female patient's sexual partner is a male by using the words he, him, his)

    e. Acknowledgment and support of the patients' feelings as valid for them throughout the time spent with them

5. Provide the necessary immediate teaching as well as identify and respond to specific informational needs

    a. Provide written as well as verbal information for later study when the patient is less stressed

    b. Role-play approaches to informing asymptomatic partners of the need to be tested or treated

    c. Explain exactly what tests are to be done, when, and *exactly* what will happen (e.g., what part of the body provides the "sample"; how it is taken; what happens to it; what cooperation is needed from the client; how long before results are available; whether it may have to be repeated; why; how soon; how often)

    d. Describe how and why a disease may be asymptomatic
       (1) How and when symptoms will change if treatment is "working"
       (2) Why treatment or medications are continued after symptoms and signs have cleared up
       (3) What to do if signs and symptoms do not go away

    e. If indicated, explain serious long-term consequences of the STD such as infertility or cancer of the cervix. In a hospital setting this is rarely a nursing responsibility, but if questions arise, they need to be answered then. In an outpatient or clinic setting, the explanation is often expected of the nurse

6. Approaches to teenage patients: The patient can be helped to get the best STD care by knowing that

    a. The clinician may need the client's help to get accurate information. The client may be embarrassed to ask about or tell things that need to be discussed

    b. The clinician may assume that the teenaged client is not sexually active or should not be

    c. Any information that the client thinks important can be shared with the clinician without being asked because this is vital in getting a complete history. The teenager can feel free to
       (1) Tell the clinician *why* he or she is there in his or her own words: "I've had a discharge." "My boyfriend's doctor says he has. . . ." "It hurts to have sex."
       (2) Tell the clinician whether he or she is having sex with more than one partner, with a male, with a female, or both

    d. The patient may ask any questions that are bothering him or her or that he or she is curious about inasmuch as this is a way to get and sometimes give information. Helpful questions for patients to ask include
       (1) Do my signs and symptoms mean STD?
       (2) Does (Do) my partner (or partners) need treatment?

(3) What are the side effects from any medications that have been prescribed?

(4) What follow-up is needed (e.g., How often will I have to come back for treatments/check-ups? How will I know when I have been cured? What do I do if the signs and symptoms recur? (Peters, 1987, pp. 1–2)

Nursing Diagnoses Related to AIDS (not prioritized)*

1. Alteration in the immune system, immunodeficiency,[†] related to
   a. Decreased number of lymphocytes
   b. Decreased number of T lymphocytes
   c. Inverted T-helper:T-suppressor ratio
   d. Increased B-lymphocyte turnover and activity
   e. Presence of recurrent opportunistic infections
2. Alteration in gas exchange, decreased, related to
   a. Presence of respiratory infections (e.g., *Mycobacterium avium, Pneumocystis carinii*)
   b. Increased oxygen requirements due to catabolic state (sepsis)
3. Alteration in nutritional status, less than body requirements, related to
   a. Catabolic status
   b. Frequent diarrhea
   c. Decreased intake secondary to anorexia, fatigue or dyspnea on exertion, decreased activity level, and possible nausea and vomiting
4. Potential impaired skin integrity, related to
   a. Decreased nutritional status or decreased available protein for maintenance of tissue integrity, decreased fatty and muscle padding of pressure points
   b. Decreased mobility due to muscle weakness, fatigue
   c. Severe night sweats
   d. Possible diarrhea
   e. Herpetic lesions and anorectal fistulas
   f. Possible Kaposi's skin lesions
5. Potential alteration in elimination (diarrhea) related to
   a. Opportunistic bowel infections (due to cryptosporidia, amoebas, salmonellae, and cytomegalo-virus)
   b. Tube feeding intolerance
6. Social isolation related to
   a. Social nonacceptance of diagnosis (fear, disgust, or anger)
   b. Previous family estrangement due to life-style differences
   c. Alterations in patterns of sexual expression
   d. Feelings of guilt or punishment
   e. Withdrawal and grieving process (fear of death)
   f. Possible alteration in communication pattern due to fatigue, intubation, sore mouth (candidial in-fection), or neural involvement

---

*The nursing diagnoses were based on a care plan developed by Robinson, 1984.

[†]This is not an accepted nursing diagnosis but is used here in the interest of clarity. With the exception of the nursing diagnosis "potential for infection," none of the accepted nursing diagnoses speak to the unique problems of the immunosuppressed patient, and the "infection" diagnosis is extremely narrow, which limits action to those that prevent infection. Such actions are few and usually not effective for AIDS patients.

P a r t

III

LABORATORY TESTS
OF SPECIFIC BODY SYSTEMS

PURPOSE OF PART III

When seemingly unrelated test results from screening procedures are considered together with clinical findings, signs, and symptoms, the body systems involved in a disorder may be indicated. Additional tests specific to that system are then in order to lead to a more definitive diagnosis related to that system or to rule the system out and provide clues to others that may be dysfunctional. The purpose of this section is to indicate the clues from screening tests that can lead to specific system testing, define and describe some of the more frequently used tests of that system, and list procedures necessary to prepare the patient for the test to prevent cross-reactions or false increases or decreases in the values obtained.

SEVEN

THE ENDOCRINE SYSTEM

RECOGNITION OF ENDOCRINE DYSFUNCTION

The endocrine and neural systems are the two major integrative or regulatory systems of the body. They work in close relationship with each other. It is not surprising, then, that endocrine disorders can present as neuropsychiatric disturbances. Because the endocrine system, through its hormones, adjusts and correlates the activities of the various body systems in adaptation to the demands of the external and internal environment, it is again not surprising that endocrine disorders are excellent imitators of many other medical disorders.

Because of this ability to look like something other than an endocrine dysfunction, the *first*, the *most critical*, and the *most difficult* clinical problem is to recognize that an endocrine disorder may be present. Endocrine disease often begins insidiously and progresses slowly. The only clue may be a single symptom or physical finding, and that perhaps amid a riot of other symptoms and signs.

Endocrine dysfunction occurs when the levels or balance of the levels of hormones produced by the endocrine glands are upset. Endocrine glands may be hyperactive or hypoactive because of a primary glandular problem or secondary to other factors; for example, the absence of the enzyme renin, elaborated by the kidney, affects the adrenal synthesis of aldosterone. Disorders can occur because the target organ is unable to respond. Disorders can be congenital, infectious, neoplastic, autoimmune, or idiopathic.

Probably the best chance of noting the presence of an endocrine disorder lies in the ability of the health care team to maintain a high index of suspicion for endocrine dysfunction as a possible cause of confusing clinical signs and symptoms.

7.1 THE ADRENAL GLAND

7.1.1 Medullary Hormones

A. *Laboratory and Clinical Indications of Adrenal Medullary Dysfunction*

1. Serum glucose: hyperglycemia due to increased epinephrine levels inhibiting insulin release; related sodium decrease
2. Urine glucose: glycosuria due to hyperglycemia

3. Serum sodium level decreases with fluid changes related to items 1 and 2
4. Increased free fatty acids due to increased epinephrine release and increased fat metabolism in the absence of insulin
5. To be compared with the presence of some or all of the following clinical features: *Clinical findings* are more definitive than the laboratory findings, so they must be assessed. Increased epinephrine or norepinephrine levels, which cause intermittent hypertension (may be persistent); signs of increased metabolism such as diaphoresis, hyperactivity, nervousness, heat intolerance, nervous exhaustion; unexplained cardiac arrhythmias; headache; paroxysmal dyspnea; weight loss. Loss of usual sympathetic postural responses, which causes orthostatic hypotension. Failure of melanin formation in the skin, which causes vitiligo (sharply demarcated, milky white patches of skin with hyperpigmented borders)

B. Tests of Medullary Function

Vanillylmandelic Acid, Urine

Synonyms: VMA, 3-methoxy-4-hydroxymandelic acid

Normal Ranges (mg/24 hr)

Adult	2.0–10.0
Pediatric	
Newborn	0–1
Neonate	0–1
Infant	0–2
Child	1–5
Adolescent	1–5

Explanation of the Test. The adrenal medulla produces catecholamines (compounds with a sympathomimetic action). An example of a sympathomimetic compound is dopamine, the precursor of epinephrine and norepinephrine. One to 5 percent of the norepinephrine and epinephrine is excreted unchanged into the urine. The rest undergoes degradation and forms derivatives, metanephrines, and vanillylmandelic acid (VMA). VMA is the principal urinary metabolite. The precursor, dopamine, is degradated to homovanillic acid (see the next test).

The VMA test is a measurement of the amount of VMA found in the urine over a 24-hour period. Assays of plasma catecholamines are available in many hospital laboratories (see the test on total urine catecholamines, later in this section). However, the 24-hour urine assay is felt to be more reliable since the secretion of VMA is sporadic and diurnal. The VMA test is, however, technically simpler than the plasma catecholamine assay.

Patient Preparation. No dietary restrictions are necessary if the test is based on the oxidation of VMA to vanillin. Certain chemicals contained in some foods distort tests based on other methods; therefore, dietary restriction of chocolate, coffee, tea, bananas, citrus fruits, nuts, and any foods containing vanilla is maintained for 3 days before the urine collection. However, certain drug restrictions may be necessary (e.g., epinephrine, lithium carbonate, nitroglycerin, chlorpromazine, guanethidine, monoamine oxidase [MAO] inhibitors, reserpine), usually for 3 days prior to the test.

Specimen Collection

1. Twenty-four-hour urine specimens are collected, usually from 8 AM to 8 AM. The patient should void at 8 AM at the beginning of the test, and this urine is discarded. All other urine is collected until 8 AM the following day, to include a final 8 AM voiding.
2. The specimen container should be refrigerated and kept at a pH of 3. In one method, 30 ml of 6 N HCl is added to the collection bottle before use, eliminating the need for refrigeration.

Related Tests of Importance or Interest. Plasma catacholamines, urine and serum glucose, and glucose tolerance test (GTT) may show a diabetic curve, and the plasma renin concentration may be increased.

VMA LEVELS INCREASED IN:

1. Tumors of the adrenal medulla or extrarenal ganglionic tissue, which cause increased secretion of epinephrine and norepinephrine, such as pheochromocytoma and neural crest tumors (e.g., ganglioneuromas). VMA levels may be normal in these tumors, but the diagnosis should not be ruled out without doing the test
2. Other conditions that increase catecholamine production (e.g., thyrotoxicosis, widespread burns, Cushing's disease and syndrome, myocardial infarct, hemolytic anemia)
3. Some muscular disorders because of an inability to use catecholamines such as some cases of muscular dystrophy and myasthenia gravis
4. Physiological conditions in some individuals. Up to a sevenfold increase has been noted when the test was done immediately after *vigorous* exercise
5. Many persons with advanced or malignant hypertension
6. False increases as a result of the use of several drugs that produce fluorescent urinary products (e.g., tetracyclines, epinephrine and epinephrinelike drugs, large doses of vitamin B complex, MAO inhibitors, nalidixic acid [NegGram], aspirin, methyldopa [Aldomet], levodopa [Sinimet], and in uremia when the test method is based on fluorescence

VMA LEVELS DECREASED IN:

1. Some cases of familial dysautomomia—Riley–Day syndrome*
2. False reaction in some patients taking clofibrate (Atromid-S)

---

*A condition present only in Askenazi Jews; an autosomal recessive trait with signs and symptoms such as dysphagia, dysphasia, decreased pain sensations, decreased gag reflex, corneal ulcerations, motor incoordination, increased sweating, progressive kyphosis, and frequent respiratory infections (Wallach, 1992, p. 441).

Homovanillic Acid, Urine

Synonym: HVA

Normal Range: 0–15 mg/24 hr

Explanation of the Test. (See also the earlier explanation of the VMA test.) The measurement of homovanillic acid (HVA) is a measurement of the products of dopamine degradation. Dopamine is present in sympathetic nervous tissue as a precursor of norepinephrine. Neuroblastomas and ganglioneuromas usually arise from the adrenal medulla and cause a significant increase in the levels of all the urinary catecholamines including HVA. The increase in HVA concentration helps to distinguish the neural crest tumors from pheochromocytoma.

Patient Preparation

1. Drugs known to interfere with the test (diuretics, nerve blockers, tranquilizers, aspirin, levodopa, reserpine, quinine, diazepam [valium], and disulfiram [Antabuse]) are held for at least 3 days before the test—the optimum time is 7 days
2. Although there is no actual dietary restriction, restraint is urged in the use of vitamin B–rich foods, coffee, alcohol, or foods high in salt or vanilla

Related Tests of Importance or Interest. Such tests include determinations of VMA, urinary and plasma total catecholamine, and metanephrine levels.

HVA LEVELS INCREASED IN:

- Neural crest tumors (neuroblastoma, ganglioneuroma). Such tumors should not be ruled out without at least one estimation of the HVA content. In certain cases of neurologic tumors, the urinary abnormality consists almost entirely of excessive dopamine secretion and its metabolite HVA

HVA LEVELS DECREASED IN:

- None

Catecholamines, Total, Urine

Synonyms: Adrenalin, noradrenaline, total, urine

Normal Ranges (μg/24 hr)

24-hr urine	0–103
Random urine	0–18

Explanation of the Test. Determination of total urine catecholamine levels measures the 1 to 5 percent of epinephrine and norepinephrine that is excreted unchanged in the urine. Increases in the concentration of degraded metabolites (VMA, HVA) correlate well with measurement of the catecholamine levels themselves. This urine test can be used to confirm the results of the VMA or the HVA tests but is not usually available in all laboratories.

Random urine total catecholamine measurements provide little useful information because of diurnal variation in excretion.

Patient Preparation

1. No dietary restriction
2. Vigorous exercise before or during urine collection for the 24-hour specimen is to be discouraged

Related Tests. See the VMA test, earlier

CATECHOLAMINE LEVELS INCREASED IN:

1. See "VMA Levels Increased in"
2. Periods of sleep, to a marked degree
3. Periods after vigorous exercise, as much as sevenfold

CATECHOLAMINE LEVELS DECREASED IN:

1. See also "VMA Decreased in," item 1
2. Malnutrition because of decreased catecholamine production
3. Transection of the cervical spinal cord, probably as a result of the loss of excitatory and inhibitory inputs, which are believed to mediate the stress response and hormone production at the hypothalamic level (Henry, 1991)

Catecholamine Fractionation, Urine

Synonyms: Epinephrine, norepinephrine fractionation, urine adrenaline-noradrenaline fractionation, urine

Normal Ranges Adult, µg/24 hr

Norepinephrine	15–80
Epinephrine	0–20
Dopamine	64–400

Definition. A catecholamine is any of a group of sympathomimetic amines, including dopamine, epinephrine, and norepinephrine, which is the aromatic (stimulant) portion of the whole.

Purpose. Usually to rule out pheochromocytoma (adrenal medullary or extraadrenal) in patients with hypertension. Plasma levels of norepinephrine and epinephrine are not as sensitive as urine measurement. For diagnosis of pheochromocytoma, a 24-hour urine specimen has 100 percent sensitivity and 98 percent specificity (plasma has 82 percent sensitivity and 95 percent specificity). Test for VMA has only 42 percent sensitivity, but its specificity is 100 percent.

There are several disadvantages in measuring *total* catecholamines levels.

1. The reference range can obscure the diagnosis of a minimally secreting tumor.

2. Dietary catecholamines, which occur in conjugated form, can interfere with total catecholamine determination (Henry, 1991, p. 323)

Logically, then, the diagnosis of pheochromocytoma is rarely ruled out by a normal level in a given test. Other tests are used to support the diagnosis. Urine catecholamine testing is most frequently used to confirm diagnosis when other tests are equivocal. Urine metanephrine (see Fig. 7–1) is considered the single most reliable screening test for pheochromocytoma with false-negative findings of only 4 percent.

URINARY CATACHOLAMINES INCREASED IN:

1. Pheochromocytoma
2. Neuroblastoma
3. Ganglioneuroma
4. Ganglioblastoma (Epinephrine excretion is *not* increased in these last three tumors)

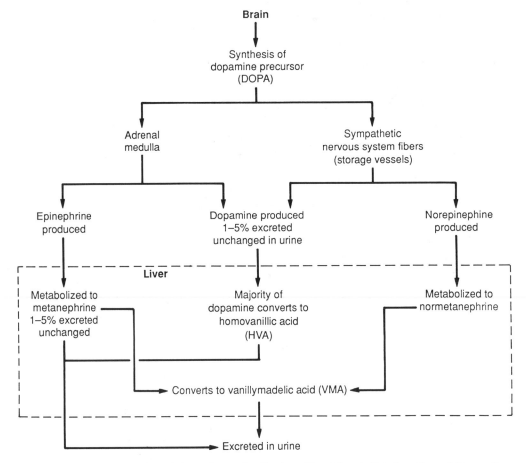

Figure 7–1. Catecholamine degradation pathways (synthesis and breakdown). *Data from Current Diagnostics, 1986, pp. 175–78, 384, and Wallack, 1992, p. 522.*

URINARY CATECHOLAMINE TEST ALSO USED IN:

1. Differential diagnosis of Ewings tumor (a.k.a. Ewings sarcoma, a round cell bone tumor, usually occurring in an extremity [Berkow, 1992, p. 1353]) versus metastatic neuroblastoma of bone
2. Determination of response to therapy

IMPLICATIONS FOR NURSING

1. Prior to the test the patient should be instructed to:
   a. Discontinue *all* medications for 3 to 7 days prior to the test (check with the laboratory doing the test for specific time frame)
   b. Follow a normal diet, being especially aware of the need to decrease intake of vitamin B–containing foods, as well as alcohol, coffee, salt, and any vanilla-containing foods because of the danger of false-positive responses on testing
   c. Eliminate any vigorous exercise within 1 hour or so prior to the test
2. Specific questioning should be done before the test to determine whether the individual has taken any of the following drugs as they will cause false elevation: adrenalin (or adrenalinlike drugs), tetracyclines, quinidine, and Aldomet
3. An increased blood pressure at the time of the test is of value during the 24-hour urine collection (Laboratory of Pathology, 1991)
4. Instruct the patient in the collection of a 24-hour urine sample (see Sections 8.1.5 or 4.7, "Implications for Nursing")

Catecholamine Fractionation, Plasma

Synonyms: Epinephrine norepinephrine fractionation, plasma; adrenaline-noradrenaline fractionation, plasma (usually includes dopamine measurement as well)

Normal Ranges (pg/ml)

Norepinephrine		Epinephrine	
Supine	70–750	Supine	Undectable–110
Standing	200–1700	Standing	200–1700
	Dopamine <30	(no postural change)	

Laboratory of Pathology, 1991

Purpose of the Test. The test measures free catecholamine metabolites and is used to confirm the diagnosis of pheochromocytoma or to avoid a false-negative diagnosis based on suggestive clinical signs and symptoms. It is less used than many other testing measures, usually only when a computerized axial tomography (CAT) scan or magnetic resonance imaging (MRI) scan fails to locate a biochemically confirmed tumor (Wallach, 1992, p. 521).

Explanation of the Test. Plasma catecholamine fractionation measures the plasma catecholamine levels individually, which assists diagnosis. The fractionation of the catecholamines into the epinephrine and norepinephrine helps localize the site of the pheochromocytoma in that adrenal tumors secrete a mixture of both; extraadrenal tumors are most often pure norepinephrine.

It is a difficult test to do and provides only limited amounts of information. It is not frequently done. Several normal physiological responses increase the secretion of catecholamines, such as postural changes or stress response, thereby altering the "normal" levels of plasma catecholamine.

The information from a controlled test is of value in confirmation of the presence of a pheochromocytoma (a tumor of the chromaffin tissue that commonly originates in the adrenal medulla but can be found [10 percent] in other tissues). Such a tumor causes excessive secretion of norepinephrine and epinephrine (see Fig. 7–1, "Catecholamine Degradation Pathways") and causes hypertension.

Patient Preparation
Outpatient:

1. One week prior to the test all drugs that can cause interference with the test results (i.e., any drugs with epinephrine or epinephrinelike qualities such as antihypertensive agents, diuretics, and sympathomimetics) should be discontinued
2. Diet: Standard daily intake of sodium for 3 days before the test. Low- or high-sodium diets affect catecholamine secretion

Inpatient:

1. No food, coffee, tea for 4 hours prior to the test
2. No smoking a minimum of 15 minutes before the test (nicotine promotes catecholamine release)
3. Insertion of an indwelling, heparinized intravenous (IV) butterfly needle (or saline lock) and catheter
4. Thirty minutes undisturbed rest in a quiet room before the test is done. Reassurance as to what to expect, and when, is valuable at this point

PLASMA CATECHOLAMINE LEVELS INCREASED IN:

- See VMA test

PLASMA CATECHOLAMINE LEVELS DECREASED IN:

- See the VMA and total urine catecholamine tests

7.1.2 Adrenocortical Hormones

A. *Expected Alterations in Screening Tests with Changes in Adrenocortical Hormone Secretion*

As the adrenal cortex secretes more than 50 hormones or their precursors, some identical to substances secreted elsewhere in the body (e.g., gonads also secrete androgens), this section must be limited. The hormones of most importance in maintaining life and health are cortisol and aldosterone. They will be covered in this discussion, with some discussion of androgens.

1. Serum glucose: fasting increased; GTT levels diabetic in pattern
2. Electrolytes
   a. Plasma sodium levels increased; serum calcium content increased
   b. Plasma potassium concentration decreased (a few persons may actually demonstrate hypokalemic alkalosis, in which case the blood gas concentration would also be altered; from screening tests, only CO_2—venous—is available, which would be increased as it represents body base); urine potassium and calcium levels increased; urine sodium concentration decreased
3. White blood cell (WBC) count. Leukocytosis with a relative lymphopenia and a decreased eosinophil count

B. Tests of Adrenocortical Function

17-Hydroxycorticosteroids, Urine

Synonyms: Porter-Silber test; 17-OHCS; 17-hydroxysteroids

Terms Used Synonymously in Glucocorticoid Terminology: *Glucocorticoids:* C_{21} steroids, corticosteroids; *Cortisol:* Compound F, hydrocortisone (the most potent glucocorticoid); *Cortisone:* Compound E (an active glucocorticoid formed in the liver from adrenal cortisol); *Corticosterone:* Compound B; *11-Deoxycortisone:* Compound S

Normal Ranges (mg/24 hr)

Female	3–10
Male	4–11

Explanation of the Test. 17-Hydroxycorticosteroids (17-OHCS) are the metabolites, or breakdown products, of hydrocortisone, cortisone, and some small amounts of aldosterone. Thus the urinary levels of these products can be used as an index of the level of cortisone and hydrocortisone production in the body and to assess the adrenocortical function. 17-OHCS levels can be measured in plasma as well, a more difficult procedure. The urine test is a 24-hour test because of the diurnal secretion of glucocorticoids.

Patient Preparation

1. As a general rule, if possible, treatment with all medications is discontinued several days before the test because there are many that interfere with the accuracy of the test. In particular, these include iodides, paraldehyde, chlorohydrate, nitrofurantoin (Furadantin), colchicine, sulfa drugs, chlorophenothiazines, spirolactones, quinine, and propoxyphene (Darvon), as well as coffee
2. Patient instruction in 24-hour urine collection and refrigeration of the urine during collection is necessary. (Refrigeration unnecessary if boric acid is present in the collecting bottle)

17-OHCS LEVELS INCREASED IN:

Any condition that increases cortisone and hydrocortisone production such as

1. Basophilic pituitary adenoma because of increased adrenocorticotropic hormonal (ACTH) secretion
2. Cushing's syndrome as a result of adrenocortical hyperplasia
3. Polycystic ovaries (Stein-Leventhal syndrome) as a result of adrenal hyperplasia or ovarian secretion
4. Late in pregnancy because of the placental secretion of glucocorticoids
5. Adrenal cancer
6. Individuals receiving therapeutic estrogen
7. Extreme stress. Moderate elevations can occur even with less than extreme stress
8. Certain nonrenal tumors (e.g., lung oat cell carcinoma) because of the secretion of an ACTH-like substance, which is known as "ectopic ACTH syndrome"

17-OHCS LEVELS DECREASED IN:

Any conditions that decrease cortisone and hydrocortisone production such as

1. Addison's disease because of adrenal atrophy
2. Hypopituitarism due to the lack of ACTH to stimulate production
3. Rarely in eclampsia and pancreatitis
4. Adrenogenital syndrome

17-Ketogenic Steroids, Urine

Synonyms: 17-KGS, total 17-OH corticosteroids

Normal Ranges (mg/24 hr)

	Female	Male
Under 1 yr	0–1	0–1
Up to 10 yr	0.1–4.0	0.1–4.0
11–14 yr	2–9	2–9
Adults	2–12	4–14
Senior adult	3–12	3–12

Explanation of the Test. The test for 17-ketogenic steroids (17-KGS) is very similar to that for 17-OHCS and is the newer of the two. It measures the concentration of 17-OHCS that can be chemically changed or converted to 17-ketosteroids (17-KS). It is used as an assessment of adrenocortical secretion even though the products measured are not metabolites of cortisone and hydrocortisone. This test is sensitive to the 17-hydroxycorticoids such as pregnanetriol, not picked up by the 17-OHCS test and frequently seen in adrenogenital syndromes. In such cases steroid synthesis is shifted toward androgen rather than cortisone production.

Patient Preparation. Although there are several compounds, including medications, that interfere with the test, no special preparation is taken before testing other than the necessary instruction in 24-hour urine collection (acetic acid rather than HCl is used as a preservative).

17-KGS EXCRETION LEVELS INCREASED IN:

1. Any conditions that increase cortisone and hydrocortisone levels (see the previous test, 17-OHCS)
2. Adrenogenital syndrome (some forms)
3. Cushing's syndrome
4. Severe burns
5. Other high-stress situations (surgical trauma, infections)

17-KGS EXCRETION LEVELS DECREASED IN:

1. Addison's disease
2. Hypopituitarism
3. Cretinism

17-Ketosteroids, Urine

Synonym: 17-KS

Normal Ranges[a] (mg/24 hr)

Adult	
Males (14+ yr)	6.0–21
Females (14+ yr)	4.0–17
Senior adult	
Values progressively decline after 60	
Pediatric (both sexes)	
Under 1 yr	0–1
1–4 yr	0–2
5–8 yr	0–3
9–12 yr	3–10
3–16 yr	5–12

[a]There are marked daily variations in 17-KS secretion.

Explanation of the Test. The test for 17-KS is a 24-hour urine test. It measures metabolites of testosterone (approximately 25 percent of the total 17-KS) and metabolites of androgens other than testosterone. This second group includes nearly 50 different compounds, the measurement of which is quite useful in androgenic and adrenal function evaluation. The adrenal cortex in the male produces some 70 percent of the 17-KS; the rest is produced in the testes. In the female the adrenal cortex produces almost all of the 17-KS. Testosterone itself is not a 17-KS. The major compound of the 17-KS group is a substance called dehydro-epiandrosterone (DHA), which is formed in the adrenal gland and has a slight androgenic effect, thus accounting for virilization syndromes in females with some adrenal tumors.

Patient Preparation. Preparation is as for the 17-KGS test.

17-KS LEVELS INCREASED IN:

1. Adrenogenital syndromes due to adrenocortical hyperplasia. In babies the condition is usually congenital. In older children and adults the syndrome is usually due to an adrenal tumor
2. Interstitial cell testicular tumors
3. Cushing's syndrome at times with a slight to moderate increase in androgen secretion due to adrenal hyperplasia
4. Adrenal carcinoma due to increased androgen metabolites, DHA (See Explanation of the Test)
5. Severe stress
6. Basophilic adenoma of the pituitary due to increased ACTH stimulation of the adrenals
7. Some patients with Stein-Leventhal syndrome (polycystic ovaries) due to adrenal androgenic hypersecretion

17-KS LEVELS DECREASED IN:

1. Conditions causing adrenal insufficiency due to decreased secretion of androgens and glucocorticoids such as
   a. Addison's disease
   b. Panhypopituitarism
   c. Severe debilitating illness
2. Pituitary hypogonadism in males due to reduced testosterone secretion
3. Castrated males because of reduced testosterone secretion
4. Nephrosis secondary to depressed urinary steroid excretion. This is not an actual decrease in hormone production but a diminished excretion by the kidney
5. Klinefelter's syndrome (a relatively common abnormality of the sex chromosomes that is typically associated with an XXY chromosome complement—polysomy X. Affecting only males and, causing infertility and a lack of development of masculine secondary sex characteristics; it may also be associated with mental deficiency). 17-KS levels decrease when testosterone production decreases

Cortisol, Plasma

Synonyms: Serum cortisol, compound F, hydrocortisone, plasma cortisol by radioimmunoassay (RIA)

Normal Ranges (µg/dl)

8:00 AM	8–24
4:00 PM	4–12

Explanation of the Test. The plasma cortisol test determines the concentration of cortisol in the blood. Cortisol is the major glucocorticoid produced by the adrenal cortex. It exists in two forms in circulation, bound and unbound: the bound being inactive, the unbound "free," analogous to thyroxine. Cortisol production is affected by a diurnal rhythm so that the peak and the nadir of secretion may both need to be determined. It is therefore of importance to know whether the person being tested has a long-term life pattern that differs from the norm (e.g., sleeping other than during the night hours). The diurnal pattern will alter in time, and testing needs to be done at different hours to reflect that person's individual rhythm. As a glucocorticoid, cortisol affects synthesis of carbohydrate from protein (gluconeogenesis). It also can act as an antiinflammatory, help maintain blood pressure, and affects renal function.

Patient Preparation

1. Specimens should be drawn at times in the diurnal rhythm for which normal levels have been established. Laboratories vary as to what hours are used.
2. No special patient preparation is necessary.

PLASMA CORTISOL LEVELS INCREASED IN:

Conditions that increase hydrocortisone, or compound F, secretion, such as

1. Hyperadrenalism—Cushing's disease and Cushing's syndrome
2. Physiological increases occurring as a result of stress or obesity
3. False increases:
    a. Occur in kidney disease because of the lack of excretion of the hormone
    b. Occur as a result of increased estrogen levels in pregnancy or individuals receiving estrogen therapy or taking birth control pills because of increased cortisol-binding protein (i.e., globulin [CBG]) levels
    c. Occur because of hepatic disease secondary to decreased hepatic metabolism

PLASMA CORTISOL LEVELS DECREASED IN:

1. Individuals taking phenytoin (Dilantin) or receiving androgen therapy because of an increase in cortisol-binding protein levels
2. Addison's disease as a result of adrenal atrophy and an inadequate response to ACTH stimulation
3. Hypopituitarism because of decreased adrenal secretion secondary to decreased release of ACTH

Cortisol, Urinary, Free

Synonym: Free cortisol, urine

Normal Range: 0–10 µg/24 hr

Explanation of the Test. A 24-hour urine specimen is collected for this test. The test measures free cortisol (not bound to CBG) in the urine, which is the only form in which cortisol can be filtered through the kidney glomerulus. The test is therefore a highly sensitive one, and free urinary cortisol levels correspond proportionately with changes in plasma cortisol levels. The test is primarily a screening one for increased corticosteroid levels, and low values are not necessarily indicators of adrenal hypofunction.

Patient Preparation. No special preparation is required.

FREE CORTISOL LEVELS INCREASED IN:

1. States with increased CBG levels as seen in pregnancy and estrogen administration
2. Cushing's syndrome because of adrenal hyperplasia. It is considered by some the most important test for hypercortisolism
3. Emotional stress with rises of 50 to 250 percent because of increased glucocorticoid production

FREE CORTISOL LEVELS DECREASED IN:

- Not clinically significant

7.1.3 Mineralocorticoid Hormones

A. *Laboratory and Clinical Indications of Mineralocorticoid Dysfunction*
Aldosterone is the major electrolyte-regulating steroid of the adrenal cortex. Indications of aldosterone dysfunctions then are primarily indications of fluid and electrolyte imbalances. Dysfunctions of other adrenocorticosteroids are frequently coexistent with aldosterone dysfunction.

CLUES TO DECREASED ALDOSTERONE LEVELS (ADDISON'S DISEASE)

1. Laboratory findings
    a. Serum electrolytes: Decreased Na^+, increased K^+ levels (aldosterone function causes Na^+ conservation, K^+ excretion); decreased pH, decreased HCO_3 concentration (or venous CO_2)—metabolic alkalosis. Electrocardiographic (ECG) changes in the adult secondary to K^+ imbalance
    b. Twenty-four-hour urine: Increased Na^+ excretion despite decreased serum Na^+ level that persists when salt intake is restricted
    c. Serum chemistry: Slight to moderate increase in serum urine nitrogen (BUN) secondary to chronic hypovolemia
    d. Evidence of other endocrine deficiency (see other tests)
2. Clinical findings
    a. Hypotension, especially postural hypotension
    b. Anorexia, nausea, changes in bowel habits, and acute or chronic abdominal or back pain because of the loss of aldosterone regulation of intestinal electrolyte balance, hypogonadism, hypothyroidism

CLUES TO INCREASED ALDOSTERONE LEVELS:

1. Laboratory findings
    a. Serum electrolytes: Na^+ levels normal or slightly increased, K^+ decreased, Cl^- decreased (in response to initiation of diuretic therapy). K^+ decrease does not respond toward normal levels with regular diet and K^+ supplements

    b. Serum chemistry: GTT result abnormal and serum glucose level increased secondarily to decreased K^+ levels. May have indications of metabolic alkalosis (e.g., increased pH, increased HCO_3 levels [or venous CO_2])

    c. Urine: Increased 24-hr K^+ excretion, which responds to sodium restriction by decreasing the amounts excreted. Sodium loading causes an increased K^+ loss in urine and a decreased plasma K^+ concentration. Decreased urine specific gravity

  2. Clinical findings: Hypertension, weakness, polyuria

B. Tests of Aldosterone Function

Serum Aldosterone

Synonym: Mineralocorticoid, electrocortin

Normal Ranges (ng/dl)

	Low Sodium Intake	Normal Sodium Intake
7:00 AM recumbent	12–36	3–9
9:00 AM upright	17–137	4–30

Explanation of the Test. Aldosterone is the most potent mineralcorticoid secreted by the zona globerulosa of the adrenal cortex. Its level in plasma is controlled by the levels of ACTH, potassium, and the enzyme renin. It is also influenced by a circadian rhythm, much like that of cortisol, with low levels (50 percent decreased) in the afternoon. Position of the body also influences plasma aldosterone levels with marked increases when the body is erect. It functions primarily on the distal convoluted tubule to promote sodium and chloride reabsorption and compensatory excretion of potassium and hydrogen. This test measures the aldosterone concentration in plasma to validate the presence of hyperaldosteronism or hypoaldosteronism. Because the serum concentration is normally low, it is more difficult to measure than is the urinary aldosterone concentration.

    Serum assays can be interpreted more readily when accompanied by a random urine sodium test. For example, a finding of less than 30 mEq/L of urinary sodium in a random sodium test (normal, 30 to 90 mEq/L) with an increased serum aldosterone value indicates a false aldosterone elevation because decreased urine sodium levels suggest decreased secretion and therefore imply a sodium deficit in the body.

    A serum renin sample is also frequently taken at the same time to help differentiate primary from secondary hyperaldosteronism (see Section 7.1.3.B, p. 282).

Patient Preparation

  1. Steroid and diuretic treatment discontinued 2 weeks before testing to establish baseline values

  2. Stable sodium diet at a known intake for 2 weeks before testing (low intake, 10 mEq/day; normal intake, 135 mEq/day)

  3. Owing to treatment, hypertensive patients may be sodium depleted despite normal plasma sodium levels. They may be placed on a high-sodium diet or salt supplements for several days before specimen collection. (*Note:* Such salt loading would invalidate a renin assay; therefore, both tests could not be done at the same time.)

4. Recumbent position for 30 minutes to 1 hour before testing
5. For an upright, usually nonfasting, specimen, the person should be *ambulatory* for 30 minutes before the sample collection

SERUM ALDOSTERONE LEVELS INCREASED IN:

1. Marked elevation in primary aldosteronism (Conn's syndrome), due to adrenocortical tumor (adenoma) or hyperplasia, which may be congenital, in which there is an overproduction of aldosterone. The release is not affected by normal feedback systems. Plasma renin levels will be decreased, an important diagnostic point.
2. Secondary aldosteronism due to excessive production of aldosterone by the adrenal glomerulosa itself, but activated by stimuli outside the adrenal, which is almost always due to increased renin angiotensin activity. Plasma renin levels will be increased, an important diagnostic point. Secondary aldosteronism is found secondary to many extra adrenal activities such as cardiac failure, nephrotic syndrome, cirrhosis, renal ischemia of any cause, essential hypertension, or Bartter's syndrome (renal juxtaglomerular hyperplasia)
3. Physiological compensatory responses as seen in normal persons with increased K^+ intake, sodium restriction (low-salt diet of less than 2 g/day), prolonged standing, diuretic therapy (furosemide [Lasix]), or stress
4. States of increased estrogen concentration such as persons receiving estrogen therapy or during pregnancy
5. Individuals taking drugs that increase plasma renin levels and thus aldosterone (e.g., hydralazine [Apresoline], diazoxide [Hyperstat], nitroprusside)

SERUM ALDOSTERONE LEVELS DECREASED IN:

1. Addison's disease (primary adrenocortical insufficiency) due to idiopathic atrophy of the adrenal, probably an autoimmune adrenalitis
2. Sheehan's syndrome (postpartum necrosis of the anterior pituitary) due to loss of ACTH stimulus
3. Adrenal destruction due to granulomatous processes such as tuberculosis, histoplasmosis, and rarely, sarcoidosis
4. Salt-losing congenital adrenocortical hyperplasia, usually in infants, due to inherited enzyme deficiencies
5. Physiological conditions in healthy subjects such as the recumbent position; high-sodium diets; decreased potassium intake; some instances of aging; and glucose ingestion, which causes a temporary decrease
6. Hypoaldosterism can be recognized by the presence of marked hyperkalemia not explained by significant renal failure

---

RELATED NURSING DIAGNOSES: CORTISOL AND ALDOSTERONE

1. With increased cortisol levels

    a. Potential for injury (trauma or infection) related to weakness secondary to protein tissue wasting or loss of muscle mass, weakness secondary to potassium depletion, and decreased immune function

    b. Potential for disturbance in self-concept (body image, self-esteem, role performance) related to physical weakness, an alteration in fat and water distribution, effects of virilism in females (skin and hair changes), and mood swings

2. With decreased cortisol and aldosterone levels

    a. Potential or actual fluid volume deficit related to active loss of fluid secondary to aldosterone deficiency

    b. Potential for injury related to postural hypotension, weakness and fatigue secondary to hyponatremia, fluid imbalance, hyperkalemia, hypoglycemia; and related to potential for addisonian crisis

    c. Disturbance in self-concept (body image, self-esteem, role performance) related to physical weakness and lethargy and alterations in pigmentation

    d. Lack of knowledge related to support or replacement hormones, administration and side effects, and self-care

Urine Aldosterone

Synonyms: Mineralocorticoids, urine aldosterone by RIA

Normal Range: 2–26 µg/24 hr

Explanation of the Test. Measurement of a 24-hour urine specimen for the aldosterone derivative concentration has the same advantages as does urine testing of other steroid hormone metabolites when done on a 24-hour sample: elimination of the short-term fluctuations occurring in response to circadian rhythms and other controlling factors such as ACTH and changes in sodium or potassium levels. There is also less overlap between normal and abnormal ranges.

    Aldosterone regulates the retention of sodium and chloride and the elimination of potassium and hydrogen ions. Comparisons of urinary aldosterone and plasma or urinary electrolyte levels are usually done with this test to validate the findings (aldosterone deficiency: hyponatremia, increased potassium levels, and low concentrations of urine and plasma aldosterone that do not rise in response to salt deprivation; primary hyperaldosteronism: normal or slightly increased levels of sodium, decreased potassium concentration, and increased levels of urine and plasma aldosterone).

Patient Preparation. No special preparation is necessary because a full 24 hours of aldosterone excretion into urine is being assayed. The patient should be instructed in the specimen collection procedure.

URINE ALDOSTERONE LEVELS INCREASED IN:

• See "Serum Aldosterone Levels Increased in" in Section 7.1.3.B, p. 280.

URINE ALDOSTERONE LEVELS DECREASED IN:

- See "Serum Aldosterone Levels Decreased in" in Section 7.1.3.B, p. 280.

Plasma Renin Activity Test; Renin, Urine Sodium/Potassium Correlation Test

Synonyms (for Plasma Renin Activity Test): PRA, peripheral renin (initial renin screen)

Normal Range

Plasma renin activity: 105–385 ng/dl/hr

Renin Urine Correlation: A special graph indicates the relationship between the PRA and the 24-hr urine values for urine electrolytes

24-hr Urine Sodium: 43–217 mEq/24 hr

24-hr Urine Potassium: 26–123 mEq/24 hr

Explanation of the Tests. Plasma renin is not directly measured; rather, plasma renin activity (PRA) is determined in a two-step process. Angiotension I, generated by the action of renin on the substrate angiotensiogen, is measured by RIA. The amount of angiotension I generated, and found in the plasma, is indicative of the plasma renin activity occurring and is expressed in nanograms of angiotension I generated per deciliter of plasma per hour (ng/dl/hr).

The renin-angiotension system is involved in the regulation of sodium balance, therefore also in fluid volume and blood pressure regulation. When circulating volume is low, kidney perfusion decreases, stimulating production and secretion of renin into the vascular system from the renal juxtaglomerular cells of the kidney. Renin acts to release angiotensin I from a plasma globulin. Pulmonary and plasma enzymes quickly hydrolyze angiotensin I to angiotensin II, which stimulates aldosterone secretion by the adrenal cortex, causing sodium and fluid retention by the kidney. Renal perfusion increases, as does blood pressure, and the renin-angiotension system is shut off (Laboratory of Pathology, 1991).

A 24-hour urine sodium or urine potassium (renin urine sodium correlation test) may be ordered at the same time and compared with the PRA. A comparison of the two or three values helps establish or rule out some nondisease causes for an elevated or depressed PRA. When kidney function is normal, urinary sodium excretion is related to the extracellular fluid (ECF) volume and inversely related to plasma concentration of renin. This information helps identify low-renin, hypertensive persons (see Section 7.1.3.A).

Patient Preparation
For PRA test:

1. Various drugs can alter PRA, especially those that affect sodium or potassium balance or blood pressure. The client should be instructed to
   a. Discontinue taking any antihypertensive or diuretic medications for 1 week before the test
   b. Discontinue birth control pills 7 to 8 weeks before the test
   c. Eat a regular diet (e.g., not low salt) for 1 week prior to the test
   d. Be ambulatory for at least 3 hours before the venipuncture

2. The client should be kept n.p.o. except for water for at least 4 hours prior to the test

For renin-urine sodium correlation test:

1. For a 1-hour sample the client should be instructed to
   a. Empty bladder 1 hour before blood sample will be taken and note the time to the minute
   b. Drink 3 large glasses of water after emptying bladder
   c. When blood is collected, again void and note time to the minute
2. For a 24-hour sample the client should be instructed to
   a. Empty bladder completely at the timed start of the test, discard the urine and record the time (most 24-hour urine samples are started in the morning at 8:00 but can start anytime. The crucial part is that the timing be accurate.) See also Section 4.7, "Implications for Nursing," item 2B
   b. All voiding during the 24 hours must be placed in a collection bottle usually containing a preservative and obtained from the laboratory. Therefore, each voiding must be caught in a clean container (bedpan, toilet "hat," urinal). If even one voiding is not collected, the test will be invalid. It is best if the urine container is kept in a cool area during the test
   c. When the 24 hours are complete, a last voiding should be done if possible and added to the storage container. Note in writing the time of the last voiding, whether it is exactly at the end of the 24 hour period or not
3. The container must then be properly labeled (minimal information needed would be the name of client, name of test to be done, exact time collection was started and completed), and finally the sample taken to the laboratory that will be doing the test

INAPPROPRIATE RENIN INCREASES OCCUR IN:

1. Malignant hypertension (50-percent increase or more) because of probable kidney damage and the consequent inability of the kidney to induce sodium retention
2. Secondary aldosteronism. An increased renin concentration is almost always the cause of increased aldosterone in this condition
3. Individuals taking oral contraceptives leading to increased blood pressure (with PRA method only) because of an increase in plasma renin substrate levels. The PRA returns to normal levels about 4 months after treatment when the medication is discontinued
4. Administration of various drugs (e.g., vasodilating antihypertensives and several diuretics)

APPROPRIATE PHYSIOLOGICAL INCREASES IN RENIN LEVELS OCCUR IN:

1. Prolonged upright posture or low-sodium diets
2. Hemorrhage
3. Severe fluid shifts or losses

INAPPROPRIATE RENIN DECREASES OCCUR IN:

1. Primary aldosteronism (Conn's syndrome) as a result of autonomous aldosterone production
2. "Low-renin" essential hypertension, cause unknown
3. Cushing's syndrome

4. Administration of various drugs (e.g., methyldopa (Aldomet), guanethidine, levodopa, propranolol)
5. Tourniquet stasis with sample collection

APPROPRIATE RENIN DECREASES OCCUR IN:

- Physiological conditions such as a high-salt diet, excess licorice ingestion, and decreased potassium levels

Adrenal Stimulation and Suppression Tests. Because the measurement of aldosterone and renin levels has been technically difficult, many tests have been developed to hasten the procedure, screen for primary hyperaldosteronism, or replace renin determinations. With the advent of simpler and more reliable aldosterone and renin measurement, the stimulation and suppression tests are rarely used. The most frequently used is the furosemide test in which the demonstration of increased aldosterone levels with a low or hyporesponsive PRA is a criterion in the diagnosis of primary aldosteronism.

Stimulation Tests

1. Furosemide (Lasix) test for aldosterone and renin (see "Patient Preparation" in Section 7.1.3.B). Renin and aldosterone secretion is stimulated by an oral dose of 80 mg of furosemide to produce acute volume depletion. The patient is kept in an erect position for 3 to 4 hours. A blood specimen is then taken and measured for plasma aldosterone levels and PRA. In primary hyperaldosteronism, plasma aldosterone levels will be inappropriately high in relation to the increase in PRA: hyporesponsiveness
2. Simplified furosemide renin stimulation test. The patient should be fasting, given 40 mg of furosemide intravenously, and 30 minutes in an upright position. The PRA is then determined. Low-renin, hypertensive patients are unable to increase the secretion to the level of the reference norm (less than 1.0 ng/ml/hr, white race; 0.5 ng/ml/hr, black race)

Suppression Tests. Suppression tests are more numerous, more time-consuming, and in most cases even less frequently used. They will be listed here by name and purpose only.

1. Deoxycorticosterone (DOCA). To demonstrate relative autonomy of aldosterone secretion in Conn's aldosteronism—nonsuppressed
2. Fludrocortisone (Florinef). Aldosterone loading, similar to DOCA
3. Saline infusion. Also similar to DOCA in purpose
4. Spironolactone (aldosterone antagonist). Measures urinary K^+ levels for changes in clearance related with aldosterone suppression
5. Saralasin test. Renin suppression is measured by decrease in blood pressure in renin-produced hypertension. Normals or nonrenin hypertension do not decrease the blood pressure

7.1.4 Pituitary Feedback Mechanism Tests

A. *Laboratory and Clinical Indications of Pituitary Feedback Dysfunction*

Any disturbance in a hormone stimulated by pituitary-stimulating hormones can be investigated by testing the negative-feedback axis between the pituitary and the target organ. The investigation can look at pituitary production of the organ-specific stimulating hormone or at the response of the target organ to the stimulation. Tests given under each endocrine gland test the response of the organ. In this section we look at the response of the pituitary to stimulation or suppression as well as measurement of plasma-stimulating hormone concentrations. Signs and symptoms of target organ dysfunction are indicators for pituitary investigation.

B. Tests of Pituitary Feedback

Dexamethasone Suppression Tests

Synonyms: DST; ACTH Suppression test

Normal Ranges (usually baseline levels)

Overnight screening test (single dose: 1 mg Dexamethasone)	8:00 AM, plasma cortisol levels suppressed to less than 10 µg/dl 4 pm levels, less than 5 µg/dl (Cushing's syndrome, greater than 10 µg/dl)
Low-dose test (total of 4 mg Dexamethasone)	Urinary free cortisol concentration suppressed to less than 20 µg/24 hr
	Urine 17-OHCS level suppressed to less than 2.5 mg/g of cretinine the second day of the test
High-dose test (total of 16 mg Dexamethasone)	Urinary free cortisol level suppressed to less than 20 µg/24 hr
	Urine 17-OHCS content suppressed to less than 2.5 mg/g of creatinine the second day of the test

Explanation of the Test. Dexamethasone (Decadron) is a highly potent synthetic steroid that is similar to cortisone in action and some 30 times more active. The small total dosage used per test (see with tests below) suppresses ACTH production from the pituitary but has little if any effect on increasing the glucocorticoid values. There are three approaches to testing.

OVERNIGHT (SINGLE DOSE). The overnight approach is an accurate and simple screening procedure to differentiate Cushing's disease and Cushing's syndrome* and can be done on an outpatient basis. A single low dose (usually 1 mg) is given by mouth at 11 PM, and the plasma cortisol concentration is measured between 8 and 9 AM. If Cushing's syndrome is present, the plasma cortisol level will not be suppressed and will exceed 10 µg/dl. If pituitary suppression is normal, Cushing's syndrome is ruled out.

Cushing's syndrome: A condition resulting from hypersecretion of cortisol over a prolonged period of time. It can be due to the therapeutic administration of glucocorticoids or ACTH, secondary to endogenous (within the body) ACTH production from an ectopic source (a source other than its usual one, the pituitary gland), or secondary to a benign cortisol-producing adrenal tumor. Mild increases in circulating cortisol levels with some signs and symptoms of Cushing's syndrome are also found in depressed or alcoholic individuals.

Cushing's disease: Overproduction of cortisol by the adrenal gland in response to pituitary stimulation. Differentiation between Cushing's syndrome and Cushing's disease determines the treatment used and depends on laboratory testing (McCance & Huether, 1990, pp. 628–630).

LOW-DOSE TEST. The low-dose approach is widely used as a confirmatory test when the overnight test produces no suppression and Cushing's syndrome is suspected. It is usually done in the hospital to control the accuracy of medicine administration and the 24-hour urine collection. A half (0.5 mg) dose of dexamethasone is given orally (or the dose is calculated by body weight: 5 μg/kg/6 hr) every 6 hours—that is, 6 AM–12 noon–6 PM–12 midnight, for 2 days, and a total of 2.0 mg. The 24-hour urine is checked each day for urinary free cortisol, 17-OHCS, and creatinine. The excretion of corticosteroids is expressed in milligrams per grams of creatinine to better discriminate between normal individuals and those with Cushing's syndrome because the creatinine value indicates whether renal function is normal. If urine free cortisol or urine 17-OHCS is not suppressed, the diagnosis of Cushing's syndrome secondary to any etiology is definitely established. The suppression has been found to be abnormal in 99 percent of patients with Cushing's syndrome.

HIGH-DOSE TEST (48-HR DEXAMETHASONE SUPPRESSION TEST). The high-dose test has been found valuable in identifying the lesion responsible for Cushing's syndrome. A dose of 1 mg of dexamethasone is given every 6 hours for 2 days to a total of 6 mg. The same testing is done as for the low-dose test. If the urinary cortisol or 17-OHCS is not suppressed adequately, the probability is that an autonomous adrenal adenoma or carcinoma exists or the ectopic ACTH syndrome is functioning. (Ectopic ACTH syndrome involves the presence of an ACTH-like hormone being produced by a tumor in tissue not considered endocrine by nature—frequently an oat cell tumor of the lung.) Cushing's disease is identified by this test (i.e., urinary-free cortisol and 17-OHCS levels are not suppressed with the low-dose test and are suppressed to less than 50 percent of the baseline values in the high-dose test).

Patient Preparation. No special preparation is needed other than an explanation of the test. Stress can negate the suppressive effects with small- or low-dose dexamethasone, and barbiturates may be given before the test for that reason.

FAILURE TO SUPPRESS CAN OCCUR IN:

Conditions other than Cushing's such as

1. Hyperthyroidism because of the high metabolic clearance of dexamethasone
2. Individuals receiving estrogen therapy as a result of increased levels of transcortin (serum transport protein for cortisol)
3. Obese individuals. They fail to suppress urinary free cortisol and serum cortisol levels in the overnight test but will suppress them in the low-dose test. 17-OHCS levels remain increased
4. Seriously stressed or seriously ill individuals because of the glucocorticoid response (see Appendix B)
5. Severe mental depression and other like psychiatric disorders because of unexplained biochemical abnormalities. The level of suppression is greater, and escapes from suppression is earlier (Henry, 1991), however, than that found with ectopic ACTH syndrome. Levels of 17-OHCS are elevated, and plasma ACTH and cortisol values lack diurnal variation
6. Individuals receiving phenytoin (Dilantin) therapy because of the increased metabolism of dexamethasone

FALSE-POSITIVE TEST RESULTS (DECREASE IN URINE 17-OHCS LEVELS):

- Occur in persons with ectopic ACTH Syndrome 2^0 bronchial or thymus carcinoids (small-cell cancer or other tumors) in 40 percent of patients. False-positive results rarely, if ever, occur in ACTH syndrome from lung small-cell cancers or other tumors (Ravel, 1989, p. 517)

Plasma ACTH Test

Synonyms: Corticotropin, adrenocorticotropic hormone; ACTH level

Normal Ranges (pg/ml)

8 AM fasting	20–100
4 PM nonfasting	10–50

Explanation of the Test. Measurement of levels of plasma ACTH, a polypeptide secreted by the anterior pituitary gland in response to corticotropin-releasing factor from the hypothalamus, can be done to further differentiate the lesion responsible for Cushing's syndrome. It identifies ectopic ACTH syndrome as opposed to adrenal adenomas or carcinomas. It is also used to establish a baseline before suppressive tests. The test is done by using a radioimmunoassay technique, which is often available only through a reference laboratory. An understanding of the pituitary-adrenal axis negative-feedback system is necessary to interpret the results. Obtaining basal AM levels prior to any stimulation or suppression test is recommended. Plasma ACTH levels peak between 8 and 10 AM and are lowest around 8 to 10 PM.

Patient Preparation. Patients should be n.p.o. except for water for 8 hours before the test except when a 4 PM sample is requested.

ACTH LEVELS INCREASED IN:

1. Primary adrenal insufficiency (Addison's disease) due to a decreased plasma cortisol concentration, which stimulates ACTH secretion if the pituitary function is intact
2. Ectopic ACTH syndrome to very high levels because of the production of an ACTH-like substance by nonendocrine malignancies that are independent of negative-feedback control and thus do not respond to increased cortisol concentrations. The ectopic focus frequently is an oat cell carcinoma of the lung. (A plasma ACTH determination may be done to confirm that diagnosis when tissue confirmation is not available.) Plasma levels are greater than 200 pg/ml, and serum cortisol levels will also be above normal
3. Stress because of an increased release of glucocorticoids

NORMAL TO LOW NORMAL ACTH CONCENTRATIONS IN:

- Individuals with Cushing's disease—pituitary-dependent adrenal hyperplasia. The plasma levels are inappropriately high for the levels of plasma cortisol, which are usually high normals. The ACTH concentration does not show diurnal variation and remains increased throughout the 24-hour cycle

DECREASED ACTH LEVELS IN:

1. Secondary adrenal insufficiency due to pituitary insufficiency (hypopituitarism), usually less than 75 pg/ml. Serum cortisol levels are also depressed. The best discrimination between normal individuals and those with adrenal insufficiency is obtained from the 8 (or 10) AM test
2. Adrenal adenomas or carcinomas (Cushing's syndrome) due to increased levels of plasma cortisol, which suppresses ACTH production at times to levels that are undetectable
3. Persons receiving glucocorticoids therapeutically (for the same reason as given in item 2). For individuals with increased glucorticoid from *any* source, blood specimens should be drawn for ACTH between 9 and 12 AM (Laboratory of Pathology, 1991)

Metyrapone Response Test

Synonyms: Cortisol/compound S—metopirone (Metyrapone) combination; compound S-metopirone (Metyrapone)/cortisol combination; cortisol/11-deoxycortisol

Normal Ranges (µg/dl)

Compound S-metyrapone,	baseline AM	0–5
	baseline PM	0–3
Cortisol,	8 AM	8–24
	4 PM	4–12

Description of the Test. This test provides information about the normality of the pituitary axis. Normal baselines of cortisol and compound S are very low. Metyrapone blocks synthesis of cortisol and removes the negative feedback on ACTH control. When cortisol measurement is combined with compound S (11-deoxycortisol, a steroid intermediate in cortisol biosynthesis normally having a very low serum level), it is possible to judge the normality of the pituitary adrenal axis. In normal function the administration of metyrapone will cause an increase of compound S and a cortisol decrease compared to baseline values (see Normal Ranges for values).

Abnormal Responses

INCREASED COMPOUND S AND DECREASED CORTISOL LEVELS IN:

1. Cushing's Syndrome due to adrenal hyperplasia, with an exaggerated rise in compound S and decreased cortisol levels
2. Pituitary hyperplasia/adenoma
3. Adrenogenital syndromes (compound S greatly increased)
4. Adrenal carcinoma (compound S greatly increased)

CORTISOL INCREASED PRIOR TO METYRAPONE, REMAINING ELEVATED AFTER METYRAPONE IN:

- Adrenal autonomous function secondary to adenoma/carcinoma

NO INCREASE IN COMPOUND S AFTER METYRAPONE IN:

- Pituitary or hypothalamic failure

DECREASED CORTISOL SECRETION; COMPOUND S GREATLY INCREASED IN:

1. Adrenogenital syndrome
2. Adrenal carcinoma
3. Pituitary autonomous function

BASELINE CORTISOL LOW IN:

1. Pituitary failure, prior to and after metyrapone
2. In pituitary or hypothalamic failure

INTERFERING FACTORS:

1. Dilantin: Invalidates the test as it interferes with absorption of metyrapone
2. Prednisone and prednisolone interfere with cortisol levels (Laboratory of Pathology, 1991)

7.2 THE PITUITARY GLAND

7.2.1 Antidiuretic Hormone*

A. *Laboratory and Clinical Indications of Antidiuretic Hormone Dysfunction*
A deficiency in antidiuretic hormone (ADH) has some relatively obvious signs and symptoms to alert one to deficiencies. The syndrome of inappropriate ADH secretion (SIADH) is less distinguishable. Both, however, require knowledge of both clinical and laboratory findings and the ability to see relationships between them.

ADH DEFICIENCY MIGHT BE SUSPECTED WITH:

1. Laboratory findings: Low morning urine specific gravity, less than 1.007 usually; high plasma sodium concentration; and the absence of indication of renal disease (e.g., normal BUN, plasma creatinine, potassium, serum calcium, and protein levels). (Hypernatremic dehydration can occur in infants and cause an increased BUN value)
2. Clinical findings: Persistent and massive diuresis (up to 12 to 15 L/day in the adult, normal value being 6 L/day), polyuria, polydipsia, nocturia, and thirst that wakes the person at night

---

Antidiuretic hormone (a.k.a. ADH or vasopressin) is an agent that suppresses secretion of urine with a specific effect on the epithelial cells of the renal tubules, stimulating reabsorption of water independently of solids and resulting in urine concentration and excess fluid retention. ADH also causes contraction of the muscular tissues of the capillaries and arteries, decreasing blood flow and increasing blood pressure. ADH is normally stored and released by the posterior lobe of the pituitary gland. Some tumors cause ectopic production of ADH, which has the same effect on urine secretion and concentration (Henry, 1991, pp. 312–13).

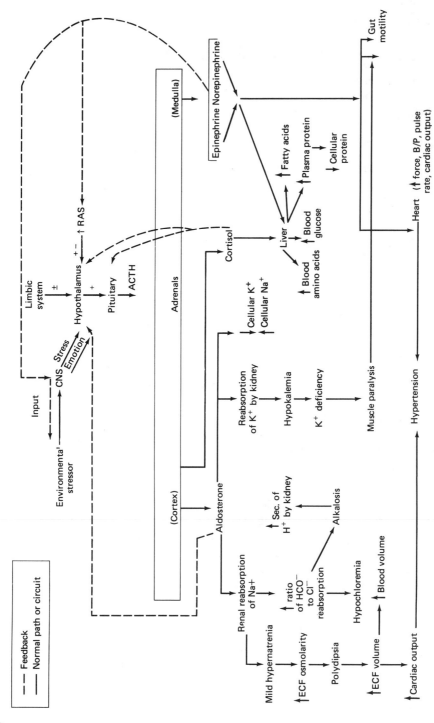

Figure 7–2. Environmental stress and the physiological response of the adrenal system with feedback channels. *(From Hazzard, M. E. [1979]. Critical care nursing—Nursing outline series. Garden City, NY: Medical Examination Publishing Company, Inc., p. 39. with permission.)*

SIADH MIGHT BE SUSPECTED WITH:

1. Laboratory findings: Decreased plasma sodium and chloride concentrations increased urinary sodium level because of water retention, dilutional changes in other values (e.g., decreased hematocrit, mean corpuscular volume [MCV], decreased mean corpuscular hemoglobin concentration [MCHC])
2. Clinical findings: Urinary output less than intake; weight gain, often 1 lb or more a day; history of trauma, surgery, cerebral lesion, lung carcinoma, or other known precipitants of SIADH as well as in early postoperative period in recovery room or intensive care unit

B. Tests of Antidiuretic Hormone Function

Serum and Urine Osmolality

Synonyms: Plasma and urine osmolality

Normal Ranges (mOsm/kg of water)

Serum	275–295
Urine	300–1000 (also expressed as mOsm/L)
Urine/plasma ratio	0.2–4.7

Explanation of the Tests. Osmolality is the measurement of the number of dissolved solute particles in a solution. It is the preferred unit of measurement for body fluids, over specific gravity or osmolarity, because it is a constant weight-to-weight relationship. Osmolarity varies with fluid volume, the expanding effect on the solution of dissolved solute, and the temperature of the solution. Specific gravity requires correction for the presence of glucose or protein as well as temperature. Osmolality can be measured over a wider range than specific gravity and with greater accuracy.

Urine osmolality gives information about a number of things: the ability of the kidney tubules to concentrate or dilute urine, the presence or absence of ADH (presumptive) for the renal tubular reabsorption of water, an indication of plasma osmolality, and assistance in the diagnosis of certain fluid and electrolyte problems as well as control of therapy. More information is available when urine osmolality is compared with plasma osmolality (U/P); electrolytes can also be compared in both solutions (U/P normal ratio). A comparison of the plasma sodium concentration to plasma osmolality is another fruitful way to use knowledge of osmolality. (Plasma sodium/plasma osmolality normal range equals 0.43 to 0.40 and remains unchanged in many dilutional and dehydration states.)

Changes in Osmolality

Condition	Urine	Plasma
Hypernatremia (increased plasma sodium level without water increase)	Increased	Increased
Hyperosmolar nonketotic hyperglycemia	Iso-osmolar or decreased	Increased

	Urine *(cont'd)*	Plasma *(cont'd)*
Hyperglycemia	Iso-osmolar or decreased	Increased
Uremia	Iso-osmolar	Increased
Diabetes insipidus	Decreased	Increased
Hypercalcemia	Decreased	Increased
Excess fluid intake (compulsive drinking)	Decreased	Decreased
SIADH	Increased	Decreased
Renal tubular necrosis	Decreased	Increased
Severe pyelonephritis	Decreased	Increased
Acidosis	Increased	Increased
Shock	Increased	Increased

Patient Preparation. No special preparation is necessary. The first-voided specimen in the morning is the most likely to demonstrate the maximum concentrating ability of the kidney.

Water Deprivation Tests

Synonyms: Mosenthal test (24 hr), Fishberg test (12 hr), renal concentration test, 14-hr deprivation test, 8-hr deprivation test

Normal Ranges

Urine osmolality greater than 800 mOsm/kg of water

Urine osmolality greater than serum osmolality

Serum osmolality unchanged

Explanation of the Tests. Water deprivation in normal persons stimulates ADH secretion through osmolar and volume stimuli. Such deprivation can be used when it is necessary to differentiate among possible causes of polyuria, particularly between nephrogenic diabetes insipidus (DI)—the inability of the renal tubules to respond to ADH—and neurohypophyseal DI, inadequate or absent ADH secretion. It also establishes the patient's ability to produce ADH.

As indicated by the number of synonyms given, there are many slightly different approaches to this test, all of which share common principles. The test is based on deprivation of *any* fluid intake over a specified length of time, until a given outcome occurs as evidenced by a change in urine osmolality to a normal concentration, to the point of a specific weight loss (e.g., greater than 3 percent of body weight), or to the point where 2- or 3-hour urine osmolality tests indicate about equal osmolality—a plateau. If the response to water deprivation is abnormal with inadequate concentration, the test can be followed by an injection of vasopressin (exogenous ADH). This will indicate whether the cause is ADH deficiency or nonresponsive kidney tubules.

The shorter tests are more frequently used because individuals with DI and polyuria exceeding 5 L/day usually reach their optimum concentrating ability, the plateau, in 4 to 8 hours, whereas normal individuals may require up to 14 hours. Plasma osmolality, plasma sodium levels, urine volume, and urine osmolality are checked at the beginning and end of the test. Urine osmolality may be checked every hour or any variation of timing, and weight is usually taken at the beginning and end as well as when indicated during the test.

Responses to Water Deprivation Tests

Condition	Osmolality Response to H_2O Deprivation	Osmolality Response to Vasopressin
Compulsive water drinking (primary polydipsia)	Normal urine and plasma osmolality	Normal; urine osmolality increases no more than 5%
Neurohypophyseal DI	Urine osmolality less than plasma; plasma osmolality greater than 300 mosm	Increased to greater than 50% of baseline and greater than plasma osmolality
Nephrogenic DI	Urine osmolality less than plasma; plasma osmolality often greater than 300 mosm	No response

Data from Henry, 1991 and Conn, 1991.

Patient Preparation

1. Conditions such as diabetes mellitus, hypercalcemia, and hyperkalemia must be ruled out by appropriate tests before starting water deprivation because they are contraindications for testing
2. The possibility of vascular collapse with water deprivation is high, and close observation is imperative. The test will be stopped at the first sign of vascular collapse (e.g., drop of 10 points in blood pressure)
3. Careful instruction and monitoring is necessary to prevent any fluid intake that would invalidate the test result

Water-Loading Tests

Synonyms: Water challenge, saline challenge, water load, Hickey-Hare osmolality test

Normal Ranges

Decrease in urine volume (flow rate in ml/min)

Urine osmolality, equal to or greater than 600 mOsm/kg (level obtained when exogenous vasopressin given)

Explanation of the Test. The purpose of the water-loading test is to establish the patient's ability to produce ADH. Some authorities believe that the information is more simply acquired by the water deprivation test (Harvey et al., 1991). Water loading is sometimes useful in the diagnosis of inappropriate ADH (IADH), but it is a dangerous test in patients with hyponatremia (less than 125 mEq/L).

The test is based on the principle that a rise in serum osmolality will stimulate ADH release, the effects of which can be measured in the increased urine concentration. Unlike water deprivation, this test also increases blood volume expansion, which alters ADH release and is a conflicting stimulus to that of increased serum osmolality.

Generally, the test is carried out as follows: Diuresis is established either by having the patient drink a 20-ml/kg load of water in 15 minutes or by intravenous infusion of 5 percent glucose at 8 to 10 ml/min, which leads to an increased glomerular filtration rate (GFR) with hypotonic fluid. When the urine flow is 5 ml/min, when over 50 percent of the initial water load is excreted, or when 1 hour has passed, an intravenous infusion of 2.5 percent saline solution (isotonic saline is 0.9 percent) is started and run at 0.25 ml/kg/min for 45 minutes. Serum osmolality is measured before and after the hypertonic intravenous infusion is given, and urine is collected every hour for 4 hours, with the volume and osmolality measured.

Vasopressin may be given as a follow-up to differentiate between the two types of DI (see the explanation under "Water Deprivation Test").

Responses to Water-Loading Tests

Condition	Response
Compulsive water drinking (primary polydipsia)	Normal (see "Normal Ranges")
DI, neurohypophyseal	No antidiuresis—urine osmolality unchanged
DI, nephrogenic	No antidiuresis—urine osmolality unchanged

Patient Preparation

1. The test is risky for patients with cardiac disease because of the initial water load given, which markedly increases the work of the heart and because of the increased chance of pulmonary edema occurring with the administration of hypotonic fluids.
2. Plasma sodium levels should be determined before the test. In some instances sodium replacement is done before the test to bring the plasma levels up to the minimum safe level (125 mEq/L).

Direct Measurement of Plasma ADH

Synonyms: ADH test, vasopressin test

Normal Ranges 1.0–13.3 pg/ml (with random hydration) (Laboratory of Pathology, 1991)

Explanation of the Test. Direct measurement of ADH levels requires a complex test using blood plasma. Because it requires multiple incubation periods with a variety of substances, it takes from 5 to 10 days or more to obtain the findings. Through the many steps of the test a precipitate is formed that contains the antibody-bound tracer, which is counted by a gamma counter. This test determines much more accurately than water loading and depriva-tion tests the ability of an individual to produce ADH and its level in the blood at the time of the test.

Purpose of the Test. The major action of ADH is that of increasing the permeability of the renal collecting ducts' membranes, thereby allowing the transfer of water and, in turn, pro-ducing urine concentration. It is a safe test for the client and consumes a great deal less of his or her time than do the tests given previously. Results take longer, and the cost is greater, but the findings are more accurate. The test is usually done in a reference lab-oratory.

ADH levels can be used in the differential diagnosis of hyponatremia and polyuric disor-ders, some of which can be caused by the inappropriate secretion of ADH.

Patient Preparation. Depending on the facility doing the test and the suspected cause of the water imbalance problem, there is usually no special preparation, or the patient may

1. Be held n.p.o. for 12 hours before the test
2. Have some limitation of physical activity before the test
3. Have certain interfering or causative substance in the form of medications withheld by physician order (e.g., estrogen, lithium)

INCREASES IN ADH LEVELS OCCUR WITH:

1. Any stressor (e.g., pain, fear)
2. Ectopic ADH production with low sodium levels, most frequently secondarily to a ma-lignancy as in small-cell cancer of the lung, also known as Syndrome of Inappropriate ADH (SIADH). This syndrome has also been known to occur with acute porphyria, hy-pothyroidism, Addison's disease, cirrhosis of the liver, and infectious hepatitis
3. Severe hemorrhage or other causes of circulatory shock
4. Many drugs, to a greater or lesser degree, such as
   a. Antineoplastic drugs (e.g., vincristine, cyclophosphamide)
   b. Antidiabetic drugs (e.g., chlorpropamide [Diabinese])
   c. Anticonvulsant drugs (e.g., carbamazepine [Tegretol])
   d. Other hormones (e.g., estrogen, oxytocin)
   e. Some tranquilizers, hypnotics, or antimaniacal drugs (e.g., lithobid)
5. Positive-pressure ventilation (perhaps related to stress?)
6. In some cases of nephrogenic DI when the pituitary tries to compensate by increased se-cretion of ADH

DECREASES IN ADH LEVELS OCCUR WITH:

1. Alcohol ingestion
2. Pituitary diabetes insipidus (DI) secondary to decreased ADH production. Pituitary DI can be caused by a large number of primary illnesses such as tumor, head trau-ma—which includes trauma secondary to neurosurgical procedures—and viral infec-tion

NORMAL OR INCREASED LEVELS OF ADH WITH SIGNS AND SYMPTOMS OF DIABETES INSIPIDUS (DI):

- Probably due to the nephrogenic type of DI in which there is renal tubular resistance to ADH action

7.2.2 Growth Hormone

A. *Laboratory and Clinical Indications of Growth Hormone Dysfunction*

Indications of secreting pituitary tumors are the decrease in all but one hormone function, most often growth hormone (GH) or ACTH, and that function shows a marked increase. Congenital, or genetic "idiopathic" pituitary deficiencies, which are presumably hypothalamic in origin, often involve GH or the gonadotropins alone.

GH DEFICIENCIES MIGHT BE SUSPECTED WITH:

1. Clinical findings. *Children*: failure to grow, with impaired linear growth within the first few months of life, delayed bone maturation, no obvious physical abnormalities other than small size. *Adults:* there are no known physical abnormalities associated with deficiency after attainment of full height
2. Laboratory findings. Usual screening test results are normal

GH EXCESS MIGHT BE SUSPECTED WITH:

1. Clinical findings. *Children:* Gigantism, overgrowth of skeleton and soft tissues with proportional overgrowth of long bones; weight and height are in proportion; may have headaches if pituitary tumor is cause. *Adults:* Early signs of acromegaly include increased size of hands, head, feet (may be noticed by gloves, hat, or shoes being too small), and facial changes (e.g., increased nose size, enlargement of forehead, jaw [dentures do not fit]); voice changes—increased resonance, lower pitch; constant perspiration; coarsening of skin; enlargement of tongue with slurring of speech; arthritic complaints.
2. Laboratory findings. *Children:* Increased serum glucose; diabetic glucose tolerance test (GTT) curve; untreated, decreased thyroid-stimulating hormone (TSH). *Adults:* Increased serum inorganic phosphorous (before GH by RIA, this was felt to be the most helpful test for acromegaly; relationship to increased GH not established, but inorganic phosphorus is also increased in growing children); increased calcium, serum, and urine; serum glucose and GTT as for child. *Related tests:* Basal metabolic rate increased; increased serum prolactin, at times urine 17-KS, 17-OHCS, or 17-KGS are increased despite normal plasma cortisol; TSH may increase.

B. *Tests of Growth Hormone Function*

Serum growth hormone, RIA

Synonyms: GH, human growth hormone: HGH, somatotropin hormone, SH, STH

Normal Ranges (ng/ml)

Adult	>18 yr	0–10
Children	<18 yr	0–20

Explanation of the Test. At the present time, GH radioimmunoassay* is the single most important test in the evaluation of GH. GH can be directly measured in the blood by RIA and can be measured equally well in either serum or plasma, although serum is preferred. GH is produced by the anterior pituitary gland in response to the hypothalamic releasing factors. Although many hormones are necessary for growth, GH is the most important. In its absence children's growth rate is decreased by one half to one third. As yet the normal function of GH in the adult is not fully understood. Measurement of GH gives information not only about its deficit or excess but also is frequently used as a guide to pituitary dysfunction, since decreases in GH values often indicate pituitary tumors (Henry, 1991).

Normal values of GH have wide variation because of the rather sporadic bursts of secretion. Levels in normal persons are often very low, and may actually be undetectable. Short bursts occur, not consistent with any pattern, but their presence is fairly consistent from day to day in a given individual. A rise in concentration occurs early in sleep (with the exception of some adults over 50 years of age). Because of the consistent secretion with sleep, basal levels would be drawn in the morning when they are most likely to be detectable—after awakening but before arising and while fasting.

Because of the overlap between the basal normal range of GH and values consistent with hypopituitarism, a definite normal is required to rule out hyposecretion of GH. This usually requires a stimulation test (see "Growth Hormone Stimulation Test," next).

Patient Preparation

1. Patients should be kept n.p.o. other than water for 8 to 10 hours before the test
2. In some methods the patient is kept recumbent for 30 minutes before blood taking to eliminate GH bursts due to exercise

INCREASED SECRETION OF GH ASSOCIATED WITH:

1. Acromegaly in the adult, usually from a pituitary tumor
2. Gigantism in children under the age of puberty, a rare occurrence that may be acquired because of a pituitary tumor or congenital "idiopathic" causes
3. Bronchogenic or gastric cancer in very rare instances as a result of ectopic GH secretion by tumors
4. Hypoglycemia
5. Physiological responses such as
   a. Sleep. There are substantial increases early in sleep, with a peak occurring between the first and second hours, and levels may peak two to three times during one night
   b. Exercise of any type, especially when fasting. Fifteen minutes of exercise in a fasting patient makes a good, easily performed, and inexpensive stimulation screening test in children of short stature (Conn, 1991)

---

*An assay is the analysis of a substance to define its nature and proportions. The assay is used in clinical laboratory testing to determine the amount of any particular substance in the mixture of substances in a body fluid. The methods used are reflected in the names of the types of assays (e.g., radioassay, competitive binding assay, radioimmunoassay, RIA). The process involves the use of a limited amount of a specific binding reagent that is held constant in the system. The binder may be an antibody (insulin assay), specific binding proteins (thyroxine assay), a cellular receptor, or an enzyme (renin assay). To complete the test, there must be a means of separating or identifying the bound and the free components (Henry, 1991).

    c. Increased levels of human placental lactogen in pregnant women

    d. After protein ingestion (e.g., a pure beefsteak meal) or the infusion of certain amino acids such as arginine

    e. Stress such as response to major surgery or even minor stressors such as anticipation of physical examination. GH levels can increase then, even in the face of hyperglycemia

6. Iatrogenic causes as with

    a. Therapeutic administration of estrogen, which elevates basal secretion

    b. Drugs such as L-dopa; however, L-dopa can also cause a paradoxical fall in GH levels in acromegalic patients

DECREASED SECRETION OF GH ASSOCIATED WITH:

1. Ateliotic (pituitary) dwarfism in children resulting from multiple, not well understood causes such as decreased secretion of GH-releasing factor; lesion of the pituitary; decreased ability of the body to respond to GH—end-organ unresponsiveness—which may in turn be due to defects in the generation of somatomedin (the GH-dependent substance in plasma that stimulates growth in responsive tissue) (Henry, 1991)

2. Ingestion of a glucose load

3. Pharmacological doses of glucocorticoid

Growth Hormone Stimulation and Suppression Tests: Overview

Introduction. GH deficiency is probably the most frequent pituitary hormone deficiency. It is due to either overall pituitary failure or to an isolated defect leading to growth retardation in childhood.

Purpose of Testing. Serum GH changes markedly from moment to moment in normal people. Therefore, single serum measurements do not provide sufficient information to distinguish normal from abnormal function. To increase accuracy in testing, either several blood draws are done 15 minutes apart (either pooling the blood from the draws, or taking an average of the findings of each draw divided by the number of draws—usually three—as the accepted GH level) or using stimulation or suppression tests.

Stimulation Test. Many substances can be used in this test as stimulators of GH production, such as arginine, clonidine, glucagon, gonadotropin-releasing factor, insulin (tolerance test), L-dopa, thyrotropin-releasing hormone, or vasopressin. Adequate growth may also depend on familial inheritance as in Turner's syndrome, trisomy (Downs') syndrome, malabsorption, malnutrition, or chronic liver or renal disease.

    Expected response with some stimulators is:

1. Arginine: Threefold increase in GH level and twofold increase in serum prolactin at 30- and 60-minute peaks

2. Insulin: Regular crystalline/intravenous (IV), 0.05–0.3 unit/kg body weight; twofold increase in GH; threefold increase in prolactin at 60-minute peak

3. Levodopa: Twofold increase in GH level at 60-minute peak

Considerable controversy surrounds the use of all GH stimulation tests (Tietz, 1990, p. 337).

Suppression Test. Glucose loading is most commonly used.

RELATED PHYSIOLOGY. GH release depends on the balance between two opposite hypothalamic hormones, that is, growth-releasing hormone (GHRH), which stimulates release of GH, and somatostatin, which inhibits that release. In turn, GH's effects occur through its stimulation of several tissues, producing a group of peptide growth factors called *somatomedins*, the most important of which is somatomedin-C, produced by the liver and acting on cartilage. Somatomedin is responsible for synthesis of collagen and other proteins by cartilage. High levels of somatomedin provide feedback to the pituitary, inhibiting pituitary release of GH and stimulating secretion of somatostatin from the hypothalamus.

Growth Hormone Stimulation Tests

Synonyms: Insulin tolerance test (ITT); GH provocation test; tolbutamide tolerance test

Normal Response Ranges

Consistent rise in GH levels to over 20 ng/ml (blood glucose concentration must decrease to less than 40 mg/dl, or less than 50% of the basal fasting level for the test to accurately assess the GH reserve)

Pediatric: Children may have no response even though GH is adequate; the combination of ITT and arginine infusion stimulation tests is felt to be the most definitive test for GH deficiency in children

Normal response to arginine test: GH levels rise to 7 ng/ml

Explanation and Purpose of the Test. The purpose of this testing approach is to maximally stimulate GH secretion because of its often extremely low or undetectable level and of its sporadic secretion. Because of the overlap between the basal normal range of GH and values consistent with hypopituitarism, a definite normal is required to rule out hyposecretion of GH.

However, the pattern of secretion is fairly consistent from day to day in a given individual. In addition, a rise in concentration occurs early in sleep (with the exception of some individuals over 50 years of age). Because of the consistent secretion during sleep, basal levels would be best drawn in the morning when they are most likely to be detectable, after awakening but before arising and while fasting.

Patient Preparation

1. Patient should be kept n.p.o. for 8 hours before the test
2. Screen for conditions contraindicating the test (ischemic heart disease, myocardial infarction, cerebrovascular disease, epilepsy, and low basal plasma cortisol levels)

Test Procedure. A basal blood sample is taken on a fasting patient for determination of the levels of serum glucose, cortisol, and GH. Insulin is given intravenously, the dosage based on 0.1 to 0.15 IU/kg of body weight, except in children, who have a tendency to severe hypoglycemia if deficient in GH. The dosage is calculated on approximately half of the adult dose in such cases. Blood samples are taken every 15 minutes for the first hour, a minimum of every 30 minutes, and every 30 minutes thereafter for 2 hours. The test is terminated immediately if any serious signs related to hypoglycemia occur (fainting, chest pain). Other tests may be run on the blood sample as well to help confirm or rule out a diagnosis:

1. Prolactin (luteotropic hormone [LTH])—most secreting tumors and half the nonsecreting tumors induce increased prolactin levels
2. Follicle-stimulating hormone (FSH)—measured when a stimulator such as clomiphene has been used because it induces an increase in FSH levels normally, which does not occur in pituitary failure
3. Thyroid-stimulating hormone (TSH)—hypothyroidism is often associated with short stature. GH levels cannot be assessed properly unless the patient has been euthyroid for a considerable time

"Failure of GH concentration to rise above the set limit after at least two stimulating tests is indicative of GH deficiency" (Henry, 1991).

Conditions Causing Possible Alterations in Results

Increased GH Response	**Decreased GH Response**
Starvation—with arginine test	Diabetes mellitus
Hyperthyroidism	Cirrhosis
	Hypothyroidism
	Obesity

Data from Henry, 1991.

Growth Hormone Suppression Test

Synonyms: GH suppression test, glucose loading test, glucose tolerance test, GTT

Normal Response (ng/ml)

Basal level GH	<10
Suppressed	<5 sometimes during the test

Abnormal Response: Found in active acromegaly or gigantism

Basal level GH	<5
With suppression	Does not suppress below 5

Explanation of the Test. The GH suppression test is a controlled effort to cause GH levels to decrease in response to the administration of glucose, a normal physiological response. The test procedure is not unlike that of the standard GTT (see Section 7.4.3), except that GH levels are the substance change evaluated. Suppression tests can be helpful in revealing abnormalities in physiological function and control. The lack of suppression of GH in conditions of hypersecretion with gigantism and acromegaly is a good example of this. Suppression testing is used less frequently than stimulation testing in the evaluation of GH.

NONSUPPRESSION OCCURRING IN CONDITIONS OTHER THAN INCREASED GH INCLUDES:

1. Known decreases in somatomedin concentration (the GH-dependent substance in plasma that stimulates growth in responsive tissue), which occurs in renal insufficiency and kwashiorkor
2. Renal failure
3. Cirrhosis
4. Starvation

7.3 THE THYROID GLAND

7.3.1 Laboratory and Clinical Indications of Thyroid Dysfunction

A. Hyperthyroidism

Clinical Findings (Adults). Hyperthyroidism is usually highly nonspecific in presentation, but if "classic" findings are present (exophthalmos, pretibial myxedema, thyroid enlargement), the diagnosis is obvious. Early symptoms include nervousness, fatigue, weight loss, and palpitations. Later, cardiovascular symptoms of angina, dyspnea, peripheral edema; emotional symptoms of instability, irritability, insomnia; gastrointestinal (GI) symptoms of increased appetite and food intake in face of weight loss and increased number of defecations, which can progress to true diarrhea; heat intolerance and increased perspiration; changes in menstrual cycle, menorrhagia, amenorrhea; muscle weakness noted particularly in stair climbing, getting out of tub, or combing hair; tremors of hands; hair fine and limp; and eye changes in Graves' disease, periorbital edema, prominent stare because of lid retraction or exophthalmos, lid lag, difficulty with vision—double vision, photophobia. After the age of 50 findings are less obvious, appetite may decrease, and cardiovascular symptoms predominate (apathetic hyperthyroidism). See Section 1.13.

Laboratory Findings. Results of laboratory tests are also nonspecific and variable. The WBC count may have a slight increase, the lymphocyte number increases, and there is mild anemia and mild hypercalcemia (to 11.5 mg/dl) in younger people as well as an increase in the alkaline phosphatase concentration. In tests other than screening tests, the creatine clearance may increase, and there is a tendency to glucose intolerance (abnormal GTT response).

B. Hypothyroidism

Clinical Findings. Hypothyroidism is often associated with hyaline membrane disease in the full-term infant; a protuberant abdomen, umbilical herniation, large tongue, hoarse cry, growth failure and mental retardation result if not treated. Infants are not usually obese. *Adults* present with nonpitting edema, both periorbital and of the face and extremities. The hair is coarse, dry, with the loss of the outer one third of the eyebrow; there is mild enlargement of the tongue, cold dry skin and cold intolerance (mottled skin), lethargy and a lethargic appearance, personality change (dulled, slowed mentation), menstrual changes with menorrhagia, cardiac enlargement and bradycardia, generalized weakness, entrapment neuropathy (carpal tunnel syndrome), and anorexia, which may be concomitant with weight gain and constipation.

Laboratory Findings. Infants show prolonged physiological indirect hyperbilirubinemia plus most of the findings in adults who present with increased serum cholesterol and triglyceride levels and anemia in 50 percent of patients, which can be macrocytic at times as well as normochromic or hypochromic. In tests other than screening tests, ECG changes with low voltage, and flattened or inverted T waves are seen.

7.3.2 Measurements of Thyroxine

A. *Thyroxine, Free Assay (by Direct Dialysis)*

Synonym: Free thyroxine; FT_4

Normal Range: 0.8–2.7 ng/dl

Explanation of the Test. This test process, a direct measurement of the physiologically active T_4, gives corrected values in patients in whom the total thyroxine (T_4) is altered because of changes in serum proteins or in binding sites (Wallach, 1992, p. 445–6). The estimation and/or indirect measurement of free T_4 by RIA is less costly and thus usually used in general screening. Only the free form can determine metabolic activity however (Laboratory of Pathology, 1991). It is a rather simple test and has almost completely supplanted the separate use of Total T_4 and T_3RU (thyroid$_3$ resin uptake) (Conn, 1991, pp. 841–42). However, some find estimation of T_4 as useful (Corbett, 1992, p. 398).

In this test, free T_4 is separated from both serum proteins and protein-bound T_4 before measurement; therefore, the results are independent of the concentration of T_4, thus unaffected by the presence of molecular variants of these proteins (Laboratory of Pathology, 1991).

LEVELS INCREASED IN:

1. Hyperthyroidism
2. Pregnancy
3. Use of some drugs (e.g., estrogens, birth control pills, T_4 replacement therapy)

LEVELS DECREASED IN:

1. Hypothyroidism
2. Hypothyroidism treated with triiodothyronine
3. Euthryoid syndrome (Wallach, 1992, pp. 445–64; Laboratory of Pathology, 1991)

B. Total T_4 Radioimmunoassay

T_4 RIA	Serum thyroxine by radioimmunoassay, previously the test of choice with satisfactory specificity and sensitivity

Normal Range: 4.5 to 12.5 µg/dl

T_4(D)	Also given as TD, T_4 Murphy-Patee. T_4 by displacement; independent of iodine content—therefore, a better choice for testing than the following tests, which are dependent on iodine content or interfered with because of iodine contamination

Normal Ranges (µg/dl)

Neonate	10.1–20.0
1–6 yr	5.6–12.6
6–10 yr	4.9–11.7
Adult	4.7–11.1

PBI	Protein-bound iodine, a measurement of all PBI, not just that bound to T_4; rarely used

Normal Range: 4–8 µg/dl

BEI	Butanol extractable iodine; T_4 measured as PBI after the removal of extraneous organically bound iodine; still altered by iodine contamination and by alterations in carrier protein levels; rarely used
T_4(C)	Also given as T_4I(C) and T_4 by column. T_4 measured as PBI after the removal of extraneous organically bound iodine; limitations as for BEI

Explanation of the Test. Determination of total T_4 is the initial screening test for most suspected thyroid disorders, particularly hyperthyroidism (see Fig. 7–3). These tests all measure total T_4, that is, both bound and free T_4, and are therefore altered by conditions altering thyroid-binding globulin (TBG). T_4 accounts for 95 percent of the total thyroid hormone output. Approximately 20 percent of T_4 produced is ultimately converted to triiodothyronine (T_3) in peripheral tissues. For some time it has been questioned whether T_4 is biologically active. Evidence indicates that it indeed is, but to a lesser degree than is T_3. Evidently, T_4 accounts for only about one third of the total biologic effect of thyroid (Farese, 1980).

T_4 exists primarily bound to TBG or in a lesser amount to thyroxine-binding prealbumin (TBPA). It is more firmly bound than T_3, which accounts, in part, for the fact that T_4 is found in higher concentrations in the plasma than is T_3.

PBI, BEI, and T_4(C) tests measure T_4 by measuring the amount of iodine present. They are then indirect estimations of T_4 and thus tend to have frequent alterations because of ingested iodine or contamination by extraneous iodine during the test procedure. They are altered as well by changes in TBG levels. For these reasons their use has been generally supplanted by the RIA test.

Patient Preparation. No special preparation is needed.

T_4 LEVELS INCREASED IN:

1. Dysfunctions of thyroid production as in hyperthyroidism and acute and subacute thyroiditis

  2. Conditions that increase the concentration or binding capacity of TBG, a transport protein for thyroid hormone, such as

    a. Increased estrogen levels found in pregnancy or the use of birth control pills

    b. Liver disease (e.g., acute viral hepatitis)

    c. Congenital increases found in familial idiopathic dysproteinemia

    d. Newborn infants

    e. Acute intermittent porphyria

    f. Some instances of hypothyroidism

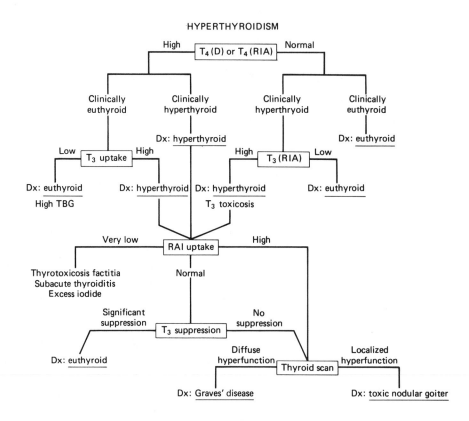

Figure 7–3. Laboratory evaluation of hyperthyroidism. T_4 determination is the initial screening test. If the level is high in a clinically euthyroid patient, a T_3 uptake test (T_3U) should be done. Either the T_3U will show that an elevated TBG level is the cause of the high T_4 value, or it will support hyperthyroidism. If the T_4 result is normal in a clinically hyperthyroid patient, a T_3 determination (RIA) will indicate whether T_3 toxicosis is present. Once the serum hormone confirmation of hyperthyroidism is completed, the radioactive iodine uptake (RAI) test will separate the various causes. If the RAIU is normal in a case of suspected Graves' disease, a T_3 suppression test should be performed. Finally, the pattern of uptake on the thyroid scan will indicate whether toxic nodular goiter or Graves' disease is the cause of the elevated or nonsuppressible RAIU. (From Marguilies, P. L, & Becker, D. V. [1977]. Hyperthyroidism. In H.F. Conn & R. B. Conn (Eds.), *Current Diagnosis 5* [p. 744]. Philadelphia: Saunders, with permission.)

T$_4$ LEVELS DECREASED IN:

1. Dysfunctions of thyroid production as in cretinism of infants and childhood myxedema, chronic thyroiditis, and occasionally subacute thyroiditis
2. Conditions that decrease the concentration or binding capacity of TBG such as
   a. Increased steroid serum levels (Cushing's disease, Cushing's syndrome, therapeutic administration of glucocorticoids)
   b. Administration of androgens therapeutically
   c. Chronic debilitating illness (multiple myeloma, leukemia, Hodgkin's disease, active acromegaly, nephrotic syndrome, nephrosis)
   d. Acute illness or with surgical stress because of increased glucocorticoid production
3. Conditions that require the administration of certain drugs that either decrease T$_4$ synthesis (salicylates, sulfonamides), increase T$_4$ destruction (reserpine), or displace T$_4$ from binding sites (aspirin, heparin)
4. Patients treated with T$_3$ alone and euthyroid (no clinical signs or symptoms of abnormal thyroid function and free thyroid index within normal limits)
5. Hashimoto's thyroiditis, radiation damage, thyroid dysgenesis. The patients may be euthyroid, however, because of increased T$_3$ secretion

7.3.3 Total T$_3$ by Radioimmunoassay (Triiodothyronine Measurement)

Synonyms: T$_3$ RIA; triiodothyronine RIA

Normal Ranges (ng/dl)

Adult	95–185
Pediatric	
Newborn/cord	15–75
1–3 day	22–216
1–2 wk	x:250
2–4 wk	160–240
1–4 mo	117–209
1–5 yr	105–269
5–10 yr	94–241
10–15 yr	82–213
Declines with aging	

(Data from Laboratory of Pathology, 1991; Tietz, 1990, pp. 556–57).

Explanation of the Test. T$_3$ is secreted by the thyroid and produced peripherally by deiodination of T$_4$. As with the serum thyroxine by RIA (T$_4$ RIA) test described previously, T$_3$ RIA measures the most metabolically active segment of thyroid hormone. Like the T$_4$ test given previously, this measures both protein-bound and free portions of T$_3$ and is therefore affected by alterations in TBG and TBPA levels. The measurement of T$_3$ is felt by some authorities to be the most sensitive test for thyrotoxicosis (Ravel, 1989). It is seldom used for the detection of hypothyroidism because of the overlap between the low–normal range and hypothyroid conditions. It is therefore not reliable for distinguishing between normal and hypothyroid states.

Patient Preparation. No special preparation is necessary.

T₃ LEVELS INCREASED IN:

1. See Section 7.3.2.B. Over 90 percent of all hyperthyroid patients have increases in both T_3 and T_4 concentrations, and the increase in T_3 is often greater than or secreted before T_4. T_3 determination may be the better diagnostic test in hyperthyroid states
2. Thyrotoxicosis. Shows persistent T_3 elevation with normal T_4
3. T_3 toxicosis. There is a significant minority of hyperthyroid patients with a normal T_4 but increased T_3, level, especially early in the course of toxic nodular goiter, in relapses after treatment of Graves' disease, and in regions of iodine deficiency
4. Overdosage with T_3 replacement (e.g., cytomel). The known time of dosage administration is important for an accurate interpretation of T_3 levels because the exogenous hormone has serum level peaks about 4 hours after administration
5. Hashimoto's thyroiditis; decreased thyroid reserve due to radiation damage to the thyroid; and thyroid dysgenesis. T_3 is secreted before T_4. The patient may be euthyroid

T₃ LEVELS DECREASED IN:

1. See Section 7.3.2.B
2. The euthyroid sick, in which T_4 is converted to a metabolically inert substance called reverse T_3 instead of active T_3 in the periphery. Reverse T_3 does not measure as T_3, thus decreasing the level (Farese, 1980). It is seen in debilitating diseases such as chronic renal failure or cirrhosis, persons being treated with glucocorticoids, gravely ill patients from any cause, starvation or during fasting, the newborn period and the elderly
3. Persons being treated with T_4
4. Persons with acute illness and after surgery because of stress effect

7.3.4 Thyroxine-Binding Globulin (Serum)

Synonym: TBG

Normal Range: (µg/dl)

Adults	16–24
Children (age 1–7, male and female)	17–26

Explanation of the Test. By most methods, thyroxine can be measured in serum in a bound state only. Therefore, serum T_4 levels are affected by changes in serum T_4 binding proteins, particularly the glycoprotein globulin, and can be misleading in diagnosis of hypothyroidism. Some drugs increase serum T_4 levels and decrease binding capacity, leading to decreased T_4 levels on most testing, but not in fact. In such cases measurement of free, or unbound, T_4 correlates better with actual thyroid status.

Evaluation of T_4 in infants is complicated because of normally increased TBG levels during the neonatal period, as well as a TSH surge during birth that increases T_4 levels for weeks after birth. Many tests have been used in this process in the past (e.g., T_3U, free thyroxine index [FTI]).

TBG is the principal protein that binds thyroxine (T_4), making it "countable." Using electrophoresis and I^{125}, unbound T_4 is removed from the serum sample in an anion exchange resin. The amount of T_4 that binds with I^{125} is then measured by counting its reactivity. The TBG is reported as micrograms of T_4 bound by the saturated protein. Actual serum T_4 levels have been found to parallel the TBG levels.

Ravel (1989) feels that with the use of " 'the corrected' thyroxine [T_4] by isotope for free T_4 index, TBG assay should rarely be needed" (p. 661).

Patient Preparation. No special preparation is required.

TBG LEVELS DECREASED IN:

Acquired conditions such as:

1. Nephrotic syndrome (through urinary excretion)
2. Marked hypoproteinemia (protein malnutrition/malabsorption)
3. Hepatic disease
4. Acidotic states (severe)
5. Steroid therapy (androgenic and/or anabolic)
6. Large-dose aspirin intake
7. Severe stress (e.g., major illness, surgical stress)

TBG FALSE LEVELS DECREASE IN:

- Dilantin therapy

TBG LEVELS INCREASED IN:

1. Pregnancy
2. Hypothyroidism
3. Acute intermittent porphyria
4. Treatment with some drugs, such as
   a. Estrogen
   b. Oral contraceptive
   c. Perphenazine (tranquilizer)
5. Infectious hepatitis

7.3.5 Measurement of "Free" Thyroid Hormone

Synonyms: By dialysis—free thyroxine (FT_4) (see also Section 7.3.2.A) and free triiodothyronine (FT_3); free thyroxine index[a]—FTI, FT_4 index, T_4 RIA or T_4 (D) and T_3 U ratio; free triiodothyronine index[a]—(FT, I, FT_3 index, T_3 RIA, and T_3 U ratio

[a]Both the free thyroxine index and the free triiodothyronine index, when combined and reported together, are called T_7 by some laboratories. T_7 is the product of the T_4 or T_3 and the T_3 U resin uptake tests.

Explanation of the Tests

DIALYSIS. It is possible to obtain accurate measurements of free T_4 and T_3. One method is equilibrium dialysis in which radioactively labeled T_4 is added to serum as a tracer. The free T_4 (or T_3) is then separated from the bound T_4, and the radioactivity of the dialysate is measured. Comparable but less precise information is available from the less expensive tests and computations of the free thyroid hormone index tests.

FREE T_4/T_3 INDEX. T_4 and T_3 are present in the circulation primarily in the bound state (99.77 and 97.0 percent, respectively). The biologic activity of both factions corresponds better with the free serum levels of the hormones because the free fractions are not tied to protein and can be used immediately. They can maintain an individual in a euthyroid state despite variations in available binding sites.

Free thyroid hormone fractions are directly proportional to the RT_3U and inversely proportional to TBG, as seen in the discussion of total thyroid hormone measurement. Usually T_4 and T_3 fluctuate together, and it is not necessary to determine both levels. In some instances (e.g., hypothyroidism), T_3 levels may be disproportionately high. The calculation called the free T_4 (or T_3) index is done according to this formula:

$$\text{Total } T_4 \text{ RIA (or } T_4 \text{ (D)} \times RT_3U = \text{free } T_4 \text{ index,}$$
$$\text{or total } T_3 \text{ RIA} \times RT_3U = \text{free } T_3.$$

Calculation of this index gives a true picture of the patient's status by compensating for TBG alterations and describing the metabolically active part of the hormone.

A method of calculating mean absolute free level of the hormone fractions makes use of the known approximate percentages of free versus bound hormone (e.g., [T_4 mean total level in mg/dl = 7.0] × [percent free = 0.03 percent] = mean absolute free level in ng/dl = 2.1).

Preparation for test. No special preparations are necessary.

INCREASES AND DECREASES IN TEST VALUES:

- These parallel those for T_4 and T_3 RIA but eliminate changes resulting from alterations in TBG values.

7.3.6 Thyroid-Stimulating Hormone (RIA), Serum

Synonyms: TSH, human thyroid-stimulating hormone, HTSH

Normal Range: 0.3–5.0 µIU/ml

Explanation of the test. TSH is a glycoprotein secreted by the pituitary gland. The serum TSH determination is not a basic thyroid diagnostic test but one that is helpful in special circumstances. Circulating serum concentrations of free thyroid hormones T_4 and T_3 regulate TSH secretion, which is released from the anterior pituitary by way of a negative-feedback cycle (e.g., increased T_3 and T_4 concentrations cause decreased TSH levels and vice versa). A second direct stimulatory control on TSH production is from thyrotropin-releasing factor

(TRF) or hormone (TRH) and is produced in the hypothalamus. Knowledge of the circulating levels of TSH can especially help differentiate between primary and secondary hypothyroidism, particularly in the milder cases. Primary hypothyroidism (e.g., myxedema) refers to thyroid gland defect—hypofunction or nonfunction—and is indicated by increased TSH levels (increased stimulation of the thyroid) resulting from the decreased circulating levels of thyroid hormone. Secondary hypothyroidism refers to a pituitary (or hypothalamic) hypofunction or nonfunction (pituitary dysfunction) and is indicated by a decreased TSH level as a result of the inability of the pituitary to produce adequate hormone. T_3 and T_4 levels have no effect in this instance. The TSH determination is considered critical in the differential diagnosis of hypothyroidism and to localize the level of dysfunction—pituitary, hypothalamic, or thyroid failure (Conn, 1991).

TSH can be stimulated to test its function by administering TRF. Its pituitary reserve is measured by the increase or lack of TSH.

Very few changes occur in TSH levels as a result of outside influences (e.g., diet, exercise, fever, diurnal factors), which makes it a quite specific test.

Patient Preparation. No special preparation is necessary.

TSH LEVELS INCREASED IN:

1. Primary hypothyroidism (e.g., myxedma), generally more than twice normal
2. Exaggerated increases may occur in response to stimulation by TRF, and the response may also be delayed
3. Clinically euthyroid persons with Hashimoto's thyroiditis
4. Physiological states such as the neonatal period (newborns, less than 3 days old). Usually a euthyroid state, but which may ultimately raise both T_3 and T_4 levels for several weeks
5. Moderate or high levels in compensated dysfunction of the thyroid (5 to 10 µIU/ml). Levels may become excessively high before failure in risk patients (goiter, chronic lymphocytic thyroiditis, after thyroidectomy or ablation of the thyroid by x-ray or radioactive iodine)

TSH LEVELS LOW NORMAL OR DECREASED IN:

1. Secondary hypothyroidism (pituitary dysfunction). An important condition to distinguish because secondary hypothyroidism almost always requires adrenal replacement as well. ACTH levels should also be evaluated. If only the thyroid dysfunction is treated, the patient may well go into adrenal crisis
2. Multinodular goiter. On rare occasions elevations do occur
3. Overdosage with thyroid replacement hormone

7.3.7 Thyroid Suppression Test

Synonym: T_3 suppression

Normal Response

TSH levels suppress below basal value

T_4 will suppress to less than 50% of the basal value

Explanation of the Test. The thyroid suppression test is based on the principle that in hyperthyroidism thyroid production and release are autonomous and that the thyroid will continue to manufacture hormone despite the administration of oral T_3 (the most active metabolic form of the hormone) in a standard dose daily over 1 week's time. It was used to confirm the diagnosis of borderline hyperthyroidism. It is seldom used at present because of the availability of T_3 RIA and TRF tests, which help define borderline cases and cause no danger to the patient. Administration of T_3 is not advised in the elderly, particularly those with cardiac disease or any person with cardiac disease or high plasma thyroid levels. If the test is performed, extreme caution must be used.

Patient Preparation. No special preparation is necessary.

FAILURE TO SUPPRESS OCCURS IN:

* Primary hyperthyroidism (e.g., multinodular goiter, Graves' disease)

7.3.8 Thyrotropin Releasing Factor Test

Synonyms: TRF, thyrotropic releasing hormone, TRH, TSH stimulation test

Normal Ranges

Prompt rise in TSH levels, peaking in 15–30 min

Women	Peak value: 16–26 µU/ml from base of 6 µU/ml
Men	Slightly lower

(Serum T_3 increases 70% above baseline 1 to 4 hr after the test but is not usually measured)[a]

[a]There is disagreement in the literature concerning how much TSH/TRF over baseline is to be considered exaggerated.

Explanation of the Test. The principle on which the TRF test, currently seldom used, is based is that TRF controls pituitary production of TSH. It is therefore primarily a pituitary stimulation test. The test is done to differentiate between hypothalamic and pituitary insufficiency in the patient with primary hypothyroidism, equivocal symptoms, and low TSH levels. An intact pituitary will respond by increasing the TSH concentration when TRF is administered.

The test supplanted the T_3 suppression test in many laboratories because the outcomes compared well with that test and it avoids the administration of T_3, which can be dangerous in the elderly, those with cardiac disease, or in those with already high levels of circulating thyroid hormone. Absent or markedly blunted responses are strongly suggestive of primary pituitary disease.

Patient Preparation. No special preparation is necessary.

NO RESPONSE IN:

1. Hypothyroidism because of pituitary failure
2. Hyperthyroidism because of functional autonomy of the thyroid as in a toxic goiter

RESPONSE LESS THAN NORMAL IN:

1. Patients who have been withdrawn from long-term thyroid therapy for a considerable time
2. Patients who have been receiving a prolonged administration of corticosteroids, L-dopa, or aspirin
3. Persons with a multinodular goiter
4. Euthyroid persons after treatment of Graves' disease

NORMAL RESPONSE IN:

1. Primary hyperthyroidism
2. Hypothyroidism because of a deficiency but not an absence of pituitary or hypothalamic function. The peak will most likely be delayed by 45 to 90 minutes

7.3.9 Thyroid Circulating Antibody Tests

Introduction. In certain thyroid disorders, those related to an autoimmune disorder, antibodies against specific thyroid constituents are formed, leading to inflammation and ultimate thyroid gland disruption, even destruction. Four separate organ-specific antigen–antibody systems have been identified in human thyroiditis.

The purpose of the following tests is to identify the cause of thyroid dysfunction related to autoimmune conditions, thereby clarifying treatment approaches.

Explanation of the Tests. There is strong evidence that the immunologic system plays a role in Hashimoto's disease (thyroiditis) and in Graves' disease. Such immunologic traits are definitely genetic in Hashimoto's disease, and the probability is for a genetic etiology in Graves' disease. The immunoglobulins produced are thought to be antibody to the TSH receptor. Some of the antibodies have been identified and are fairly widely known such as the long-acting thyroid stimulator (LATS), LATS protector (LATS-P), and human thyroid stimulator. (LATS at one time was thought to be implicated in the exophthalmos of Graves' disease; that belief is now uncertain at best [Krupp, et al., 1987; Phipps et al., 1983]). Four separate organ-specific antigen-antibody systems have been identified in human thyroiditis.

The two aforementioned serum tests help diagnose the autoimmune thyroid conditions, which also include lymphadenoid goiter, and can be useful in following treatment responses. Several different types of organ-specific autoantibodies exist in almost all patients with thyroid disease and some nonsymptomatic, but genetically related individuals. Extremely high titers are inconsistent with most thyroid diagnoses other than Hashimoto's thyroiditis, Graves' disease, and lymphadenoid goiter. Lymph node enlargement and lymphocytosis are frequent concomitant signs occurring with Graves' disease that reinforce its autoimmune origin.

Patient Preparation. No special preparation is necessary.

HIGH TITERS OCCUR IN:

• Hashimoto's and Graves' diseases primarily

LOW TITERS OCCUR IN:

1. Almost all thyroid disorders and in some nonaffected but related persons. The elevations are due principally to an increase in antithyroglobulin antibody levels
2. Some patients with pernicious anemia and myasthenia gravis (with some regularity) and without evidence of thyroid dysfunction. Over 50 percent of all patients tested with pernicious anemia demonstrated detectable thyroid antibodies (Seigler, 1978)
3. Approximately 10 percent of all persons with juvenile-onset diabetes
4. Patients with primary myxedema (hypothyroidism), primarily of the antithyroid antibody

A. Antimicrosomal Antibody Titer, Serum

Synonyms: Microsomal antibody; antithyroid microsomal antibody

Normal Range: <1:100

(may be nondetectable; low titers occur in 5–10% of normal individuals with no signs or symptoms of disease)

Explanation of the Test. This test has been found to be more sensitive than the thyroglobulin antibody assay (see Section 7.3.9.B) for Hashimoto's thyroiditis. Microsomal antigen is isolated from human thyrotoxic thyroid glands and used to sensitize red blood cells (RBCs) (usually turkey). When exposed to serum containing the autoantibody, the RBCs agglutinate, a positive response.

Patient Preparation. No special preparation is necessary. (Serum sample should be frozen if not to be examined within 24 hours.)

HIGH TITERS OCCUR IN:

1. Eighty percent of persons with Hashimoto's thyroiditis/disease (positive at 1:200 dilution)
2. Graves' disease (80 percent)

PERSISTENT PRESENCE

- May be predictive of increased thyroid stimulating hormone

PRESENT IN:

1. Some persons with other thyroid disorders (low incidence)
2. In some normal subjects at low titer levels in the general population; lower incidence in males

B. Antithyroglobulin Antibody Titer

Synonyms: Thyroid autoantibodies; antithyroid antibody; thyroglobulin antibody titer

Normal Range: <1:10

Explanation of the Test. Human thyroglobin is used to coat RBCs, (as described in Section 7.3.9.A). Antithyroglobulin antibody in the individual's serum being tested causes cells to agglutinate. An assay is then done on serial dilutions, determining a titer.

Patient Preparation. None.

HIGH TITERS OCCUR IN:

1. Hashimoto's disease (80 percent of cases)
2. Lymphadenoid goiter (80 percent of cases)

LOW TITERS OCCUR IN:

1. Hashimoto's disease (10–20 percent)
2. Lymphadenoid goiter (16–20 percent)
3. Some persons with pernicious anemia or no disorders

HIGH TITERS—BOTH MICROSOMAL AND ANTITHYROGLOBULIN ANTIBODIES:*

1. Primary myxedema (11 percent of cases)
2. Graves' disease (5 percent of cases)

7.3.10 Serum Calcitonin

Synonyms: Thyrocalcitonin; CT

Normal Ranges (pg/ml)	*Males*	*Females*
Basal	≤19	<14
Calcium infusion	≤190	≤130
Pentagastrin infusion	≤110	≤30

Definition. Calcitonin is a hormone (polypeptide) secreted from the parafollicular C cells of the thyroid. The major action of the hormone is to inhibit bone resorption. It also promotes excretion of calcium and phosphate in the urine.

CALCITONIN LEVELS INCREASED IN:

1. Medullary carcinoma of the thyroid
2. Response to circadian rhythm

Explanation of the Test. Measurement of the hormone calcitonin from a serum (not plasma) sample helps in the detection of medullary carcinoma (MTC) of the thyroid. This tumor produces excess thyrocalcitonin and usually elevates the serum levels before there are other evidences of the cancer.

*Absence of both antibodies is strong evidence against autoimmune thyroiditis (Wallach, 1992, p. 22).

Calcium administration by infusion will stimulate calcitonin production, increasing the blood levels, which assists in early diagnosis of the tumor. Other stimulants in use include pentagastrin by injection or a combination of both calcium and pentagastrin. Normal increases in response to the stimulants should be no more than 0.2 ng/ml (Wallach, 1992).

Patient Preparation. Usually the individual is kept n.p.o. for 8 hours prior to the test. The blood collection is most frequently done in the early morning, as that sample provides the best comparison with normal values. Stimulants are often used (see Explanation of Test, paragraph 2).

IMPLICATIONS FOR NURSING

1. Recording to be done by nurse or laboratory personnel and sent with the serum sample to be tested includes:
   a. The name of the stimulant used, if any
   b. The time of administration of the stimulant
   c. The time of the blood draw
   d. The name and amount of the stimulant used
2. Explain these to the client to ensure understanding and compliance

---

7.4 THE PANCREAS

The pancreas functions in a dual role, one of which is endocrine, the production of the hormones glucagon and insulin that is the focus of this section. The second role is as an exocrine organ producing digestive enzymes (amylase, lipase, and trypsin), which is discussed in Chapter 9.

7.4.1 Laboratory and Clinical Indications of Pancreatic Endocrine Dysfunction

A. Hyposecretion of Insulin
Hyperglycemia may be due to other causes than the direct effect of decreased insulin levels, but insulin change is the major offender.

Laboratory Findings. In hyposecretion of insulin, laboratory findings include fasting serum glucose levels of more than 110 mg/dl or a 2-hour postprandial (p.p.) level between 120 and 140 mg/dl; glycosuria occurring in the presence of "normal" levels of fasting blood sugar (FBS); glycosuria or hyperglycemia with stress (surgery, trauma, stroke, myocardial infarction [MI], adrenal steroid administration); hyperlipoproteinemia (lactescent serum); ketonuria; increased serum cholesterol levels; increased serum uric acid concentration; presence of gallstones (cholelithiasis); and the presence of Charcot's joint (a neuropathic arthropathy with degeneration of the bone and cartilage of a joint and hypertrophic changes at the joint edge that cause deformity and instability of the joint; found most commonly in diabetic polyneuritis, syringomyelia, and tabes dorsalis).

Clinical Findings. Other than the most obvious signs and symptoms of polyuria, polydipsia, and polyphagia, clinical findings include a family history of diabetes mellitus; personal history of hypoglycemia, vascular disease, pruritus, or impotence; a history in females of having been pregnant or borne children or a history of spontaneous abortion, toxemia, hydramnios, or congenital defects in an infant; obesity and orthostatic hypotension in adults; eye changes (cataracts, retinopathy); frequent infections; vascular disease (peripheral, coronary, or cerebral); sensory changes primarily in the feet or hands (glove and stocking); plantar abscesses; and periodontal disease.

B. Hypersecretion of Insulin
Hypoglycemia may be due to causes other than the direct effect of increased insulin levels, but insulin change is the major offender.

Laboratory Findings. Indications of hypersecretion of insulin include serum glucose levels under 60 mg/dl (by more recent and liberal standards under 46 mg/dl is the criterion), either fasting or postprandial. It can occur in infants or adults but is usually transient when postprandial.

Clinical Findings. In infants, risk groups include low-birthweight babies, diabetic mother, and many hereditary conditions such as galactosemia. In adults, there are signs and symptoms related to increased epinephrine release, frequently postprandial (e.g., hunger, nervousness, feelings of anxiety, tachycardia), and signs and symptoms related to central nervous system (CNS) response (e.g., decreased attention span, headache, bizarre behavior, convulsions). Although an individual patient may have any or all of the possible signs and symptoms, the same set of symptoms tends to recur in the same individual.

7.4.2 Hemoglobin A$_{1C}$, Whole Blood

Synonyms: Glycohemoglobin HbA$_{1C}$; glyconated hemoglobin; glycosolated hemoglobin; "fast" hemoglobin

Normal Range: 3.4–6.0 percent (of total hemoglobin)

Explanation of the Test. HBA$_{1C}$ (HbgA$_{1C}$) is a minor component of hemoglobin (Hbg) found in normal individuals (3 to 6 percent of total Hbg), but it is elevated two- to threefold in patients with uncontrolled diabetes mellitus. The component increases at a slow and constant rate in response to physiological occurrences of hyperglycemia during the 120-day life span of the red cell. Measurement of the component provides a picture of the state of hyperglycemia over time in the individual (the life span of the RBC) and correlates with glucose intolerance in diabetics. With good diabetic control the concentration of HbA$_{1C}$ returns to the normal range as the RBCs with increased concentrations die off.

Relationships have been established between the increase in HBA$_{1C}$ levels and basement membrane thickening, functional abnormalities of leukocytes and platelets, and the increased incidence of infection, lipoproteinemia, and thrombotic complications in diabetics. A more useful approach for assessing diabetic control than measurement of urine glucose, this test is specific for HBA$_{1C}$, which is the major component of the glycosolated Hbgs and the one directly affected by blood glucose alterations. (In earlier tests of this kind, all glycohemoglobin was measured.) The other Hbg variants, HbgA$_{1A}$ and HbgA$_{1B}$, account for 1.6 and 0.8 percent, respectively. HbgA$_{1B}$ undergoes a slow nonenzymatic reaction with glucose throughout the life span of the RBC.

Increased synthesis of HBA$_{1C}$ has been shown to correlate with glucose control.

Fast hemoglobin refers to measurement of the total fractions of all three glycohemoglobins as a group.

Patient Preparation. None. (Hemolysis of the whole-blood sample will require a second whole-blood draw, however.)

HBA$_{1C}$ LEVELS INCREASED IN:

- Hyperglycemic states such as uncontrolled diabetes mellitus, two to three times normal.

HBA$_{1C}$ LEVELS DECREASED IN:

- Conditions leading to loss of Hbg rather than decreased production, such as massive blood loss (see also Section 2.1.2, "Hemoglobin Levels Decreased in")

7.4.3 Glucose Tolerance Test, Plasma, Oral*

Synonyms: GTT; OGTT

Diagnostic Ranges (mg/dl)

Criteria for diagnosis of gestational diabetes mellitus. At least two values must exceed the following:

Pregnant	Fasting	105
	1 hr	190 (peak level)
	2 hr	165
	3 hr	145
Nonpregnant	2-hr glucose	>200 and minimum of one other value over 200

Laboratory of Pathology, 1991.

Explanation of the Test. The purpose of the test is to define diabetes chemically by using the response of the patient to a glucose load or challenge, after which plasma values are determined at specific time intervals. (See Table 7–1.)

Individuals with diabetes evidence higher glucose levels (curves) than normal that remain high for a longer period of time. Individuals with hypoglycemia may show an initial high level that eventually falls below 50 mg/dl and is usually, although not always, symptomatic. With abnormal intestinal absorption of the glucose there may be no elevation, a so-called flat curve. The test is very sensitive but lacks specificity and will give abnormal findings in a large number of

---

*The IV glucose tolerance test GTT (IVGTT) with cortisone and glucose is not included in this edition as it is seldom used. Cortisone promotes gluconeogenesis and tends to accentuate carbohydrate (CHO) intolerance in latent or mild diabetes (Henry, 1991). The IVGTT has been found to be much less sensitive than the OGTT and can cause painful venous thrombosis. The prognostic implications of the test are uncertain in all age groups (McCance & Huether, 1990).

TABLE 7-1. CRITERIA FOR DIAGNOSIS OF IMPAIRED GLUCOSE TOLERANCE

Author	Plasma Glucose (mg/dl)	Diagnostic Criteria
Fajans & Conn[a]—1.75 g/kg	1-hr >185 1½-hr >160 2-hr >140	All three values abnormal
U.S. Public Health Service, Wilkerson[b]—100 g	Fasting >130 = 1 point 1-hr >195 = ½ point 2-hr >140 = ½ point 3-hr >130 = 1 point	Two points or more
O'Sullivan & Mahon[c] (for use in pregnancy)—100 g	Fasting >110 1-hr >195 2-hr >175 3-hr >150	Two or more values abnormal
American Diabetes Association[d]—40 g/m[b]	Fasting >115 1-hr >185 1½-hr >165 2-hr >140	Elevated fasting or all three posttest values abnormal
Danowski, glucose tolerance sum[e]—1.75 g/kg	Venous whole blood	Sum = fasting + 1 hr + 2 hr + 3 hr 　　　　　　 *Adults*　*Children* Normal　　<450　　<450 Borderline 450–700　450–700 Diabetic　>600　　>650
Seltzer[f] (for children)—1.75 g/kg	Capillary whole blood Fasting >115 1-hr >175 2-hr >140 3-hr >125	Elevated fasting or two of three posttest values abnormal

[a](1959). *Annals of the New York Academy of Sciences,* 82, 208.
[b](1961). *Journal of Chronic Diseases,* 13, 6.
[c](1964). *Diabetes,* 13, 278.
[d](1969). *Diabetes,* 18, 299.
[e](1973). *Metabolism,* 22, 295.
[f](1970). In M. Ellenberg & H. Rifkin (Eds.), *Diabetes Mellitus: Theory and Practice* (p. 480). New York: McGraw-Hill.
From Shipp, J. C., & Lourien, F. C. (1977). Diabetes mellitus. In H. F. Conn & R. B. Conn (Eds.), *Current Diagnosis* 5th ed. (p. 734). Philadelphia: Saunders, with permission.

diseases, and diet influences results. The use of guidelines set by the American Diabetes Association can assist in standardizing the test, making accurate interpretation possible.

Patient Preparation

1. A minimum of 10 hours but no more than 16 hours of fasting before the test is required. (Water is permitted.) Pregnant women usually fast no more than 8 to 14 hours
2. Diet for 3 days prior to the fasting period must include at least 150 g of CHOs daily. (Inadequate CHO intake may produce false-positive glucose intolerance findings)
3. Certain drugs must be eliminated because of their ability to elevate plasma glucose (e.g., anticonvulsants, corticosteroids, diphenylhydantoid, estrogens, salicylates, thiazide diuretics, propranolol)
4. Oral contraceptives should not be taken for one full menstrual cycle before the test

5. Review of history should include any history of endocrine disorders associated with abnormal glucose tolerance (e.g., acromegaly, Cushing's syndrome, hyperthyroidism) unless the condition has been evaluated and corrected

---

IMPLICATIONS FOR NURSING

1. Make sure that the patient is informed of the preparations for the test and understands the underlying rationale of the requirements in order to decrease anxiety and increase compliance during the test
2. The test is usually performed in the morning. If it is offered on an outpatient basis, provide the patient with preparation information in writing
3. Depending on the laboratory doing the test, some of the following instructions may need to be included:
   a. Smoking is often prohibited before the test
   b. Limit exercise to a minimal level: no unnecessary activity such as jogging
   c. Test may be canceled if there has been an intervening illness in the 2 weeks prior to its schedule
4. Also provide information as to:
   a. Time required for the test: usually 2 hours for men and nonpregnant women and 3 hours for pregnant women
   b. Glucose dosage: determined by the physician depending on variables such as the client's age, body weight, and whether the client is pregnant. (A frequently used measurement is that of the National Diabetes Data Group [endorsed by the American Diabetes Association]: all nonpregnant subjects: 75 g; diabetes: fasting ≥140 mg/dl)
5. Pure glucose is unpalatable for most individuals. Commercial products can be used (e.g., 7 oz. of "Glucola," a combination of hydrolyzed saccharide of corn syrup with carbonated water and flavoring, which provides 75 g of glucose)
6. Criteria for a diagnosis of diabetes mellitus is based on:
   a. Unequivocal increase in plasma glucose with classic signs and symptoms
   b. More than a single increased fasting plasma glucose level
   c. More than one elevated plasma glucose level in response to an oral glucose challenge. Insulin levels done with the glucose measurements are rarely used at present for several reasons: (1) expense; (2) difficulty in the interpretation of the data; and (3) extreme variability of insulin response to identical glucose loads

Data from Henry, 1991; Laboratory of Pathology, 1991; McCance & Huether, 1990.

DECREASED GLUCOSE TOLERANCE FOUND IN (DIABETIC-TYPE CURVE):

1. Diabetes mellitus, assuming that all variables are controlled
2. Physiological conditions such as
   a. Inadequate carbohydrate intake before the test. Obesity causes peripheral resistance to insulin secondary to increases in GH and catecholamine output
   b. Increased age. Otherwise, normal individuals' GTT will increase approximately 1 mg/dl/yr or 7 mg/dl/decade from ages 20 to 80. The degree of the abnormality is not severe enough to affect the fasting serum glucose level
   c. Inactivity (bed rest)
   d. Fever

    e. Diurnal variation with decreased carbohydrate tolerance in the afternoon and normal tolerance in the morning

    f. Emotional stress, probably secondary to catecholamine release and steroid gluconeogenesis

    g. Pregnancy because of increased estrogen and progesterone levels; the mechanism is unclear

    h. Race. Oriental races have significantly higher glucose levels than either white or black races

3. Individuals receiving a number of different drugs (e.g., xanthines, nicotine): diuretics, especially thiazides, furosemide, and ethacrynic acid; hormones (oral contraceptives—adrenocortical steroids—excessive thyroid dosage); nicotinic acid; chlorpromazine; phenytoin [Dilantin]; sympathomimetic amines (epinephrine, ephedrine, most decongestants); diazoxide (Hyperstat) and salicylates

4. Other diseases such as

    a. Adrenal, thyroid, and pituitary dysfunctions resulting from the hormonal influence on tissue response to changes in serum glucose concentrations, for example

        (1) Cushing's syndrome because of increased gluconeogenesis

        (2) Pheochromocytoma because of an increase in epinephrine production

        (3) Primary aldosteronism as a result of potassium (K^+) depletion, which affects the pancreatic beta-cell response to hyperglycemia, mechanism unknown. This mechanism relates also to thiazide's effect on glucose tolerance (item 3)

        (4) Hyperthyroidism with variable effect and without relation to the severity of the hyperthyroidism, which is due in part to increased glucose absorption. The IVGTT response is normal

        (5) Hypothyroidism with variable effect, from a diabetic curve to a "flat" oral GTT response

        (6) Hyperpituitarism, especially acromegaly, because of increased GH levels

    b. Pancreatitis; abnormal GTT result extremely common because of beta-cell dysfunction

    c. Chronic renal disease with azotemia, reason not known

    d. Cerebral lesions, mechanisms not known, possibly as a result of the presence of a medullary glucose regulation center that is injured

    e. Severe carbon monoxide poisoning because of a direct cerebral effect

    f. Malignancies—may be due to secondary effects of the malignancy (e.g., fever, starvation, inactivity, or liver dysfunction)

    g. Liver disease (e.g., cirrhosis). GTT response abnormality correlates with the severity of the disease because of the amount of disruption of glucose homeostasis

    h. Stressful or stress-related conditions such as MI, surgery, "strokes"

INCREASED GLUCOSE TOLERANCE IN (FLAT CURVE):

1. Some cases of hypothyroidism
2. Any condition that decreases glucose absorption from the GI tract (e.g., severe diarrhea—infectious or stress related)
3. The black race, who tends to have lower glucose values than does the white race
4. Idiopathic

7.4.4 Lactose Tolerance Test, Oral

Synonyms: Lactase deficiency test; oral disaccharide absorption test

Normal Range: Serum: Blood glucose level: 20 mg/dl above fasting level

Diagnostic Range: An increase of <20 mg/dl of blood glucose drawn at set intervals (e.g., 15, 30, 60, and 120 min) after administration of lactose/"milk sugar" (1 g/kg body weight)

Purpose of the Test. Used to diagnose congenital intestinal malabsorption due to specific or generalized disaccharidase deficiencies or true "milk allergy."

Explanation of the Test. The presence of the enzyme lactase in the intestinal mucosa is indicated by a rise in blood glucose level following administration of lactose. In order for lactose to be hydrolyzed into the disaccharides glucose and galactose, the enzyme lactase must be present. The lack, or deficiency, of lactase is the most common intestinal disaccharide deficiency and can be due to congenital or acquired malabsorption.* With such a deficiency, the intestinal tract is unable to convert adequate amounts of lactose and galactose into blood glucose (known as glucose, or milk sugar, intolerance) (Wallach, 1992). Depending on protein intake, it can cause hypoglycemia (Laboratory of Pathology, 1991). The ability of the affected person to digest milk sugar is affected and is a common cause of osmotic diarrhea in children.

Patient Preparation

1. No food or drink (n.p.o.) other than water for 8 hours before the start of the test
2. Nothing by mouth for the duration of the test
3. Urine samples are not required

Test Procedure

1. A fasting 1.5-ml serum sample is drawn at the start of the test
2. Fifty grams of lactose in water is given orally
3. Blood specimens (1.5-ml serum) are taken at 15, 30, 60, and 120 minutes after the sugar (lactose) solution is administered
4. No urine specimens are collected

DECREASED LACTOSE TOLERANCE OCCURS IN:

1. Genetic lactose deficiency/inherited recessive defect, such as malabsorption due to deficiency of a single, or all, brush border oligosaccharides. Found in greater incidence in certain races or ethnic groups, such as Native Americans, Arabs, Asians, Blacks, Inuit eskimos, Jews, and develops in childhood/early adulthood
2. Acquired/secondary lactose deficiency related to intestinal mucosal damage or dysfunction due to:

---

*Speculation among scientists suggests that the cause may lie in the fact that humans were not meant to drink milk after infancy but adapted over time as humans began to herd milk cows and developed dairying (Lehman, 1987; Levine, 1987).

  a. Chronic intestinal diseases (gluten-sensitive enteropathy), such as tropical sprue, celiac, and/or Crohn's disease
  b. Acute gastroenteritis
  c. Deficiency of a single, or all, brush borders
3. Isolated lactose deficiency (milk allergy or intolerance), affecting 10 percent of the white population

Patient Teaching. The following points should be considered when the nursing diagnosis is a lack of knowledge related to diet management:

1. Determine the individual's and his or her families' previous level of knowledge, accuracy of that knowledge, as well as what she or he wants to learn first, and start there
2. Assess the level of difficulty the client has with lactose intolerance, what milk or milk products can be taken, if any. (Usually, when given milk, half of all people with lactose intolerance will have symptoms; given yogurt, none will have symptoms; given ice cream or frozen yogurt, a quarter will have symptoms)
3. Suggest using the following approaches if patients have been able to take *any* milk products in the past
  a. Limit quantities. Most lactose-intolerant people can handle a small amount of lactose
  b. Slow the emptying time of the stomach by increasing fat intake when taking milk products. (This will decrease the lactose load in the small intestine at any one time. If any lactase is produced, it will then have a better chance of coping with the lactose.) This can be done by
    (1) Using whole milk instead of skim
    (2) Eating high-fat foods with milk or milk products, e.g., chocolate, eggs
    (3) Eating high-fat ice cream rather than taking milk
  c. Eat fresh yogurt. The active bacterial cultures used to make yogurt contain lactase. (Acidophilus milk also contains lactase but not in a form the human intestine can use. Frozen yogurt does not contain active bacterial culture)
  d. Eat hard cheeses rather than soft because they contain lactase
4. If money or access to markets with special foods is not a problem
  a. Lactose-free milk, cheese, and ice cream may be purchased
  b. A semipurified yeast lactase preparation called Lact-Aid may be purchased and added to milk. The milk must be allowed to sit for 24 hours before one drinks it while a majority of the lactose is converted to galactose and glucose
5. Individuals who decide or prefer to limit or completely omit milk and its products from their diet should be counseled about the importance of taking in adequate amounts of vitamin D and calcium (e.g., for middle-aged, postmenopausal women, calcium carbonate, 500 mg two to three times daily, plus vitamin D, 400 units daily) to maintain bone structure and prevent osteoporosis

7.4.5 Serum Insulin

Synonyms: Immunoreactive insulin (IRI), insulin assay (values tend to be higher in plasma)

Normal Range: 0–20 µU/ml; borderline: 21–25 µU/ml[a]

Newborn	3–20
>60 yr	6–35

[a]UU stands for microunit, as does µU. One unit of insulin = 0.04167 mg (Tietz, 1990).
Data from Laboratory of Pathology, 1991; Tietz, 1990.

Explanation of the Test. Insulin was the first substance successfully measured in radioisotope immunoassay. It is a small polypeptide hormone produced by the pancreatic beta-cells of the islets of Langerhans in response to increased blood glucose levels. During fasting states, serum insulin levels decline and are particularly helpful in detecting insulin-producing tumors with high levels of insulin and severe hypoglycemia.

Serum insulin determinations are used as the diagnostic tool of choice in evaluating fasting hypoglycemia. They are of little value in diagnosis of postprandial or reactive hypoglycemia. Insulin concentrations may be more useful there in looking at groups of people rather than individuals because of the variability in normal responses. Serum insulin determination is not used at present in the diagnosis of diabetes mellitus, probably for the same reason.

The insulin assay can be used with the glucose tolerance test (GTT) to show characteristic curves in given conditions (e.g., early type I, insulin-dependent diabetes mellitus [IDDM]—flat curve—little or no increase in insulin concentrations; mild diabetes, delayed rise in insulin). The insulin GTT has been found to be no more efficient than the serum glucose GTT in the diagnosis of subclinical diabetes.

Ratio of Insulin to Glucose. The insulin/glucose ratio (IRI/G) is important in defining inappropriate insulin secretions. The normal ratio is usually less than 0.30 μIU (microunit of insulin) to 1 mg of glucose in normal, nonobese, fasting individuals. In obese persons the ratio is abnormal if greater than 0.3 μIU compared with a serum glucose level below 60 mg/dl. Inappropriate insulin secretion is most often due to the presence of an insulinoma (a pancreatic beta [islet]-cell tumor). Even with an insulinoma, actual insulin serum concentrations may be within the normal range. The concentration will be excessively high for the degree of hypoglycemia present, however, which demonstrates the usefulness of the IRI/G ratio.

Insulin secretion from normal beta cells is at basal level (4 μIU/ml) in the presence of hypoglycemia in the normal person. When glucose concentrations decline to a value of 30 mg/dl, insulin levels cannot be detected by RIA. Thus in making the equation for the IRI/G, a value of 30 mg/dl is subtracted from the glucose level. The IRI/G is then calculated by this formula (Henry, 1991):

$$\frac{IRI}{G} = \frac{100 \times \text{insulin level (μIU/mL)}}{\text{glucose (mg/dl)} - 30 \text{ mg/dl}}$$

Patient Preparation. Patients should remain n.p.o. except for water for 8 hours before blood sampling.

SERUM INSULIN LEVELS INCREASED IN:

1. Insulinoma, a pancreatic islet cell, insulin-producing tumor. Such tumors can produce insulin to a concentration of 20 to 30 μIU/ml when the serum glucose level is less than 30 mg/dl (inappropriate insulin secretion)
2. Conditions causing reactive hypoglycemia—postprandial—such as
   a. Early diabetes, mild type II (NIDDM)
   b. Alimentary hypoglycemia, most frequently found after gastric surgery
   c. Idiopathic (functional) hypoglycemia. Insulin secretory patterns vary widely in these conditions and may be normal despite hypoglycemic symptoms. The condition may be

due to early impaired glucose tolerance (IGT), an alimentary disorder, or psychological problems, in which case the symptoms are usually due to a stress response rather than true hypoglycemia. A combination of causes can also occur (Permutt, 1980).

   d. Idiopathic hypoglycemia of childhood is often considered a separate nonreactive hypoglycemia

   e. Abrupt termination of prolonged glucose infusion

   f. After ingestion of alcohol. Alcohol can potentiate hypoglycemia, even in normal subjects

3. *Persons being treated with insulin* for a period greater than 6 weeks. Insulin antibodies developed in the body may not be distinguished from those used in the insulin RIA test (see "Serum Insulin Levels Decreased in," item 4)

4. Acromegaly, active disease after glucose ingestion

SERUM INSULIN LEVELS DECREASED IN:

1. Type I/IDDM and may be nondetectable

2. Type II/Non–insulin-dependent diabetes mellitus (NIDDM)

3. Obesity. The decrease may be relative, however, not necessarily an absolute deficiency; that is, the insulin level is low in comparison to the amount of glucose present; the IRIG ratio is out of balance

4. Some persons being treated with insulin for a period greater than 6 weeks. The formation of insulin antibodies interferes by competing with insulin antibodies used in the RIA test. Depending on the method used for testing, the insulin level can be either falsely decreased or falsely increased (see preceding list).

7.4.6 Tolbutamide Tolerance Test

Synonyms: Insulin tolerance, Orinase diagnostic, TTT, insulin stimulation

Normal Ranges

Maximum fall of serum glucose level at 30 to 45 min, usually to slightly higher than 50% of fasting blood sugar (FBS) level

Serum glucose level returns to fasting, basal values in 1½ to 3 hr

Serum insulin level decreases to basal level (4 µU/ml) or lower depending on the degree of hypoglycemia

Explanation of the Test. Tolbutamide (Orinase) is a sulfonylurea drug that apparently stimulates insulin production of the pancreatic beta cells. The drug is used therapeutically in the treatment of many cases of type II diabetes (NIDDM) in which pancreatic function exists but is reduced. In this test, it is used to stimulate insulin secretion, the levels and effects of which can be measured. The test is thought by some to be one of the more specific tests for diabetes mellitus. Others feel that there are too many false-positive responses. The TTT has been found to be somewhat less sensitive than the oral GTT. The TTT has been used most frequently in determining the presence of an insulinoma. Manifestations of inappropriate insulin release are exaggerated in response to tolbutamide. *Diagnostic criteria* for the presence of an insulinoma are serum glucose levels decreased more than 65 percent or to less than 30 mg/dl; glucose depression persisting up to 2 hours or longer; and serum insulin levels increased beyond upper limits of normal (over 24 mU/ml) (Henry, 1984). The persistence of the hypoglycemia is thought to be more diagnostic than its level of decrease, and the decrease usually persists over 3 hours.

The test process begins with a FBS sample taken and 1 g of a water-soluble Orinase sodium solution (20 cc), tolbutamide, given rapidly over 2 or 3 minutes by intravenous injection. The response to the tolbutamide stimulus is observed by taking blood samples for glucose and/or insulin determinations every 15 minutes for the first hour and every 30 minutes thereafter. The test is discontinued when severe hypoglycemic symptoms occur and intravenous glucose is administered to reverse the process. *(Caution:* The physician must differentiate between hypoglycemic symptoms and symptoms resulting from hyperventilation and therefore needs to be present throughout.)

A diabetic response is identified by a diminished response to the tolbutamide. Maximum serum glucose decreases are also delayed, occurring after 45 minutes. There is, however, considerable overlap between mild diabetic and normal responses.

Patient Preparation

1. A high-carbohydrate diet (150 to 300 g/day) for 3 days before the test
2. Patient should be kept n.p.o. except for water for 8 hours before the test
3. No smoking, drinking, or eating for the duration of the test
4. A fasting blood specimen is collected and sent to the laboratory
5. A physician should administer the IV tolbutamide, supervise during the test, and assume responsibility for the effects of the tolbutamide. The tolbutamide is usually given at a constant rate, IV, over 2 to 3 minutes
6. The test is not used or used with extreme caution in the last trimester of pregnancy with individuals having a history of heart disease, in the elderly, and in many severe acute illnesses or chronic disease. Hypoglycemia resulting from intravenous tolbutamide can be fatal
7. Specimens (blood) are collected at 15-minute intervals for the first hour postinjection and at 30-minute intervals for the next 2 hours

FALSE-POSITIVE RESPONSES OCCUR IN:

1. Reactive hypoglycemia, although the blood glucose level returns to 80 percent of normal in 3 hours
2. Adrenal insufficiency, with an initial decrease as low as that in an insulinoma, but the serum glucose level returns to 80 percent of normal in 3 hours
3. Some types of liver disease, although the occurrence is rare. The pattern is very similar to that of an insulinoma
4. Obese individuals
5. Conditions of starvation and alcoholism

FALSE-NEGATIVE RESPONSES OCCUR IN:

- Approximately 50 percent of patients with insulinomas

INSULINOMA—DIAGNOSTIC RESPONSE

1. Blood glucose decrease distinctly greater than normal
2. Hypoglycemia persistence for 3 hours after tolbutamide administration

7.5 THE PARATHYROID GLANDS

7.5.1 Laboratory and Clinical Indications of Parathyroid Dysfunction

A. Hyperfunction

Laboratory Findings. Levels of serum calcium are increased. There are decreased serum inorganic phosphate levels, uric acid levels may increase, and there is an increased concentration of alkaline phosphatase; BUN levels and hematology are normal (anemia may occur and BUN levels increase with long-standing hyperfunction). Urine calcium levels are increased in a 24-hour sample—hypercalciuria.

Clinical Findings. There are many nonspecific and variable findings: (clinical "pearl": bones, groans, stones, psychiatric overtones). Also present may be hypertension; recent weight loss; dry skin; mental changes (depression, anxiety, emotional lability); neurological changes (increased fatigability, proximal muscle weakness, hypotonia, slight to moderate muscle wasting, hyperreflexia, loss of vibratory sense in the feet); if taking digitalis, patients may experience an increased incidence of intoxication; renal symptoms (polyuria, nocturia, renal colic with renal stones); polydipsia; skeletal symptoms (bone pain, joint pain, tooth loss, bone cysts, arthritis, arthralgia); and possibly symptoms of a peptic ulcer.

B. Hypofunction

Laboratory Findings. Serum calcium levels are decreased, and there are increased levels of serum inorganic phosphorus; BUN and total protein or serum albumin levels are normal (important to differential diagnosis). Other pertinent tests reveal normal serum magnesium (Mg) levels. Urine calcium levels are decreased (hypocalciuria).

Clinical Findings. There are increased muscle tone and irritability—may be slight or overt. Latent symptoms include elicited spasm (Chvostek's sign: twitching of facial muscle when facial nerve is tapped; Trousseau's sign: carpopedal spasm with inflation of the blood pressure cuff above systolic pressure for 3 minutes); early symptoms include neuromuscular irritability, feelings of "needles and pins" in extremities or circumorally, twitching, muscle spasms causing laryngeal stridor, dysphagia, wheezing (bronchospasm), carpopedal spasm, photophobia, and blepharospasm. As for general symptoms, lenticular cataracts are common, and the skin is coarse and scaly and may have patches of brown pigmentation and exfoliative dermatitis. Fingernails are brittle and horizontally ridged. Moniliasis is common. An ECG, if done, may show a prolonged ST segment. In infants and young children, teeth may be hypoplastic with enamel deficits. Presenting symptom may be bowed legs only.

7.5.2 Serum Calcium

Synonyms: Ca, serum; calcium, total serum

Normal Ranges (mg/dl)

Cord	8.2–11.2
Premature	6.2–11.0
0–10 days	7.6–10.4
10 days–24 mo	9.0–11.0
24 mo–12 yr	8.8–10.8
12 yr–60 yr	8.4–10.2
>60 yr	8.8–10.0

Data from Tietz, 1990.

Explanation of the Test. Calcium ions (Ca^{++}) are essential for preservation of bone structure, activation of certain enzymes, blood coagulation, muscle contraction, and transmission of nerve impulses (Laboratory of Pathology, 1991). Measurement of serum calcium levels includes both the active fraction (ionized calcium), which makes up approximately 50 percent of the total calcium, and the inactive fraction bound to protein, also about 50 percent of the total. The serum levels then depend in part on the serum levels of protein, particularly albumin. When the calcium concentration decreases secondarily to a decrease in serum protein levels, tetany rarely occurs because such a decrease involves only the metabolically inactive fraction, or bound calcium. Ionized serum calcium (Ca^{2+}) levels are not affected. An increase in total protein levels (as in some cases of multiple myeloma or sarcoidosis) will increase the total serum calcium concentration but will not significantly alter the amount of ionized calcium present. Therefore, it is important to know the total protein values of serum to interpret the results of total serum calcium tests.

Calcium levels are regulated and influenced by several things, the major regulator being parathyroid hormone (PTH). Increased amounts of PTH will increase serum calcium levels. If renal function is normal, an increase in serum calcium levels will be accompanied by a decrease in the serum inorganic phosphate concentration and vice versa.

Acid-base balance affects protein binding of free calcium, increasing binding of calcium with increased pH.

Patient Preparation. Depending on the laboratory being used, there may be no special preparation, or the patient may be required to fast for 12 hours before the test. In either case it is important that the blood sample be removed with minimal venous stasis or hemolysis.

SERUM CALCIUM LEVELS INCREASED IN:

1. Primary hyperparathyroidism because of (in order of frequency of occurrence) single parathyroid adenoma, multiple adenomas, and hyperplasia
2. Conditions causing increased concentrations of total protein and albumin (a fairly rare occurrence) such as multiple myeloma or sarcoidosis
3. Conditions causing increased bony resorption (osteoclasia) such as
   a. Invasive bone disease
   b. Disuse atrophy of bone

    c. Osteoporosis or osteomalacia. Over time the presence of increased serum calcium levels can also *cause* so-called renal rickets and lead to osteoporosis and osteomalacia

4. Excess intake of vitamin A, which increases bone resorption
5. Excess intake or absorption of vitamin D, which increases calcium absorption from the gut
6. Carcinoma with metastases to the bone, particularly in the elderly, because of increased bony breakdown
7. Carcinoma with PTH-like production from the tumor (ectopic PTH syndrome), which is found most frequently in cancers of the lung
8. Milk-alkali syndrome (Burnett's syndrome) as a result of intensive antacid therapy and milk ingestion; infrequent cause now
9. Physiological causes such as dehydration (relative increase) or the prolonged use of a tourniquet when drawing blood (hemoconcentration)

SERUM CALCIUM LEVELS DECREASED IN:

1. Hypoparathyroidism. Primary hypoparathyroidism is due to postthyroidectomy, either temporarily, probably because of gland injury, or permanently because of total removal; primary hypoparathyroidism can also be due to an idiopathic cause—heredity, which is rare. Secondary hypoparathyroidism may be due to severe hypomagnesemia, which decreases body tissues' ability to respond to PTH and ultimately parathyroid loss of the capacity to produce/release PTH; other causes of secondary hypoparathyroidism include irradiation, hypoalbuminemia (nephrotic syndrome, starvation, cachexia, celiac disease, cystic fibrosis of the pancreas), chronic renal disease with uremia or azotemia with phosphate retention and a decreased production of the active metabolite of vitamin D by the kidney, vitamin D deficiency rickets (rickets of childhood); de Toni-Fanconi's syndrome because of a renal tubular defect; and hyperinsulinism
2. Conditions causing increased osteoblastic (bone-building) activity such as with healing of fractures
3. Physiological conditions such as recumbent posture or insufficient ingestion of calcium or vitamin D (late pregnancy)
4. Neonates whose mothers have hyperparathyroidism because of the suppression of fetal parathyroid activity
5. Individuals receiving long-term therapy with phenytoin (Dilantin) by increasing the metabolic inactivation of vitamin D
6. Any patient with a decreased serum albumin level because the albumin is the carrier protein for bound calcium (the majority of calcium found in the serum). However, if the decrease is due solely to the lack of transport albumin, the ionized serum calcium (see Section 7.5.3) will be within normal limits, and no sign of tetany would be expected to be present

7.5.3 Serum Calcium, Ionized

Synonyms: Ca, I; Ca^{2+}; Ca^{++}

Normal Ranges (mg/dl)

Adult	4.75–5.20 at pH 7.4
Child	2.10–2.60

Explanation of the Test. Measurement of this relatively stable, metabolically active (free) fraction of serum calcium is believed to be a better indicator of calcium metabolism than total serum calcium levels and is not influenced by changes in total protein or serum albumin levels. The ionized calcium fraction is pH-dependent, however, whereas protein-bound calcium is not. (An increase in pH equals a decrease in ionized calcium at 0.2 mg/dl per 0.1 pH unit and vice versa.) Very slight variations in serum pH will produce changes in ionized calcium concentrations (e.g., hyperventilation sufficient to increase the serum pH 0.1 to 0.2 pH units of blood pH will cause up to a 10-percent decrease in the ionized calcium concentration) (Henry, 1991).

This test is specific for metabolically active calcium and is useful in persons with increases or decreases in serum protein levels. It should be accompanied by a pH measurement as well.

Patient Preparation. Preparation is as for total serum calcium.

IONIZED SERUM CALCIUM LEVELS INCREASED IN:

1. All conditions listed under total serum calcium except those related to increased serum total protein or albumin concentrations
2. Acidotic conditions (e.g., diabetic ketoacidosis, hyperosmolar nonketotic acidosis, respiratory acidosis, renal acidosis)

IONIZED SERUM CALCIUM LEVELS DECREASED IN:

1. All conditions listed under total serum calcium except those related to decreased serum total protein or albumin concentrations
2. Alkalotic conditions, metabolic or respiratory, that cause ionized serum calcium to become bound to protein in greater concentrations
3. Serum samples exposed to air or allowed to stand

7.5.4 Serum Phosphorus

Synonyms: Inorganic phosphorus, phosphate; PO_4

Normal Ranges (mg/dl)

Adult	2.5–4.7
Senior Adult (>60 yr)	2.3–3.7
Pediatric	4.0–7.0
Newborn	4.0–9.0
Infants	4.5–6.7
Child	4.0–6.0

Explanation of the Test. Under optimum conditions ionized calcium and serum phosphorus exist in a reciprocal balance in the blood. Increases in calcium levels due to an increased release of PTH result in decreases in serum inorganic phosphorus levels and vice versa. The balance is evidently maintained by selective reabsorption or filtration and excretion of phosphorus by the renal tubules under the influence of PTH. Excretion is also increased or decreased by the level of calcium mobilization from other causes. The excretion of phosphorus is referred to as a phosphate diuresis.

Patient Preparation. Patients should be n.p.o. except for water for 8 hours before a blood sample is taken.

SERUM PHOSPHORUS LEVELS INCREASED IN:

1. Any chronic renal failure, most commonly chronic glomerulonephritis
2. Hypoparathyroidism, primary or secondary (see "Serum Total Calcium Levels Decreased In") due to increased renal reabsorption of phosphate
3. Prolonged or massive administration of antacids, vitamin D, heparin, tetracycline, Pituitrin (a pituitary extract), and salicylates
4. In GH excess (e.g., gigantism)

SERUM PHOSPHORUS LEVELS DECREASED IN:

1. See "Serum Calcium Levels Increased in" in Section 7.5.2
2. Women during menstrual periods
3. The time immediately after meals
4. Persons receiving aluminum hydroxide, epinephrine, parathyroid by injection, insulin or who received a general anesthesia
5. Vitamin deficiency (rickets)

7.5.5 Intact Parathyroid Hormone, Serum

Synonyms: Immunoreactive parathyroid hormone (immunoradiometric assay/IMRA); PTH; parathormone; PTH and Ca^{++}; parathyrin;

Normal Range: 10–65 pg/ml

(normal levels depend on the serum calcium levels, which should always be determined simultaneously)

Physiology. PTH is a polypeptide whose production is stimulated and maintained within specific limits by the level of ionized calcium.

INTACT PARATHYROID HORMONE. There is a wide variation among individuals in both the metabolism of the intact, biologically active PTH (half-life 5 minutes) into its fragments and the speed with which the fragments are cleared from circulation. In circulation, the polypeptide splits into two inactive fragments, which are difficult to measure reliably because they are also quickly cleared from circulation (half-lives of 5- to 15-fold longer than intact PTH).

PTH has a major role in calcium homeostasis, that of maintaining the concentration of ionized calcium within the precise limits necessary to maintain its functions (metabolic and neuroregulatory). Parathyroid hormone secretion is increased or decreased based on the levels of ionized calcium present.

Purpose of the Test. PTH measurements aid in the assessment of calcium metabolism disorders, especially when evaluated along with calcium level changes. PTH measurement is vital to establish the cause for hypercalcemia.

Patient Preparation

1. No food or drink (other than water) for 8 hours prior to taking blood samples
2. Morning blood sampling preferred for comparison with normal levels usually calculated for that time

Uses of the Test

PTH immunoassay: Diagnosis of primary hyperparathyroidism, secondary hyperparathyroidism in renal failure, and hypoparathyroidism with hypercalcemia due to nonparathyroid malignancy.

PTH LEVELS INCREASED IN:

1. Primary hyperparathyroidism
2. Secondary hyperparathyroidism (e.g., chronic renal disease)
3. Pseudohypoparathyroidism
4. Hereditary vitamin D dependency, types I and II
5. Zollinger-Epstein syndrome
6. Spinal cord trauma
7. Pseudogout
8. Familial medullary thyroid carcinoma
9. Acromegaly

PTH LEVELS DECREASED IN:

1. Autoimmune hypoparathyroidism
2. Hypoparathyroidism due to thyroidectomy (often transient)
3. Sarcoidosis (even in the presence of renal failure)
4. Hypomagnesemia
5. Neonatal hypocalcemia (transient)
6. Postthyroidectomy, probably because of transient trauma to the parathyroid
7. Postparathyroidectomy: intentional, for removal of a tumor, or to control calcium levels in some forms of renal disease
8. The morning hours because of the normal diurnal rhythm
9. False decrease in presence of gross lipemia (specimen should be ultracentrifuged to prevent this from occurring)

7.5.6 Tubular Phosphate Reabsorption

Synonyms: TPR, parathyroid function test, tubular reabsorption of phosphate (TRP)

Normal Ranges

TRP[a]	78–90%
Serum creatinine	0.7–1.5 mg/dl

Serum phosphorus	2.3–4.3 mg/dl
Creatinine clearance	70–130 ml clearance/min
Phosphate excretion index (PEI)	0 ± 0.12%

[a]TRP is calculated by using serum creatinine, serum phosphorus, and the creatinine clearance rate. A rough formula can approximate the process (Ravel, 1989):

$$\text{Percent TRP} = \frac{\text{Urine } PO_4 \text{ concentration} \times \text{serum creatinine concentration}}{\text{Urine creatinine concentration} \times \text{serum } PO_4 \text{ concentration}} \times 100$$

Explanation of the Test. Tubular phosphate resorption is an indirect measurement of PTH by measuring its effect on phosphate reabsorption; it is done to help distinguish hypercalcemia due to hyperparathyroidism from that due to other etiologies by demonstrating the presence or absence of a phosphate diuresis. Normally, about two thirds of the dietary phosphate appears in the urine (5 to 15 mg/min), except when intake is low. Phosphate clearance and reabsorption is not solely under the control of PTH; serum calcium levels, potassium depletion, calcitonin secretion, changes in certain hormone levels (estrogen, adrenal steroids, GH), and renal defects also play roles.

Despite the many variables and related problems (inability to void, inability to completely empty the bladder, timing inaccuracies of sample collection), the TRP seems to be one of the better *simple* diagnostic tests for primary hyperparathyroidism.

The test can be done in 2 ways by using a 24-hour urine specimen or by taking an hourly sample. The 24-hour test is preferred by many facilities because it eliminates many of the inaccuracies inherent in the need for precise timing of the hourly test; however, the hourly test can be done more easily on an outpatient basis.

Patient Preparation and Test Procedure

1. Diet. Normal phosphate intake (more than 500 mg/day and less than 3000 mg/day). Excessive amounts of coffee, tea, and meat to be avoided for 24 hours before the test
2. Patient should be kept n.p.o. other than water for 8 hours before blood drawing with a 24-hour urine specimen test. The patient is not required to be n.p.o. the full 24 hours—n.p.o. 8 to 12 hours before the test beginning with the hourly test
3. Twenty-four-hour test. Follow the usual procedure for a 24-hour urine collection; urine is not to be refrigerated. The patient fasts until the blood sample is taken. The sample can be drawn at any time during the 24 hours, but it is usually done as soon as possible for comfort of the patient
4. Hourly test. Complete emptying of the bladder is essential with each urine collection. Timing of each step of the test must be accurate for the test to be reliable
   a. Patient drinks a minimum of two 8-oz glasses of water
   b. One hour later the bladder is emptied, and another full glass of water is taken. The time of voiding must be noted exactly and the lab notified; the urine is discarded
   c. One hour after first voiding, the patient voids completely again, and the exact time is noted. The urine is saved (in some facilities the urine is sent to the lab with each voiding; at others it is sent only at the end of the test). If the urine volume is less than 120 ml, the test should be restarted. A full glass of water is taken

   d. One hour later (2 hours after the first voiding), the patient completely empties the bladder, the urine is saved (exact time noted), the patient drinks a full glass of water, and a blood sample is taken

   e. Again in 1 hour, the patient voids completely and drinks a full glass of water, a blood sample is taken, and the test is complete. All urine is examined for urine creatinine and phosphorus; the blood sample examined for serum creatinine and phosphorus. Urine volume is also measured

LOW TRP INDEX VALUES (LESS THAN 80 PERCENT) OCCUR IN (INCREASED SERUM PTH, INCREASED CA^{2+}, DECREASED PO$_4$ LEVELS): Related to:

1. Primary hyperparathyroidism
2. Hypercalcemia because of a PTH-secreting malignancy
3. Some patients with sarcoidosis or myeloma
4. Five percent of patients with renal stones but without a parathyroid tumor
5. Serum elevations of estrogen or adrenal steroids because of disease or the administration of the substances therapeutically. Administered calcium has the same effect
6. Renal defects causing increased creatinine clearance. (The test is not reliable in the face of renal insufficiency)

FALSE NORMAL TRP VALUES (OVER 80 PERCENT) OCCUR IN (DECREASED PTH, DECREASED CA^{2+}, INCREASED SERUM PO$_4$ LEVELS): Related to:

1. Increased circulating levels of GH or thyroid
2. Prolonged heparin administration

7.5.7 Urine Calcium

A. Qualitative

Synonym: Sulkowitch's qualitative test, urine

Normal Range: 1+ to 2+

(also reported as negative, moderately positive, and strongly positive)

Explanation of the Test. A substance called Sulkowitch's reagent is used to test the urine for calcium, hence the test name. It is a quick, simple precipitation test that is relatively inexpensive and is used more often than the more complex and costly urine calcium test in medical offices and clinics.

   Under normal conditions calcium is excreted in the urine at about 2.5 to 15 mEq/day. That output depends on skeletal weight, many endocrine factors, and the intake of calcium. Given a normal physiological state with an adequate calcium intake and adequate renal function, urine calcium concentrations reflect serum calcium levels. If the serum calcium concentration falls to 7.5 mg/dl or below, almost none is excreted in the urine.

Patient Preparation. No special preparation is necessary.

URINE CALCIUM LEVELS INCREASED IN:

1. Physiological conditions such as concentrated urine
2. Hyperparathyroidism
3. Conditions causing bony reabsorption without repair such as osteolytic bone disease and osteoporosis
4. Renal tubular acidosis
5. Hyperthyroidism
6. Vitamin D intoxication
7. Increased intake of dietary calcium

URINE CALCIUM LEVELS DECREASED IN:

1. Physiological conditions such as dilute urine
2. Hypoparathyroidism; hypothyroidism
3. Malabsorption disorders such as steatorrhea because of inadequate calcium or vitamin D absorption, even with normal intake
4. Vitamin D deficiency because of the need for the vitamin in the absorption of calcium in the gut

B. Quantitative, Urine Calcium

Synonym: Ca, urine

Normal Range: 100–300 mg/24 hr

Explanation of the Test. The quantitative urine calcium test is used when knowledge of the precise amount of calcium being excreted is important. It requires collection of a 24-hour urine specimen. Urinary calcium excretion mirrors serum calcium levels as long as renal function is normal (Laboratory of Pathology, 1991).

Patient Preparation

1. Because a more precise measurement of the calcium concentration is needed, the patient is usually placed on a controlled diet of 100 mg calcium for 3 days before urine collection and testing.
2. The 24-hour urine specimen container should be kept at room temperature rather than refrigerated to prevent insoluble calcium sediment from precipitating. The urine is preserved with 6 N HCl, a strong acid; caution in handling is advised.
3. At start of urine collection, the 8 AM void is discarded. All samples thereafter, including the 8 AM void the following morning, are saved.

URINE CALCIUM LEVELS INCREASED IN/DECREASED IN:

- Changes in values are the same as those given in the Sulkowitch test except that large amounts of phosphate in the urine can lower the values

7.5.8 Serum Magnesium/Urine Magnesium

Synonym: Mg

Normal Ranges (mEq/L)

Serum	1.5–1.95
Urine	1.0–24.0
24-hour random urine	None established

Explanation of the Test. The test to determine serum and urine Mg levels fits equally well with a number of systems (neural, GI) but is placed with the endocrine parathyroid section because deficiencies of the substance produce a tetany that cannot be differentiated from hypocalcemic tetany except by laboratory examination. Although the test itself is relatively expensive and not applicable to many other laboratory tests, the occurrence of magnesium deficiency in the hospitalized surgical patient is frequent enough to warrant attention being directed to it. It is also of importance because of the use of total parenteral nutrition (TPN)—hyperalimentation—which does not always provide magnesium supplementation. Deficiencies occur more frequently than excesses but rarely occur in individuals who are eating.

Magnesium is the second most plentiful intracellular cation after potassium. It works primarily as an activator of various enzymes and is essential to the preservation of DNA/RNA structure. It is absorbed in the intestine and excreted in the urine, so that defects in those systems can cause changes in the body's concentration of magnesium. Preservation of serum levels is accomplished by renal tubular absorption.

Serum levels do not always reflect the total body magnesium. Two suggested testing approaches that may give more accurate findings are:

1. Collection of a 24-hour urine specimen after the injection of 2 ml of 50 percent magnesium sulfate solution. Body retention of more than 25 percent of the magnesium appears to indicate a magnesium deficiency
2. WBC magnesium levels may also be a more accurate indicator of total body magnesium and is more convenient than gathering a 24-hour urine specimen (Carrol, 1986, p. 4)

Patient Preparation. No special preparation is necessary.

Mg LEVELS INCREASED IN (RARELY ENCOUNTERED):

1. Serum
   a. Decreased Mg^+ excretion secondary to
      (1) Renal retention due to renal defects, primarily loss of glomerular function (e.g., uremia)
      (2) Physiological conditions such as dehydration
   b. Increased intake or absorption secondary to
      (1) Overadministration therapeutically (e.g., intravenous line replacement, overuse of Mg^+-containing cathartics, or of excess Mg^+ in dialysis fluid)
      (2) Untreated diabetic coma

      (3) Aspiration of sea water (rare)
  2. Urine: Rarely demonstrates increased levels

Mg LEVELS DECREASED IN:

Decreased Mg levels are relatively uncommon, especially in individuals who are eating but are clinically more significant than increases. Signs and symptoms do not usually occur until the serum level is less than 1 mEq/L.

  1. Serum
    a. Secondary to decreased absorption in
      (1) Patients receiving TPN. Mg concentrations must be followed intermittently
      (2) Malabsorption problems such as steatorrhea
      (3) Rapid transit of chyme through intestine (e.g., diarrhea)
      (4) Patients having nasogastric suction and fluid replacement without magnesium replacement, usually postoperatively
    b. Conditions interfering with metabolism of magnesium, such as hepatic cirrhosis and pancreatitis
    c. Excessive excretion, as in early chronic renal disease (diuretic stage), diuretic therapy, and chronic alcoholism
    d. Response to effects of hormonal influence
      (1) Hyperaldosteronism: Aldosterone facilitates renal excretion of Mg^+ ions
      (2) Decrease in ADH levels: *Excessive* loss of all substances excreted in the urine
    e. Patients with decreased serum albumin levels because Mg uses albumin as its carrier protein
  2. Urine
    a. Serum magnesium deficiency which causes a urine magnesium deficiency
    b. Conditions that destroy renal glomerular function

IMPLICATIONS FOR NURSING

1. In patients at risk, check for signs and symptoms (see previously mentioned conditions and 3 below) of imbalance (e.g., patients taking magnesium-containing medications)
  a. Check *all* medications for inclusion of magnesium
  b. Check the diet for high Mg^+-content foods (green vegetables, fresh milk, fruit, and nuts). Teach the patient about diet
2. Suspect a magnesium deficiency if any patient is not eating for long periods and is without Mg replacement
3. Signs and symptoms of imbalance
  a. Hypomagnesia
    (1) Weakness, tremor
    (2) Dizziness, convulsions, confusion
    (3) Hyperreactive reflexes
  b. Hypermagnesia
    (1) Decreased blood pressure secondary to vasodilation
    (2) Nausea, vomiting
    (3) Drowsiness, hyperreflexia
    (4) Muscular weakness

RELATED NURSING DIAGNOSES IN ENDOCRINE DYSFUNCTION

Despite the disparity of body functions linked to the various endocrine glands, patients with endocrine dysfunctions share a remarkable number of actual or potential nursing diagnoses.

The following list is submitted as a tool for primary nursing assessment of the patient with suspected or diagnosed endocrine dysfunction. Representative data from five of the most common endocrine disorders are presented with each of the nursing diagnoses selected as being the most likely to be common problems with all endocrine patients.

Activity Intolerance Related to Inadequate Rest, Sleep, or Exercise

1. Hyperthyroidism secondary to decreased metabolic and arousal rate, anemia, and hypotonia of muscles (hypothyroidism)
2. Hyperthyroidism secondary to physical exhaustion due to increased metabolic rate and inability to replace nutritional stores by ordinary food intake, which is accompanied by weight loss, loss of muscle mass, weakness, rapid fatigue, and an increased response to sensory stimuli
3. Hypercortisolism—Cushing's disease or syndrome—secondary to protein tissue wasting, loss of muscle mass, hypokalemia, and a disturbance in sleep patterns related to the elevated concentration of circulating cortisol
4. Hypocortisolism and hypoaldosteronism—Addison's Disease—secondary to hyponatremia, hyperkalemia, dehydration, and hypoglycemia
5. Hyperglycemia—diabetes mellitus—secondary to potential or actual fluid and electrolyte imbalances, such as hyperkalemia, hypovolemia due to osmotic diuresis; acid-base imbalance, (i.e., metabolic acidosis [noncarbonic acidosis]); and intracellular hypoglycemia due to lack of insulin

Potential or Actual Disturbance in Self-Concept Related to Alterations in Body Image/Self-Esteem and Role Performance Secondary to

1. Hypothyroidism: Mucosaccharide deposits causing thickening or dulling of facial characteristics; dry brittle hair, male hair pattern in females, premature greying; presence of goiter (rare); decreased mental acuity, weight gain due to decreased metabolic activity and poor food selection (high caloric, easily digested foods); decreased or absent libido
2. Hyperthyroidism: Awareness of decreased emotional control due to increased sensitivity to environmental and physical stimuli; negative body changes, such as severe weight loss, exophthalmos (limited), increased oil production of hair follicles and skin with acne; inability to concentrate
3. Hypocortisolism: Physical weakness and lethargy; pigmentation changes
4. Hypercortisolism: Alterations in fat and water distribution, effects of virilism (skin and hair changes), and mood swings
5. Hyperglycemia: Adaptation to chronic illness as change in self-image, alteration in daily schedule for self-care and body monitoring, consideration of possible complications and their effects on quality of life

Potential for Injury (Falls, Trauma, Infection, or Bleeding) Related to

1. Hypothyroidism: Decreased nutritional status with weakness and hypotension (see diagnosis, decreased skin integrity) due to dry skin and decreased peripheral circulation, decreased phagocytic activity of leukocytes (cause?), potential for arrhythmias because of potassium imbalance
2. Hyperthyroidism: Physical weakness (see first Diagnosis, Activity, Intolerance), elevated blood pressure, potential for cardiac arrhythmias because of potassium imbalance, decreased attention span and hyperactivity
3. Hypocortisolism Postural hypotension due to hyponatremia/fluid loss; potential for addisonian crisis
4. Hypercortisolism: Weakness due to loss of muscle mass and potential for fractures due to decreased calcium storage in bones and demineralization, potential for cardiac arrhythmias because of potassium imbalance, potential for bleeding due to stress ulcer formation, decreased effectiveness of leukocytes, decreased effectiveness of skin barrier due to thinning

5. Hyperglycemia: Blood pressure instability due to possible sudden fluid loss with hyperglycemia, decreased sensation (balance, pain, pressure) in lower extremities due to diabetic neuropathy, possible visual impairment (blurring with hyperglycemia, retinal damage or cataracts, long term;), decreased effective bacterial resistance due to high blood glucose levels

Lack of Knowledge Related to

1. Hypothyroidism: Reversibility of physical changes with treatment over time; time frame for changes; lifelong hormone replacement, expected effects, side effects to be monitored or reported
2. Hyperthyroidism: Disease process, such as reversibility of physical changes with treatment over time; time frame for changes; medication: antithyroid, side effects to be noted or reported; preparation for surgical treatment if needed, risks versus benefits; self-care postsurgery (hormone replacement)
3. Hypocortisolism: Purpose and effect of support or replacement hormones, how administered, monitoring or reporting changes and/or side effects
4. Hypercortisolism: Treatment options (depending on cause); monitoring and reporting possible secondary or side effects of decreasing hormone levels as well as signs and symptoms of complications due to increased levels (e.g., hypertension, peptic ulcer disease, bone fractures)
5. Diabetes: Disease process, complications, prevention of complications, self-care procedures (body monitoring, foot care, insulin or hypoglycemic medication administration, testing for glucose, diet and exercise management)

The nursing diagnoses used are presented as *broad concepts*, That is, many other nursing diagnoses may be subsumed under the one given. These diagnoses are interdependent under the broad conceptual statement because, if the broad (or primary) diagnosis is resolved, the dependent diagnoses will also be resolved. For example, a patient is returned from the recovery room to the surgical nursing unit after having had a cholecystectomy. The primary nurse for the patient does a brief, but thorough, primary assessment of the patient's status and identifies the following nursing diagnoses:

- Pain related to surgical trauma
- Impaired gas exchange related to increased pain on deep breathing
- Ineffective individual coping related to the inability to accept the level of pain and discomfort
- Activity intolerance related to increased pain on movement
- Potential impairment of skin integrity related to a probably inadequate nutritional level before admission and to a lack of positional change secondary to pain

All are legitimate nursing diagnoses that need the nurse's attention. If, however, the nurse looks at care planning from a broad conceptual view, she or he will be able to incorporate all under one nursing diagnosis for immediate care, that is, pain related to surgical trauma. If the *pain* is managed, it is more than likely the patient will be able to breathe deeply enough for adequate gas exchange; change position often enough to be able to prevent skin breakdown on pressure points; and cope with the pain, which will be bearable with a well-planned medication regimen. Later, when pain control is established or not a problem, the originally identified nursing diagnosis in the areas of coping and nutritional deficit, if still present, will emerge as independent nursing diagnoses or perhaps again as subproblems related to the nursing diagnosis "Lack of Knowledge."

This example is fairly evident; all cases are not quite so clear, and determining the primary or broad conceptual problem becomes a judgment call on the part of the nurse, which must be well supported with subjective and objective data as well as logical reasoning.

E I G H T

THE RENAL SYSTEM

RECOGNITION OF RENAL DYSFUNCTION

The evaluation of kidney function is still relatively crude, relying as it does on measurement of what passes into and out of the kidney. What goes on inside the kidney can only be speculated. Such speculation requires careful correlation with other clinical and laboratory data and a thorough understanding of the actual physiological basis for each test. (See also Section 4.1 for the physiology of urine production.)

Renal function tests look at two specific areas of the kidney nephron:

1. *The glomerulus:* A tuft of capillaries invaginated into the dilated, blind end of the nephron (Bowman's capsule) whose purpose is to filter water and solutes from the blood plasma presented to it. Normal glomerular filtration depends on adequate hydrostatic pressure in the glomerulus (60 to 70 mm Hg), colloid osmotic pressure of plasma proteins (30 mm Hg), pressure in the glomerular capsule itself surrounding the capillaries (5 to 10 mm Hg), and an intact glomerular membrane. Glomerular function tests look at the glomerular filtration rate (GFR), which is the amount of a substance filtered through the glomerulus in a given time. The normal filtration rate of plasma is approximately 125 ml/min, or 25 percent of the cardiac output. The GFR increases with increased glomerular pressure and decreases with increased colloid osmotic pressure and decreased cardiac output.

2. *The tubules:* Proximal, loop of Henle, and distal portions. Both proximal and distal tubules have convoluted sections. The tubules empty into a collecting duct in the kidney cortex. Tubular function includes active and passive reabsorption of the glomerular filtrate from the tubules to the systemic circulation and tubular secretion—active transport from the peritubular capillaries to the tubular lumen—to maintain acid-base, water, and electrolyte balance (see Table 4–1 and Fig. 4–1).

8.1 TESTS OF GLOMERULAR FUNCTION

8.1.1 Laboratory and Clinical Indications of Glomerular Dysfunction

Laboratory Findings. In the urine, the major clue to glomerular dysfunction is the presence of proteinuria (which may include hematuria), increased specific gravity, a cloudy or smokey gross appearance of the urine, and increased uric acid levels (normally the glomerular filter does not allow protein, especially large protein, to pass). Increased numbers of casts of all types, increased WBC count, increased numbers of oval fat bodies, and lipiduria may also appear, depending on the cause of glomerular dysfunction. In blood glomerular dysfunction is manifested by hypoalbuminemia because of a loss in urine, dilutional anemia because of the decreased glomerular filtration of water, electrolyte concentrations usually within normal limits (WNL) but a possibly decreased total serum calcium level (lost with protein), and normal levels of ionized calcium. There may also be increased total cholesterol levels, hyperlipidemia and cholesterolemia, increased blood urea nitrogen (BUN) concentration, true anemia with severe renal insufficiency because of a decreased erythropoietin concentration (normocytic, normochronic), and the hallmark of severe renal disease, increased serum creatinine level.

Clinical Findings. The symptoms of glomerular dysfunction depend in part on the cause of glomerular function loss and in part on the total renal status. The most common symptoms of glomerulopathies are slight to moderate hypertension, edema, and oliguria. Headache may occur. Edema is often periorbital, especially in the morning; later it is dependent. The urine is excessively foamy; there is growth failure in children; vague signs and symptoms of malaise, fatigue, and irritability are evident; ascites may be present; and signs and symptoms of congestive heart failure occur.

8.1.2 Creatinine Clearance Test

Synonyms: None

Normal Ranges[a] (70–130 ml cl/min—ml clearance/min)

Serum creatinine	
Adult	0.7–1.5 mg/dl
Senior adult	0.6–1.2 mg/dl
Child	0.3–1.1 mg/dl
Urine creatinine	
Adult	
Female	16–22 mg/kg/24 hr
Male	21–26 mg/kg/24 hr

[a]The clearance rate decreases after approximately 40 years of age, because of a decreased GFR and renal plasma flow. In some facilities 10 ml/min is subtracted from the normal value for every 10-year period after 40 (Kagan, 1979).

Explanation of the Test. Because there is little tubular excretion or reabsorption of creatinine, using creatinine measurements in the blood and in the urine appears to be a valid measure of the GFR. The creatinine clearance test is used most frequently as an indicator of total renal status rather than just a valid measure of glomerular status. The values of creatinine clearance closely parallel the percentage of functioning nephrons. The serum creatinine concentration rises when the GFR declines and creatinine clearance into the urine decreases, whereas the creatinine clearance increases with increased GFR. The creatinine clearance test has been found to be the most practical of the clearance tests, since creatinine is endogenous to the body and is formed at a fairly constant rate. Values can vary with age (see Figure 8–1).

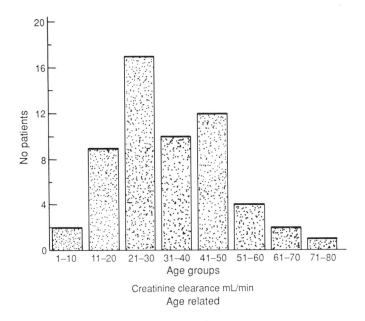

Creatinine clearance mL/min
Age related

Figure 8–1. Age-related creatinine clearance levels (ml/min). (Mary Reynolds Morrissey, R.Ph., F.A.S.C.P., Joy B. Plein, R.Ph., Ph.D., and Elmer M. Plein, R.Ph., Ph.D., "The Study and Implementation of a System to Prospectively Review Dosing of Renally Eliminated Medications for Nursing Home Patients." (Presented at the 19th Annual Meeting of the American Society of Consultant Pharmacists, Las Vegas, Nevada, November, 1988. Used with permission.)

The test can be used to determine long-term management of patients with chronic disorders of renal function and to calculate appropriate fluid and electrolyte replacement therapy. Changes are more significant over time.

Clearance is calculated by multiplying the concentration of measured urine creatinine by the volume of urine in a set time interval (converted to milliliters per minute) and dividing the product by the serum concentration of creatinine. The outcome of the calculation is corrected when necessary for differing kidney masses by using a body surface nomogram (Henry, 1991).

Creatinine clearance tests are best compared sequentially in the seriously ill patient with an increased serum creatinine content because impaired renal function may be one of the factors increasing plasma levels and absolute normal values may not be an accurate reference for the measurement of increased tubular secretion of creatinine.

The dosage of some medications may need to be adjusted depending on creatinine clearance values (see Table 8–1).

Patient Preparation

1. The test can be done as an 8-hour or 24-hour test. The 24-hour test is preferred. The hourly test requires extreme accuracy in timing, complete collection of urine specimens, as well as adequate hydration and renal blood flow

TABLE 8–1. EXAMPLES OF MEDICATIONS REQUIRING ADJUSTMENT OF DOSAGE IN ACCORDANCE WITH RENAL FUNCTION

Medication	Creatinine Clearance (CLCR)	Adjustment to Dose
Amantadine	30	200 mg twice weekly (usual adult dose 100 mg twice daily)
Ciprofloxacin	<30	1/2 of usual adult dose
Norfloxacin	<30	1/2 of usual adult dose
Macrodantin	<50	Avoid
Thiazide diuretics	<30	Ineffective when creatinine clearance level is above 30
Trimethoprim-sulfamethoxazole	15–30	1/2 usual adult dose
	<15	Avoid

Data from Mary Reynolds Morrissey, R.Ph., F.A.S.C.P., Joy B. Plein, R.Ph., Ph.D., and Elmer M. Plein, R.PH., Ph.D., "The Study and Implementation of a System to Prospectively Review Dosing of Renally Eliminated Medications for Nursing Home Patients." Presented at the 19th Annual Meeting of the American Society of Consultant Pharmacists, Las Vegas, November, 1988. Used with permission.

2. The process for hourly collection of urine and blood sampling is the same as that described for the urea clearance test (see "Patient Preparation and Test Process," in Section 8.1.3)
3. The patient remains fasting for 8 hours prior to blood drawing in the 24-hour test and for 8 hours prior to the test start in the 8-hour test, fasts for the duration of the 8-hour test, and is kept at rest to decrease the amount of creatinine formed by the body
4. Excessive amounts of tea, coffee, or meat must be avoided for 24 hours before either test
5. Timing of the 24-hour test *must* be exact. At the beginning of the 24-hour test, have the patient void. Discard that sample. Save *all* urine thereafter (refrigerate or keep on ice). A blood specimen will be taken as well (fasting patient).

CREATININE CLEARANCE RATES INCREASED IN:

1. Renal disease after clearance values fall to 50 to 60 percent of normal
2. Severe renal impairment; the level is factitiously higher than true clearance value

CREATININE CLEARANCE RATES DECREASED IN:

1. Falsely low values because of nonrefrigerated specimens or specimens tested over 24 hours after collection
2. Any significant renal disease, regardless of cause (Sodeman & Sodeman, 1982)
   a. Glomerulonephritis as a result of destruction of the glomeruli
   b. Nephrosis because of an increased permeability of the glomeruli
3. Any condition that decreases the GFR, such as congestive heart failure, cirrhosis with ascites, shock, dehydration. With a normal BUN concentration, normal blood pressure, and an absence of anemia, diffuse bilateral renal disease is suspected; with an increased BUN level, the prognosis is guarded

8.1.3 Urea Clearance Test

Synonyms: None

Normal Ranges (ml cl/min—ml clearance/min)

Standard clearance	40–68
Maximum clearance	64–99
Minimum clearance	24–40
Urine urea nitrogen	10–20 gm/24 hr per specimen
Serum urea nitrogen	4–22 mg/dl per specimen

Explanation of the Test. Urea is a nitrogen-containing waste product of protein metabolism, made up of ammonia and various amino acids, alanine being the most important. It is both filtered and reabsorbed by the kidney and varies with the state of hydration and diet. No tubular adaptation modifies urea levels, as happens with creatinine, because it is excreted primarily by glomerular filtration.

Urea clearance (removal) rates are determined by the rate of urine flow based on millimeters per minute. At low flow levels (<2 ml/minute), the values are very inaccurate. Levels of blood urea also change to some extent during the day and vary with diet. Anything that reduces the renal plasma flow also reduces the clearance rate.

The test can be of two types, an hourly or a 24-hour test. The 24-hour test is preferred. A serum urea and urine urea are also done routinely with the clearance test.

When urine clearance averages 2 ml/min, the clearance rate is at the maximum clearance level. With less urine flow (<0.35–2.0 ml/min), a larger portion of the urea in the glomerular filtrate diffuses passively into the tubules, decreasing clearance. Urea clearance values done when urine flow is decreased (<2 ml/min) are less useful than those determined at higher flow rates.

Currently, creatinine clearance determinations are preferred over this test for indication of renal function status.

Patient Preparation and Test Process. If the patient is unable to void voluntarily or is unable to completely empty the bladder, catheterization can be done with physician approval.

24-hour Urine Test (Preferred Test)

1. Explain the steps in the test and the patient's responsibility in urine collection, if any. Written instructions and verbal reminders are suggested
2. The urine is collected in a sterile container with a preservative (5 ml toluene). At the beginning of the test (usually 8:00 AM), the patient voids, and that sample is discarded. Thereafter, all urine voided is placed in the container, up to, and including, an 8:00 AM void the following morning. If possible, the container should be refrigerated
3. Sometime during the 24-hour collection period, when the patient is in a 8-hour fasting state (usually before breakfast), 2 ml of blood will be collected by the laboratory for the serum urea measurement.

Hourly Test. Urine specimens may be collected other than exactly on the hour. The exact *elapsed time* must be noted, however. The patient must remain fasting throughout this test. It is important to follow the procedure exactly to obtain reliable test results.

1. One hour before the test starts, usually 7:00 AM, the person drinks two glasses of water
2. At start time of test (8:00 AM), the person voids (if possible), saves the sample, and drinks an 8-oz glass of water. If the laboratory is to collect the blood samples, it should be notified at this time. A record should be kept, by the client if practical, of the exact time and amount of each voiding in the next 24 hours
3. At 9:00 AM the patient voids, notes the time, saves the sample, and drinks one glass of water. If the void is less than 120 ml, the patient should notify the responsible staff, and the test should be restarted
4. At 10:00 AM, again the person voids, saving the sample, drinks a glass of water, and notes the exact time. Usually, a blood sample is taken at this time as well
5. At 11:00 AM, the end of the test, the person voids and saves the sample. All urine samples are carefully labeled and sent to the laboratory

8.1.4 Inulin Clearance Test

Synonyms: None

Normal Ranges (ml/min)

Adult
Male	124 ± 15 (corrected to 1.73 m² of body surface)
Female	110 ± 15

Lower in children up to 2 yr

Explanation of the Test. Inulin is a polysaccharide of fructose that is freely filtered by the glomerulus and neither reabsorbed nor secreted by the tubules. Inulin clearance is therefore equal to the GFR. Because inulin is not normally present in the body, it must be infused to maintain a constant plasma level. It is not used for routine laboratory work because of the need to monitor plasma levels frequently and the need for extremely careful urine collection. The test has, however, provided information in research studies about the relative accuracies or shortcomings of other clearance tests used clinically. It is also used to calculate tubular transport capacity (T_m). See Section 8.2.2.

Patient Preparation. The inulin clearance test is not used clinically.

INULIN LEVELS DECREASED IN:

• See Section 8.1.2.

8.1.5 Uric Acid, Urine

Synonym: Urate

Normal Ranges

Standard clearance	24 hr: 250–750 mg per 24-hr sample
Random	Not established

Data from Laboratory of Pathology, 1991.

Definition. Uric acid is found normally in the urine as the final waste product of dietary and endogenous purine metabolism, the end product of nucleic acid metabolism. This test is often used as a supplemental test with serum uric acid (more commonly known as BUN).

Physiology. The excretion of urea depends on the amount of protein metabolism; therefore, a single, isolated test would be useful only if the protein intake in known (Laboratory of Pathology, 1991). Protein is released from muscle at a continuous rate. Urea is both filtered and reabsorbed by the kidney; thus, levels will vary with diet and hydration. There is no tubular adaptation to modify urea levels (urea is excreted primarily by glomerular filtration), and plasma levels will increase as the glomerular filtration decreases if protein intake and metabolism are constant (McCance & Huether, 1990, pp. 1154–55). Approximately 60 percent of the uric acid pool is replaced daily through formation and excretion (Henry, 1991, pp. 145).

Pathophysiology. Any condition that affects the rate of urine flow will decrease urea clearance outcomes. The uric acid content of urine is important to identify people at risk for uric acid urinary calculi. In gout there is actual overproduction of uric acid. *Primary gout* is due to overproduction of uric acid secondary to enzyme defects and has been found only in men. *Secondary gout* occurs in both men and women, usually after age 30. In this pathology hyperuricemia is the result of an acquired chronic disease (for example, psoriasis, leukemia, multiple myeloma) or is due to a drug that interferes with normal balance between production and excretion of uric acid (i.e., diuretics) (McCance & Huether, 1990, pp. 1348–49).

Increased levels of uric acid are much more frequent than decreased levels and clinically more significant (Henry, 1991, pp. 145).

URINE URIC ACID DECREASED IN:

1. Gout, preceding an attack; increasing during the attack, a characteristic pattern (Laboratory of Pathology, 1991)
2. Any disorder that will disrupt renal filtration, such as renal tubular defects—congenital: Fanconi's syndrome or Wilson's disease: acquired: toxic damage; in association with some malignant disorders as in Hodgkin's disease, multiple myeloma; bronchogenic carcinoma; acute liver failure (Henry, 1991, p. 145)
3. Some drugs, such as allopurinol, Diamox, or long-term, low-dose use of salicylates
4. Preeclampsia or eclampsia due to decreased glomerular filtration

URINE URIC ACID LEVELS INCREASED IN:

1. Gout (see "Levels Decreased in," item 1)
2. Inadequate renal function with multiple causes, the most frequent cause of dysfunction. The level of increase does not correlate with the severity of the renal disease (Corbett, 1987). Examples are uremia and urinary obstruction
3. When kidney function is normal, elevations are of diagnostic value for gout, prior to formation of tophi (the chalky urate deposits in tissue around joints)
4. Conditions causing increased cellular breakdown or destruction such as
   a. Increased cell destruction (leukemia, multiple myeloma, polycythemia vera)
   b. Treatment of neoplastic disease
   c. Prolonged fasting or malnutrition
   d. Patients being treated with adrenocorticotropic hormone (ACTH)

5. Use of most diuretics (e.g., furosemide, bezthiazide) secondary to decreased plasma volume, a form of the syndrome of inappropriate antidiuretic hormone (ADH) (SIADH) (McCance & Huether, 1990)
6. Administration of a diet high in purines (liver, dried beans, some fish and meat) (Harvey, et al., 1991; McCance & Huether, 1990)
7. The use or administration of many uricosuric drugs (e.g., Benemid) secondary to blocking active reabsorption of uric acid (Harvey, et al., 1991, p. 434)

IMPLICATIONS FOR NURSING

See also Section 1.7, "Serum Uric Acid"

1. This test is done using a 24-hour urine sample (see process under 1.6, "Serum Urea Nitrogen")
2. Uric acid is stable in both serum and urine for about 3 days at room temperature (refrigeration of the urine should not be necessary) (Henry, 1991)
3. There are usually no physical preparations for patients having this test
4. The major obligation of the nurse in care of a patient having this test is to provide information about the purpose and process of the test, so that anxiety is not increased and the test does not have to be repeated (e.g., keep the collection bottle at room temperature, not refrigerated)
5. A diagnosis of gout may have already been made or may only be suspected. If only suspected, the nurse should include assessment of the client for possible signs or symptoms of the disorder and adaptation of care and teaching to best meet his or her present needs and plan for the future (see "Implications for Nursing, Serum Uric Acid," in Section 1.7)
6. Urine pH checks may also be requested, or the nurse may wish to test this independently. Should the urine alkaline level be high, the chance of stone formation is increased, and preventative measures are necessary

---

8.1.5 Urea Nitrogen, Urine

Synonyms: Urate; Urea Clearance

Normal Ranges

Standard clearance: 24 hr: 10–20 gm/24-hr sample

Data from Laboratory of Pathology, 1991.

Definition. This test is primarily a renal function test for urea clearance. It is most often used as a supplemental test with serum uric acid (also known as BUN, or blood urine nitrogen).

Physiology. Urea is filtered at the glomerulus, and about 40 percent is reabsorbed in the tubules. Therefore, given usual conditions, urea clearance values parallel true glomerular filtration rates (Ravel, 1989, p. 175). The excretion of urea depends on the amount of protein metabolism; therefore, a single, isolated test would be useful only if the protein oral intake is known (Laboratory of Pathology, 1991). Protein is released from muscle at a continuous rate. Urea is both filtered and reabsorbed, and it will vary with diet and hydration. There is no tubular adaptation to modify urea levels (urea is excreted primarily by glomerular filtration); thus, plasma levels will increase as the glomerular filtration decreases if protein intake and metabolism are constant (McCance & Huether, 1990, pp. 1154–55). At low filtration levels (<2 ml/min), the findings are inaccurate, even when correction formulas are used (Ravel, 1989, p. 175).

Pathophysiology. Any condition that affects the rate of blood flow through the kidney, therefore affecting the rate of urine flow, will affect urea nitrogen clearance outcomes.

EXCRETION INCREASED IN:

- Disease states associated with increased tissue catabolism, as in fevers (Laboratory of Pathology, 1991)

IMPLICATIONS FOR NURSING

1. Because urea excretion very closely depends on protein metabolism, a single urine test would not provide adequate information, and a 24-hour specimen is collected. Preservatives are usually added to the collection container by the laboratory
2. Twenty-four-hour urine collection process: An arbitrary 24-hour period is selected, usually from 8:00 AM to 8:00 AM. The person given the test is asked to completely empty his or her bladder at 8:00 AM, day 1, and discard that specimen. All subsequent specimens are to be collected in a large, sterile container with a preservative added. The container needs to be kept cool, refrigerated if at all possible, during collection and should be brought to the laboratory promptly at the end of the test period (8:00 AM, day 2). It will need to be labeled with:
   a. The name of the client
   b. Title of test to be performed (24-hour urine)
   c. Hospital room number (or address if done on an outpatient basis)
   d. Physician's full name
   e. Dates and times of each collection
   Check for any discrepancies between the label on the collection container and the laboratory requisition slip that must accompany the specimen to the lab
3. Provide the client with clear, written instructions for the test procedure process at the outset, especially if the test is being done on an outpatient basis
4. Go over the instructions with the client and, if possible, another family member or friend
   a. If protein intake is to be assessed, ensure that the dietician is informed and will do an ongoing diet assessment during the test or will teach the client to do so
   b. The nurse (or the patient if the test is done on an outpatient basis) is ultimately responsible to see that an accurate record is kept of all food and fluid intake. In either case, the patient should be informed as much as possible about the purpose and process of data collection and involved as much as possible, especially for tests done on an outpatient basis

---

8.2 TESTS OF TUBULAR FUNCTION

8.2.1 Laboratory and Clinical Indications of Tubular Dysfunction

Laboratory Findings. In the urine, tubular dysfunction is evidenced by a decreased specific gravity and, with severe tubular dysfunction, a fixed specific gravity of 1.010; also seen are an increased pH (alkaline urine may be due in part to NH_3 production by urea-splitting bacteria

(*Proteus*), glycosuria, aminoaciduria (general or specific to a few), white blood cell (WBC) casts, pyuria, bacteriuria, increased urinary sodium concentration in salt-losing conditions, and an increased K+ level. In the blood, tubular dysfunction is manifested by increased BUN increased H+ (decreased pH), and decreased HCO_3 levels; increased phosphorus and decreased calcium concentrations (vice versa in nephrogenic diabetes insipidus); decreased potassium (K+) level, decreased sodium content in salt-losing conditions, increased in uremia; serum creatinine value increased when 50 percent or more of renal function is lost; and anemia—normocytic, normochromic.

Clinical Findings. In tubular dysfunction the clinical findings are specific to the underlying problems. Children show inadequate growth and rickets. In general, there may be polyuria (nephrogenic diabetes insipidus and acute pyelonephritis); polydipsia; oliguria (with acute tubular necrosis); bruising, purpuric lesions; increased susceptibility to infections; complaints of burning feet, pruritus, nausea; vomiting and diarrhea; changes in level of consciousness; changes in muscle tone and function (twitching, tremors, weakness); functional abnormalities (e.g., urinary incontinence in children); and anatomic abnormalities of the genitourinary tract (e.g., spraying of urinary stream, enuresis).

8.2.2 Excretion Tests

A. *Para-aminohippuric Acid Clearance Test, Urine*

Synonyms: PAH clearance; sodium *p*-aminohippurate clearance

Normal Ranges

Depends on venous plasma PAH concentration—90% clearance

With 0.02 mg/ml venous plasma concentration, 600–700 ml/min; effective renal plasma flow (ERPF): what is in contact with the tubules; normal RPF would be higher (Sodeman & Sodeman, 1982)

Explanation of the Test. Para-aminohippuric acid (PAH) is excreted primarily by tubular secretion (that bound by plasma proteins) and to a limited extent by glomerular filtration (unbound PAH). The total urinary excretion is measured and compared with the GFR obtained by inulin clearance. Clearance of PAH from low plasma levels is almost total, but clearance is self-suppressed with high plasma values because the excess saturates the transfer system (plasma proteins).

Because the test is technically and clinically difficult, it is not widely used. When done in a normally functioning kidney with intact tubular function, the test indicates renal plasma flow.

Patient Preparation

1. A baseline, or control, blood and urine specimen is collected
2. PAH is given in an intravenous priming dose and then by slow continuous infusion in a low concentration
3. Three timed urine specimens are collected, and blood samples are taken at the beginning and end of each urine collection. All three clearance values are averaged
4. Adequate hydration is important

PAH LEVELS DECREASED IN:

- See Section 8.1.2

B. *Phenolsulfonphthalein Test*

Synonyms: PSP test; PSP excretion test

Normal Range

25–35%	excretion in 15 min
40–60%	total excretion in 1 hr
60–75%	total excretion in 2 hr

Explanation of the Test. The phenolsulfonphthalein (PSP) test is an older test of renal function that provides much the same information as the creatinine clearance test and has been mostly replaced by it in practice. Its purpose is to indicate the secretory ability of the renal tubules. Ninety-five percent of the PSP injected intravenously is actively secreted by the tubules and cleared (excreted) from the kidney. The excretion is proportional to renal blood flow. It is a simpler measurement of secretory function than the PAH test.

Decreased, or depressed, 15-minute excretion rates are usually due to impaired renal perfusion rather than decreased tubular function and indicate the need to explore for cardiac failure or renal vascular disease.

Patient Preparation and Test Procedure

1. The bladder is emptied. Catheterization as necessary if approved by the physician in charge
2. Hydration with 600 to 800 ml of water
3. Dye injected in 20 minutes, usually by lab personnel
4. Postinjection urine samples collected at 15 and 30 minutes and 1 and 2 hours. All urine voided during the time of testing must be saved, collected in separate bottles, and labeled with the time of collection
5. The test is not used if increases in BUN and creatinine levels or other indicators of severely diminished renal functions are present because of the danger resulting from the rapid hydration used with this test

PSP EXCRETION INCREASED IN:

1. False elevations because of hypoalbuminemia. Normally 80 percent of the PSP is protein bound and therefore slowed in clearance
2. Liver disease with an excess of 90 percent excretion. A small percentage is usually excreted by the liver; excess renal excretion may indicate a lack of that function by the liver

PSP EXCRETION DECREASED IN:

1. Acute tubular necrosis, idiopathic and acquired
2. de Toni-Fanconi's syndrome, secondary and idiopathic

3. Chronic pyelonephritis
4. Galactosemia
5. Idiopathic hypercalcemia
6. Vitamin D–resistant rickets
7. Any severe, diffuse kidney disease

8.2.3 Concentration Tests

See Section 7.2.1.B ("Serum and Urine Osmolality," and "Water Deprivation Tests.")

8.2.4 Tests Done in Specific Renal Conditions

A. Renal Transplant, All Patients

The following tests are those done most frequently during hospitalization as well as at postdischarge follow-up. The test selection may vary from hospital to hospital but will include many of those given here (Table 8–2).

B. Renal Transplants, Selected Patients

Daily Laboratory Tests

1. Glucose: If the transplant patient is also a diabetic, glucose levels will be checked at least once a day. Good control of serum glucose is imperative for wound healing and maintaining fluid balance
2. Cyclosporine trough levels: Taken daily for any renal transplant patient who is being given this immunosuppressant

C. Renal Dialysis, All Patients

All of the aforementioned tests, with the exception of the cyclosporine trough levels, may be done for the patient receiving any kind of dialysis. While the patient is hospitalized, the tendency is to individualize the laboratory work to the needs of the specific patient on the basis of past medical history, related current medical treatment, and clinical signs and symptoms. After discharge from the hospital whether dialysis occurs at a center or at home, routine laboratory work is generally done once a month, depending on the patient's previous history or present condition. The tests most frequently done at that time are one or more of the following:

1. CBC
2. Creatinine
3. Alkaline phosphatase (Alk. PO_4)
4. BUN
5. Uric acid
6. Plasma sodium (Na^+)
7. Plasma chloride (Cl^-) (HCO3)
8. Plasma potassium (K^+)

TABLE 8–2. RENAL TRANSPLANT TESTS

Name of Test	Findings Related to Renal Transplantation
Complete blood count (CBC) (or just hematocrit)	The ability of the kidney to produce erythropoietin is depressed or absent in renal failure. Increasing levels of red blood cells (RBCs), hematocrit, and hemoglobin help indicate a functioning kidney. The use of cyclosporine as an immunosuppressive agent (which is a frequent method) also decreases RBC production; the dosage may need to be altered
WBC count and differential	These values give information about a number of possible occurrences in the transplanted kidney. An increased total WBC count can indicate stress, infection, or an immune response. Increased polymorphonuclear cells with a shift to the left usually indicates acute infection. If this were a renal infection, expectation of failure of the transplant occurs. Increased numbers of lymphocytes may indicate a viral infection. Decreased numbers of lymphocytes, especially T4 cells, relates to an immunodeficiency. When the number of "polys" increases, a decrease in the number of lymphocytes always occurs unless a total count is done. (This is not a *real* loss of lymphocytes.) The use of cyclosporine decreases WBC production; the use of glucocorticoid immunosuppressants tend to increase WBC production (polys)
Platelet count	(This is a count, not an estimation.) Platelets become dysfunctional in uremic states with decreased aggregation, decreased adhesiveness, and decreased release of platelet factor 3. If no improvement is seen in hematopoiesis after transplantation, rejection may be occurring. Platelet production can also be suppressed by the use of chemotherapeutic drugs such as cyclosporin
BUN	An increase in BUN levels posttransplant can be a sign of transplant rejection. It will also increase with anything that increases catabolism (e.g., fever, bleeding, severe stress)
Creatinine	An increase may be a sign of transplant rejection[a]. An increase in both BUN and creatinine levels with a decrease in creatinine clearance are strong indicators of azotemia and transplant failure
Electrolytes	
Sodium	Sodium levels may be increased, decreased, or within normal limits. Sodium restriction depends on the excretion ability of the kidney and can vary from having only to avoid "salty" foods or adding salt to cooked foods to limits of 1500–2500 mg/day of sodium. Water restriction is based on daily urine output
Potassium	An increased level can indicate failure of the transplant. It is also dangerous because of the potential for cardiac arrythmia production
Chloride	Changes that are proportional to sodium changes indicate changes in fluid balance. Changes unrelated to sodium change may indicate acid-base imbalances, especially metabolic acidosis when bicarbonate is selectively reabsorbed over chloride, assuming a functioning kidney
Bicarbonate	The bicarbonate concentration is also a major indicator of acid-base balance (see chloride) and useful for differential diagnosis as to the cause of altered sensorium (e.g., uremia versus acidosis)
Beta-2-microglobulin (B-2-microglobulin)	B-2 microglobulin is a small peptide, released by cells into body fluid at a fairly constant rate, proportional to cellular turnover. Because it is

(continued)

TABLE 8–2. *(continued)*

Name of Test	Findings Related to Renal Transplantation
	eliminated from the kidney by glomerular filtration and reabsorbed by the proximal tubules, it reflects glomerular filtration even more accurately than does serum creatinine. The concentration of B-2 microglobulin increases with acute renal allograft rejection. Its concentration is also related to tumor burden and disease activity in malignant lymphoma and myeloma. It has been found to change concentration in response to disease activity with rheumatoid arthritis, sarcoidosis, and systemic lupus erythematosus.
	Recently, elevations of B-2-microglobulin concentrations were thought to mark early stages of AIDS. However, they would seem to represent a general response to viral infections

[a]Clinical signs and symptoms of kidney transplant rejection also include fever, decreased urine output, increased blood pressure, and painful swelling at the transplant site.
Data from Laboratory of Pathology, 1991.

9. Serum bicarbonate
10. BUN-to-creatinine ratio*

The reference range (normal value) of the BUN-to-creatinine ratio is 20:1.

RATIO INCREASED IN (BUN INCREASE):

1. Volume deficit related to an actual decreased intake or a decreased cardiac output
2. Catabolic states (e.g., stress, infection, starvation)
3. Loss of lean body mass through a lack of muscular activity and/or a strict diet regimen

RATIO DECREASED IN (CREATININE INCREASE):

1. Renal filtration dysfunction
2. Increased lean body mass
3. Increased level of exercise

D. Renal Stones

The appearance of casts in the urine (other than infrequent hyaline casts) is one of the early warning signs of renal stone (calculus) formation. (See Section 8.1.1, "Laboratory Findings"; Section 4.12, "Pathophysiology," Fig. 4–2, and "Implications for Nursing")

Cause. As yet unknown. Some people form stones, and others do not, in an identical physiological state.

Predisposing Factors

1. Dehydration
2. Urinary tract infections (in part related to a pH change in the urine)

---

*For both renal transplant and dialysis patients a calculation based on the BUN and creatinine concentrations is frequently useful.

3. Obstruction of urinary flow from whatever cause, including immobility
4. Specific diseases that increase levels of stone-forming material in urinary filtrate (e.g., hyperparathyroidism [calcium], gout [uric acid], genetic defects [cystinuria])
5. Excessive dietary intake of stone-forming material (calcium, vitamin D, oxalates)
6. Absence of inhibitors to stone formation (e.g., citrate, pyrophosphates, magnesium, glycoaminoglycans)
7. Fixation of pH over a narrow range for at least a 24-hour period with a loss of normal acid-alkaline fluctuations, that is, tides (Laboratory of Pathology, 1991)
8. Mucosal metaplasia such as occurs in vitamin A deficiency (Laboratory of Pathology, 1991)
9. Accumulation of debris, normal and abnormal, in urine (nidus formation), such as epithelial cells, blood clot, mucoproteins, and/or bacteria around which the aforementioned inorganic materials crystallize

Diagnostic Tests (In Order of Usual Use)

1. Urinalysis (see Chapter 4, "Urinalysis Screen")
2. X ray: kidney-ureter-bladder (KUB) (see Section 17.2.2, "Plain Film of the Abdomen")
3. Renal sonogram (see Section 17.6.1.G)
4. Stone analysis to determine the mineral content of the stone (see discussion that follows)
5. Intravenous pyelogram (see Section 17.2.9)
6. Retrograde pyelogram (see Section 17.2.8, item 4)

RELATED NURSING DIAGNOSES

The Renal Transplant Patient

1. Anticipatory grieving related to fear of transplant rejection
2. Lack of knowledge related to purpose, effect, or schedule of medications and fluid and diet restrictions
3. Self-care deficit related to fatigue resulting from inadequate gas exchange (anemia), stress, pain, and lack of knowledge
4. Potential/actual alteration in fluid/electrolyte balance related to decreased renal function, alteration in nutritional status (decreased secondary to anorexia), and dietary restrictions
5. Potential ineffectual coping (individual) related to possible sense of obligation and/or guilt (if live kidney donor), uncertain outcome of transplant, economic burden, and loss of usual role function (family/work/social) for undetermined length of time

The Renal Dialysis Patient

1. Alteration in fluid balance (excess) and electrolyte balance related to inadequate filtration or excretion by the kidney
2. Alteration in nutrition (less than body requirements) related to
   a. Unwelcome dietary changes
   b. Anorexia related to disease process (e.g., increased BUN concentration)
   c. Gastric discomfort related to uremia
   d. Anorexia due to anxiety/fear
   e. Decreased activity level
   f. Presence of constipation or diarrhea related to uremia or medications

(continued)

3. Potential for injury (trauma or falls, bleeding, dialysis disequilibrium [see Appendix C]) related to infection secondary to decreased immune response with uremia, related to potential medication overdosage/toxicity due to inadequate elimination and related to potential decreased awareness with uremia
4. Activity intolerance related to weakness and fatigue secondary to inadequate nutritional status, hypoxia due to anemia, loss of muscle mass with enforced bed rest; and electrolyte imbalance (particularly K^+ increases)
5. Grieving related to loss of life expectations due to chronic illness causing life-style changes (role, economic, social)
6. Pain and discomfort related to process of hemodialysis (especially with a fistula) secondary to headaches, peripheral neuropathy

Renal Calculi (Stones)

1. Pain related to pressure or colic due to obstruction or distention by stone(s) or due to infection secondary to obstruction or trauma; intensified by fear
2. Lack of knowledge related to cause and prevention of calculi, self-care to evaluate progress (intake and output recording, urine straining, checking pH)
3. Anxiety related to unknown outcomes (potential surgery, potential recurrence)

E. Stone Analysis

Synonyms: Renal calculus analysis, spectrophotometric; crystalography

Normal Range: Presence of calculus is abnormal. There is no "normal" stone

Explanation of the Test. Unless a single stone has been passed that is visible to the naked eye, a 24-hour urine sample is collected and screened for stones. (Any volume of urine can be screened, but the 24-hour specimen is most likely to yield stones.) The urine is filtered through a large paper and gauze funnel, which traps the stones (gravel). This process is called a 24-hour stone screen and may be ordered as a separate test in itself.

Any calculi retrieved are examined for color, shape, and weight. Some of the outside of each different type of stone is crushed to a powder and analyzed, and each of these stones is then cut in half and the center pulverized and analyzed using a polarizing microscope. Each of the chemical compounds has a recognizable index of refraction that is used to identify the compounds. X-ray diffraction can be used to confirm the findings, if needed. (Laboratory of Pathology, 1991)

Patient Preparation. If the patient is ambulatory and therefore able to go to the bathroom, she or he will need instruction about saving the 24-hour urine specimen. A large, clean collection bottle free of any acid or alkali is obtained (usually from the laboratory), to be placed in the bathroom after being labeled with the patient's name, time, date of the test start, and type of test to be done. (If the patient is in the hospital, the room number is also included.) The patient is instructed to void at 8:00 AM, and discard that urine. Thereafter, all urine voided until and including an 8:00 AM void the following day is saved. The urine is voided into a clean urinal, in the case of a male, or a clean receptacle placed under the toilet seat (often called a urinary "hat") for a female and then poured into the collection container. It is not necessary to keep the container cool or in a dark place.

TABLE 8–3. PAIN WITH RENAL CALCULI (STONES)

Pain Location	Type	Probable Stone Location
May be none, in back if present	If present, dull	Renal pelves and calyces
Back or abdomen or both	Dull to colicky	Calyx or ureteropelvic junction
Abdominal (costovertebral tenderness may be present)	Intense, severe, colicky	Calculi traveling down ureter
Costovertebral angle to the flank, to the suprapubic area, and to the external genitalia	Intense, severe, may be colicky	Calculi that produce an obstruction within the kidney

Data from Lewis & Collier, 1983; and Stark, 1983.

Related Urine Sediment Abnormalities

1. RBCs present because of injury to urinary tract
2. WBCs present because of inflammation/infection secondary to injury, urine stasis, or stress
3. Protein present because of infection, injury to glomerular basement membrane or primary renal dysfunction per se
4. Pus, bacteria (>1,000,000 organisms/ml) related to infection
5. Crystals present because of urinary stasis (see Section 4.12, "Physiology"). The type is pH-dependent

Signs and Symptoms

1. Alteration in urinalysis or urine culture consistent with causative factors (e.g., bacteria or RBCs with infection, increased specific gravity with decreased filtrate, presence of crystals or casts related to decreased urinary flow)
2. Alterations in blood test results consistent with causative factors (e.g., increased uric acid, chloride, and/or bicarbonate levels; increased total protein/albumin concentration)
3. May have hematuria secondary to abrasion of the ureter, pyuria and possible increased WBC count with infective source, nausea and/or vomiting in response to pain
4. Pain, the key and major symptom. The severity and type of pain depend on the size, location, and cause of the calculi. The pain can be excruciating at its peak and tends to be colicky in nature (Tables 8–3 and 8–4)

TABLE 8–4. RENAL AND URINARY CALCULI[a]

Type and Mineral Content	Formation Factors	Characteristics
Calcium oxalate	Unknown; may be due to Ca^+ increase or hyperoxaluria	Small stones; tend to be trapped in the ureters
Calcium phosphate	Alkaline urine; primary hyper-parathyroidism	Usually found with other types of renal stones
Cystine	Genetic defect of gastrointestinal absorbtion with increased concentration presented to the kidney	Infrequent—2% or less of all renal stone events

(continued)

TABLE 8–4. (Continued)

Type and Mineral Content	Formation Factors	Characteristics
Struvite	Occurs with urinary tract infections; usually combined with milligrams of ammonium and/or phosphate.	Only renal stone occurring more often in women; often the staghorn type
Uric acid	Gout	Found most frequently in Jewish males

[a]Most renal calculi are made up of a number of different cations, e.g., calcium, magnesium or ammonium combined with phosphate, oxalate, uric acid, or carbonate (SHMC, 1984). *Data from Lewis & Collier, 1983; Stark, 1983; and SHMC, 1984.*

NINE

THE GASTROINTESTINAL SYSTEM

RECOGNITION OF GASTROINTESTINAL DYSFUNCTION

Because gastrointestinal (GI) symptoms are so often a part of the prodromal symptoms of other diseases, their occurrence is likely to be discounted as "not serious" until rather marked dysfunction is present. Therefore, assessment for familial gastrointestinal disease and the presence of factors in life-style or environment that predispose to gastrointestinal problems are particularly important.

9.1 LABORATORY AND CLINICAL INDICATIONS OF GASTROINTESTINAL DYSFUNCTION

Laboratory Findings. GI dysfunction may be noted by the presence of occult blood in the stool, chronic iron deficiency anemia (hypochromic, microcytic) or macrocytic anemia (normochromic with an increased mean corpuscular volume [MCV], mean corpuscular hemoglobin [MCH], and mean corpuscular hemoglobin concentration [MCHC]), anisocytosis, poikilocytosis, neutropenia, hypersegmented white blood cell (WBC) nuclei (four to six lobes), thrombocytopenia, and in many instances an increased lactic dehydrogenase (LDH) level. Other tests: decreased serum haptoglobin.

Clinical Findings. Clinical findings of GI dysfunction include complaints of "ulcerlike" pain (pinpoint, periodic, which is decreased in the morning, increased in the afternoon, and is relieved by eating or vomiting; there is a return of pain 30 to 90 minutes after eating); hemoptysis and dark, tarry stools; glossitis (red, smooth, painful tongue); easy bruising; paresthesias; impaired vibratory sense; premature graying; signs and symptoms of anemia (e.g., fatigue, pallor, shortness of breath, lassitude, angina); complaints of indigestion, anorexia; history of recent weight loss (some of these symptoms in persons of Japanese, Finnish, or Icelandic heritage should increase the index of suspicion for gastric cancer); family history of pernicious anemia, gastric cancer, or gastric-duodenal ulcer; self-history of previous peptic ulcer; and a consistent use of antacids.

9.2 TESTS OF GASTRIC SECRETION

9.2.1 Basal Secretory Test

Synonyms: Gastric secretory test, basal gastric secretion, 1-hr morning aspiration

Normal Range: 0–5 mEq HCL/hr (females and senior adults tend to be within the lower ranges of normal)

Normal Fasting Volume: 20–100 ml. A volume greater than this could indicate obstruction or increased secretion.

Explanation of the Test. Basal gastric secretion under fasting conditions is the response of the secretory cells of the stomach to endogenous stimuli continually present. The test can be used to determine gastric acidity or to obtain material for exfoliative cytology. Differences in basal secretion rates, rarely diagnostic in themselves, can be helpful in the differential diagnosis of several conditions (gastric versus duodenal ulcer). There is considerable overlap among the responses. No pathognomonic range exists for any of the disease states linked with basal gastric secretion rates, with the exception of the very high acid output of Zollinger-Ellison (Z-E) syndrome. If there is no evidence of basal secretion or the results of the test are ambiguous, stimulation tests are done. Since the advent of the fiberoptic gastroscope, gastric analysis is rarely done.

Patient Preparation and Test Procedure

1. Any medications or foods that might influence gastric secretions should be held for 24 hours before the test (e.g., alcohol, anticholinergics, adrenergics, alcohol, corticosteroids, reserpine); no antacids or coffee
2. Patient should be fasting for 12 hours before the test
3. Water may be taken until 8 hours before intubation
4. No smoking the morning of the test
5. Basal physiological and environmental conditions maintained; quiet, stress-free environment with no odor or sight of food; (saliva should be expectorated, not swallowed, during the test)
6. An upper GI series should not precede this test
7. In the fasting patient a gastric tube is inserted, often by a gastroenterology nurse. Sampling is done as follows:
   a. The patient is seated in an upright position as the tube is inserted (usually 55 cm are introduced—tube length needed is measured by the length from the nose, or teeth, to the stomach)
   b. If the patient has a history of partial gastrectomy, only 50 cm of the tube is introduced with the patient supine
   c. All five sample secretions are collected by aspiration (syringe suction). The first fasting gastric specimen is collected and discarded, thereafter, *all* of the secretions, aspirated at 15 minute intervals, are collected in four separate bottles with appropriate labels (e.g., test name, patient name, time of collection)
   d. In collection of specimens, the syringe plunger should be pulled briefly every few minutes, rather than one prolonged pull

e. The tube must be kept open by introducing small amounts of air briefly every few minutes

SIGNIFICANCE OF RESPONSES:

1. Basal secretion within normal limits will rule out the presence of pernicious anemia, in which true achlorhydria exists
2. A high basal secretion (15 to 20 mEq/hr, as high as 60 mEq/hr at times) is strongly suggestive of Z-E syndrome
3. Benign gastric ulcers usually have normal or even low rates. Basal secretion greater than 10 mEq/hr is strong evidence against their existence
4. Duodenal ulcers tend toward basal secretion rates of 5 to 15 mEq/hr. Low acid secretion is evidence against their existence
5. Gastric cancer is often concurrent with somewhat lower than normal basal secretion or can be suspected with a total absence of acid secretion, particularly if pernicious anemia is ruled out

9.2.2 Gastric Stimulation Test

Synonyms: Free and total acid; Histalog stimulation test; pentagastrin stimulation test

Normal Range (1–50 mEq/hr)

Basal acid output (BAO—response of the stomach to the continuous presence of endogenous stimuli)	0–5
Maximal acid output (MAO—total acid excreted in hour after stimulation)	0–20
Peak acid output (PAO—the highest acid output for two successive specimens, adjusted to the hourly rate × 2)	1–50

Explanation of the Test. As noted in Test 9.2.1, "Basal Secretory Test," there is a basal level of gastric juice secretion continually present in the stomach in response to endogenous stimuli. Only in Zollinger-Ellison (Z-E) syndrome is a specific, pathognomonic basal acid secretion present.

Maximal acid output is based on the acid output of the four collection samples, poststimulation.

Peak acid output is the highest total output of two specimens (adjusted to an hourly rate, i.e., total/30 minutes × 2).

This test is usually done following the gastric secretion test. A drug (Histalog, pentagastrin) is used to stimulate gastric acid secretion.

Patient Preparation

1. As with the basal secretory test, any medications that might influence gastric secretions are held for 24 hours prior to the test
2. The person being tested must fast for 12 hours, refraining from ingesting aspirin and coffee
3. No smoking the morning of, or during the test
4. No upper GI test prior to the test

5. Provide as stress-free an environment as possible. In particular, eliminate any chance that the person to be tested is exposed to the *smell of food*
6. Position the patient for the test to allow him or her to be sitting up or lying on the left side in bed to prevent regurgitation

Test Process

1. A nasogastric tube is inserted, usually though the nares, and taped in position
2. Gastric juices are removed by suction from the fasting stomach over a period of 1 hour to obtain a basal acid level
3. A stimulant drug is administered (currently, pentagastrin or Histalog are the drugs of choice). The nurse should be alert to side-effects to the drug. Reactions are many and vary in severity. Any reaction should be noted and reported immediately. Reactions can include abdominal pain, nausea, vomiting, flushing, transitory dizziness, faintness and numbness of extremities
4. pH measurements are converted to hydrogen ion concentration in mEq/hr and reported as basal, intermediate, or extremely high values

Significance of Findings

1. Basal/lower values (0–5 mEq/hr) occur in:
   a. Achlorhydria
   b. Elderly persons: Considered normal in patients older than 60 years
   c. Gastric carcinoma
   d. Gastric ulcer, benign (normal or low rates; secretion >10 mEq is strong evidence *against* gastric ulcer)
   e. Pernicious anemia (may show total absence of acid secretion)
2. Intermediate values (5–15 mEq/hr) may be associated with duodenal ulcers
3. Extremely high values (>20 mEq/hr); can reach 80 mEq/hr; Z-E syndrome

9.2.3 Serum Gastrin

Synonyms: None

Normal Range: 0–100 pg/ml (a level of 101–150 pg/ml is considered borderline)

Explanation of the Test. Plasma gastrin determination is a sensitive, and specific, double anti-body radioimmunoassay (RIA) test. Gastrin is a peptide hormone that acts on the parietal cells of the stomach's fundal mucosa and of the duodenum. Measurement of its concentration is of particular use in the diagnosis of Z-E syndrome (gastrinoma) and pernicious anemia, both of which are associated with marked increases in gastric acid secretion.

Patient Preparation

1. No food or drink other than water for 10 hours prior to the test
2. No anticholinergic drugs and/or histamine antagonists (e.g., cimetidine) for several days before the test

Physiology. Gastrin is a hormone (polypeptide) secretion by endocrine cells called "G-cells" found in the gastric antrum primarily, but also in the proximal duodenum. Its function is to increase acid secretion from parietal cells of the fundus. It is released by the presence of protein and amino acids, coupled with an alkaline gastric pH, cholinergic stimulation and distension of the gastric antrum.

PLASMA GASTRIN LEVELS INCREASED IN:

1. Postprandial tests in normal individuals because of physiological gastrin secretion, presence of proteins and amino acids, alkaline gastric pH, and distension of gastric antrum
2. Peptic ulcer disease caused by pancreatic islet cell tumors (Z-E syndrome). Serum gastrin levels may be very high, 800 to 1000 pg/ml. When levels are in lower ranges, 200 to 400 pg/ml, stimulation by infusion of calcium or secretin will induce high levels
3. Pernicious anemia with very high levels in the presence of achlorhydria
4. Gastric ulcer, gastric carcinoma (gastrinoma), and GI obstruction with slight to moderate elevations (levels of 500 pg/ml have a high predictive value for gastrinoma)
5. Aging, with slight to moderate elevations
6. Individuals who had a vagotomy
7. Individuals taking cimetidine
8. Z-E syndrome

9.3 TESTS OF DIGESTIVE FUNCTION (PANCREATIC EXOCRINE FUNCTION)

9.3.1 Laboratory and Clinical Indications of Pancreatic Exocrine Dysfunction

Laboratory Findings. Pancreatic exocrine function refers to glands excreting externally via a duct. Laboratory findings in pancreatic exocrine dysfunction include hyperglycemia (moderate to frank diabetes). With acute pancreatitis, findings include moderate leukocytosis with a shift to the left, increased serum glutamic-oxaloacetic transaminase (SGOT) and alkaline phosphatase levels, transient hyperlipidemia, possible glucose in the urine, and aminoaciduria (cystine, lysine). With chronic pancreatitis, findings of postprandial (p.p.) hypoglycemia and decreased serum calcium levels (may be due to malabsorption of vitamin D or increased combining of calcium with fat) are seen.

Clinical Findings. Acute clinical findings of pancreatic exocrine dysfunction are severe epigastric pain with a sudden onset and radiating, nausea and vomiting, abdominal distension, mild jaundice, decreased urine output, fever, signs of dehydration, hypovolemia, and shock. Chronic findings include steatorrhea, bleeding tendencies, and osteomalacia.

9.3.2 Amylase, Serum and Urine

Synonyms: Alpha-amylase, diastase, AMY, 1,4-α-D-glucan-glucanohydrolase

Normal Ranges

Serum, total
Adult   40–220 U/l

(continued)

Pancreatic	
Newborn, 2–4 days	5–65 U/l (serum)[a]
Adult	17–115 U/l
Timed Urine	
Neonatal	1–17 U/hr
Adult	5–50 U/hr

[a]Reaches adult levels at the end of the first year.
Data from Tietz, 1990.

Explanation of the Test. Amylases are enzymes that catalyze the hydrolysis of polysaccharides. Serum and urine amylase tests are quantitative measurements of the amount of that enzyme found in the blood or urine. This test is most important in evaluating acute pancreatitis. Amylase found in the blood is produced primarily in the salivary glands and the pancreas. Damage to the glandular cells (as in acute pancreatitis) will liberate large amounts of amylase. The enzyme rapidly enters the blood and increases its serum levels. Urine amylase levels also increase promptly, often within several hours of the serum increase. Urine increase often occurs as the serum levels begin to decrease. The ratio between urine amylase levels and creatinine clearance (expressed as a percentage or as units per hour) is used diagnostically. Urine testing can be done on random urine, but no normal values have been established for a random urine specimen.

Serial determinations at 4- to 6-hour intervals often provide more helpful information than a single determination.

Patient Preparation

1. No special preparation is necessary for serum tests
2. Blood should be taken 1 to 2 hours after eating (p.p.), and preferably not when intravenous glucose is being administered
3. Urine tests are usually done on 24- or 2-hour specimens
   a. Twenty-four-hour specimens are collected after voiding and discarding 8:00 AM specimen. The urine must have a preservative in the collection bottle (5 ml toluene) and be refrigerated, if possible
   b. Two-hour specimens start with initial urine discarded and the exact time noted. Two hours later the person will void again and that total sample is collected and sent to the laboratory immediately

AMYLASE LEVELS INCREASED IN:

1. Acute pancreatitis. Serum values over five times the upper limit of normal are highly suggestive of this diagnosis. The levels fall abruptly, within 2 to 3 days after onset, even though active inflammation persists. Urinary amylase levels may be diagnostic at such a time. A continued increase in serum levels suggests continuing pancreatic necrosis or formation of a pseudocyst
2. Chronic, relapsing pancreatitis, but to a much less marked degree. It may be associated with trauma, alcohol, viral hepatitis, or hyperparathyroidism or may be idiopathic in origin

3. Conditions causing obstruction of the sphincter of Oddi (e.g., cholecystitis, biliary tract stones, tumor, or spasm secondary to the use of morphine, meperidine [Demerol], or biliary tract cannulation)
4. Pancreatic carcinoma, only late in the progress of the disease, if at all
5. Miscellaneous conditions such as renal failure as a result of decreased excretion, pregnancy, burns, drug hypersensitivity (thiazides, ethacrynic acid, oral contraceptives), and diabetic ketoacidosis in some 60 percent of patients (salivary amylase is predominant in this rise—cause not clear)
6. Some diseases of the parotid glands such as mumps. This determination can be useful in diagnosing cases of mumps orchitis or encephalitis when there is little salivary gland involvement noted
7. Conditions causing chemical irritation of the pancreas such as peptic ulcer, postoperatively after gastric resection, or with intestinal obstruction, mesenteric thrombosis, peritonitis, and ruptured ectopic pregnancy
8. Individuals with a protein abnormality (macroamylasemia). It is found in persons with malabsorption or alcoholism and who have normal pancreatic function. Urine levels are normal, however, because the protein is too large to pass the renal glomerulus

AMYLASE LEVELS DECREASED IN:

1. Physiological situations such as after a meal or the administration of glucose intravenously
2. Conditions associated with a decrease in the number of functioning pancreatic cells such as in some cases of chronic pancreatitis, pancreatic cancer, and massive hemorrhagic pancreatic necrosis
3. Infrequently in miscellaneous conditions such as congestive heart failure, GI cancer, bone fractures, and pleurisy. It is due to multiple and, in some cases, not clearly understood mechanisms

9.3.3 Serum Lipase

Synonyms: None

Normal Ranges

Adult	0–27 IU/dl
Pediatric	8–35 IU/ml (olive oil, 37°C)

Explanation of the Test. Lipases are enzymes that hydrolyze (or split) emulsified fats from fatty acids to triglycerides. Bile salts, calcium, and albumin are lipase activators and necessary to that activity. Lipase is found primarily in the pancreas but is also present in stomach, intestine, WBCs, fat cells, milk, and ascitic fluid in pancreatitis. There are also other related but different forms of lipase in the body. Measurement of serum lipase is considered more specific but less sensitive for pancreatic damage than is amylase. Like amylase, lipase is released into the bloodstream after damage to the pancreatic secretory cell. Its levels rise later than do those of amylase, within 24 to 48 hours, and stay elevated longer, 7 to 10 days, usually peaking on day 4. Urine lipase measurement, although available, is not currently used.

Patient Preparation. No special preparation is necessary.

SERUM LIPASE LEVELS INCREASED IN:

1. Acute pancreatitis with levels up to four times the upper limit of normal. It is helpful in diagnosis to look at serum lipase when amylase levels have already returned to normal limits
2. Conditions leading to obstruction of the ampulla of Vater (e.g., some cases of pancreatic carcinoma, carcinoma of the ampulla of Vater, chronic biliary disease)
3. Some cases of mumps when there is significant secondary pancreatic involvement as well

9.3.4 Serum Carotene

Synonyms: Plasma carotene, serum carotenoids

Normal Range: 50–100 µg/dl

Explanation of the Test. Carotene is a fat-soluble precursor (provitamin) of vitamin A. Its absorption from the intestine depends on the presence of dietary fat and the normal absorption of that fat. It is not stored by the body. Carotene is found in green or yellow vegetables and in some animal protein. Measurement of serum carotene levels is useful in establishing the presence of intestinal malabsorption conditions and as a screening test for steatorrhea.

SERUM CAROTENE LEVELS INCREASED IN:

1. Excessive intake of carotene (e.g., carrots)
2. Increased absorption as in pregnancy
3. Hyperlipidemia and hypocholesterolemia, associated with diabetes mellitus

SERUM CAROTENE LEVELS DECREASED IN:

1. States of lipid malabsorption (steatorrhea)
2. Conditions of inadequate intake of either fat (e.g., individuals on low-fat diets) or carotene (green or yellow vegetables)
3. Severe liver disease
4. States with high fevers

9.3.5 Secretin Stimulation Test

Synonyms: Pancreatic stimulation test, augmented secretin test

Normal Ranges (Adult)[a]

	Standard	Augmented
Volume	Increased volume of clear watery secretion; 2 ml/kg of body weight	4.5–8.1 ml/kg

Bicarbonate concentration (HCO₃)	Marked increase; peak of 90–100 mEq/L	93–141 mEq/L
Sodium	Increased	
Chloride	Decreased–reciprocal to HCO₃ increase	
pH	Increased; greater than 8.0	

[a]Values less than those given are significant of decreased pancreatic activity. Values greater than those given are not useful for determining pancreatic status because hypersecretion of pancreatic fluid is not known.

Explanation of the Test. Secretin is a hormone known to stimulate secretion of pancreatic fluid and bile. A standard (1.0 IU/kg) or augmented dose (4.0 to 5.0 IU/kg) of secretin is given intravenously after the stomach and duodenal contents have been aspirated until clear through a double-lumen tube. Pancreatic secretions are then collected for 60 to 80 minutes and the aspirate measured at 20-minute intervals for volume, bicarbonate content, and other measurements as dictated by the facility's procedure or doctor's request. There is controversy over the usefulness of the measurement of serum amylase by the stimulation of secretin. Secretin is not known to stimulate the release of pancreatic enzymes. Pancreozymin is used for this purpose.

The test is useful in the differentiation of causes of malabsorption by designating pancreatic hypofunction. The augmented test is done when the standard test result is equivocal.

Patient Preparation

1. Patient should be kept n.p.o. other than water for 8 hours before the test
2. Treatment with all anticholinergic drugs discontinued 48 hours before the test (e.g., atropine, Pro-Banthine)
3. Patient teaching before the test should be done about the need for and process of a double-lumen gastric tube insertion and the usual length of the test (3 hours). Three or four continuous 20-minute collections of duodenal secretions are done

EXPECTED (NORMAL) RESPONSE:

1. Increased volume of clear watery secretion
2. Marked increase of bicarbonate concentration
3. Increased sodium concentration
4. Reciprocal fall in chloride to sodium rise
5. pH increase above 8.0

SECRETION RATE INCREASED IN (HYPERSECRETION RATE NOT KNOWN):

1. Biliary cirrhosis and nonalcoholic cirrhosis. Increased volume and high normal bicarbonate secretion occurs
2. Z-E syndrome, hemochromatosis, and alcoholic cirrhosis with a marked volume increase and a lesser increase in bicarbonate secretion

SECRETION RATE DECREASED IN:

1. Conditions causing a mechanical decrease in the excretion of pancreatic juice such as cystic fibrosis and edema of the pancreas

2. Conditions causing decreased secretion of pancreatic juice because of cell injury or loss such as chronic pancreatitis, pancreatic cysts, pancreatic calcification, and cancer of the pancreas

9.4 LIVER FUNCTION TESTS

9.4.1 Laboratory and Clinical Indications of Liver Dysfunction

Laboratory Findings. Liver dysfunction findings in blood include increased total bilirubin levels, direct and indirect in most cases; increased serum cholesterol and alkaline phosphatase concentrations (especially with biliary obstruction); decreased total protein levels because of decreased albumin with prolonged disease (total protein levels could be normal or elevated with increases in the gammaglobulin fraction); high elevations of serum aspartate transaminase (SAST) and slight increases in LDH levels; dilutional decrease in serum sodium; serum potassium levels decreased; with viral hepatitis or cirrhosis, increased number of WBCs with atypical lymphocytes; decreased platelet count; prothrombin time (PT) 1 to 2 seconds above normal or control; and mild to moderate anemia, which may be normocytic to macrocytic and normochromic to hyperchromic. In urine, bilirubin levels are increased, and feces may be positive for occult blood or be blood streaked because of a rupture of hemorrhoids.

Clinical Findings. Clinical liver dysfunction findings include clay-colored stools, jaundice, dark urine, anorexia, fatigue, ascites, edema, spider angiomas, muscle wasting, virilization or feminization with changes in hair pattern, varicose veins of the legs and/or periumbilical area, increased susceptibility to infections, and an enlarged tender liver.

9.4.2 Serum Alanine Aminotransferase (ALT)

Synonym: glutamic pyruvic transaminase (SGPT)

Normal Range: 0–50 U/l*

Explanation of the Test. Serum alanine transaminase (ALT) is found most often, but not exclusively, in the liver. Because of this, serum increases are seldom seen without involvement of the liver. More severe or more extensive liver damage is necessary to cause abnormal values than is the case with aspartate aminotransferase (AST) (previously known as SGOT). It can be said that the ALT test is less sensitive but much more specific than the AST test. Tissues of the kidney, heart, and skeletal muscle have significant amounts of ALT in descending order as just listed. ALT levels usually return to normal* before AST, probably because most tissues containing

---

*Previously the reader has been warned of the danger of comparing reference ranges (normal ranges), especially when dealing with serum enzymes. Because of the multiple variations in methods of measurement and the variations intrinsic to even the same methods done in different settings, values are *not* comparable. The reader should use as a guide the normal reference range supplied by the laboratory doing the test. See the discussion in Section 1.12.

both enzymes contain proportionately more AST than ALT. It is often helpful to compare the two in a differential diagnosis.

Patient Preparation

1. If possible in cases of suspected hepatic disease, treatment with hepatotoxic drugs should be stopped about 12 hours before testing.
2. See "Implications for Nursing: SAST and LDH" in Section 1.12.3

ALT LEVELS INCREASED IN:

1. Acute hepatocellular injury with a tenfold or higher increase over normal values. The increase is greater than that of AST. Increases are seen in viral A or B, and with less marked elevations, type C hepatitis. In hepatitis C there are very notable patterns of elevation: monophasic, biphasic, and plateau (Jensen & Koff, 1992, p. 144)
2. Extrahepatic jaundice resulting from biliary obstruction with up to a tenfold increase. AST levels are increased about the same or slightly less
3. Primary or secondary carcinoma of the liver with a fivefold increase. The AST increase is seven- to tenfold
4. Primary biliary cirrhosis with a fivefold increase. The AST increase is about the same
5. Alcoholic hepatitis with a threefold increase. The AST concentration has a five- to sixfold increase
6. Alcoholic cirrhosis with a slight, one- to twofold increase. The AST concentration has a three- to fourfold increase. In fatty liver secondary to alcoholism but without cirrhosis, the rise is very slight or may be within normal limits. The AST concentration is slightly above normal
7. Chronic active hepatitis with or without cirrhosis with an increase from 1 to 12 times normal. The AST level rises to 15 to 75 times normal
8. Infectious mononucleosis with an increase about 15 times normal. The AST concentration rises approximately 10 times normal (Henry, 1991)
9. Use of many therapeutic drugs: acetometophen; amiodarone hydrochloride (Cordarone); carbamazepin (Tegretol); hydralazine hydrochloride (Apresoline); isoniazid (Laniazid/Teebaconin); methyldopa (Aldomet); nonsteroidal antiinflammatory drugs are associated with minimal elevations of ALT, AST, or both in 1 to 10 percent of patients; valproic acid (Depakene) can cause elevation of AST (as well as blood ammonia). ALT level may remain normal (Jensen & Koff, 1992, p. 149)
10. Individuals after strenuous and prolonged exercise
11. Obesity due to fatty liver, mechanism unknown (Jensen & Koff, 1992, p. 149)

9.4.3 Gamma-Glutamyl Transferase, Serum

Synonyms: GGT, gamma-glutamyl transpeptidase. γ-glutamyl transferase, GGTP[a]

Normal Ranges (U/L)

Female	8–55
Male	10–65

[a]The test can be done on plasma, but serum is preferred.

Explanation of the Test. GGT is a microsomal enzyme. It is found in an almost identical intracellular distribution as that of alkaline phosphatase (AP) in the liver, biliary system, and pancreas. The two enzymes rise roughly in parallel in hepatobiliary and pancreatic disease. Although GGT is found in its greatest concentrations in the liver and kidney, with smaller amounts in heart muscle, that found in circulation derives from cells that line the small branches of the biliary tract. The feature that distinguishes GGT from other enzymes used in assessing liver function is its response to alcohol. Alcohol apparently stimulates rapid GGT elevations (within 18 hours), even with a relatively small intake and without other evidence of hepatocellular damage such as an increase in the levels of other liver enzymes. It provides objective evidence of recent drinking. For this reason it has been recommended for use in the evaluation of patients with alcoholism. In normal persons the GGT serum level varies little from day to day.

Patient Preparation

1. The test is not interfered with by hemolysis as are LDH and AST (GOT) determinations
2. No special preparation is necessary

GGT LEVELS INCREASED IN:

1. Hepatobiliary obstructive disease and pancreatic obstructive disease to its highest recorded levels. Because their intracellular distribution is nearly identical, increases are roughly parallel to the degree of increase in levels of alkaline phosphatase (AP) and serve as an estimate for the level of the hepatic isoenzyme of AP
2. Neoplastic or granulomatous hepatic infiltrates to levels greater than ten times the upper limit of the normal range. GGT is a more sensitive detector of hepatic metastases
3. All diseases with hepatic involvement of lesser magnitude (e.g., hepatitis, biliary tract disease, cirrhosis), with early and persistent increases as long as cellular damage exists
4. Alcohol ingestion and are elevated before AST levels. Usually elevated in 75 percent of all chronic alcoholics
5. Patients receiving certain drugs (e.g., phenytoin [Dilantin], phenobarbital), possibly because of induction of the microsomal enzyme system by such drugs
6. Neonates to rather high levels. The cause is unknown, thus not useful in diagnosis
7. Mild to moderate amounts in renal disease and congestive heart failure
8. Congestive heart failure

GGT LEVELS NORMAL IN:

- Metabolic or bone disease. The test is therefore useful in differentiating bone disease from hepatobiliary disease when the AP concentration is increased

9.4.4 Serum Ammonia

Synonyms: NH_4, plasma ammonia

Normal Range: 0–150 µg N (nitrogen)/dl (values with plasma are somewhat lower than with serum)

Explanation of the Test. The ammonia found in the blood is derived primarily from bacterial action on nitrogen-containing materials such as food in the intestine. Some ammonia comes from the kidney, from hydrolysis of glutamine—a temporary storage substance for ammonia. Blood ammonia is presumed to be in transit to the liver, where it is synthesized to urea. Elevations do not usually occur without some degree of hepatic failure, causing shunting of portal blood past the liver and impaired hepatic parenchymal function.

Patient Preparation

1. Patient should be kept n.p.o. other than water for 8 to 12 hours before the test
2. Patient activity should be minimized. Blood should not be drawn after vigorous muscular activity
3. Ammonia is highly unstable. The blood sample must be iced and tested immediately

NH LEVELS INCREASED IN:

1. Some instances of hepatic cirrhosis because of impaired hepatocyte function and shunting of the blood past the liver secondarily to congestion and portal hypertension
2. Some instances of hepatitis as a result of incomplete removal of ammonia because of defective urea synthesis
3. GI bleeding, usually from esophageal varices, that is associated with hepatic cirrhosis because of an increased load of ammonia being delivered to a compromised liver
4. Severe heart failure, or cor pulmonale, because of hepatic congestion and possible hepatic damage
5. Metabolic acidosis with renal failure, or azotemia, because of decreased excretion of renal hydrogen
6. Reye's syndrome as a result of diffuse hepatic dysfunction with peculiar accumulation of microvacuoles of fat (may be virally induced)
7. Stored blood, which may reach five to ten times normal ammonia levels. The use of such blood, especially in large volumes, is particularly dangerous in liver disease

9.4.5 Hepatitis Tests

A. Hepatitis A IgM

Synonyms: Anti-HAV; anti HA; Hep antibody IgM; IgM anti-HAV; Hep-A AB antibody (McCance & Huether, 1990, p. 1245)

Normal Response: Negative (usually requires 2–4 days for report) (Laboratory of Pathology, 1991)

Type of Test. Serological, competitive binding.

Patient Preparation. None.

Discussion. Hepatitis A occurs epidemically with multiple outbreaks (known in the past as epidemic hepatitis). It occurs most frequently in children and young adults and is caused by an

RNA enterovirus (genome single-strand RNA).* The condition is often so mild, and the duration so short (as brief as 2 weeks prodromal; 2 weeks after peak abnormal enzyme levels) that the diagnosis of hepatitis can easily be overlooked unless testing is done. It is not known to cause a chronic hepatitis, but a fulminant form of hepatitis A develops in a very small number of cases (0.1 percent) and is often fatal. There is no known prevention or known carrier states.

Transmission. Transmission is via fecal/oral routes or a common oral source such as contaminated food or water; it is rarely a source of posttransfusion hepatitis.

Diagnosis. The presence of Hep. A antibody IgM (IgM anti-HAV) confirms the diagnosis of a *recent* acute infection of the hepatitis A virus. Presence of total antibodies to hepatitis A (IgM anti-HAV and IgG anti-HAV) does not discriminate between active disease and immunity resulting from past infection. IgM antibodies disappear within 6 months; IgG antibodies last for many years and provide immunity to reinfection.

Testing. An antigen to the hepatitis A virus is always present during the course of the disease. The Hep-A antibody (anti-HAV) produced by Hep-A antigen Ig is detectable with the onset of hepatitis A symptoms and rises rapidly. Early in the infectious state the antigen for the hepatitis A virus (anti-HAV) is produced entirely by this IgM antibody at very high levels. Thereafter, anti-HAV IgG antigen levels rise as IgM levels decrease. Usually IgM antibodies disappear within 6 months of infection (a range of 3 to 12 months). IgG may be detectable for months, years, often a lifetime, providing protection from reinfection. However, both antigens *can* be totally absent from the blood in 3 to 6 months, although such an event is the exception. Of the two antigens, only the presence of anti-HAV IgM can distinguish acute infection from previous infection. There is no carrier state in hepatitis A.

B.1 Hepatitis B Surface Antigen

Synonyms: HBsAg; hepatitis B associated antigen (HBAg, HAA); serum hepatitis antigen; Australia antigen (AA)

Normal Response: Negative (may require 2–4 days for report)

Type of Test. Serological, RIA using monoclonal IgM anti-HBs to detect hepatitis surface antigen.

Patient Preparation. None.

Discussion. Disease process: Hepatitis B (hep. B) is caused by a DNA virus (hepadnavirus) and has a long incubation period. It is more prevalent and much more contagious than AIDS.

HBsAg, a protein envelope found on the outside of the virus (which is thought to be the "Dane particle") is the first serological marker of hepatitis B to appear after infection. It is pre-

---

*A genome is the complete set of hereditary factors contained in the set of 46 chromosomes. Somatic cells (diploid cells) have a pair of each chromosomal characteristic of a species. A gamete is referred to as a haploid, having only one member of each chromosomal pair.

sent (positive) for 2 weeks to 2 months before symptoms occur (Price & Wilson, 1992, p. 349). Chronic fatigue may be the initial symptom. The disease is infectious as long as HBsAg or HBeAg (see 6.4.5.B.3) is present in the blood, which may be months or years. These factors make it the most important follow-up serological test in hepatitis B. Retesting at 3 months and again at 6 months can determine if the person has become a carrier (5 to 10 percent of adults who have the acute disease become carriers in the western hemisphere [Aach, 1992, p. 38]). It is found only in the blood, not in stool.

The infection can become chronic (approximately 20 percent of patients), which may result in an asymptomatic carrier state or chronic active hepatitis (Aach, 1992, p. 35) with potential for sequelae of cirrhosis or hepatocellular cancer. These last are more frequently found in endemic areas such as Asia and Africa and in immunocompromised individuals (Bonacini, 1991, p. 125). A carrier is usually defined as one in whom HBsAg persists for more than 6 months (Price & Wilson, 1992, p. 349).

Transmission. Transmission is predominantly parenteral via blood, blood products (transfusion hepatitis), mucous secretions, and transplacentally. A recent study showed that anal intercourse is a risk factor for HBV in women (Rosenblum et al., 1992, p. 2481).

Diagnosis. Presence of recent infection with hepatitis B virus is confirmed by HBsAg's presence in the blood. It *may* be negative because of early loss of the antigen, in which case the presence of IgM anti-HBc (core antibody) will confirm the diagnosis (Wilson, 1992, p. 4).

There are three distinct antigen–antibody systems associated with hepatitis B: the surface (HBsAg), the core (HBcAg) and the "e" (HBeAg), along with the individual antibody. *Early* diagnosis depends on antigen measurement. Presence of antibodies (anti-HBs) can be delayed for weeks, months, and, in rare cases, up to 1 year, at times even after the antigen clears from the plasma. Development of antibodies indicates recovery and immunity. Continued presence of antigen may indicate a carrier state. A better test for carrier state is HbeAg, the presence of which indicates chronic active hepatitis (Laboratory of Pathology, 1991).

B.2 Hepatitis B Surface Antibody

Synonyms: Anti-HBs; Australian antibody (AA); antibody to hepatitis surface antigen; HB

Normal Response: Negative

Type of Test. Serological radiometricassay indicating antibody levels

Patient Preparation. None.

Discussion. Development of this antibody is usually delayed for several weeks, months, or 1 year after the antigen (HBsAg) disappears from the plasma. Individuals who have been immunized against hepatitis B demonstrate positive anti-HBs as well, but the pattern differs from that of natural immunity. Natural immunity usually develops both anti-HBs *and* anti-HBc markers (Aach, 1992, p. 38).

Diagnosis. Development of anti-HBs indicates a recent infection and recovery from the hepatitis B infection. The individual is no longer infectious to others and is immune to any future hepatitis B infection (Laboratory of Pathology, 1991).

B.3 Hepatitis Be Antigen and Antibody

Synonyms: Antibody: anti-E; anti-HBe
Antigen: HBeAg

Normal Response: Negative for both antigen and antibody

Type of Test. Serological solid-phase RIA.

Patient Preparation. None.

Discussion. Found only in individuals with hepatitis B infection, that is, only HBsAg-positive persons (Burdash & Fernandes, 1992, p. 1037).

Hepatitis Be Antigen (HBeAg). HBeAg is considered a marker of high infectivity and is present in individuals only during acute hepatitis B virus (HBV) infection or during the early phase of chronic hepatitis. Thus, its presence and rate of increase are useful in determining the infectivity or transmissibility of the virus. It is present during the early stages of the disease, following the rise in HBsAg (see 6.4.5.B.1), and increases rapidly as the virus replicates itself. The rise provides information about the risk of viral transmission to others. *Chronic active hepatitis* is indicated by the persistence of HBeAg in the hepatitis-B carrier 6 months after infection.

Hepatitis Be Antibody (Anti-HBe). Anti-HBe begins to appear as the HBeAg level decreases, indicating decrease in viral replication and, usually, resolution of the disease process. Antibody to HBeAg (anti-HBe) when found in carriers generally indicates lower infectivity and disease remission (Burdash & Fernandes, 1992, p. 1037).

B.4 Hepatitis B Core Antibody

Synonym: Anti-HBc

Normal Response: Negative

Type of Test. Serological, competitive binding.

Patient Preparation. None.

Discussion. Hepatitis B core antibody is the inner shell, or core, of protein that surrounds the nucleic acid of the hepatitis B virus ("Dane" particle?) (Laboratory of Pathology, 1991). It does not become available for testing until 12 through 20 weeks after exposure. Its appearance often accompanies or shortly follows the appearance of hepatitis B antigen in the blood (anti-genemia).

It is also thought to be produced in response to the active replication of the virus as its presence is also associated with prolonged circulation of HBsAg (hepatitis surface antigen) and is the hallmark of ongoing HBV infection.

Diagnosis. The presence of IgM anti-HBc indicates convalescence or recent infection rather than immunity (Aach, 1992, p. 37). It can also be used to gauge the course of HBV infection, along with the appearance or disappearance of HBsAg, anti-HBs, and HBc (Laboratory of Pathology, 1991). During acute infection HBsAg may be undetectable, producing the so-called window effect. During this period, testing for antibody to core antigen of the B virus (anti-HBc) is used to identify the presence of the virus (Burdahs & Fernandes, 1992, p. 1037).

C. Hepatitis C

Synonym: Previously called Non-A, Non-B (NANB) hepatitis

Normal Response: Negative

Tests available: Serological

1. HCV enzyme immunoassay (HCV EIA) (Laboratory of Pathology, 1991)
2. Anti-HCV enzyme-linked immunoassay (ELISA) (Conn, 1991, p. 731), multiantigen (Aach, 1992, pp. 45–46)
3. Recombinant immunoblot assay (RIBA), the most advanced clinical test available, primarily used as confirmatory test for a positive ELISA (Kucera, 1992, p. 20). (The RIBA test is most specific but does not distinguish active from chronic or inactive infection. It confirms exposure with fewer false positives or negatives than other tests ["Hepatitis C: A Potential Perinatal Menace," 1992].
4. The polymerase chain reaction (PCR) test detects the HCV genome RNA as well as active Hep-C viremia (Kucera, 1992, p. 21)

Patient Preparation. None.

Incidence. Ninety percent of cases of posttransfusion hepatitis have been found to be related to HCV. HCV also accounts for 25 percent of nontransfusion-associated hepatitis in the United States, making it fairly common (Henry, 1991, p. 1253).

Transmission. Parenteral. HCV is primarily blood-borne, especially via drug abuse (Aach, 1992, p. 46), but it has also been found to spread through sexual contact (Price & Wilson, 1992, p. 350). The risk of perinatal transmission is unknown but thought to be considerable ("Hepatitis C: A Potential Perinatal Menace," 1992, pp. 231–32).

Diagnosis. Seroconversion doesn't usually occur during the symptomatic phase of this disease, making diagnosis difficult (Kucera, 1992, p. 22). The disease itself is often inapparent, without any noted jaundice or other specific signs or symptoms (Conn, 1991, p. 731).

Antibodies to HCV usually appear in serum between the first and the fourth month after exposure, but it can appear as late as 12 months (Kucera, 1992, p. 21) or may not appear at all in patients with acute, resolving infection (Conn, 1992, p. 732). Once developed, antibodies to HCV (Anti-HCV) persist up to 12 years (Aach, 1992, p. 46).

Discussion. Identification of HCV (an RNA virus of the flavivirus group) required major advances in molecular-biological cloning techniques. There are a significant number of false positives even when one uses the ELISA test.

Symptoms vary widely and may be related to the severity of the hepatic inflammation and fibrosis. Frequent physical complaints include fatigue, fever, abdominal pain, pleurisy, dermatosis (skin disorder not characterized by inflammation), arthralgias, amenorrhea, and/or chronic diarrhea. Hepatomegaly, splenomegaly, jaundice (recurring or persistent), and a variety of signs or symptoms indicating cirrhosis (e.g., ascites, spider angiomas) are also found (Kucera, 1992, p. 21).

About 50 percent of HCV infections are likely to develop chronic liver disease. This progression is not predictable as yet, but aminotransferase has been found to increase, as it does in all chronic liver disease.

It has been suggested that supplemental testing be done on all positive screening tests, especially since treatment is available for hepatitis C ("Sees Much Room for Improvement in Hepatitis C Detection, Care," 1992).

Chronic carrier state development has been at a greater than 50 percent level (Conn, 1991, p. 731).

D. Hepatitis D Antibody

Synonyms: Hepatitis delta antibody; anti-HD virus (anti-HDV)

Normal Response: Negative

Type of Test. Serological, antibody assay.

Patient Preparation. None.

Incidence. Hepatitis D virus (HDV) causes infection only in persons with coexisting acute or chronic hepatitis B and who are HBsAg positive (see Section 6.4.5.B.1). HDV is found most frequently in the blood of intravenous (IV) (parenteral) drug abusers, but it can also be found in patients with hemophilia.

Transmission. Parenteral.

Diagnosis. The HBV-infected individual who is HBsAg positive can, and *must*, be tested for the presence of antibodies to HDV (Burdash & Fernandes, 1992, p. 1037). Other populations that should be tested include any individual with known HBV infection who is at risk for hepatitis D (see Incidence) and who develops acute hepatitis that cannot be serologically identified as hepatitis A. Diagnosis can also be made by liver biopsy (Laboratory of Pathology, 1991).

Discussion. HDV, or delta agent, is a defective/incomplete RNA virus that requires the presence of the outer shell of the hepatitis B surface antigen (HBsAg) to replicate. As a consequence, HDV causes infection only as coinfector. Only individuals positive for HsAg are infected by HDV (Aach, 1992, p. 50).

E. Hepatitis E

Synonyms: Hepatitis E virus, HEV; enteric non-A, non-B hepatitis

Normal Response: Negative

Transmission. Fecal/oral.

Discussion. An enteric non-A, non-B virus originating in Asia but now found in the western hemisphere and now called hepatitis E virus appears to account for some cases of hepatitis that cannot be attributed to any of the known viral agents. Only indirect evidence exists to support its existence, but the subject is under study. The HEV appears to occur only in the acute infection state. Testing is not yet available (Henry, 1991, p. 240). Antigen and antibody responses have been identified (HEVag, anti-HEV), as has the viral marker, calcivirus, which is made up of viruslike particles (Burdash & Fernandes, 1992, pp. 1037–38).

Further *potential* human hepatitis viruses are also being investigated, such as hepatitis F (a non-HCV form of parenteral, non-A, non-B hepatitis [NANBNC]) and hepatitis G (a paramyxovirus infection with severe hepatitis)(Wilson, 1992, p. 2).

F. Hepatitis Screen

Synonyms: Includes hepatitis A antibody-IgM specific; hepatitis B surface antibody; hepatitis B surface antigen; hepatitis B core antibody

Normal Response: Negative

Purpose. With clinical symptoms that are not diagnostically specific, the screen is used to identify the type of hepatitis and the stage of the disease process. Hepatitis A antibody identifies *recent* infection with hepatitis A. Hepatitis B surface antigen diagnoses *recent* hepatitis B infection. Hepatitis B core antibody identifies HBV in the convalescent stage and may be positive after the antigen is negative. Hepatitis B surface antibody can identify an HBV infection after both the antigen and core antibody to hepatitis B have been found negative (Laboratory of Pathology, 1991).

IMPLICATIONS FOR NURSING: Hepatitis

1. Nosocomial transmission prevention:
   a. Spring-loaded fingerstick devices for test blood sampling must be properly disinfected between uses. The device platform, the lancet, and the worker's gloves must also be changed between patients. If practical, a separate device for use with each individual is ideal. Protection of both patient and nurse requires these preventative steps.

The mandate applies universally in high-risk situations (as with known hepatitis infections) as well as any testing of "well" populations

b. Reinforce the importance of personal and environmental hygiene with the patient, family, or significant others

2. Teaching:

a. Hepatitis A: In caring for the client with hepatitis A, it is important that information about safe sex and the process of the disease be clarified and reinforced

   (1) Incidence of Hepatitis A has risen in the homosexual population, possibly because of confusion about the safety of oral-anal sexual contact. Clarify the client's understanding about transmission of hepatitis A (i.e., fecal/oral) and that there is no protection in anal or oral sex

   (2) Supply information related to:

       (a) The infective periods of the disease (i.e., during late incubation, early acute illness phases, and, usually, ending by the time jaundice occurs, if it does) (Aach et al., 1992, p. 34)

       (b) The appearance of hepatitis A IgG antibody (IgG anti-HAV) about 6 to 12 months after resolution of the acute stage appears to confer lifelong immunity

       (c) Passive prophylaxis is recommended for people who have had close personal contact with the infected individual (standard immunoglobulin) within 2 weeks of exposure (e.g., all household contacts)

   (3) Preventative immunoglobulin prophylaxis is also recommended for people planning to travel in hepatitis A endemic areas, especially if a prolonged stay is planned (several months) or if traveling out of usual "tourist" areas

   (4) In the rare instance of fulminant hepatitis A, protein restriction helps prevent increased hepatitis encephalopathy; other medications are used to control hepatic coma (e.g., lactulose) (Aach, 1992, p. 37)

b. Hepatitis B

   (1) Laboratory indicators of resolution of hepatitis B and full recovery include:

       (a) Transaminase values within normal limits

       (b) Negative tests for HBsG

       (c) Appearance of anti-HB (the major protective mechanism for persons who have had hepatitis B), an indicator of lifelong immunity

   (2) Prevention:

       (a) Condom use and avoidance of intercourse during menstruation or when intermenstrual bleeding occurs are of major preventative importance with known or suspected carriers

       (b) Because hepatitis B is easier to prevent than it is to treat, *all* people at risk (exposure to blood or body fluids; occupation; lifestyle) should be vaccinated. People at risk include:

           • All pregnant women and infants (with special precautions for infants born to HBsAg-positive mothers. Immediately after birth the infant should receive hepatitis B immunoglobulin, followed by the vaccine)

           • All HIV-positive patients

           • Anyone practicing unprotected sex

       (c) A series of three doses of vaccine (in the *deltoid* muscle) will afford protection in more than 90 percent of those immunized

   (3) Other immunization recommendations:

       (a) The special precaution of routine serological testing after immunization is only recommended if:

           • The vaccine was given in the gluteus maximus rather than in the deltoid muscle

           • The person is over 50 years of age

           • The person is at a high risk of exposure

       (b) Check the immunity pattern:

           • After deltoid immunization a positive anti-HBs (surface) marker appears, indicating immunity

           • Natural immunity is indicated by the presence of both anti-HBs and anti-HBc (core) markers (Aach, 1992, p. 38)

       (c) Cost may be a negative factor for many who need immunization, which as of this writing, is $150 for the series of three for an adult and $60 for a child. The effects of the disease and the expense of care, treatment, lost time at work can be more costly and should be pointed out

Immunization is strongly recommended for those at risk. However, some 30 percent of cases come from groups not obviously at risk. A small drop of contaminated blood can contain billions of particles, and contaminated blood can spread easily among children through simple rough play.

There have been an estimated 200,000 to 300,000 new cases of Hepatitis B a year. Only one drug (interferon alfa-2B) has been approved to date for treatment, and little is known about its long-term effects (Hepatitis B: The Sneaky Virus, 1992, p. 9)

    (4) History taking: Areas to be explored to help identify individuals at risk for hepatitis B include:

        (a) Chronic recipients of blood products

        (b) Presence or history of multiple tattoos/acupuncture

        (c) Health care workers

        (d) Past history of other risk factors

- Previous hepatitis
- IV drug abuse
- Mental handicap (risk increased in institutionalized)
- History of or documented sexually transmitted disease (multiple diseases?) (Bonacine, 1991, p. 125; Mangle et al, 1992, p. 51)

c. Hepatitis C

    (1) Identified risk factors include IV drug abuse; reception of blood products; alcohol abuse or dependence; sexual intercourse with infected partner ("Sees Much Room for Improvement in Hepatic C Detection, Care," 1992)

    (2) Laboratory data of importance: elevated liver enzymes, (i.e., ALT, AST, gamma-glutamyl transpeptidase (GGT); serum alkaline phosphatase) ("Sees Much Room for Improvement in Hepatic C Detection, Care," 1992)

    (3) *Chronic* hepatitis C has been treated experimentally with recombinant alfa interferon with clinical improvement in all of the 10 controlled trials over a 2-month treatment period. Treatment is usually recommended, and the possibility should be explored. There were variable relapses in each trial with a mean of 57 percent among the total group. Acceptable side effects include fatigue, fever, chills, myalgia, arthalgias, anorexia, nausea, insomnia, and difficulty concentrating. Treatment was stopped with evidence of bone marrow (neutrophil and platelet) suppression, infection, autoimmune disorders, or psychiatric response (Wilson, 1992, p. 13)

3. Generalities related to care of the hepatitis patient:

  a. If a diagnosis has not been established, or if there is a question concerning a differential diagnosis between a viral infection and alcoholic hepatitis, some laboratory findings can be helpful

    (1) In acute *viral* hepatitis the AST to ALT ratio is usually less than 1

    (2) In *alcoholic* hepatitis the ratio is often greater than 2, and peak aminotransferase levels are rarely over 500 U/l

  b. Plan nursing care to avoid any unnecessary needle sticks or bruising because of the increased bleeding tendency in individuals with any liver disease

  c. Especially during, but also after, the acute stage of illness, hydration and nutrition are major concerns in nursing care because of the presence of anorexia, nausea, vomiting, and the probable onset of aversion to some foods, as well as the inability to digest or retain others

    (1) Diet should be high in calories and protein, low in fat, and based on patient preference as much as possible. Consult with dietician and see that the patient or home caretaker learn how to plan meals and assess adequacy of intake

    (2) Frequent small feedings are preferable as they are more readily retained and absorbed

    (3) In the adult, an oral fluid intake goal of 3,500 ml/24 hr should be maintained if consistent with the patient's overall condition (e.g., no cardiovascular difficulties). Keep 24-hour intake and output records

  d. Use adequate measures to prevent fatigue, yet promote muscle strength and safety

  e. Provide the family or caretakers with specific information in writing for home care, based on the patient's actual or expected stamina and physical strength at the time of discharge

  f. Review and reinforce information related to the prevention of the spread of hepatic infection to family or friends or a reinfection of the patient, necessary at the time of discharge and consistent with the type of hepatitis involved

g. Keep informed on related laboratory findings daily in order to monitor the disease status as well as possible complications and total health of the patient. Tests of value include ALT(SGPT), AST(SGOT) (Section 9.4.2), AP (Section 1.12.1); serum bilirubin (Section 1.10); serum albumin (Section 1.9.1); and urine urobilinogen (Section 9.5.3). Liver cell dysfunction can affect clotting mechanisms; therefore, follow laboratory findings related to prothrombin time (PT) or partial thromboplastin time (PTT) (Section 3.5) for prolonged bleeding potential, and carefully assess for petechiae and increased bleeding (e.g., postinjection)

h. Be aware of potential for altered mentation or other indicators of liver cell necrosis, and include mentation status in daily assessment

4. NURSING DIAGNOSES (active disease stage)*

a. Pain, discomfort related to inflammation, enlargement of the liver

b. Altered nutritional status, less than body requirements, related to:

(1) Decreased liver metabolism of nutrients

(2) Decreased intake of nutrients due to nausea, vomiting, or anorexia

c. Activity intolerance related to:

(1) Inadequate nutritional status

(2) Increased metabolic rate secondary to infectious process

(3) Early fatigue (see items a and b)

(4) Pain secondary to inflamed and or enlarged liver

d. Alteration in body image related to:

(1) Activity intolerance

(2) Possible jaundice

(3) Potential restrictions or changes in life-style (e.g., sexual practices, drug or alcohol use, diet alterations)

(4) Prolonged inability to function as a well person

(5) Possible sense of guilt related to cause(s) of illness

*Adapted from Lewis & Collier, 1992, pp. 1128–29

9.5 TESTS OF GALLBLADDER FUNCTION

9.5.1 Laboratory and Clinical Indications of Gallbladder Dysfunction

Laboratory Findings. In many cases the findings are very similar to dysfunction of the liver; many liver function test results may be abnormal: increased total bilirubin, increased direct conjugated fraction most frequently; increased WBCs to 12,000 to 15,000 mm^3 in acute cholecystitis; increased AP levels; possibly increased SAST (SGOT) levels; bilirubinuria.

Clinical Findings. Clinical gallbladder dysfunction findings include possible jaundice; right upper quadrant pain/tenderness, which may be first noted by awareness of decreased respiratory excursion; with acute cholecystitis, possible vomiting and a slight temperature elevation that can progress to a marked elevation with chills and fever spikes; and chronic cholecystitis, dyspepsia, intolerance of fatty foods, heart burn. There should be an increased index of suspicion if these symptoms occur in a fair, fat, fortyish female.

9.5.2 Visualization Tests

At present specific diagnostic tests for gallbladder dysfunction tend to fall more in the field of x-ray or other visualizing diagnostic methods. The reader is urged to check any complete medical-surgical text or other laboratory texts for information on endoscopy. Chapter 17 in this text

(Diagnostic Modalities) gives fairly complete coverage of many of the other diagnostic tests used in gallbladder dysfunctions.

9.5.3 Urobilinogen, Urine and Fecal

Synonyms: Mesobilirubinogen, stercobilinogen

Normal Ranges

Urine	
2 hr	0–1.0 EU (Ehrlich units)/2 hr
24 hr	0.5–4.0 EU/24 hr
	(values of 5–10 are borderline)
Fecal	75–275 EU/100 g

Explanation of the Test. The urobilinogens (mesobilirubin, stercobilinogen, and urobilinogen) are formed by reduction of bilirubin and released as bile into the intestinal tract. The vast majority of the urobilinogen formed is excreted in the feces. A smaller portion is reabsorbed into the portal circulation (see Fig. 1–3, Bilirubin Metabolism) and is excreted into the urine. The major portion is extracted by the liver cells and is again excreted as bile. Increases in direct, conjugated bilirubin levels will increase the amounts excreted into feces and urine. Increases in indirect, unconjugated bilirubin levels, when due to the breakdown of RBCs only, as in hemolytic disease, increase fecal urobilinogen levels only. Other increases in indirect, unconjugated bilirubin levels cause an increased production of conjugated bilirubin, ultimately increasing urobilinogen levels in both urine and feces.

Patient Preparation. No special preparation is necessary.

CHANGES IN UROBILINOGEN LEVELS

Condition	Urine Urobilinogen	Fecal Urobilinogen
Hemolytic anemia	Normal	Increased markedly
Biliary obstruction	Decreased markedly	Decreased markedly
Liver parenchymal disease	Increased	Normal or slightly decreased

9.6 STOOL EXAMINATIONS*

9.6.1 Fecal Occult Blood Test: A Preliminary Screening Test

Synonyms: FOBT; Hemoccult

Normal Reaction: Hemoccult, negative
HemeQuant, 0.10–2.67 mg/g of stool

---

*See also steatorrhea listing in the index and Sections 5.1.2, "Specimen Collections," item b; 17.2.5, "Barium Enema"; 17.2.7, "Cholecystograms/Cholangiograms"; and 17.2.10, "Upper Gastrointestinal Series."

Explanation of the Test. Blood is not a normal constituent of stool. Frank blood, visible to the naked eye, may be present with hemorrhoids or anal fissures. Occult (hidden) blood in the stool can only be "seen" through testing. It can be suspected with a stool color change to a very dark brown or black. Hemoglobin causes this color change; however, there are many other substances that will also cause a dark, "tarry" stool such as large quantities of raw green vegetables, rare red meat, numerous root and "flower" vegetables (e.g., carrots, red radishes, parsnips, potatoes, turnips, Jerusalem artichokes, cabbage, cauliflower) as well as many fruits. Oral medications such as iron also darken the stool.

Hemoglobin entering the alimentary tract is attacked by digestive enzymes and bacterial degradation, which converts it to protoporphyrins; this gives a negative reaction on testing for peroxidase activity, the basis for guaiac testing. However, inhibitory substances appear to be present in the stool that make such testing possible. The peroxidaselike enzymatic activity of the hemoglobin, or hematin, is what causes the positive response in the Hemoccult test. The HemeQuant test reacts not only to heme but also identifies the fraction of heme already converted to porphyrin during fecal transit; therefore it is felt to be a more sensitive measure of GI bleeding. Although Hemoccult testing is less sensitive and less likely to have false-positive reactions, it is also more likely to miss lesions of the right side of the colon since it does not identify degraded heme (porphyrin).

Purpose of the Test. The age-specific risk for colon or rectal cancer, as presented by Nord (1992, p. 243), indicates that the risk becomes consistently greater with age, approximately 0.06 percent at age 50, 3 percent at age 70, and 5 percent at age 80. He also reports that individuals with a positive fecal occult blood test have only a 0.2 percent risk of colorectal carcinoma and a 0.7 percent risk of polyp formation in the following 2 years. However, more than 50 percent of lesions are undetected if only fecal occult blood testing is done. Checking the stool for occult blood is one of the major, first screening tests recommended for early colorectal neoplasia, a matter of continued interest. Any cause of GI bleeding will, of course, produce positive results if there is sufficient blood and if the testing procedure is carefully selected. The most frequently used test, at present, is the guaiac-impregnated filter paper slide, sold under many brand names. The most used of these slides is the Hemoccult II.

METHODS TO IMPROVE TEST RESULT ACCURACY WITH HEMOCCULT II:

1. Extend the testing period. At present testing of persons considered at risk is done over a period of 3 days; it is recommended that the tests be done over a 6-day period
2. Increase the number of samples tested from each stool. No truly optimal number of samples has been determined, but two will measurably increase the likelihood of finding occult blood. (The Hemoccult II test slide provides for two samples to be tested from different areas of each stool)
3. Cover the *full* test area with fecal sample
4. Store the test slides in a cool (not refrigerated), dry, and dark area. (Rehydration of the slide sample was found to increase the sensitivity of the test but also produce more false-positive test results, so it is not recommended)

COLORECTAL SCREENING RECOMMENDATIONS (HOPKINS, 1984)

Digital rectal examination	After age 40, every year
Hemoccult slides	After age 50, every year
Sigmoidoscopy	After age 50, every 3 years after two consecutive annual
(flexible only)	negative exams

Self-testing. With minimal instruction, individuals in need of frequent stool testing, especially at home, are able to make their own stool slides and, when necessary and with more specific instruction, may also be able to read their own slides and report their findings to the physician. The importance of total population screening with this test has become a national issue, and testing materials are available through health departments, hospital outpatient departments, and individual physicians' offices as well as sold in pharmacies.

Procedure (For Patient-Administered Test)

1. Making a slide
   a. Collect a small stool sample on the end of an applicator stick
      (1) The sample should be taken from an inner portion of the stool. This requires that the stool be collected in a container rather than discharged into the toilet. (Check with a pharmacy or physician's office for a plastic liner "hat" that fits under the toilet seat)
      (2) With no history of frank rectal bleeding the sample can be collected from toilet paper used to cleanse the rectum if a large, intact specimen can be collected
      (3) Apply a *thin* smear *covering* the small box on the slide. (If there are two such boxes, two samplings from different sections of the stool should be done)
   b. Close the cover, and either do the testing or return the test slide to the physician for testing. Protect it from heat and return it as soon as possible if it is a Hemoccult slide (see "Purpose of Test," earlier in this section)
2. Preparing and reading the test
   a. Open the flap on the back of the slide
   b. Place a watch with a second hand in easy sight
   c. Place two drops of developer fluid directly on the stool smear area
   d. Start timing immediately for 60 seconds
   e. Check the slide for color change at exactly 60 seconds. If positive, the test area will turn blue. If the full area has not been covered, note especially whether the space between the stool and edge is also blue
   f. If the slide has "Performance Monitors," place *one* drop of developer fluid on each opening. One (the positive monitor) should turn blue; the other (the negative monitor) should not change. If this does not occur, the solution is no longer usable and should be replaced and the stool retested

FALSE-NEGATIVE RESULTS DUE TO (RELATIVELY UNCOMMON; HEMOCCULT TEST ONLY; NONE WITH HEMEQUANT):

1. Blood ununiformly distributed throughout the stool and samples taken from non-bloody areas. Bleeding from the left side of the colon causes this inconsistent pattern especially (Gnauck et al., 1984, p. 137)

2. Bleeding inconsistent or not persistent, even with the largest cancers of the colon
3. Blood not accessible for sampling, as in a very constipated stool

FALSE-POSITIVE RESULTS DUE TO (HEMOCCULT):

- Ingestion of different compounds with high peroxidase contents such as vegetables, meat, iron tablets, vitamin C, cimetidine and nonsteroidal antiinflammatory agents. (See "Explanation of the Test," this section, second paragraph)

FALSE-POSITIVE RESULTS DUE TO (HEMEQUANT):

1. Dry stool
2. Consumption of aspirin
3. Ingestion of red meat

9.6.2 Ova and Parasites—Stool

Synonyms: Stool for parasites, O&P, rule out giardiasis

Normal Findings: No ova or parasites[a]

[a]Ova and parasite testing is also done on sputum and gastric contents.

Explanation of the Test. Many parasitic infections are "silent" or produce only mild symptoms. Half of all human parasitic infections can be diagnosed through a stool examination (Fischbach, 1984, p. 370) because they inhabit the GI tract. Very few protozoa that infest humans cause clinical problems, but almost all worm infestations cause disease states. Two organisms are most responsible for diarrhea states related to parasites in the United States: *Giardia lamblia* and *Entamoeba histolytica*. *Giardia lamblia* (not an officially reportable disease) is probably the most frequently occurring of the two. Amebiasis, caused by *Entamoeba histolytica*, is a more severe disease. Both organisms are resistant to gastric acidity, and their cysts or trophozoites can be found in various areas of the GI tract (e.g., *Giardia* cysts are found in stool specimens). The major symptom of both conditions is diarrhea or foul-smelling, bulky stools (Heitkemper & Martin, 1986, p. 1216).

Purpose of the Test. The O&P test is used to make a differential diagnosis as to the cause of protracted diarrhea with the aforementioned characteristics.

Significant Findings

1. Trophozoites of *Entamoeba histolytica*
2. Cysts of *Giardia lamblia*
3. Presence of helminth larvae, ova, or proglottids
4. *Iodamoeba bütschlii* and *Endolimax nana* (recently associated with a diarrheal disease)
5. Large numbers of *Cryptosporidium* and *Blastocytis hominis* if other organisms have been ruled out

6. *Cryptosporidium* has been associated with diarrhea in immunocompromised hosts (Laboratory of Pathology, 1991)

Sample Collection

1. Fresh, warm, nonformed stools are usually required for protozoan screening
2. Examination for helminths (parasitic worms) can be done with formed stool
3. The first stool in the morning is usually preferred
4. *Stool must be delivered to the laboratory in 30 minutes or less after defecation*
5. Collections cups should be filled only one fourth full; cap and keep in an upright position. (Keep the lid clean to protect the laboratory worker)
6. To prevent the spread of infection wear gloves when filling the collection cup or whenever in contact with the stool and wash hands at least on beginning and when ending patient contact
7. For maximum detection of parasites, three nonformed stools should be collected over a 5-day period, every other day
8. Label the sample container with the patient's name, type of test, room number (if hospitalized), physician's name, and the date and time

Patient Preparation

Pretest Assessment. Check whether the patient has received mineral oil, a waxy suppository, or a barium x-ray within the 4 days before this test. If so, notify the laboratory and physician because the test will probably have to be delayed.

Patient Teaching

1. Explain what day(s) the sample(s) will be collected and the preferred time for stool collection, based on the presumed type of infection and laboratory scheduling. Stress the importance of samples being sent to the laboratory *immediately*
2. If a dependent
    a. Explain why anything that might be contaminated with stool is best handled with gloves, both by the patient and the health care worker, and why handwashing is necessary as well
    b. Explain the mechanism for spread of infection and/or reinfection and ways to prevent it
        (1) Wash hands well after any defecation
        (2) Wear disposable gloves whenever there is expectation of contact with stool, bedpan, or toilet seat
        (3) The patient should alert anyone assisting him or her of any bedding or clothing that is soiled by stool so that it may be changed, placed in a laundry bag, and washed as soon as possible
3. If ambulatory and capable of self-care and/or not hospitalized
    a. Provide with or tell where toilet collection containers (hats) are available, and explain how to use it in the toilet for collecting the stool specimen
    b. Inform the person that the collection cup should be filled only one fourth full (more than one sample may be requested) and that it is important to keep the lid clean of any

feces. (Instructions as to amount may vary depending on the laboratory, but keeping the lid clean protects others from contamination)

c. Provide with disposable gloves to use when cleaning self after defecating, collecting fecal samples, and cleaning toilet seat after use, and explain how all this will help protect from reinfection

d. Stress the importance of handwashing after urinating and defecation even with the use of gloves

---

RELATED NURSING DIAGNOSES

These are general diagnoses used in almost all GI disturbances. The signs and symptoms and medical diagnoses provided in parentheses throughout are restricted for the most part to those having to do with the GI system and provide examples only, not the full range of possible causes of the problem. The reader is cautioned to keep in mind that almost all disease has an impact on nutritional status.

Alteration in Nutrition

Less than body requirements, related to

1. Inadequate intake secondary to
   a. Embarrassment, anxiety, fear of pain/discomfort with food intake (dumping syndrome after gastrectomy, overdistention of pouch after stomach stapling, diarrhea with lactase deficiency)
   b. Easy fatigue with activity (long-term nutritional deficit)
   c. Anorexia and nausea (e.g., most people after abdominal surgery, infectious hepatitis, severe pain)
   d. Dislike of or nutritional inadequacies in prescribed diet
   e. Disabilities in the mechanics of mastication, swallowing (extensive, destructive, or long-term facial or oral surgery, oral-facial cancer, postcerebral vascular accidents, lack of dentures, presence of dysphagia)
   f. Eating disorders (anorexia nervosa, anorexia nervosa/bulimia)
2. Inadequate metabolism of nutrients (cirrhosis, pancreatitis, intestinal enzyme deficiencies/lactase deficiency, decreased bile production due to liver disease, or decreased bile excretion due to biliary stones or obstruction of ducts by cancer)
3. Decreased absorption of nutrients due to *decreased* transit time of chyme in the alimentary canal (Crohn's disease, ulcerative colitis, and/or all diarrhea whatever the cause); due to *increased* transit time of chyme in alimentary canal (bowel obstruction, "silent bowel" secondary to trauma [abdominal surgery, penetrating wounds]), and lack of available body water for transport of nutrients (dehydration, third spacing)
4. Increased or long-term actual loss of nutrients (diarrhea and vomiting)

Alteration in Nutrition

Greater than body requirements, related to

1. Increased food intake secondary to
   a. Learned behavior (cultural/family beliefs)
   b. Psychological dependence on food for satisfaction/comfort/stress relief
   c. Psychophysiological basis—inappropriate setting of or damage to satiation center ("set point") in the hypothalamus (brain tumor or head injury) (Lewis & Collier, 1983, p. 1683; Heitkemper & Brubacher, 1986, p. 166; Rakel, 1987, p. 460)
   d. Lack of adequate motivation to decrease food intake
2. Decreased activity level without dietary changes
3. Lack of knowledge of balanced nutritional diet
4. Genetic (developmental) predisposition (childhood obesity secondary to increased number of fat cells in body [hyperplastic obesity, Frölich's syndrome] [Rakel, 1987, p. 460]); adult obesity sec-

ondary to increased amount of fat per cell (hypertrophic obesity) (Heitkemper & Brubacher, 1986, p. 1165; Rakel, 1987)

Potential for Impairment of Skin Integrity Related to

1. Decreased available nutrients (primarily protein) for wound healing, lesion repair (See first diagnosis above)
2. Obesity secondary to reduced vascularity of skin, which retards wound healing; decreased free body movement leading to chafing and/or prolonged weight bearing on pressure points
3. Increased exposure of skin/mucous membranes to irritating or digestive body fluids (ileostomy drainage, diarrhea, bile drainage postcholecystectomy)
4. Itching/scratching of skin due to presence of irritating chemicals in the skin cells (bile backup into blood in cholelithiasis of the biliary tree, increased serum ammonia in hepatic cirrhosis)
5. Lesions of oral mucous membrane (stomatitis, protracted vomiting of stomach acid/duodenal alkali)
6. Loss of protective skin barriers—oil/tissue elasticity (any malnutrition/dehydration)
7. Presence of tissue edema (cirrhosis with third spacing)
8. Increased risk of bruising (thrombocytopenia in hepatic disease)

Potential for Infection Related to

1. Decreased immune competency secondary to
   a. Decrease in salivary immunoglobulin (Crohn's disease [Ulrich, Canale, Wendell, 1986, p. 520])
   b. Decreased available protein for production of WBCs (decreased phagocytosis) and immunoglobulins (decreased cell-mediated immunity)
   c. Decreased movement of WBCs out of the vascular space in stress (increased cortisol levels)
2. Increased mucous membrane and skin fragility (see third diagnosis), decreasing the efficacy of normal barriers to infection
3. Poor wound healing with obesity (see diagnosis concerning skin integrity)
4. Movement of irritating or infective fluids into normally sterile body cavities (transudation with bowel obstruction; rupture of infected appendix, peptic ulcer, or diverticula; blunt abdominal trauma; potential with all bowel resections)

Potential and Actual Activity Intolerance Related to

If actual and *severe*, the diagnosis would be potential for injury (trauma)

1. Physical weakness secondary to a loss of muscle mass (nutritional deficit, decreased activity, see first diagnosis above)
2. Early fatigue with activity secondary to tissue hypoxia due to nutritional anemias (decreased iron/folic acid stores and decreased available vitamin B_{12} in peptic ulcer) or anemias secondary to blood loss due to decreased platelet and fibrinogen production (liver disease) or traumatic bleeding (esophageal or rectal varices, peptic ulcer)
3. Decreased awareness or level of consciousness secondary to impaired oxygenation of brain (anemias, see earlier) or clouded sensorium (increased NH_4 levels with hepatic coma)
4. Depression secondary to prolonged fatigue, lack of any sense of accomplishment, and general discomfort

Alteration in Bowel Elimination

Constipation Related to
1. Marked decrease in physical activity or prolonged immobility
2. Inadequate fluid intake
3. Inadequate intake of dietary fiber
4. Barium (diagnostic testing)
5. Side effects of medications, prescribed or over the counter (narcotics, sedatives, excessive use of laxatives or cathartics)
6. Psychological factors (inadequate toilet facilities, lack of privacy, changes in environment, and/or emotional or physical stress) (Kelley, 1985, pp. 88–89)

Diarrhea Related to

1. Side effects of medications (antibiotic therapy, excessive use of laxatives)
2. Hyperosmolar tube feedings
3. Acute inflammation of the GI tract (diverticulitis, acute flare-ups of chronic inflammations, e.g., gastritis)
4. Chronic inflammation of the GI tract (ulcerative colitis, Crohn's disease)
5. Specific food intolerances or allergies (sprue, celiac disease)
6. Bacterial infections
7. Stress (Kelley, 1985, pp. 91–92)

Fecal Incontinence Related to

1. Weakened anal sphincter (aging)
2. Excessive use of laxatives
3. Altered level of awareness (oversedation, cerebral injury or cerebrovascular accident [CVA], extreme anxiety)
4. Spinal cord injury
5. GI obstruction with rectal oozing (tumor) (Kelley, 1985, p. 95)

T E N

THE RESPIRATORY SYSTEM

RECOGNITION OF RESPIRATORY DYSFUNCTION

Because the functions of the respiratory and cardiovascular systems are so closely connected, what affects one in time usually affects the other. There is, therefore, considerable overlap in the clues indicating a need to investigate the function of these systems.

10.1 LABORATORY AND CLINICAL INDICATIONS OF RESPIRATORY SYSTEM DYSFUNCTION

Laboratory Findings. In blood there may be an increased white blood cell (WBC) count and a slight shift to the left (infectious processes), an increased erythrocyte sedimentation rate, and eosinophilia with allergic processes (with sputum culture, gram-positive organisms such as *Streptococcus pneumoniae* or *Haemophilus influenzae*, and increased WBC count on gross examination). Chronic infections may be accompanied by a normochromic, normocytic anemia. Electrolyte imbalances can occur with chronic obstructive pulmonary disease (COPD) (e.g., decreased potassium and chloride levels; venous CO_2 concentration may increase, which indicates compensation for respiratory acidosis). Polycythemia is secondary to decreased arterial O_2. An increased WBC count without a shift to the left may be found with pulmonary emboli and increased lactic dehydrogenase (LDH) and glutamic-oxaloacetic transaminase (GOT) (aspartate transaminase [AST]) levels. There may be a change in the total protein concentration—it may decrease in chronic disease with a long-term decrease in albumin production or may increase with hypersensitivity pneumonitis because of increased gamma-globulin production. In urine there are changes in pH that depend on the acid-base and compensatory status of the body; changes in volume and specific gravity depend on the effect of pulmonary changes on cardiac action.

Clinical Findings. Clinical findings in respiratory system dysfunction include changes in respirations: increased rate, shallow, gasping; asymmetrical chest movement, use of accessory muscles, chest retraction between the ribs and at the sternal notch—particularly in children—shortness of breath (SOB), pursed lip breathing, complaint of dyspnea, orthopnea, and dyspnea on exertion. Changes in skin color include pallor with chronic anemia, lividity with polycythemia, and cyanosis with cardiac involvement (may not occur if anemia is severe). Changes in the level of consciousness (LOC) can include hyperirritability, decreased attention span, vertigo, increased sleeping during day, and difficulty in arousal. Changes in neuromuscular activity can include hyperreflexia and twitching. Changes in breath sounds can be heard: rales not cleared by a cough, rhonchi, decreased or absence of breath sounds, friction rub, stridor, and wheezing. Cough may be persistent, nonproductive or productive of secretion that may be mucoid or purulent. A barrel chest, hunched shoulders, and sitting positions that support the arms away from the chest may be noted. There may be increased complaints of severe fatigue, which may be picked up in children by their voluntary limitation of activity and squatting to catch their breath. A history of repeated respiratory infections or a family history of COPD may be present.

10.2 BLOOD GASES

10.2.1 Carbon Dioxide, Venous, Serum

Synonyms: Plasma carbon dioxide; CO_2, venous; total CO_2; CO_2 combining power

Normal Range: 23–30 mEq/L

Explanation of the Test. CO_2 is the by-product of cellular aerobic metabolism and is excreted through the lungs. Most often the plasma carbon dioxide test is done as part of a routine screening of serum electrolytes. It provides a reflection of overall acid-base balance and is useful in checking and corroborating arterial blood gases such as those of P_{CO_2} and pH. Venous CO_2 determination is actually an indirect measurement of blood base, specifically bicarbonate (HCO_3). All of the aforementioned test titles are measurements of this value. Although venous HCO_3 can be measured more directly, most commonly it is measured as total CO_2, that is, with the other combined and dissolved CO_2 in the blood. The value reached approximates that of serum HCO_3 very closely because 89 to 90 percent of all CO_2 in serum is in the form of HCO_3. Levels of total CO_2 (measured as HCO_3) are slightly lower in arterial blood.

CO_2 combining power is used less frequently than total CO_2 because the process is more difficult, it excludes the respiratory contribution to the acid-base status, and it is more subject to error.

VENOUS CO$_2$ INCREASED IN:

1. Metabolic alkalosis
2. Compensation of respiratory acidosis secondary to significant respiratory pathology or decreased respiratory rate.

VENOUS CO$_2$ DECREASED IN:

1. Metabolic acidosis
2. Compensation of respiratory alkalosis

10.2.2 Total Arterial and Venous Blood Gases

Synonyms: Arterial blood gases (ABG), venous blood gases (VBG)

Normal Ranges

	Arterial	Venous
pH[a]	7.35–7.45	7.31–7.42
Pco_2 (mm Hg)	35–45	39–55
Po_2 (mm Hg)	80–100	30–50
HCO_3 (mEq/L)	22–29	22–28
O_2 saturation (SaO_2) (%)	95–100	75
		(SvO_2)
Base excess/deficit (mEq/L)	0 ± 2.3	
O_2 content (vol %)	15.0–23.0	11–16
Hb (g/dl)		
Female	12–15	
Male	13–17	

[a]pH range compatible with life, 6.8–7.8.

Explanation of the Tests. The "routine" blood gas test usually includes only the pH, Pco_2, PO_2, and HCO_3, but some laboratories routinely include one or more of the other determinations as well, for example, base excess/deficit (see Table 10–1). The combination of blood gases (arterial) and spirometry is considered adequate for the assessment of most problems in clinical medicine involving the lungs. Arterial blood gas measurements are the most accurate, but venous blood is much more readily attainable. Arterial capillary blood from the finger can be used for pH and Pco_2 determinations when conditions make acquisition of arterial blood too difficult. Such a sample is not acceptable for PO_2 measurement, but in some cases, arterialized capillary blood from an earlobe can be used for PO_2 values. Although arterial blood gases are much preferred for the diagnosis and management of acute disease, venous blood gas samples are often used in conjunction with serum electrolytes in the management of chronic conditions that can be followed on an outpatient basis.

It is important to remember that all factors involved in acid-base balance are in dynamic interchange, attempting to maintain equilibrium. Therefore, the more factors that are known, the better the basis for health care. This includes not only the blood gases but also the clinical history and present signs and symptoms.

Expected Changes in Arterial Acid-Base Factors in Given Conditions

Primary Respiratory Acidosis. Primary respiratory acidosis is due to airway obstruction (severe COPD, severe asthma), neuromuscular disorders (myasthenia gravis, poliomyelitis, amyotrophic lateral sclerosis), and respiratory center depression (trauma, narcotics, sedatives).

Respiratory Acidosis (Carbonic Acid Excess)	pH	Pco_2	HCO_3	Base Excess/Deficit
Acute uncompensated	D	I	N	N
Early compensation	D	I	I	I (excess)
Chronic compensated	N	I	I	I (excess)

(D, decreased from lower limits of norm; I, increased from upper limits of norm; N, within normal limits.)

(continued)

TABLE 10–1. INDIVIDUAL ARTERIAL BLOOD GASES

Substance Tested	Definition	Significance in Interpretation	Compensatory Mechanism and Discussion
pH	From a chemical point of view, it is the expression of the ratio between bicarbonate and carbonic acid: 20:1 = pH of 7.4; an expression of the hydrogen ion (H^+) in the blood	Low values indicate acid state (less than 7.35); high values indicate an alkalotic state (more than 7.45); the body adjusts (compensates) better with slow changes in pH than with rapid ones, which can be fatal; the body cannot tolerate for prolonged periods values beyond the normal range but still compatible with life (extremes compatible with life: 6.8–7.8)	(See Pco_2 and HCO_3 for compensatory mechanism) pH measurement is unreliable in blood drawn more than ½ hr before testing and not refrigerated or in blood allowed to contact ambient air
Pco_2	A measurement of dissolved carbon dioxide's tension (partial pressure[a]) in the blood	CO_2 unites with water in the extracellular fluid (ECF) to form carbonic acid (H_2CO_3); measurement of CO_2 tension is, in effect, measuring the H_2CO_3, its level being directly proportional to H_2CO_3, and it is thus considered an acid (volatile) that indicates lung status; increased Pco_2 = respiratory acidosis; decreased Pco_2 = respiratory alkalosis	The rate and depth of respirations affect the increase or decrease in Pco_2 but are not useful for compensation because the problem is respiratory in primary respiratory acidosis or alkalosis; increased renal secretion and/or reabsorption of H^+ or HCO_3 is the primary compensatory mechanism (see Table 10–2 for the relationship between pH and Pco_2 in primary respiratory disease)
Po_2	A measurement of dissolved oxygen tension in the blood	The partial pressure (pp) of a gas is what determines the force it exerts; the pp of O_2 determines how rapidly and to what extent it can diffuse from the alveoli into the blood and from the blood to body cells; changes in pp can be due to decreased available oxygen and/or decreased available hemoglobin	Oxygen lack is compensated for, to some extent, by an increased rate and depth of breathing; in chronic O_2 lack, red blood cell (RBC) production increases to increase oxygen carring capacity, which causes a secondary polycythemia; usually, O_2 pp is decreased to some degree in all restrictive or obstructive pulmonary disease, depending on the extent and severity of the disease process

(continued)

HCO_3	Bicarbonate; the principle buffer substance in the plasma; calculated from known values of pH and Pco_2 by using the Henderson-Hasselbalch equation or a nomogram based on it	Decrease in HCO_3 levels usually indicates primary base deficit called metabolic acidosis; increase in HCO_3 levels is usually due to a base excess (metabolic alkalosis) in ratio to H^+ available; HCO_3 also increases or decreases as a compensatory response to other imbalances, especially Pco_2	Primary mechanism is respiratory, with excess H^+ being blown off by increased respiratory rate and depth, thereby usually restoring the 20:1 ratio; if not, and given adequate kidney function, compensation for severe acid-base imbalances can usually be achieved by increased kidney tubule secretion or reabsorption of either H^+ and HCO_3
O_2 saturation	A measurement of the amount of O_2 being carried by the hemoglobin; O_2 saturation is the value used when plotting the oxyhemoglobin dissociation curve (see "Physiology," Section 2.1.2)	Decreased values indicate the lack of available O_2 or the lack of hemoglobin; the percentage of saturation is limited by the capacity of the blood to bind O_2; thus increased administration of O_2 is useless in the face of inadequate hemoglobin stores	See Po_2 above
Base excess or deficit	A measurement of all buffers available in the blood, including both volatile (HCO_3) and nonvolatile (hemoglobin, Cl^-, PO_4, SO_4, protein), which are usually not measured (see Appendix A)	Base excess or deficit provides a more complete picture of the individual's acid-base status than does just the information available from the pH, Pco_2, and HCO_3	The compensatory mechanisms depend on the basic dysfunction causing the excess or deficit (see Pco_2 and HCO_3 above); base excess or deficit is calculated by plotting measurements of pH, Pco_2, and hematocrit on a nomogram
O_2 content	A measurement of the total amount of O_2 in the blood, including that bound to hemoglobin (O_2 saturation) and that dissolved or "free" in the plasma	O_2 content varies directly with Po_2, but not in a linear relationship; its measurement helps explain differences that can occur between Po_2 and O_2 saturation.	See Po_2 above

aPartial pressure is defined as the pressure exerted by one of the gases in a mixture of gases in a liquid. Each partial pressure is exerted independently of the pressure of other gases.

Primary Respiratory Alkalosis. Primary respiratory alkalosis is due to hyperventilation (anxiety, fever, artificial ventilation), hypoxemia (high altitudes, moderate COPD, moderate asthma, pulmonary embolism), and early salicylate poisoning.

Respiratory Alkalosis (Carbonic Acid Deficit)	pH	P_{CO_2}	HCO_3	Base Excess/Deficit
Acute uncompensated	I	D	N	N
Early compensation	I	D	D	D (deficit)
Chronic compensated	N	D	D	D (deficit)

Primary Metabolic Acidosis. Primary metabolic acidosis is caused by an increase in nonvolatile H^+ levels (ingestion of ammonium chloride, diabetic ketoacidosis, lactic acidosis, renal failure), exogenous poisoning (salicylates, late), and a loss of HCO_3 (diarrhea, renal tubular acidosis, prolonged intestinal suctioning, use of carbonic anhydrase inhibitors).

Metabolic Acidosis (Base Bicarbonate Deficit)	pH	P_{CO_2}	HCO_3	Base Excess/Deficit
Acute uncompensated	D	N	D	D (deficit)
Early compensation	D	D	D	D (deficit)
Chronic compensated	N	D	D	D or N

Primary Metabolic Alkalosis. Primary metabolic alkalosis is due to a loss of H^+ (prolonged vomiting, prolonged nasogastric suctioning, diuretic therapy, hyperadrenocorticism [Cushing's disease or Cushing's syndrome, adrenal steroid therapy, aldosteronism]), and increased bicarbonate levels (excessive intake).

Metabolic Alkalosis (Base Bicarbonate Excess)	pH	P_{CO_2}	HCO_3	Base Excess/Deficit
Acute uncompensated	I	N	I	I (excess)
Early compensation	I	I	I	I (excess)
Chronic compensated	N	I	I	I or N

Mixed Acid-Base Imbalances. The older the individual or the more seriously ill he or she is, the less likely it is that the aforementioned "pure" imbalances are to be found. Besides being under attack with the primary problem, most persons found in hospital settings are also doing battle to maintain acid-base equilibrium in other areas because of chronic or superimposed illnesses. For example, a respiratory and metabolic acidosis can coexist (COPD–diabetic ketoacidosis [DKA]). To discover whether the respiratory problem is primary in origin, the relative change of relationships between P_{CO_2} and pH (see Table 10–2) can be plotted over a series of arterial blood gas (ABG) measurements to see whether the changes follow the "rule." Nothing is of more value, however, than a thorough understanding of the patient's past and present history and general status.

TABLE 10–2. CHANGES IN pH RELATIVE TO Pco$_2$ IN PRIMARY ACUTE RESPIRATORY ACID-BASE IMBALANCES[a]

Pco$_2$ (mm Hg)	pH
10	7.7
20	7.6
30	7.5
40	7.4 normal
60	7.3
80	7.2
100	7.1

[a]There is an inverse relationship between pH and Pco$_2$ in acid-base imbalances as a result of primary (pure) acute respiratory problems. For each 0.1 decrease in pH below 7.4, a 20-mm Hg increase in Pco$_2$ occurs. For each 0.1 increase in pH above 7.4, a 10-mm Hg decrease in Pco$_2$ should occur (Milhorn, 1980).

Special Pediatric Procedures

Transcutaneous PO$_2$ Monitoring (Normal Range, 50 to 100 mm Hg). A miniature oxygen-measuring electrode with a built-in warmer that is placed on the infant's chest or thigh is used to monitor transcutaneous Po$_2$ levels. As the skin warms, O$_2$ diffuses out of the capillaries. The electrode measures the amount of oxygen at the skin surface, which is proportional to the Po$_2$ of the blood. The amount of heat necessary to keep the infant's skin at 43°C is also recorded, which is said to correlate with blood tissue perfusion.

Scalp pH (Blood Sample from a Scalp Vein; Normal Range, 7.25 to 7.40). Scalp pH is used together with other clinical data to help determine the need for a cesarean section in some situations. A fetal scalp pH of less than 7.15 in the face of a normal arterial pH in the maternal blood indicates serious fetal acidosis and the need for an immediate cesarean. A scalp pH of 7.15 to 7.24 is considered ambiguous and requires further close monitoring (SHMC, 1984).

10.2.3 Pleural Fluid Analysis and Examination

Synonym: Diagnostic thoracentesis

Normal Range: Negative findings

Explanation of the Test. A thoracentesis is a surgical (invasive) procedure involving a needle insertion and drainage of the pleural space. With the advent of noninvasive diagnostic measures, this test is used less often for diagnosis.

It can be indicated in the diagnostic evaluation of pneumonia; for removal of a pleural effusion when the cause of a pleural effusion is not known or the degree of pleural effusion is severe enough to impair breathing; or for confirmation of suspected malignancy.

Purpose. To determine the etiology or the appropriate treatment of fluid effusion into the pleural space, as well as to facilitate adequate respiration, relieve pain or dyspnea.

It is used as a diagnostic aid in neoplastic, inflammatory, or pleural lung disease. It is also used therapeutically in the prevention of lung collapse by the removal of fluid accumulated in the pleural space of the thoracic cavity. It is usually preceded by chest x-ray and/or ultrasound study of the chest to locate the fluid and lessen the risk of puncture of vital organs (e.g., lung, liver, spleen).

Process. Examination of gross appearance and constituents of the excess pleural fluid.

1. Gross appearance:
   a. Empyema: foul odor, thick fluid with appearance of pus
   b. Chylothorax: fluid has an opalescent appearance (A total lipid and cholesterol count is usually done if chylothorax is suspected)
2. Tests of pleural fluid:
   a. Cell counts:
      (1) WBC: >1000/mm^3 suggestive of exudate
      (2) Inc. polymorphonuclear leukocytes: indicative of acute inflammatory condition
      (3) >1/2 WBC's small lymphocytes: exudate or effusion usually secondary to tumor or tuberculosis
   b. Pleural protein content:
      (1) Exudate: >3g/dl, usually due to infectious disease or neoplastic disorders
      (2) Transudate: <3g/dl, usually due to congestive heart disease, cirrhosis, nephrotic syndrome, decreased thyroid (myxedema), peritoneal dialysis, or glomerular nephritis
   c. Serum lactate dehydrogenase/pleural fluid ratio: >0.6, typical of an exudate
   d. Pleural fluid/serum protein ratio: >0.5, with findings of item "c" above identifies an exudate with a high degree of accuracy
   e. Pleural glucose: Decreased below serum levels, due to impaired glucose diffusion secondary to damage to the pleural membrane, as well as glycolysis by the extra cells
   f. Pleural amylase: Slight elevation in effusion due to malignancy. Very high elevations when cause of effusion is pancreatitis or esophageal rupture with release of salivary amylase
   g. Pleural fluid pH: Normal level: 7.4 or above; <7.2 with empyema; similar decreases in cancer and tuberculosis

Patient Preparation and Teaching
1. Determine early on whether the subject is allergic to local anesthetics used during this procedure
2. Make sure that the patient knows the general, if not specific, purpose for his or her thoracentesis before the procedure
3. Clarify as necessary for the patient's psychological comfort the relationship and purpose of preliminary tests, such as chest x ray (to identify area of fluid accumulation), to the goal of this test (e.g., to increase respiratory depth by fluid removal)
4. Depending on the individual patient's interest in, concern about, and ability to cope with information, provide or see that information about the process of this study is provided
5. No food or fluid restriction (a cough suppressant may be administered if indicated)

6. Positioning for the test (usually done in the patient's room of the hospital or on an outpatient basis):
   a. In bed: may be sitting up, leaning forward on forearms, supported by pillows on the overbed table
   b. Lying on the unaffected side with chest on pillows and upper arm elevated over the head
7. Instruct and remind the individual that he or she cannot move, cough, or deep-breathe during the actual sample taking
8. Vital signs are taken and recorded before and after the test
9. During the test, observe for indications of respiratory distress, such as complaints of dyspnea, feeling of weakness and presence of pallor, rapid breathing, decreased blood pressure, or changes of heart rate, both increased or decreased
10. If x ray, ultrasound, or fluoroscopy are expected to be necessary to assist in locating the pleural fluid, the procedure would not be done in bed
11. Time involved depends on difficulty in locating the fluid deposit and the need to use other diagnostic tests. It can take as little as half an hour if only a cell count is done. If other tests are done with it (see below), the time could extend markedly, 2 to 3 hours.

10.2.4. Other Respiratory Function and Diagnostic Tests

The reader is referred to other tests of the respiratory system in this text: Sections 17.2.1, "Chest Film"; 17.2.4, "Bronchogram"; 17.4.5, "Pulmonary Arteriogram"; and 17.6.1, "Lung Scan."

The scope of this book does not allow for the inclusion of tests of pulmonary function, which does not minimize their importance. Such tests include spirometry, or flow volume loops (i.e., vital capacity [VC], forced vital capacity [FVC], residual volume [RV], functional residual volume [FRV], total lung capacity [TLC], expiratory reserve volume [ERV], forced expiratory volume [FEV], maximal midexpiratory flow [MMEF], peak inspiratory/expiratory flow rate [PlFR/PEFR], inspiratory capacity [IC], maximal voluntary ventilation [MVV], and maximal breathing capacity [MBCO]).

NURSING DIAGNOSES RELATED TO THE RESPIRATORY SYSTEM

1. Impaired gas exchange related to
   a. Decreased effective lung surface secondary to
      (1) Tissue damage (pneumothorax, atelectasis, adult respiratory distress syndrome [ARDS], cancer)
      (2) Hyperinflation of alveoli with decreased surface area (COPD)
      (3) Decreased depth and length of respiration secondary to pain and/or abdominal distention
      (4) Rapid, shallow breathing secondary to anxiety
2. Ineffective breathing patterns related to
   a. Pain restriction related to
      (1) Anxiety
      (2) Flattened diaphragm (chronic, long-term COPD)
3. Anxiety related to
   a. Feelings of suffocation or dyspnea related to
      (1) Poor prognosis
      (2) Unacceptable nature of diagnosis secondary to requirements for change in total life-style

(3) Anticipation of noxious medical treatment or surgery
(4) Lack of understanding of purpose for, or necessity of diagnostic tests, therapy regimen
(5) Loss of control over daily life patterns

4. Ineffective airway clearance related to
   a. Increased, retained, or tenacious secretions (bronchiectasis of upper respiratory infections) related to
      (1) Increased viscosity of secretions (dehydration/third spacing)
      (2) Ineffective cough secondary to pain or altered level of consciousness secondary to selected medications (narcotics)

5. Potential or actual increased risk of injury (physiological) related to
   a. Cerebral hypoxia and/or muscular weakness (falls)
   b. Increased risk of complications (infection and suprainfection secondary to decreased immune competence with chronic disease, thrombus formation secondary to hypercoagulability of the blood with slowed circulation, bleeding secondary to formation of stress ulcer)

6. Activity intolerance and/or self-care deficit related to
   a. Tissue hypoxia
   b. Loss of muscle mass secondary to decreased mobility and decreased nutritional status
   c. Fear/anxiety related to falls/injury

7. Alteration in nutrition (less than body requirements) related to
   a. Anorexia secondary to increased secretions, dry mucous membrane related to
      (1) Dyspnea on exertion (eating)
      (2) Loss of nutrients with vomiting
      (3) Increased nutritional requirements secondary to fever and other catabolic processes

8. Impaired communication related to
   a. Shortness of breath or dyspnea
   b. Physical loss of, or loss of the use of the vocal cords (laryngectomy, tracheostomy)

9. Alteration in tissue perfusion related to
   a. Decreased gas exchange
   b. Potential or actual decreased cardiac output secondary to hypoxia of cardiac muscle

10. Self-care deficit related to
    a. Impaired mobility with weakness
    b. Shortness of breath and dyspnea
    c. Fatigue secondary to sleep loss

11. Alteration in comfort related to
    a. All of the above
    b. Dry mucous membranes with oxygen therapy
    c. Positional dyspnea limiting postural change

E L E V E N

THE CARDIOVASCULAR SYSTEM

RECOGNITION OF CARDIOVASCULAR DYSFUNCTION

The individual experiencing repetition of alterations in heart rate, presence of syncope, or chest pain is apt to attribute the symptoms to cardiac dysfunction. Part of the management of such patients may involve close assessment of psychogenic aspects as well as laboratory and clinical findings.

11.1 LABORATORY AND CLINICAL INDICATIONS OF CARDIOVASCULAR SYSTEM DYSFUNCTION*

Laboratory Findings. Indications of cardiovascular system dysfunction as pertains to blood include findings of increased levels of aspartate transaminase (AST) and lactic dehydrogenase (LDH). The alanine transaminase (ALT) concentration may be elevated as well if there is liver involvement due to congestion. Increased serum cholesterol* and glucose levels,* and decreased plasma potassium levels as well as some changes in sodium—either increased or decreased—may be seen. Indications in the urine include increased uric acid* and blood urine nitrogen (BUN) levels, proteinuria, an increase in the number of white blood cells (WBCs) with granular casts seen by gross examination. Creatinine levels are usually within normal limits except in badly decompensated cardiac conditions or those with concomitant renal disease. The specific gravity may increase with a decreased circulating volume.

Clinical Findings. The presence of edema (dependent), increased fatigue (in children evidenced by a voluntary limitation of activity and squatting to rest), and complaints of dyspnea or overt shortness of breath are hallmark signs of cardiovascular dysfunction. Also found are clubbing of fingernails and toenails, poor peripheral perfusion with cold extremities, mottling of the skin of the extremities, and xanthomas on the skin.* The presence of heart murmurs, S_3 and S_4 heart sounds (except in children where they may be normal), increased strength of the point of maximal impulse (PMI) may be visible on the chest wall (myocardial hypertrophy), hepatomegaly and a tender liver can be noted. There may be complaints of anginal pain and pain on exertion or after eating. Dizziness, fainting, and premature vascular disease are indications. There is often a

---

*Findings indicated by asterisks in this section have been identified as known risk factors.

history of hypertension,* heavy cigarette smoking,* diabetes mellitus in the family* and/or diagnosed in the patient,* obesity,* oral contraceptive use,* hypothyroidism, excessive intake of saturated fats, renal disease, or alcoholism.* Cardiovascular system dysfunction is more common with increased age,* and there may be evidence of retinal lipemia. A family history of death from heart disease before the age of 60* is not common but of great importance.

Other Diagnostic Tests. See Sections 17.2.6, "Cardiac Series"; 17.3.6, "Cardiac Catheterization"; 17.4., "Millisecond CT Scans"; 17.4.1, "Cardiac Scans"; 17.8, "Electrodiagnostic Tests"; and 17.8.1, MRI, "Purpose of the Test."

11.2 CARDIOVASCULAR LIPID PROFILE

Synonyms: Lipid profile, lipid fractionation, plasma lipoproteins, includes (varies with the laboratory) total cholesterol (see Section 1.11), total lipid, phospholipid, triglycerides, high-density-lipoprotein cholesterol (HDL-cholesterol), low-density-lipoprotein cholesterol (LDL-cholesterol), "standing" plasma test (lipid phenotyping may be included but generally has not proved useful)

Normal Ranges (plasma or serum may be used) (mg/dl)

Total lipids	500–1000
Phospholipids	180–320
Triglycerides	30–175
Cholesterol—total	
Desirable:	<200
Borderline:	200–329
High Risk:	>329
(For a more complete breakdown, see Section 1.11)	
HDL-cholesterol	
Female	Mean, 55
Male	Mean, 45
LDL-cholesterol	
Desirable:	<130
Borderline:	130–159
High Risk:	>159

Explanation of the Test. Plasma lipids travel as complex molecules combined with several proteins, so the lipid profile tests actually measure lipids and proteins. These lipoproteins appear in five classes in the plasma: chylomicrons, consisting almost entirely of *dietary* triglycerides; very low density lipoproteins (VLDL); intermediate-density lipoproteins (IDL); low-density lipoproteins (LDL), also known as beta lipoproteins; and high-density lipoproteins (HDL), also known as alpha lipoprotein. All five classes contain varying amounts of the different lipoproteins, as depicted in Figure 11–1. The purpose of the lipid profile or fractionation is to characterize more clearly the various components that make up hyperlipidemic states and to identify the increased-risk patient.

The test discussed in this section is the *lipid profile test*, the purpose of which is the identification of the type of lipoprotein disorder, including those disorders associated with increased risk of cardiovascular disease—familial or secondary to acquired disease states (e.g., alcoholism, diabetes mellitus, excess dietary cholesterol, hypothyroidism).

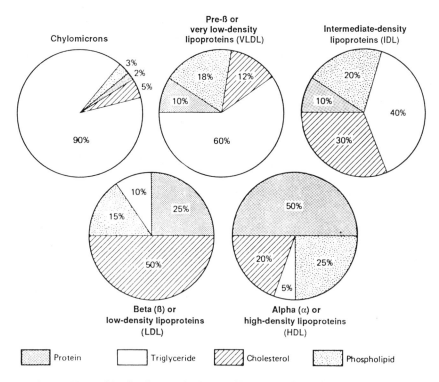

Figure 11–1. Compositions of the five lipoprotein classes. (From Levy, R. I. [May, 1980]. Hyperlipoproteinemia and its management. *Journal of Cardiovascular Medicine*, p. 436, with permission.)

Another test, not frequently used now, is that of phenotyping the plasma lipoproteins (Fig. 11–1). This test, usually called *complete lipid fractionation*, uses lipoprotein electrophoresis to distribute the lipoproteins into beta (low-density), pre-beta (very-low-density), and alpha (high-density) lipoprotein. The process was developed when inherited hyperlipoproteinemia identification was considered the best approach to identification of all cases of hyperlipoproteinemia, and for establishing prognosis of, and treatment for hyperlipoproteinemia (Lab. of Pathology, 1991).

With the knowledge that many instances of hyperlipoproteinemia were secondary to acquired disease states, phenotyping has proved to be less useful and is less often done (Lab. of Pathology, 1991). The information provided by the lipid profile test is preferred in terms of cost and response time, and provides sufficient information for most purposes.

Significance of the Tests

Total lipids. The total lipid concentration increases when there is an increase in any fraction of the plasma lipids (except triglycerides), as in nephrotic syndrome, ketosis, and cardiovascular disease (atherosclerosis). Decreased total lipid concentrations may be found in malabsorption syndromes. A physiological increase occurs after a fatty meal, and several drugs will elevate the total lipid (e.g., oral contraceptives, estrogen).

Phospholipids. Phospholipid levels increase with biliary obstruction concentration biliary cirrhosis. There is a decrease in the ratio of phospholipid to cholesterol in atherosclerosis.

Triglycerides. Triglycerides are composed of glycerol and fatty acids. (Their concentration in the five classes of lipoproteins is shown in Fig. 11–1.) Conditions in which triglyceride lipids predominate can be derived from Tables 11–1 and 11–2 with the knowledge that the triglyceride content is greatest in chylomicrons, VLDL and IDL. Increases in triglyceride levels with myocardial infarction may last as long as a year. Triglyceride levels by themselves have very little predictive value and will increase after fat intake.

Cholesterol total. See Section 1.11.

HDL-Cholesterol, LDL-Cholesterol. Currently, it is thought that LDL, made up primarily of cholesterol, relates *directly* with the risk of coronary artery disease (high LDL, high risk; low LDL, low risk) and that HDL-cholesterol relates *inversely* with that risk (high HDL, low risk; low HDL, high risk). It is postulated that the measurement of HDL and LDL-cholesterol levels is more important in the diagnosis of atherosclerosis development than is the measurement of total cholesterol levels. HDL increases with exercise training and is believed to be protective against atherosclerosis.

"Standing" Plasma Test. This test consists of observing a serum sample that has been refrigerated overnight for the presence of lactescence, or fatty turbidity, a positive response in which indicates excess VLDL, primarily triglycerides, in the sample. Normally, the serum is clear. If a creamy layer appears on the top of the serum, it indicates either an abnormality in the VLDL content or that the sample taken was from a patient who was not fasting. With excessive VLDL, the refrigerated sample will be uniformly turbid. Cholesterol and LDL levels cannot be demonstrated by this approach.

There are both primary (genetic) and secondary hyperlipoproteinemias. A classification was developed by Frederickson et al. to identify types of hyperlipoproteinemias (grouping of disorders that affect plasma lipid and lipoprotein concentrations in a similar manner) (see Table 11–1). The classification is limited in genetic analysis, and the process of classification is elaborate. At present the use of the varying densities of the lipoproteins as organizational threads has been more widely accepted (Henry, 1991).

Patient Preparation for Lipid Profile Tests

1. Patient should be n.p.o. other than water for 12 to 14 hours before the test
2. The patient should be in a physiological steady state (no vigorous exercise) and on his or her usual diet the day before the test

11.3 TESTS FOR CARDIAC MUSCLE CELL DAMAGE

11.3.1 Creatine Phosphokinase, Serum

Synonyms: creatine kinase, CK, creatine, CPK

Normal Ranges (IU/L)

Female	8–150
Male	10–190

TABLE 11–1. BIOCHEMICAL AND CLINICAL FEATURES OF THE LIPOPROTEIN CLASSES

Class	Origin	Function	Catabolism	Plasma Appearance in Elevation	Clinical Correlates of Elevation
Chylomicrons	Intestine, from dietary fat	Transport dietary fat	Lipoprotein lipase at tissue sites degrade chylomicron, remnants cleared by liver	Creamy, supernate, clear infranate	Eruptive xanthoma, lipemia retinalis, organomegaly pancreatitis
VLDLs	Liver and small bowel, from carbohydrates, free fatty acids, medium-chain triglycerides	Transport endogenous triglycerides	Complex, probably requires lipoprotein lipase for degradation	Turbid	Glucose intolerance, hyperuricemia
IDLs	VLDLs	Unknown	(?) Degradation to LDL	Turbid	Glucose intolerance, hyperuricemia; premature atherosclerosis; tuboeruptive, tendinous, palmar planar xanthoma
LDLs	VLDL and IDL, (?) alternative source	Unknown	Primary site of removal unclear	Clear	Premature atherosclerosis, corneal arcus, tendinous and tuberous xanthoma, xanthelasma
HDLs	(?) Intestine, liver	(?) Facilitate cholesterol ester and triglyceride metabolism	(?) Liver	Clear	No associated abnormality

From Levy, R. I. (May, 1980). Hyperlipoproteinemia and its management. *Journal of Cardiovascular Medicine*, 438, with permission.

TABLE 11–2. TYPES OF HYPERLIPOPROTEINEMIA

Type	Features	Possible Secondary Causes
I	↑Chylomicrons	Insulinopenic diabetes mellitus, dysglobulinemia, lupus erythematosus
IIa	↑LDL	Nephrotic syndrome, hypothyroidism
IIb	↑LDL and VLDL	Obstructive liver disease, porphyria, multiple myeloma
III	↑IDL, sometimes with ↑chylomicrons	Hypothyroidism, dysgammaglobulinemia
IV	↑VLDL	Diabetes mellitus, nephrotic syndrome, pregnancy, hormone use, glycogen storage disease, alcoholism, Gaucher's disease, Niemann-Pick disease
V	↑Chylomicrons and ↑VLDL	Insulinopenic diabetes mellitus, nephrotic syndrome, alcoholism, myeloma, idiopathic hypercalcemia

From Levy, R. I. (May, 1980). Hyperlipoproteinemia and its management. *Journal of Cardiovascular Medicine*, 439, with permission.

Explanation of the Test. CK is primarily an intracellular enzyme that plays a major role in the energy-storing functions of cells. It is found primarily in cardiac, smooth muscle, skeletal, and brain tissue. CK is released from the cell after irreversible injury, which is the major source for the increase in serum levels of CK after cardiac injury (myocardial infarction [MI], surgery). The CK test is sensitive to but not specific for MI. Before the general availability of CK isoenzyme fractionation, the CK measurement was considered a criterion essential to the diagnosis of MI, even though its lack of specificity was known. The duration of its elevation was felt to correlate with the extent and severity of the infarct (see Fig. 1–2, elevation of enzymes in MI). Serum CK levels increase early—within 6 hours—in myocardial damage. Peaks occur at about 18 hours and return to normal in 3 to 4 days if no further damage occurs (Grenadier et al., 1980).

Patient Preparation. No special preparation is necessary.

CK LEVELS INCREASED IN:

1. Muscle disorders (skeletal) such as muscular dystrophy, polymyositis, alcoholic myopathies, and dermatomyositis because of the increased permeability of the cell membrane. The increases are persistent and remarkably high
2. Cardiac cell injury or destruction as in angina, MI
3. Conditions causing dysfunction of neural tissues such as meningitis, encephalitis, cerebral tumors, acute cerebral vascular accidents, convulsions, head trauma, and subarachnoid hemorrhage
4. Muscular trauma such as with repeated intramuscular (IM) injections, vigorous exercise, surgical incisions through muscle (especially in heart surgery)
5. Hypothyroidism, believed to be due to skeletal muscle deterioration

11.3.2 Isoenzyme M-B, Serum[a]

Synonyms: CK-2 (MB); CPK isoenzymes; CPK$_2$; creatine kinase isoenzymes; phosphokinase isoenzymes

Normal Range (ng/mL)

CK	
Female	0–5.5
Male	0–7.5
CK_2	0–10 U/l (cardiac fraction)

[a]Total CK and the isoezymes (CK_1, CK_2) are determined in this test.

Explanation of the Test. CK has three isoenzymes: CPK_1, found primarily in the brain and smooth muscle; CPK_2 found primarily in cardiac cells (they were once thought to be contained exclusively in cardiac cells, but are now known to also occur in some skeletal muscle, the brain, the tongue, and various viscera); and CK_3, found in both cardiac and skeletal muscle with a small amount (5 percent) in smooth muscle (Bauman, 1980; Laboratory of Pathology, 1991).

When CK_2 was first used as the "ideal MI marker," it was thought not only to be exclusive to cardiac cells but also to be released only when there was irreversible destruction of the cell; however, increases in CK_2 levels have been found with such conditions as unstable angina, sustained supraventricular arrhythmias, and ischemia resulting from coronary insufficiency, with no evidence of MI. However, within 4 to 8 hours after an MI, CK_2 should be present in *100 percent* of MI patients. It rapidly disappears after 72 hours. CK_2 is also found to be present in differing concentrations in various parts of the myocardium, so the locale of the infarct may influence the level of CK_2 activity in the serum. Therefore, although the test is a useful adjunct to the diagnosis of MI, it can have elevated levels in the absence of an MI, as with significant skeletal muscle injury, or normal ones in the presence of an MI (Bauman, 1980). At present, the concentration of CK_2 relates most closely to the extent of, and the time after, a cardiac insult (Laboratory of Pathology, 1991).

The CK_2 level can be of particular use in many instances of differential diagnosis. It has been found to be the most sensitive indicator of cardiac contusion after automobile accidents. It is more sensitive to an MI than is the total CK concentration (Grenadier & Palant, 1980). CK_2 does not elevate in response to IM infections, congestive heart failure, nonischemic arrhythmias, seizures, or strokes (Laboratory of Pathology, 1991).

Patient Preparation. No special preparation is necessary.

11.3.3 Myoglobin, Serum and Urine

Synonyms: None

Normal Ranges

Serum	0–90 ng/ml
Urine	Negative

Explanation of the Test. Myoglobin is a globin complex similar to hemoglobin but present in muscle tissue. It is excreted in the urine by way of glomerular filtration. Its excretion increases in circumstances involving any muscle cell damage. Serum and urine myoglobin measurements are used in the differential diagnosis of darkly pigmented urines and to help substantiate or rule out a diagnosis of MI. In the presence of a normal total CK concentration, normal serum and urine myoglobin levels, and electrocardiogram (ECG) findings limited to short-lived ST and T wave changes, MI can usually be ruled out in patients with unstable angina.

Serum myoglobin levels peak approximately 8 to 12 hours after an MI and return to normal—or nondetectable levels—as early as 12 hours after rise. More frequently, a return to normal takes at least 24 hours. Serum myoglobin may appear intermittently in the first 6 to 18 hours after an MI, and serial determinations may be indicated.

Myoglobin increases can appear in the urine within 3 hours after an MI. Levels may return to high normal in 30 hours; usually, however, a return to normal takes 72 hours or longer (Ravel, 1989).

MYOGLOBIN LEVELS INCREASED IN:

1. Cardiac muscle damage (trauma, ischemia, inflammation, necrosis)
2. Skeletal muscle damage, most frequently in crushing injuries
3. Familial myoglobinuria (Meyer-Betz disease)
4. High fevers, stress (e.g., hyperthermia and vigorous physical activity. In susceptible persons, fever can cause muscle destruction)
5. Uncommon occurrences with diabetic acidosis, hypokalemia, or barbiturate poisoning

11.3.4 Cardiac Enzyme Tests

A. Lactic Acid Dehydrogenase Electrophoresis

Synonyms: LD electrophoresis, LD fractionation (includes total LD and isoenzyme fractions I, II, III, IV, V)

Normal Ranges[a] (IU)

I	14–38
II	33–73
III	23–43
IV	15–31
V	14–34

---

[a]Serum enzyme normal-range values are not comparable between laboratories. Use the reference ranges provided by the laboratory that does the test. Usually in known cardiac diagnostic cases the LD-1 or enzyme battery tests are ordered.

Explanation of the Test. Normally, most of the circulating LD isoenzymes come from the heart and kidney (fractions I and II). Less is found in fraction III with only traces in IV and V.

The LD isoenzymes are numbered sequentially, beginning with the most rapidly moving one and ending with the slowest moving. The individual LD isoenzymes have different concentrations in different tissues, which provides a way to identify the tissues responsible for an elevated total LD level. A separation, or fractionation, of the isoenzymes measures the individual concentrations of each isoenzyme. Measurement of the fractions is often done, even if the total LD concentration is normal, when a condition usually causing an increase in a given fraction is suspected. Because the range of normal for total LD is quite broad, it is possible for the level of one or more isoenzymes to be increased with a total LD value within normal limits.

General Interpretation of Isoenzyme Elevations. LD_1 is found primarily in heart muscle and red blood cells (RBCs) and found in moderate amounts in the kidney. Its level increases long before a total LD increase is seen in MI (within 4 hours). By 24 hours there is a definite reversal of the normal LD_1/LD_2 ratio (normally LD_2 has higher levels than does LD_1), often referred to as the *LD flip* or "flipped LD." This flip is of significant importance as evidence of MI, renal infarct, or erythrocyte disease. The inverse ratio lasts longer in myocardial problems, but the initial increase in level is greater in hematologic problems. It can be strikingly elevated in megoblastic anemia.

Because of its close correlation with MI, "mini tests" measuring LD_1 only and technically simple are available.

Other conditions increasing LD_1 levels include active myocarditis following heart surgery (if the elevation persists more than 5 to 6 days postsurgery, a postoperative MI should be suspected), megaloblastic anemia (pernicious anemia, folate deficiency anemia), hemolytic anemias, and muscular dystrophy (MD). (MD causes a relative increase because levels of LD_4 and LD_5 are depressed.)

LD_2 is found primarily in the kidney, heart, and in moderate amounts in brain tissue, blood cells, both white and red, and probably in the cells of the reticuloendothelial system as well. LD_2 levels are increased in MI and other cardiac inflammatory conditions (LD_2 does not increase as high as does LD_1) such as granulocytic leukemia, pancreatitis, hemolytic and megoblastic anemias, some lymphomas, and MD (see the note regarding MD increase in the preceding paragraph).

LD_3 is primarily of pulmonary origin but is also found in moderate amounts in adrenal tissue, lymphocytes, skeletal muscles, brain, and kidney. Its levels are also increased in pulmonary infarction and other pulmonary destruction, granulocytic leukemia, and pancreatitis. An increase in the LD_1 concentration may confuse the picture in pulmonary infarct because of the frequency with which that condition is accompanied by hemorrhage (Widmann, 1983).

LD_4 is found in about equal but moderate concentrations in the liver, skeletal muscle, brain, and kidney. Increased levels are seen in pulmonary infarct (may be due to subsequent circulatory collapse), congestive heart failure (CHF), viral and toxic hepatitis, and cirrhosis (Henry, 1991).

LD_5 is found primarily in the liver. Just as LD_1 is the "heart" enzyme, LD is the "liver" enzyme. It is found in significant amounts in skeletal muscle as well as in moderate amounts in kidney tissue. Increased levels are noted in cirrhosis, toxic and viral hepatitis, CHF, and pulmonary infarct (as with LD_4, probably because of circulatory collapse). Increases in LD_5 levels in viral and drug-associated hepatitis can be enormous. Increases usually precede jaundice, and decreases occur before bilirubin or ALT (GPT) levels fall. Moderate rises are found in LD_5 levels in hepatitis associated with infectious mononucleosis, but total LDH increases are often very high in that disease.

At present this test is used primarily for noncardiac cases. The tests that follow (LD_1 and cardiac enzyme battery) are more specific for cardiac dysfunction.

Patient Preparation. No special preparation is required.

FALSE INCREASES IN LD LEVELS ARE SEEN IN:

- LD_1 and LD_2 levels if the blood sample is allowed to hemolyze

B. Lactate Dehydrogenase, Isoenzyme 1

Synonym: LD$_1$

Normal Range (12–18 U/l—total LD included) (Laboratory of Pathology, 1991)

Explanation of the Test. (See also "LD Electrophoresis Test," Section 11.3.4.A.). This test is useful in the diagnosis of cardiac disease. Five major lactic acid dehydrogenase enzymes exist in normal serum and are numbered according to their electrophoretic activity. The most active is designated LD$_1$, the least LD$_5$. Each cardiac cell (myocardial cell) contains large amounts of LD$_1$. (Red blood vessels also contain large amounts.) With damage to myocardial tissue, whatever the cause, the serum isoenzyme patterns change with increased LD$_1$ from the damaged tissue.

Since LD$_1$ enzyme is also found in substantial amounts in other tissues (primarily RBCs and kidney tissue), serum increases are not absolutely diagnostic of a cardiac disorder, neither does the increase exclude a nonmyocardial source. Differential diagnosis, requires using this test with other data (clinical signs, symptoms, ECG findings, other enzymatic findings characteristic) to rule out hemolytic or kidney disorder.

Patient Preparation. None, other than explanation of the purpose for the venipuncture. Hemolyzed blood sample cannot be used for testing because of the high levels of LD$_1$ in RBCs.

LD$_1$ LEVELS INCREASED IN:

- Myocardial infarction, 10 to 12 hours after the event, peaking (approximately three times normal) in 48 to 72 hours with prolonged elevation. The prolonged elevation is useful in delayed diagnosis.

C. Cardiac Enzyme Battery

Synonyms: Creatinine kinase isoenzymes; cardiac isoenzymes (includes total LD, LD$_1$, total CK, CK-2)

Normal Range*

CK Total	
Male	10–190 U/l
Female	8–150 U/l
CK-2	
Male	0–7.5 ng/ml
Female	0–5.5 ng/ml
LD total	60–220 U/l
LD$_1$	12–81 U/l

*Laboratory of Pathology

Explanation of the Test. Creatinine kinase (CK) and lactic dehydrogenase (LD) are enzymes found in cardiac muscle, as well as many other tissues. The isoenzyme CK-2 is found in the myocardium. LD$_1$ is found in large amounts in cardiac tissue. Any injury to the myocardium that causes necrosis, whether due to disease or trauma (as in cardiac surgery), will cause an increase in LD_1, CK, and CK-2.

The rate at which they rise, stay at maximum levels, and clear provides diagnostic information:

1. LD_1: Rises within 24 hours after myocardial injury, returning to normal in 2 to 3 days
2. Total LD: Rises to a maximum level in 3 to 4 days after injury, staying increased for 7 to 10 days
3. CK-2: Rises at the same rate as total CK but is cleared more rapidly

Findings. The cardiac diagnosis is based on correlation of the enzymatic findings with ECG and clinical data. The total data are interpreted by a pathologist who considers such factors such as the amount the enzymes are above the upper limits of normal and the presence of hemolysis. Because other tissues are also rich in LD_1 (liver, kidneys, hematopoietic tissue, skeletal muscle), use of this enzyme alone is inadequate for diagnosis. (Data from Laboratory of Pathology, 1991; Tietz, 1990)

RELATED NURSING DIAGNOSES

The following diagnoses were selected for their close relationship to cardiovascular function. There are, however, other nursing diagnoses that may well be used more frequently. They are no less important than the ones given with this chapter, but they are more "generic" by nature—problems that almost all patients share. These diagnoses are a potential or actual knowledge deficit (everyone has some learning needs); potential or actual noncompliance (no medical or nursing care will be very effective unless the recipient believes in its importance; teaching does not mean learning); potential and actual anxiety (illness or dysfunction is usually the unknown in some respect for all patients, and their future with it is always unknown); and potential and actual pain or discomfort, which more often than not accompanies illness/dysfunction and can also be eased more often than not, if not wholly removed.

Alteration in Cardiac Output*

Actual, Decrease Related to
1. Cardiac muscle damage (MI), aneurysm of the heart wall with possible paradoxical movement
2. Altered conductivity and contractibility of the heart secondary to hypoxia (respiratory arrest, atherosclerotic coronary artery disease, digitalis toxicity)
3. Vascular collapse secondary to anaphylaxis (drug sensitivity)
4. Hypovolemia (hemorrhage)
5. External constriction of the heart's pumping action (tamponade)
6. Severe hypotension secondary to medication therapy (narcotics, inotropic agents, anesthesia) (See "Potential," following)
7. Regurgitation of blood flow within the heart (valvular incompetence)
8. Prolonged increase in metabolic rate (hyperthyroidism)

---

*This nursing diagnosis is rather ambiguous. Most of the truly critical judgments and nursing actions related to it are either interdependent or wholly dependent on medical judgments and orders. Therefore, only if treatment is prescribed through the use of nursing judgment and without reference to medical protocols of care should the nursing diagnosis be used. Rather, the medical diagnosis would be the operating one. In actual practice, however, to communicate the *total* plan of care to all nursing personnel involved, the nursing diagnosis is used for both dependent and independent activities (Kelley, 1985, p. 111).

Potential, Decrease Related to

Side effect with hypertensive drug therapy (vasodilators, arterial and venous)

Alteration in Tissue Perfusion, Related to

1. Decreased cardiac output (see Diagnosis 1)
2. Edema, dependent and pulmonary (CHF), causing decreased gas exchange or hypoxemia
3. Increased peripheral resistance (hypertension)
4. Thrombosis/embolization secondary to compensatory increase in RBC count in hypoxemia (CHF), slowing/partial obstruction of blood flow (atherosclerosis or varicose veins), immobilization
5. Vasoconstriction secondary to smoking, anxiety, tight clothing—especially in dependent body areas (legs/thighs)
6. Increased body fat
7. Venous stasis with prolonged standing and sitting
8. Hypovolemia (dehydration, blood loss)
9. Decreased oxygen carrying capacity of the blood (decreased hematocrit/anemias, decreased gas exchange/pulmonary edema due to CHF)
10. Diminished venous return (thrombophlebitis/varicose veins)

Alteration in Fluid Volume

Deficit, Related to

1. Fluid loss secondary to prolonged or excessive diuresis (diuretic therapy in CHF; diuresis period postoperatively in cardiac surgery)
2. Third spacing secondary to increased intravascular pressure (decreased cardiac output leads to increased aldosterone levels, which leads to decreased renal output, which leads to increased intravascular pressure over time)

Excess, Related to

1. Increased ADH levels with severe stress (immediate postoperative period/heart surgery)
2. Increased aldosterone/ADH levels with inadequate renal perfusion (CHF)

Alteration in Electrolyte Balance, Related to

1. Digitalis toxicity due to competition between potassium (K^+) and digitalis for cardiac muscle receptor sites
2. Sodium retention or loss with associated fluid volume changes secondary to decreased cardiac output (CHF, cardiogenic shock)
3. Potassium loss in severe stress or sodium or water retention

Activity Intolerance, Related to

1. Postural instability due to postural hypotension (hemorrhage, hypertension)
2. Decreased level of consciousness or level of awareness due to cerebral hypoxia (hypertension)
3. Fear and anxiety due to pain on exertion or fear of pain (angina, peripheral arterial disease)
4. Exhaustion due to fear/anxiety/muscular hypoxia
5. Loss of muscle mass due to prolonged activity restrictions
6. Muscle weakness due to electrolyte imbalance (decreased or increased potassium levels). See diagnosis for "Alterations in Electrolyte Balance"

TWELVE

COLLAGEN-VASCULAR DISEASES OR SYNDROMES

INTRODUCTION

The conditions addressed in this chapter are a group of disorders with multisystem manifestation in which, despite the title, *primary* involvement of collagen is rare and blood vessel involvement is unusual.

The disorders share a potential for involvement of *any* organ system, inflammatory reactions, and merging of one clinical representation into another. Awareness of these facts should be kept in mind when weighing the single, or multiple immunologic findings that the collagen-vascular disorders present in terms of diagnosis and/or prognosis.

Survival depends on the immunosystem's ability to recognize and respond to many foreign substances (antigens). This defense mechanism becomes an obstacle when immune recognition triggers autoaggressive reactions.

Essential proteins for immune recognition are encoded by the major histocompatibility complex (MHC) genes and produce three classes based on structure, function, and genetic origin. In humans, class I molecules include HLA-A, HLA-B, and HLA-C. Human MHC studies made their first contribution in tissue transplantation.

In actuality, the results of any *one* laboratory finding can only be considered partial evidence, not diagnosis (Harvey et al., 1991).

RECOGNITION OF COLLAGEN-VASCULAR DISEASES OR SYNDROMES

As indicated in the chapter title, collagen-vascular diseases or syndromes are not considered a body system per se. They are, instead, an ill-defined collection of disorders involving many systems that share certain points. One of these is the tendency of the disorders included in this group to involve collagenous tissue in a fibrinoid necrosis, so the disorders are considered to be diseases of the connective tissue. A second shared trait is their collective tendency to involve various subdivisions of arteries in an inflammatory process, so the disorders can be properly considered vascular disorders, hence the title "collagen-vascular." Some investigators prefer the term "rheumatoid-collagen diseases." Another major connection among these dissimilar conditions has been identified. The probability is that the group of disorders share an etiology based on immunologic hypersensitivity (Ravel, 1989). Therefore, in many texts the diseases and/or syndromes will be found in the discussion of immunologic problems. For the purposes of this text it seems less confusing to use the older designation, collagen-vascular, because the immunologic testing process itself could be mistaken for a discussion of immunologic disorders.

The most common disorders included in this group are rheumatoid arthritis (RA), systemic lupus erythematosus (SLE), polyarteritis nodosa (PAN), and systemic sclerosis (SS; also known as scleroderma). Rather specific tests for acute rheumatic fever are included as well because the disease demonstrates some similarity with the rheumatoid collagen-vascular group and may well be one of them.

12.1 LABORATORY AND CLINICAL INDICATIONS OF COLLAGEN-VASCULAR DISEASES OR SYNDROMES

The major clues indicating possible collagen-vascular syndrome or disease are the presence of otherwise unexplained skin manifestations (rash, nodules), proteinuria or other abnormality of urine, polyarthralgia or arthritis, and less frequently, unexplained pleural effusion inflammation. (See Table 12–1 for occurrence in specific diseases.)

Fibromyalgia, a musculoskeletal pain syndrome, is a good example of collagen-vascular disorder. Fibromyalgia, or fibromyalgia syndrome, rather than fibrositis, is now the preferred term for this probable collagen-vascular condition. It is often also referred to as soft-tissue rheumatism. Even though the underlying mechanisms are still uncertain, it is now recognized as a discrete and legitimate medical entity (Wallace, 1993, p. 14).

The term fibromyalgia refers to pain (*-algia*) in muscle (*-my-*) and fibrous tissue (*fibro-*), which is characteristic of the condition, as is fatigue. The painful areas (trigger points/tender points) are found on the neck, trunk, and hips. That discomfort disrupts sleep, particularly the deep, nonrapid eye movement stage 4, involving a burst of alpha brain activity leading to even more intense fatigue.

Diagnosis is usually symptomatic, including:

1. Elicited pain in 11 of 18 tender point sites on palpation (also known as trigger points). The tender points are no more than a few millimeters in diameter and reproducible in specific anatomic locations:
   a. Bilaterally at the suboccipital muscle insertion
   b. Low cervical at the anterior aspects of the intertransverse spaces/C5–C7
   c. Trapezius, bilateral, midpoint upper border
   d. Supraspinatus, bilateral at origins and near the medial border above the scapula
   e. Second rib, bilateral, at second costochondral junctions
   f. Lateral epicondyle, bilateral, 2 cm distal to the epicondyles
   g. Gluteal, bilateral, upper outer quadrants, anterior muscle fold of buttock
   h. Greater trochanter, bilateral, posterior to trochanteric prominence
   i. Knee, bilateral, medial fat pad, proximal to joint line
2. The subject must indicate that the palpation was "*painful*," not just "tender."

TABLE 12-1. CLINICAL MANIFESTATIONS IN COLLAGEN-VASCULAR DISORDERS

Common Sign or Symptom	Collagen-Vascular Disorders				
	SLE[a]	PSS[b]	Polymyositis	PAN[c]	RA[d]
Fever	++	−	+	++	±
Unexplained skin eruptions	++	−	++	±	−
Muscle weakness/soreness	+	+	++	+	+
Joint pain/stiffness	+	+	+	+	++
Dry eyes/dry mouth (sicca syndrome)	±	±	±	±	+
Pulmonary/cardiac inflammation	++	+	−	±	+
Pulmonary fibrosis	−	+	±	±	±
Myocardial hypoxia/angina	+	+	−	+	±
Hypertension	+	+	−	+	−
Raynaud's phenomenon	+	++	±	±	+
Abnormalities in urine	++	+	−	++	−
Altered esophageal intestinal motility	±	++	+	±	±
Focal brain involvement	+	−	−	+	−
Leukopenia	++	−	−	−	±
Anemia (hemolytic)	+	±	−	−	−
Thrombocytosis	−	±	±	−	−

Legend: ++, greater than 50 percent; +, greater than 10 percent; ±, less than 10 percent; −, not present.
[a]SLE, syptemic lupus erythematosis; [b]PSS, progressive systemic sclerosis; [c]PAN, periarteritis nodosa; [d]RA, rheumatoid arthritis
Data from Hanson, 1987; Katz, 1987; Lauter, 1987; Madaio, 1987; SHMC, 1984; Speed, 1987; and Tuffanelli, 1987.

3. The pain must be widespread in both left and right sides of the body, as well as above and below the waist.

To date there is no totally accepted and specific laboratory or diagnostic testing available for this disorder. Laboratory tests, such as autoantibody tests, that would seem to be related and therefore useful, are more often normal than abnormal. There are some specific tests, however (i.e., sleeping electroencephalograms; alpha wave intrusion into delta wave; elevation of substance P in spinal fluid; decreased activity of natural killer cells; decreased spinal fluid levels of metabolites of biogenic amines), but they are too expensive or impractical for everyday use (Wallace, 1993, p. 14).

Treatment is usually highly individualized. The major focus is on restoring normal sleep patterns.

A test developed to identify chronic fatigue syndrome (also sometimes known as *chronic fatigue immune dysfunction syndrome—CFIDS*), which focuses on one particular cytotoxic T cell (CD_{8+}), may at least eliminate that diagnosis from consideration.

Laboratory Findings (General). The following findings for SLE may or may not occur: false-positive test for syphilis (Venereal Disease Research Laboratory antigen [VDRL]) or rapid plasma reagin (RPR),* profuse proteinuria (greater than 3.5 g/day,* cellular casts in the urine,* hemolytic anemia,* leukopenia, thrombocytopenia*) and normocytic anemia.* Findings indicative of periarteritis nodosa (PAN) include anemia with a very low hemoglobin content, leukocytosis, eosinophilia, increased erythrocyte sedimentation rate (ESR), proteinuria at 0.5 to 2.5 g/day, and hematuria. SS findings include hypergammaglobulinemia—abnormal urine sediment and renal involvement. Juvenile rheumatoid arthritis (JRA) shows anemia, at times profound. Findings indicative of acute rheumatoid arthritis (RA), include hypergammaglobulinemia, an increased ESR, mild anemia, and possible leukopenia and thrombocytopenia.

Clinical Findings. Clinical indications of SLE are a skin rash in a butterfly distribution over the cheeks and nose that is sensitive to sunlight (photosensitivity)—also known as focal erythema*—and occurs in greatest frequency in females between the ages of 12 and 45 and in the black race; Raynaud's phenomenon* (arterial vasoconstriction causing blanching of the fingers and hands, loss of sensation and pain, usually triggered by contact with cold); oral or nasopharyngeal ulceration*; polyarthritis without deformity*; evidence of pleuritis (pleural effusion) or pericarditis*; psychosis*; convulsions*; alopecia*; discoid lupus* (cutaneous lesions—sharply circumscribed erythematous macules and plaques—disk shaped); urticaria; and purpura. For PAN, polyarthralgias, hypertension, and abnormal urine in a middle-aged person are cardinal signs. Other skin manifestations include subcutaneous nodules and peripheral gangrene of the fingers and toes; gastrointestinal manifestations are cramping, abdominal bleeding, and a bleeding ulcer; renal manifestations include flank pain and abnormal urine; and respiratory manifestations are bronchitis and possible pleural effusions. In progressive systemic sclerosis (PSS), skin manifestations, are purplish indurated plaques that become waxy, smooth, shiny, devoid of hair, and linear on extremities, possibly on the trunk; if muscle or bone is involved, growth disturbances occur or muscular atrophy or flexion contractions; if systemic, the initial symptom is usually Raynaud's phenomenon, swelling and sclerosis of distal extremities, pain, stiffness, and weakness of joints and muscles. In juvenile rheumatoid arthritis (JRA), a rheumatoid rash may be present anywhere on body as well as the presence of myalgia, arthralgia, polyarthritis, fever, possible pleural effusion, and growth retardation. Clinical indications of RA include polyarthritis and persistent, prolonged morning stiffness.

12.2 ANTINUCLEAR ACTIVITY TESTS

Antinuclear antibodies (ANA) are antibodies against cell nuclear constituents that act as antigens. These antibodies are produced as common findings in systemic rheumatic diseases, many of which are collagen-vascular in type. They can also be seen occasionally in otherwise seemingly healthy persons.

ANA-positive diseases include RA, Sjögren's syndrome (keratoconjunctivitis sicca, dry eyes, xerostomia, and a connective tissue disease, usually RA), polymyositis, scleroderma, mixed connective tissue disease (MCTD), and lupus erythematosus (LE). These diseases may present

---

*Findings indicated by asterisks are criteria for the diagnosis of SLE. The patient must have at least four of the findings marked with an asterisk presenting serially or simultaneously over any period of observation (American Rheumatism Association Criteria, 1971).

with similar symptoms, although they vary greatly in both treatment and prognosis. Determination of the presence of certain ANAs can be useful in the differential diagnosis of these conditions.

Antibodies to DNA and to the soluble nucleoproteins were determined some time ago. An area of antibody testing discovered later is that of antibodies against the nonhistone acidic nucleoproteins. Histone proteins provide the base, or core, around which DNA is wound; nonhistone nucleoproteins serve more specific regulatory and catalytic roles in genetic expression.

12.2.1 Screening Tests

A. Immunofluorescent Antibodies, Indirect

Synonym: Autoantibody screen

Includes screening of:

Antimitochondrial antibody (AMA)

Antinuclear antibody (ANA) or antinuclear factor (ANF)

Antismooth muscle antibody (ASmA)

Intercellular antibody (IC [Pemphigus])

Basement membrane zone antibodies (bullous pemphigoid)

Anticentromere

Normal Range: Negative (elderly may have a 1:20 ratio for ANA)

Explanation of the Test. All the tests are done on serum samples taken at the same time. The test is a screening test that looks at each of the conditions individually. Separate tubes (red top) are used for each antibody to be tested. Each test requires 1 or 2 ml of serum.

The blood samples are allowed to react with specific animal tissue components, and reactions are made visible by rinsing off unreacted serum proteins and adding fluorescein-labeled antihuman immunoglobulins and complement. These react with the person's antibodies that have fixed to tissue sections.

Examination for specific immunofluorescence and pattern is done with a fluorescent microscope.

Findings. A positive test is defined as one in which "serum diluted 1:20 yields nuclear fluorescence regardless of pattern" (Laboratory of Pathology, 1991):

1. ANA in titers less than 1:10 occur in approximately 30% of healthy blood donors. Healthy older adults often have an elevated ANA titer, but in the low range (e.g., 1:40 or 1:80)
2. More than one pattern of nuclear staining can be found in positive sera
3. Although there is no single pattern found to be diagnostic of any one disease, certain patterns tend to occur more frequently in certain disorders (see Table 12–2)

TABLE 12–2. APPROXIMATE PREVALENCE, TITER AND NUCLEAR STAINING PATTERN OF ANA

Disease	% Positive	Titer	Homogenous	Speckled	Rim or Peripheral	Nucleolar
SLE: active	98–100	High	+++	±	+++	+
SLE: remission	90	Low-mod.	+++	+	+	+
DLE	20–50	Low-mod.	++	±	–	+
PSS	45–90	Mod.-high	+	++	Rare	++
RA	30–50	Low-mod.	+++	+	–	+
JRA	–	Low-mod.	+	–	–	+
Sjögren's syndrome	25–30	Mod.	++	+++	+	+
MCTD	100	Mod.-high	±	+++	±	+
Raynaud's disease	63	–	–	+	–	–
Polymyositis	25–75	Mod.	–	+	–	–
DIL	–	–	+++	±	–	–
PBC[a]	35–45	–	+	+	–	–
CAH[b]	65–75	–	+++	+	–	–

[a]Antimitochondrial antibody (AMA) is positive in 90–100% of cases of PBC.
[b]Antismooth muscle antibody (ASmA) is positive in 60–80% of cases of CAH.
Abbreviations: SLE, systemic lupus erythematosus; DLE, discoid lupus erythematosus; PSS, progressive systemic sclerosis; RA, rheumatoid arthritis; JRA, juvenile rheumatoid arthritis; MCTD, mixed connective tissue disease; DIL, drug induced lupus; PBC, primary biliary cirrhosis; CAH, chronic active hepatitis.
Table used with permission, Laboratory of Pathology, Seattle, WA, 1991.

B. Antiextractable Nuclear Antigen

Antigens tested: Antinuclear antibody (ANA); Antiextractable nuclear antigen (Anti-ENA); Extractable Nuclear Antigen (ENA); Antiribonucleoprotein (ARNP)

Includes screening of anti-ENA, anti-Sm (Smith), antiribonucleoprotein (anti-RNP), anti-SSA (Sjögren's syndrome A antibody), anti-SSB (Sjögren's syndrome B antibody); anti-RO, anti-LA

Normal Range: Negative

Explanation of the Test. Each specimen is run against all of the listed antigens found normally in the human spleen (Sm, RNP, SSB, SSA) as well as rabbit thymus extract treated with DNASE-containing Sm, RNP, and SSB, and RNASE-containing Sm and SSB. The antibodies can be detected by a number of techniques (Laboratory of Pathology, 1991).

TEST ADVANTAGES:

1. Immunofluorescence tests (ANA, FANA, Immunofluorescent ANA) provide the advantage of high sensitivity, especially with tissue cultures. For example, a persistently negative outcome would be strong evidence against a diagnosis of SLE
2. ANA tests provide almost immediate findings
3. Large amounts of sera can be screened at one time

TEST DISADVANTAGES:

1. Not very specific, especially for SLE
2. Does not allow a consistent distinction among antibodies against *specific* nuclear components
3. The high sensitivity can cause inconsistency when used as a parameter to follow the disease process because of response to treatment
4. There is considerable overlap in test responses among SLE, RA, and Sjögren's syndrome (Henry, 1991, pp. 887–888)

ENA ANTIBODY POSITIVE IN:

1. Eighty-six percent of individuals responsive to treatment for SLE (8% in nonresponsive individuals)
2. High titers in mixed connective tissue disease also associated with signs or symptoms of SLE and scleroderma
3. Anti-SM (antibodies to RNASE-resistant ENA) found in 74% of individuals demonstrating signs or symptoms of mixed connective tissue disease

SSA AND SSB ANTIBODIES POSITIVE IN:

- Diagnosis of Sjögren's syndrome and some forms of LE

12.2.2 Specific Tests

A. Antigen Test: Human Lymphocyte Antigen B27

Synonyms: Lymphocyte antigen B27; HLA B27*

Normal Range

Both positive and negative responses can be normal; positive in 7% of the caucasians

---

Explanation of the Test. The HLA complex is a major histocompatibility complex (MHC)* that controls many important immune functions in man. It is located on the short arm of chromosome 6 and is polymorphic (occurring in several different forms in different developmental stages). HLA antigens are present in lymphocytes and in most body tissues in varying densities (Henry, 1991, p. 775).

In transplantation of human tissue, identification of compatible HLA is essential. The test is also used for paternity testing.

Many disease processes are associated directly with certain positive HLA antigens (Henry, 1991, p. 775).

---

*Survival depends on the immunosystem's ability to recognize and respond to many foreign substances (antigens). This defense mechanism becomes an obstacle when immune recognition triggers autoaggressive reactions. Essential proteins for immune recognition are encoded by the major MHC genes and produce three classes based on structure. function, and genetic origin. In humans, class I molecules include HLA-A, HLA-B, and HLA-C. Human MHC studies made their first contribution in tissue transplantation (Kee, 1991, pp. 761–63; Lab. of Pathology, 1991).

POSITIVE RESPONSES OCCUR IN:

1. Ankylosing spondylitis (Marie Strumple disease). In caucasians, a positive B-27 occurs in over 90% of cases. A negative reaction virtually rules out the disease
2. Uveitis; indicates increased susceptibility
3. Other spondyloarthopathies:
   a. Juvenile rheumatoid arthritis (>50 percent)
   b. Arthritis associated with Reiter's syndrome (79 percent)
   c. Arthritis associated with psoriases
   d. Enteropathic arthritis: arthritis associated with ulcerative colitis, Crohn's disease or Yersinia entercolitica

FREQUENCY OF POSITIVE REACTIONS GREATER IN:

1. The white race
2. Men rather than women. Symptoms tend to be milder and progression less rapid in women

B. Antibody Tests

B1. Anti-n-DNA (Crithidia)

Synonyms: Anti-DS-DNA antibody (antibody to double-stranded DNA); double-stranded anti-DNA; Antinative DNA antibody

Normal Range

Negative at 1:10 screening dilution (a positive response indicated by a bright apple green within the *Crithidia luciliae* organism) (Laboratory of Pathology, 1991)

Explanation of the Test. This test (assay) is the most specific test for anti-n-DNA (antinative DNA), but it is less sensitive than the two other tests in frequent use (Farr-radioimmunoassay [RIA] and solid-phase enzyme immunoassay [EIA]), thereby ruling out more false-positive responses. Antibodies levels to native DNA occur in high titer and correlate with disease activity. They are therefore important in disease management, especially with SLE.

POSITIVE RESPONSES OCCUR IN:

1. High levels almost exclusively in SLE. The occurrence of native DNA antibodies are thought to be involved in the pathogenesis of the most severe variants of SLE when deposited as immune complexes (Laboratory of Pathology, 1991)
2. Low levels in dermatomyositis, discoid lupus erythematosus, mixed connective tissue disease, progressive systemic sclerosis, rheumatoid arthritis and Sjögren's syndrome (Tietz, 1990, p. 63)

B2. Antibodies to Other Nonhistone Acidic Nucleoproteins

Anti-RNP (antiribonucleoprotein). An increase in anti-RNP is usually found with an increase in anti-Sm. Anti-RNP may increase to high levels even in the absence of an anti-Sm increase.

Increased levels are seen in a variety of rheumatic diseases, including systemic lupus erythematosus (SLE), Rheumatoid arthritis (RA), Sjögren's syndrome, systemic scleroderma (SS), discoid (cutaneous) lupus erythematosus (LE), and mixed connective tissue disease (MCTD) with high titers (Henry, 1990, pp. 890–891).

Anti-Sm. Anti-Sm is sometimes referred to as antismooth muscle antigen, but it is actually named for the person in whom the antibody was first identified (Smith). Anti-Sm is present in 30 percent of systemic lupus erythematosus (SLE) patients, along with an increase in RNP, usually found in active disease and with renal involvement. It is rarely positive in other disorders, such as rheumatoid arthritis (RA), but can be present in sera of patients with scleroderma, polymyositis (often in atypical presentations with photosensitivity), subacute cutaneous lupus, or in neonatal lupus with congenital heart block.

Anti-Ro (SSA). Anti-Ro is a small cytoplasmic RNA protein whose function is unknown. It is found mostly in systemic lupus erythematosus (SLE) and Sjögren's syndrome. In some testing methods the antinuclear antigen (ANA) findings will be negative.

Anti-La (SSB). The simultaneous appearance of anti-Ro and a positive anti-La in SLE is generally associated with a milder disease than in the appearance of anti-Ro alone, and it is referred to as Sjögren's SLE.

ScL-70. ScL-70 (DNA topoisomerase; involved in DNA supercoiling) is found in system sclerosis (20 percent) and CREST patients. (CREST is an acronym used to describe the syndrome of *c*alcinosis cutis, *R*aynaud's phenomenon, *e*sophageal dysfunction, *s*clerodactylia and *t*elangiectasis [Henry, 1991, p. 891].)

Explanation of Nonhistone Acidic Nucleoprotein Antibody Tests. The listed antibodies are often considered more specific, even highly specific, in some collagen diseases, such as mixed connective tissue disease (MCTD). In that disease there is low incidence of renal and central nervous system (CNS) complications. It also responds well to corticosteroid treatment. Therefore, early diagnosis can be followed with early effective treatment.

Antibody and antigen screening tests (given in Section 12.2.2.A) usually precede specific testing. Specific testing (assays) is more expensive and, as the name implies, specific to a limited range of diseases. Such testing is usually performed only on those patients likely to have positive findings.

Patient Preparation. No special preparation is required.

C. Rheumatoid Arthritis (RA) Latex Test

Synonyms: RA latex; latex fixation; rheumatoid factor; RF

Reactions Reported:

Negative reaction	Normal
Positive	Titer of 80 or greater

Laboratory of Pathology, 1991

Explanation of the Test. The major use for this test at this time is in diagnosing rheumatoid arthritis (RA). The test is done on serum (*not* plasma) or synovial fluid. Rheumatoid factors exist in IgG, and IgM. In rheumatoid arthritis the IgM immunoglobulin is most common with IgG a rather distant second. The appearance of these macroglobulins in RA are believed to be a secondary manifestation of the disease (Tietz, p. 493).

The term *latex* refers to a suspension of latex that serves as an antigen after being coated with albumin and denatured human gamma globulin. (Body fluids other than serum that contain rheumatoid factors [RFs] include joint, tissue, and spinal fluid of most individuals.) The suspension detects RFs, indicating their presence. If specific dilutions of the factors are desired or confirmation of positive results needed, tube tests, rather than the slide test, can be done, which will provide the titer of the highest agglutination factor.

POSITIVE REACTIONS OCCUR IN:

1. Rheumatoid arthritis (85 percent)
2. Sclerodema
3. Systemic lupus erythematosus
4. Sjögren's syndrome (80–90 percent positive with high titers)
5. Dermatomyositis
6. Sarcoidosis

TITERS LESS THAN 80 FOUND IN:

1. Infectious mononucleosis
2. The elderly, with or without signs or symptoms of RA
3. Juvenile rheumatoid arthritis has only a 20-percent positive response

FALSE-POSITIVE REACTIONS CAN OCCUR IN:

- Individuals with hyperlipid serum

FALSE-NEGATIVE REACTIONS CAN OCCUR IN:

- Some individuals with definite clinical diagnostic signs and symptoms, cause unknown

D. *Tests Used for Differential Diagnosis of Rheumatoid or Muscular Disease*

D1. *Serum Aldolase*

Synonym: ALD

Normal Range: 2.5–7 U/l

Laboratory of Pathology, 1991

Explanation of the Test. Although the serum aldolase test is used only infrequently in the area of rheumatoid or muscular disease, it is particularly sensitive to detection of early skeletal muscle disease and is therefore occasionally used as a marker for muscle disease. Its "A" isoenzyme is found largely in skeletal muscle. It is useful in differential diagnosis among muscular disorders because serum levels of aldolase are *normal* in patients with neurogenic muscle disease.

Hemolyzed serum samples cannot be used as they contain high levels of aldolase from the red cell, producing false elevations.

Patient Preparation. n.p.o. except for water for 8 hours prior to serum collection.

SERUM ALDOLASE LEVELS INCREASED IN:

1. Muscular diseases:
   a. Duchenne's muscular dystrophy and dermatomyositis (high levels) as well as slight to moderate increase in female carriers of either of these disorders
   b. Lower-level increases occur in neurogenic muscle disease or motor endplate disease (e.g., myasthenia gravis/myotonic dystrophy)
2. Nonmuscular diseases:
   a. Carcinomatosis
   b. Granulocytic/chronic myelogenous leukemias
   c. Megaloblastic anemia
   d. Hepatitis
   e. Myocardial infarction
   f. Myotonic dystrophy
3. Normal development:
   • Newborn infants (levels four times that of adults; two times adult range in early childhood; gradual decrease to adult range by age 18–20)
4. Secondary to use of certain medication:
   • ACTH, cortisone, deoxycorticosterone (injected)

(Tietz, 1990, pp. 30–31)

D2. Synovial Fluid Analysis

Synonyms: Synovial analysis, joint fluid exam, joint tap[a]

Normal Range: See specific tests in Table 12–3

Includes one or all of the following:

Routine	Cell count (white blood cell [WBC], differential [if WBCs greater than 5] and red blood cells [RBCs])
	Gross appearance—clarity, color, viscosity
	Mucin clot formation
	Polarized light microscopy
Special	Complement level
	RFs
	Glucose
	Total protein (TP)
	Culture and Gram's stain

---

[a]See also Section 17.2.3, Arthrogram.

TABLE 12–3. GENERAL INTERPRETATION OF JOINT TAP TESTS

Test	Normal	Deviations from Normal, Possible Significance
Cell Count		
WBC	Less than 5 cells/ml (or 200/µL; usually flattened, lining cells and lymphocytes)	
RBC	None formed	Presence indicates hemorrhage or traumatic tap
Differential	Granulocytes less than 25% of nucleated cells	Polys: inflammatory septic arthritis; increased lymphocyte or monocyte counts: viral infections, foreign body reaction
Other	Lining cells: mesothelial	With any injury, these cells react by becoming stratified and change from flat to cuboidal; usually accompanied by a protective effusion Can mimic benign or malignant cells Malignancy involving serosal surfaces usually metastatic except for rare primary mesothelioma and a few sarcomas In RA: superficial synovial cells proliferate; marked villous hypertrophy; marked infiltration of chronic inflammatory cells (lymphocytes/plasma cells) tending to form "lymphoid nodules"; compact fibrin deposited on surface or interstitially; necrosis
Gross appearance	Crystal clear; straw color (pale yellow); transparent; turbidity reported as 1+ to 4+[a]	Turbid yellow; increased leukocyte count secondary to infection or inflammation Milky (pseudochylous); tuberculous arthritis, chronic arthritis, acute gouty arthritis, or SLE Grossly purulent: acute septic arthritis, late stages Greenish tinged: influenza septic arthritis; chronic RA; in some instances of gout or pseudogout
String test[b] (viscosity)	Viscosity reported as normal or "high"; normal string test result: formation of a string 4–6 cm in length; if string breaks before 3-cm length is reached, viscosity is below normal	Viscosity is decreased in a wide variety of inflammatory conditions (e.g., septic, gouty, or rheumatoid arthritis); decreased viscosity can also occur following trauma or with fever
Mucin clot test (Rope's test)	A firm clot forms rapidly after a drop of synovial fluid (SF) is placed in an acetic acid solution Reported as: Good or abundant Fair: soft clot in slightly turbid solution	Generally as for viscosity above, with exceptions of acute effusions (e.g., rheumatic fever, sepsis, trauma, overuse); although viscosity is decreased by fever, clot formation remains normal

(continued)

TABLE 12–3. (Continued)

Test	Normal	Deviations from Normal, Possible Significance
	Poor: friable clot in turbid solution; shreds on agitation Very poor: no clot formation; flakes in cloudy suspension	
Polarized light microscopy	No crystals	Simple, precise, definitive test; aids in differential diagnosis of gout and pseudogout by demonstrating urate (gout) and phosphate (pseudogout) crystals Phosphate: calcium pyrophosphate dihydrate (CPPD) Urate: monosodium urate (MSU) Apatite crystals: rare form of arthritis Talcum crystals: rare form of arthritis secondary to joint surgery Crystalline: secondary to therapeutic injection of corticosteroids Osteo- or traumatic arthritis: fragments of cartilage and collagen fibrils
Complement	Varies with the concentration of SF protein; expressed in relationship to total protein	Decreased in RA and SLE Occasionally decreased in rheumatic fever, bacterial arthritis, gout, pseudogout, and other types of inflammatory arthritis Total hemolytic complement increased in arthritis of Reiter's syndrome
Rhumatoid factors (RFs)	Absent	Present in about 60% of patients with RA; may be present before becoming measurable in serum; high incidence of false positives
Glucose	70–110 mg/dl; concentration identical or slightly less than plasma glucose (usually within 10 mg/dl)	If patient not fasting 6–12 hr before test, SF glucose may be lower than that in plasma; under 40 mg/dl suggests decreased SF glucose in this instance Noninflammatory arthritis: SF glucose level decreased10 mg/dl Inflammatory arthritis: SF glucose level decreased more than 25 or 50 mg/dl
Total protein (TP)	1–3 g/dl; often expressed as spinal fluid (SF)/plasma ratio	Levels of individual proteins in SF change with changes in plasma proteins Increased SF/plasma TP ratio occurs with inflammation resulting from increased permeability of synovial membrane Therefore, increased SF/plasma TP = evidence of inflammation

[a]0, Crystal clear fluid; 1+, faintly "cloudy," "smoky," "hazy" with slight (barely visible) turbidity; 2+, turbidity clearly present—newsprint easily read through the tube; 3+, newsprint not easily read through the tube; 4+, newsprint cannot be seen through the tube.
[b]A string test is an estimate of viscosity done by allowing SF to form a string by dropping from a syringe into a beaker (Henry, 1991).
Data from Bienenstock, 1980; Henry, 1991; Laboratory of Pathology, 1991; and Wenig, 1980.

Explanation of the Test. Because there is little fluid in any joint (0.1 to 2.0 ml), a "dry" tap is common unless an effusion is present. For this test, joint fluid is aspirated from an involved joint by a process known as *arthrocentesis,* that is, withdrawal of fluid by way of a sterile needle and syringe. The area to be aspirated is generally prepared as for orthopedic surgery, and strict sterile technique is used to prevent infection of the joint. The test is a fairly simple one, it provides substantial information, and the cost is relatively low. Therefore, it can be used for the initial evaluation or differential diagnosis of possible arthritis, suspected infection, or other inflammatory rheumatoid conditions (Christian, 1980); see Table 12–3.

Patient Preparation

1. Fasting for at least 6 to 8 hours if glucose concentration is to be measured
2. If infectious arthritis is suspected, a Gram's stain and culture are usually carried out as well

---

RELATED NURSING DIAGNOSES

The nursing diagnoses selected for this chapter are those that most often affect patients with active juvenile and adult RA, SLE, PAN, and SS (or scleroderma) because these are the most frequently seen disorders of this rather imprecise body system. Table 12–1 provides some insights into the variety of signs and symptoms these disorders share.

The nursing diagnosis knowledge deficit is not addressed here because it is seen as a universal diagnosis that applies to all people who are ill.

Alteration in Comfort: Pain, Acute and Chronic, Related to:*

1. Inflammation and/or swelling of joints (synovitis due to RA; inflammation because of SLE, PAN), known as arthralgia
2. Inflammation and/or swelling of skeletal muscles (myalgia) due to PAN, SLE, RA
3. Dry mucous membrane (sicca or Sjögren's syndrome)
4. Peripheral arterial spasm (Raynaud's phenomenon)
5. Severe headache
6. Peripheral neuritis

Impaired Mobility Related to

(Depending on the severity and duration of the following conditions, the differential nursing diagnoses here would be activity intolerance and self-care deficit)

1. Progressive muscle weakness due to disease process (polymyositis) or prescribed rest with a loss of muscle mass
2. Pain on movement (see diagnosis 1)
3. Stiffness after periods of inactivity, e.g., on rising in the morning (SLE, RA)
4. Skin fibrosis (PSS) causing thickening, painless swelling, flexion contractures, soft tissue atrophy
5. Proximal muscle weakness of the shoulder and pelvic girdles (polymyositis)
6. Excessive fatigue (SLE)
7. Joint deformity (RA)
8. Contractures (RA, PSS {see item 4})
9. Decreased nutritional status (all)
10. Prescribed prolonged rest
11. Possible hemiplegia (complication of PAN, dependent on site)

---

*Rheumatoid disorders tend to fluctuate between acute and chronic episodes, but the individuals afflicted with these disorders almost always have *some* degree of pain.

Disturbance in Self-concept

Body Image, Related to

1. Skin lesions (SLE)
2. Disfigurement as with swollen joints, contractures (RA, SLE), fibrosis of facial skin (PSS)
3. Bloodshot eyes (sicca syndrome, PSS)
4. Need for assistive devices, e.g., splints, wheelchairs

Self-esteem, Related to

1. Increased dependence on others
2. Mood swings (SLE, therapy with corticosteroids)

Role Performance (Social, Work, and Family), Related to

1. Dyspareunia (sicca syndrome, PSS)
2. Disability discharge (loss of job due to poor health)
3. Displacement from family activities

Injury: Potential for

Trauma/Falls, Related to

1. Decreased muscle strength due to inactivity
2. Lack of ability to maintain balance due to pain on movement, contractures
3. Orthostatic hypotension due to
   a. Difficulty in or inability to change position independently or change position frequently
   b. Blood pooling in dependent areas with muscle wasting (loss of somatic pump effect)
4. Behavioral disturbance/convulsions with CNS involvement (PAN)

Trauma/Skin Breakdown, Related to

1. Decreased mobility (see Trauma/Falls, item 3)
2. Increased dependency on others for skin care
3. Decreased nutritional status (inadequate nutrients and/or obesity)

Side Effects of Long-term Medication Use

1. Bleeding secondary to long-term aspirin use (gastritis, peptic ulcer disease [PUD])
2. Fluid/electrolyte imbalance secondary to long-term ibuprofen administration
3. Infection secondary to decreased immune response with administration of glucocorticoids. (WBC production also decreases with long-term decreased mobility)
4. Fractures secondary to long-term glucocorticoid use

Altered Growth and Development, Related to

In Children, Motor, Social, or Emotional Retardation Due to

1. Decreased mobility (may be totally dependent) secondary to pain, muscle weakness
2. Environmental deprivation secondary to
   a. Prolonged hospitalization (separation from family)
   b. Activity restriction (isolation from peer group)
   c. Potential for impaired bonding with parents

In Adults, Developmental Tasks Incomplete

1. Social isolation secondary to
   a. Withdrawal because of, or in fear of rejection
   b. Fear of being a burden on others
   c. Lack of mutual interests and abilities with peer group
   d. Prescribed activity limitations
2. Physical or social constraints on long-term planning, secondary to
   a. Early retirement (voluntary or forced)
   b. Economic constraints with unknown future costs of illness
   c. Unknown future level of function

T H I R T E E N

THE HEMATOLOGIC SYSTEM

RECOGNITION OF HEMATOLOGIC DYSFUNCTION

Disorders of the red blood cells (RBCs), hemoglobin (Hgb), or white blood cells (WBCs) are usually diagnosed in a stepwise fashion. The basic screening tests are done first (see Part I) as well as a thorough history and physical examination. If anemia is evident but a definitive diagnosis is still lacking, a reticulocyte count is usually done to roughly determine marrow function. At this point most anemias can be identified. Only after a tentative diagnosis is determined are further tests usually ordered, because the tests tend to be specific to given foci or etiologies and are more expensive.

13.1 LABORATORY OR CLINICAL INDICATIONS OF HEMATOLOGIC SYSTEM DYSFUNCTION

Laboratory Findings. Indications of hematologic system dysfunction include evidence of anemia that is persistent and/or nonresponsive to therapy; decreased number of reticulocytes present, given the severity of the anemia (the percentage may increase but not to appropriate levels); pancytopenia; poikilocytosis, anisocytosis, stippling, or polychromatophilia in RBCs; presence of target cells; WBC count increased above 25,000/mm^3 or decreased below 1000/mm^3, decreased neutrophil count, and wide shift to the left with large numbers of blast cells. In urine, persistent hemoglobinuria or hemosiderinuria is found.

Clinical Findings. Clinical indications of hematologic system dysfunction include chronic, progressive fatigue, pallor, weakness; dyspnea; bleeding such as petechiae in the lower extremities, small retinal hemorrhages, oozing from mucous membranes; lemon-yellow jaundice; splenomegaly; decreased resistance to infection with recurrent infections, especially of mucous membranes (e.g., oral cavity, anorectal area, genitourinary tract, and respiratory tract); neurologic symptoms such as headache, vertigo, tinnitus; and joint pain (acute with disability), swelling of hands and feet otherwise unexplained.

13.2 TESTS OF HEMATOLOGIC PRODUCTION

13.2.1 Bone Marrow Examination

Synonyms: None

Includes: Bone marrow aspiration, bone marrow biopsy

Normal Range: See Table 13–1

Explanation of the Test. Bone marrow aspiration is one of the nine basic tests of hematology, not in the sense of a screening test, but rather as a keystone of diagnosis. Marrow cells are either aspirated or removed by biopsy (percutaneous needle biopsy is the most common method). If the marrow cannot be aspirated (dry tap), a biopsy is required. There is a technique that permits both aspiration and biopsy, which provides more information and is endorsed by many practitioners (Harvey et al., 1988). A biopsy specimen includes both bone and marrow. An aspiration provides marrow only. The most accessible marrow-containing bone is the sternum, but in adults the iliac crest is used primarily. Marrow cellularity (the ratio of volume of hematopoietic cells to total marrow space volume) decreases with age and varies with the site. Marrow-containing bones in the adult, in decreasing order of marrow cellularity, are the vertebrae, sternum, iliac crest, and the ribs. Once the specimen is obtained, smears are made and examined, or a clot section (clotted marrow) is processed like an ordinary histological specimen. The specimens are examined for the presence, number, and developmental, or maturational, stage of each type of cell. A differential count of the cells may be done and the myeloid (leukocytes of the myeloid or nucleated series)/erythroid (nucleated erythrocytic cells) (M/E) ratio determined. Iron stores can also be determined by a staining process when requested.

Normal values for the differential count vary widely depending on the source used (see Table 13–1). Variation occurs because of differing cell classification, the type of process used, the wide range of normal values, and the fact that reliable data regarding normal bone marrow are scarce (Widmann, 1983).

INDICATIONS FOR USE:

1. Diagnosis of megaloblastic anemias, leukemia, or multiple myeloma
2. To demonstrate bone marrow cellular precursor deficiency (hypoplasia) as the cause of decreased levels of one or more cellular elements of the blood
3. To document a decrease in body iron stores in certain iron deficiency anemias
4. To demonstrate metastatic neoplasm
5. To demonstrate certain types of infectious disease (tuberculosis, histoplasmosis)
6. To determine the existence of diseases that affect macrophages (e.g., lipid or glycogen storage diseases)

CHANGES IN BONE MARROW

Interpretation is ordinarily done by a hemotologist or a clinical pathologist.

1. Hypoplasia (decreased cellular production) as a result of
   a. Chronic infection

TABLE 13–1. DIFFERENTIAL CELL COUNTS OF BONE MARROW (PERCENTAGE OF TOTAL NUCLEATED CELLS)

| | Rosse et al. (1977) | | | | | | Mauer (1969) | | Wintrobe et al. (1974) | |
| | Birth | | | 1 month | | | Over 4 months | | Adult | |
	Mean	±	SD	Mean	±	SD	Mean	Range	Mean	Range
Normoblasts, total	14.5	±	7.2	8.0	±	5.0	23.1		25.6	(18.4–33.8)
Pronormoblasts	0.02	±	0.06	0.10	±	0.14	0.5	(0–1.5)		(0.2–1.3)
Basophilic normoblasts	0.24	±	0.24	0.34	±	0.33	1.7	(0.2–4.8)		(0.5–2.4)
Polychromatophilic normoblasts	13.1	±	6.8	6.9	±	4.4	18.2	(4.8–34.0)		(17.9–29.2)
Orthochromatic normoblasts	0.69	±	0.73	0.54	±	1.88	2.7	(0–7.8)		(0.4–4.6)
Neutrophils, total	60.4	±	8.7	32.4	±	7.7	57.1		53.6	(49.2–65.0)
Myeloblasts	0.31	±	0.31	0.62	±	0.50	1.2	(0–3.2)		(0.2–1.5)
Promyelocytes	0.79	±	0.91	0.76	±	0.65	1.4	(0–4.0)		(2.1–4.4)
Myelocytes	3.9	±	2.9	2.5	±	1.5	18.3	(8.5–29.7)		(8.2–15.7)
Metamyelocytes	19.4	±	4.8	11.3	±	3.6	23.3	(14.0–34.2)		(9.5–24.6)
Bands	28.4	±	7.6	14.1	±	4.6				(9.5–15.3)
Segmented	7.4	±	4.6	3.6	±	3.0	12.9	(4.5–29.0)		(6.0–12.0)
Eosinophils	2.7	±	1.3	2.6	±	1.4	3.6	(1.0–9.0)	3.1	(1.2–5.3)
Basophils	0.12	±	0.20	0.07	±	0.16	0.06	(0–0.8)	0.1	(0–0.2)
Lymphocytes, total	15.6			49.0			16.0	(4.8–35.8)	16.2	(11.1–23.2)
Transitional	1.2	±	1.1	2.0	±	0.9				
Small (mature)	14.4	±	5.5	47.0	±	9.2				
Plasma cells	0.00	±	0.02	0.02	±	0.06	0.4	(0.2–0.6)	1.3	(0.4–3.9)
Monocytes	0.88	±	0.85	1.01	±	0.89			0.3	(0–0.8)
Megakaryocytes	0.06	±	0.15	0.05	±	0.09			0.1	(0–0.4)
Reticulum cells									0.3	(0–0.9)
M/E ratio	4.4			4.4			2.9	(1.2–5.2)	2.3	(1.5–2.3)

Gross appearance: dark blood with greater viscosity than blood

From Nelson, D. A. (1969). Hematopoiesis. In J. B. Henry (Ed.), *Clinical diagnosis and management by laboratory methods* (16th ed.), p. 958. Philadelphia: Saunders, with permission. Data from Mauer, A. M. (1969); Rosse, C. et al. (1977); and Wintrobe, M. M. et al. (1974).

   b. Hypothyroidism (present in one third of patients with macrocytic anemia)
   c. Chronic renal failure because of decreased erythropoietin production
   d. Advanced liver disease such as far-advanced cirrhosis
   e. Marrow replacement because of fibrosis (myelofibrosis) or neoplasm
   f. Aplastic anemia because of toxic destruction or idiosyncratic reaction (Ravel, 1989)
2. Hyperplasia (increased cellular production) as a result of
   a. Anemias such as iron deficiency or pernicious, other folate and vitamin B_{12} metabolic disease with peculiar RBC appearance as well as megaloblastic maturation, thalassemias as a compensatory response to inadequate or ineffective peripheral blood cells
   b. Hemoglobinopathies
   c. Hypersplenism, because of increased cell sequestration or destruction
   d. Enzyme deficiencies (e.g., glucose-6-phosphate dehydrogenase [G-6-PD]) because of ineffective cellular activity
   e. Red cell membrane abnormalities (e.g., hereditary spherocytosis [as for item d])
   f. Destructive processes (e.g., antibody-mediated, bacterial, or chemical hemolysis) because of increased cell loss
3. Appearance of abnormal or rare cell types in marrow, found in

Cell	Associated Disorder	Comment
Tissue mast cells	Increase in number in aplastic or refractory anemias and macroglobulinemia	Occur frequently
Osteoblasts, osteoclasts	Occur in adult marrow with hyperparathyroidism, Paget's disease, metastatic tumor, or after a recent biopsy at the same site	Occur normally in small numbers in infants and children
Metastatic neoplastic cells	Metastic tumor at site of biopsy sample; resemble primitive blast cells	Usually appear in clusters or clumps

Data from Henry, 1984.

4. Increases and decreases in M/E ratio (normal range, 2:1 to 4:1)
   a. Increases in (increased number of myeloid cells or decreased number of nucleated RBCs)
      (1) Normal newborns and infants, only slightly higher than the norm and less than 4:1
      (2) Infection, chronic myelogenous leukemia, and erythroid hypoplasia
   b. Decreased in polycythemia vera (less than 2:1; greater than normal proportion of nucleated red cells because of depression of leukopoiesis or increased number of nucleated RBCs)
5. Iron stain for siderocytes (synonyms: siderocyte stain, sideroblast stain)
   a. Explanation of the test: normoblasts (marrow RBCs) in the bone marrow that contain iron granules can be demonstrated by special staining. The stained cells, called sideroblasts, are a normal and expected inhabitant of bone marrow
   b. Deviations from normal
      (1) Sideroblasts are totally absent or greatly reduced in patients with iron deficiency anemias

(2) The number of granules per cell (sideroblast) is greatly increased in sideroblastic anemias and forms a ring around the nucleus

See also Section 13.2.3.

Patient Preparation/Teaching: Bone Marrow Test. Except for skin preparation and psychological support, no special preparation is necessary. Iliac crest taps are painful, and the patient will need advance warning and instruction in methods of coping (e.g., instructions and assistance in place-ment to maintain position during the tap so that a second puncture will not be necessary; pain control by way of arranging for availability of sedatives before the procedure and analgesics at the time of marrow aspiration).

If a bone marrow biopsy is done with a local anesthetic, a small incision is made in the skin to allow introduction of the large-bone needle used. The procedure is done only in the iliac bone in adults because the sternum is too thin and will follow the aspiration if both are being per-formed. A biopsy is more painful than an aspiration and may require the use of narcotic anal-gesics before the procedure.

Postprocedure Care: Bone Marrow Test. Pressure should be applied to the site for several min-utes to prevent any hemorrhage. Usually there is no discomfort after a bone marrow aspira-tion. If a bone marrow biopsy is done (usually of the iliac crest), pressure should be applied for 60 minutes by using both a pressure dressing and having the patient lie recumbent on the site.

13.2.2 Schilling Test

Synonym: Vitamin B_{12} uptake

Normal Value: Values are dose dependent; 7% excretion/24 hr with 0.5-μg dose

Range: 8–40%/24 hr

Explanation of the Test. The Schilling test is used to further define the cause of a macrocytic or megaloblastic anemia—for the differential diagnosis of pernicious anemia and various other malabsorption syndromes. The person with pernicious anemia does not absorb vitamin B_{12} be-cause of the lack of intrinsic factor in gastric secretions. Intrinsic factor is essential to vitamin B_{12} absorption from the terminal end of the ileum. The Schilling test is the most convenient method for determining the ability of the patient to absorb an oral dose (0.5 to 2.0 μg) of ra-dioactive vitamin B_{12}. This is done by measuring the radioactivity in a 24-hour urine sample. To ensure that the labeled vitamin B_{12} absorbed will be excreted into the urine and not bound to protein in the body, a parenteral dose of unlabeled vitamin B_{12} is given as a large flushing dose. It is given parenterally for quicker absorption and will saturate tissue-binding sites, thereby al-lowing the labeled vitamin B_{12} to be excreted into the urine. The timing of this dose varies with the facility using the test. It has been given before the labeled dose of vitamin B_{12}, at the same time, or 1 or 2 hours after.

If the test response is abnormal, that is, less than 7 percent excretion in 24 hours, it is re-peated, usually after 3 days. The test is then identical except that hog intrinsic factor is given in adequate amounts together with the oral labeled vitamin B_{12}. If excretion is within normal limits on the second test, the diagnosis of pernicious anemia is made because supplying the missing factor normalized the response. If the 24-hour excretion is still below or at the lower limit of normal, something other than intrinsic factor lack is the cause (e.g., folate deficiency or malabsorption), and further tests are indicated.

BELOW-NORMAL REACTIONS OCCUR IN:

Conditions other than pernicious anemia such as in

1. Individuals with poor renal function. The test is usually prolonged to 48- or 72-hour collection in known cases of reduced urine production or when blood urine nitrogen (BUN) is elevated
2. A considerable number of patients with sprue because of malabsorption
3. The elderly. This is usually a physiological and normal finding
4. Incomplete urine collection for the test—a falsely low value. Measurement of urine creatinine levels may be helpful in checking on the completeness of urine collection

Patient Preparation/Teaching

1. The patient should be kept n.p.o. except for water 12 hours before the test and maintained until the "flushing dose" of nonlabeled vitamin B_{12} has been given
2. Thorough patient instruction with follow-up observation and reminders are indicated when the patient is responsible for collecting the urine. Written instructions should also be supplied
3. If a bone marrow examination is planned, it should precede this test because the large dose of vitamin B_{12} given in the second step of the test can quickly convert the megaloblastic changes to a normal picture
4. The test may be done even though treatment for pernicious anemia has already begun as long as intrinsic factor itself is not given

13.2.3 Iron Studies

A. *Total Iron*

Synonyms: Serum iron concentration, serum iron, SI

Normal Ranges (µg/dl)

Adult	65–175
Senior adult	As for adult
Pediatric	
Newborn	100–200
4 mo.–2 years	40–100
Thereafter	85–150

Explanation of the Test. Iron studies, in general, are undertaken when a microcytic, hypochromic anemia has been discovered and blood loss cannot be documented. Iron deficiency is the most common cause of that type of anemia (mean corpuscular volume [MCV] less than 80 fl; mean corpuscular Hgb concentration [MCHC] less than 32 percent—on a Coulter counter it may be within normal limits or only slightly hypochromic). Knowledge of serum iron levels and the total iron-binding capacity (TIBC) usually permits discrimination between iron deficiency anemia and the second most commonly occurring anemia, that associated with chronic disorders.

Iron deficiency anemia resulting from dietary lack is very rare in adults but not uncommon in infants and the elderly. The anemia of chronic illness with a slow, gradual onset is not uncommon in the adult.

Serum iron levels are often decreased in anemias other than pure iron deficiency. Iron deficiency anemia is almost always due to one of three factors or a combination of the three factors: inadequate dietary iron intake, poor absorption of iron from the intestine, and chronic blood loss—probably in reverse order of occurrence.

Other tests of importance in the diagnosis and follow-up of iron deficiency anemia are MCV, TIBC, erythrocyte sedimentation rate (ESR), and serum bilirubin (helpful in patients with liver disease: bilirubin is a normal endproduct of RBC destruction, and when cells are lost from the body before the end of their life span, serum bilirubin levels will decrease and can be totally absent).

SERUM IRON LEVELS DECREASED IN:

See also Table 13–2 in the next section, Total Iron-Binding Capacity.

1. Physiological diurnal variation with a decrease of as much as 100 mg/dl in evening levels over morning levels
2. The nephrotic syndrome because of the urinary loss of protein, to include transferrin, the transport plasma protein for iron. Transferrin is also sometimes called siderophilin
3. Response to long-term chronic blood loss. In the adult over 40 years of age, gastrointestinal cancer should be ruled out. Other causes include heavy menstrual flow, peptic ulcer, ulcerative colitis, Crohn's disease, diverticulitis, and hemorrhoids
4. Periods of rapid growth such as in the infant aged 6 months to 2 years—particularly the premature and the infant on a prolonged milk-only diet
5. Decreased intake at any age over a prolonged period of time—2 to 3 months
6. Some malabsorption syndromes or other disorders of the digestive tract such as achlorhydria (an acid environment is necessary for iron absorption)
7. Repeated pregnancies, especially when coexisting with a marginal intake. Each pregnancy causes 600 to 900 mg of iron loss, which is due in part to fetal demand for iron
8. Conditions leading to chronic slight hematuria such as tumors, stones, or inflammatory disease. Rarely, large amounts of iron are lost in the urine of patients with a chronic hemolytic disorder
9. Infection. Occurs rarely in adults, frequently in children who have repeated infections such as upper respiratory or chronic inflammatory processes (e.g., rheumatic fever). Other factors are also instrumental in the occurrence of iron deficiency anemia in children with rheumatic fever
10. Individuals receiving certain drugs therapeutically (e.g., adrenocorticotropic hormones [ACTH], steroids, hydroxyurea)

SERUM IRON LEVELS INCREASED IN:

1. Sideroblastic anemias* such as thalassemia because of the decreased synthesis of available iron in Hgb (Miale, 1972)
2. Increased intake
3. Increased Hgb breakdown as in the hemolysis of sickle cell anemia
4. Individuals who are being treated with a number of drugs (e.g., estrogen, oral contraceptives, chloramphenicol)
5. Hemochromatosis as a result of a highly increased rate of iron absorption by the intestinal mucosal cell

Patient Preparation. No special preparation is necessary; however, a fasting specimen is preferred.

B. Total Iron-binding Capacity

Synonyms: Iron-binding capacity, IBC, TIBC, human transferrin test

Normal Ranges (μg/dl)

Adults	250–450
Senior adults	As for adults
Pediatric	
Newborn	60–175
4 mo.–2 years	100–400
Thereafter	350–450

Explanation of the Test. Iron enters the body in a ferrous state. Once absorbed, it is transported by a plasma protein called transferrin, or siderophilin, which combines avidly with the iron. Once combined, the iron is converted to its ferric state. The capacity of transferrin to combine with iron is measured as iron-binding capacity, and its concentration is markedly consistent. Generally but not always, conditions that decrease serum iron levels increase total iron binding, that is, the less iron available to be bound, the greater the number of empty binding sites. The capacity of transferrin to bind iron is about three times as great as the normal serum concentration of iron.

Usually the *percent saturation of TIBC* is calculated when the TIBC determination is done. Percent saturation represents the ratio of serum iron to the TIBC concentration (Table 13–2). It follows a diurnal pattern much as serum iron does, being highest in the morning and lowest in later afternoon and early evening. Values below 15 percent indicate an iron deficiency anemia or iron deficient erythropoiesis (Henry, 1991).

---

*Conditions in which the body is unable to incorporate iron into Hgb and when iron granules are found ringing the nucleus of marrow RBCs (normoblasts), in peripheral erythrocytes, and in diffuse body tissues. Siderocytes are nonnucleated red blood cells (RBCs); sideroblasts are nucleated red blood cells, the immature forms of the siderocyte. Laboratory of Pathology, 1991.

TABLE 13–2. COMPARISON OF CHANGES IN TIBC, SERUM IRON, AND PERCENT SATURATION IN SELECTED DISORDERS

Pathology	TIBC	Serum Iron	Percent Saturation
Iron deficiency anemia	Increased	Decreased	Decreased
Thalassemia, trait	Normal	Normal or increased	—
Thalassemia	Decreased	Increased	Increased
Anemia of chronic disease	Normal or decreased	Decreased	—
Sideroblastic anemia	Decreased	Increased	—
Nephrosis	Decreased	Increased	Increased
Chronic infections	Decreased	Decreased	Decreased
Menses, heavy	Normal	Decreased	Decreased
Hemolytic anemia	Normal or decreased	Increased	Increased
Hemochromatosis	Normal or decreased	Increased	Increased
Oral contraceptives, use of	Increased	Normal or increased	Normal
Acute hepatitis, viral	Increased	Increased	Normal or increased
Chronic renal disease	Decreased	Decreased	Normal or decreased
Pregnancy	Increased	Normal or decreased	Decreased

Data from Henry, 1984; Miale, 1972; and Widmann, 1983.

Patient Preparation. No special preparation is necessary.

C. Serum Ferritin Concentration

Synonym: Iron stores

Normal Range: 12 to 300 µg/L—radioimmunoassay (RIA)

Male mean	130 ng/ml
Female mean	59 ng/ml radiometric assay
Iron depletion at less than 31 ng/ml	
Absent iron stores at less than 10 ng/ml	

Laboratory of Pathology, 1991

Explanation of the Test. Ferritin is the body's major iron storage protein, a high-molecular-weight protein and correlates with total body iron stores. It is found in almost all body tissue but is located primarily in reticuloendothelial cells and liver cytoplasm. Its measurement (quantitation) accurately reflects intracellular iron stores. When done together with serum iron and TIBC measurements, a more complete diagnostic picture is available and may eliminate the need for bone marrow examination for the diagnosis of iron deficiency.

The test is used mainly for differentiating iron deficiency anemia from other microcytic, hypochromic anemias because it is a more specific indicator than the other standard tests. It can also be used for monitoring iron stores in hemodialysis patients with chronic renal failure or for monitoring therapy for patients with iron deficiency or overload (Detmer, et al., 1992, p. 78).

IRON LEVELS DECREASED IN:

• Iron deficiency anemia

IRON LEVELS NORMAL OR INCREASED IN:

1. Some other forms of anemia, e.g., Thalassemia minor
2. Conditions that disturb erythropoiesis such as liver disease (e.g., infectious hepatitis, cirrhosis, cancer, Hodgkin's disease with liver involvement) and leukemia

POSSIBLE FALSE ELEVATIONS IN:

• Active liver disease because a protein, not iron, is measured (Laboratory of Pathology, 1991)

13.3 TESTS OF HEMOGLOBIN

13.3.1 Hemoglobin Electrophoresis

Synonym: Hgb Electrophoresis

Normal Ranges (%)

Hgb A + F	96.5–98.2
Hgb A$_2$	1.8–3.5
Hgb F (fetal Hgb, alkali-resistant Hgb) (% of total)	
Adult	0
Adolescent	0–2
Newborn	40–70
Neonatal	20–40
Infant	2–10
Abnormal Hgbs	
Hgb S, adult (sickle cell test)	0
Methemoglobin, adult (Hgb M)	2
Carboxyhemoglobin	
Adult	0–2.3
Smoker	2.1–4.2
Hgb C, adult	0

Explanation of the Test. Electrophoresis shows the movement of particles of different isoelectric points in an electric field at controlled pH. In this test the differing molecular structure of the various Hgbs are identified by the rate and direction in which they travel. Although there are many different methods of electrophoretic separation, none are able to separate *all* the Hgbs. The methods most frequently used for routine Hgb electrophoresis separate Hgbs S, F, C, A, and A$_2$, which identifies normal Hgbs and those Hgbs most commonly abnormal in humans as well as most important in the western hemisphere (Ravel, 1989).

Hgb electrophoresis is used as a screening test for patients believed to have one of the many hemoglobinopathies. By characterizing the presence of one or more abnormal Hgb, or the presence of abnormally large or small amounts of normal Hgbs, the specific disorder or disorders can be diagnosed. Most abnormal Hgbs result from the substitution of a single amino acid for another one on the four globin polypeptide chains of the Hgb molecule but do not always result in hemolytic anemias. Hemoglobinopathies can also be due to a deficient synthesis of normal Hgb such as in thalassemia (Laboratory of Pathology, 1991).

Table 13–3 lists the clinical syndromes associated with hemoglobinopathies.

TABLE 13–3. CLINICAL SYNDROMES IN HEMOGLOBINOPATHIES

Syndrome	Abnormal Hgb	Comments
Sickle cell anemia	Hgb-S present (60%); SS—homozygote; Hgb F (10%)	Infants protected by presence of Hgb F; can become anemic, however; causing crises because of intravascular sickling of RBCs and decreased blood flow to the part
Sickle cell trait	Hgb S present; AS—heterozygote	Usually no clinical disease; provides protection against malarial infection *(Plasmodium falciparum)*
Hgb C disease	Hgb C present; CC—homozygote	Rare; mild chronic anemia usually, but can be quite severe; large number of target cells present
Hgb C trait	Hgb C present; AC—heterozygote	Usually asymptomatic; occurs in 2–5% of black Americans; target cells present
Sickle cell–Hgb C disease	SC; both Hgb C and S present	Causes moderate to severe hemolytic disease; many target cells; hematuria, splenomegaly (contrasts with pure sickle cell anemia), necrosis of bone even more common than in pure sickle cell disease
Beta-thalassemia major (Cooley's anemia, Mediterranean anemia)	No abnormal Hgb in any pure thalassemias; beta-chain defect with decreased synthesis rate; two patterns: increased % Hgb F + Hgb A_2 levels normal or decreased; Hgb F levels normal, Hgb A_2 greater than normal	Usually detected in childhood, thus the normal Hgb F; found primarily in Mediterranean races; most severe of the thalassemias; Howell-Jolly bodies often present in RBCs; severe anemia; often increased WBC count; splenomegaly
Beta thalassemia minor	Hgb F levels decreased or normal or may even be higher than normal; increased Hgb A_2 content	Usually asymptomatic; mild anemia of iron deficient type but nonresponsive to iron; serum iron concentration is high normal or above normal; decreased TIBC
Alpha thalassemia major and minor	Alpha-chain defect causing slowed synthesis	Homozygous, or major, incompatible with life, heterozygous: may be asymptomatic or have a mild hemolytic anemia
Hgb C thalassemia	Presence of Hgb C; Hgb F level may be increased (severe cases); Hgb A_2 cannot be measured—moves in same pattern as Hgb C	Mild in American blacks; more severe in Mediterranean races; target cells present in peripheral smear; RBC crystals

(continued)

TABLE 13–3. (Continued)

Syndrome	Abnormal Hgb	Comments
Sickle cell thalassamia	Presence of Hgb S with beta-chain defect and decrease in Hgb A$_1$; % of Hgb S greater than that of Hgb A$_1$	Can occur as a severe sickling disease or a mild hemolytic anemia; target cells present; because Hgb A may be entirely absent, requires measurement of Hgb F and S for diagnosis; easily misdiagnosed as sickle cell disease without such tests
Hereditary persistence of fetal Hgb (HPFH)	Defect in "switching mechanism"; high levels of Hgb F persist into adult life: 15–35%; Homozygous: only Hgb F; no Hgb A present	Usually heterozygous and usually occurs in the black race; Hgb F found equally in all body cells, which helps distinguish it from beta thalassamia

Data from Conn & Conn, 1980; Frolich, 1976; Groer & Shekleton, 1983; Luckman & Sorensen, 1974; and Miale, 1972.

Patient Preparation. No special preparation is necessary.

13.3.2 Serum Haptoglobin

Synonyms: None

Reactions Reported

Normal	
Adult	100–150 mg/dl
Newborn	0–10 mg/dl
Critical value (probable)	<40 mg/dl

Explanation of the Test. This test is most useful in detecting intravascular hemolysis (RBC destruction). Haptoglobins are alpha$_2$-globulins, produced by the liver, that bind any free Hgb in the plasma to the amount of 100 mg/dl. Once its binding capacity is exceeded, the free Hgb is excreted into the urine (hemoglobinuria). The complex formed by Hgb and haptoglobin is cleared from the plasma by the liver. The presence of free Hgb in plasma is a sure indicator of pathological red cell destruction (Widmann, 1983), and decreases in serum haptoglobin levels are a fairly sensitive indicator of that hemolysis. In cases where haptoglobin levels are increased, however, hemolysis cannot be ruled out by a normal haptoglobin finding.

Haptoglobins can be estimated by haptoglobin-binding capacity (electrophoresis or chemical methods) or measured directly as total haptoglobin (immunologic antibody test). The binding capacity is more sensitive to decreases in the haptoglobin concentration because it responds more rapidly than does the assay.

SERUM HAPTOGLOBIN LEVELS INCREASED IN:

1. Many inflammatory diseases and many infectious inflammatory diseases
2. Patients receiving androgen or steroid therapy
3. Use of some drugs such as oral contraceptives, streptomycin

SERUM HAPTOGLOBIN LEVELS DECREASED OR ABSENT IN:

1. Hemolysis, regardless of cause
2. Severe liver disease because of decreased production of haptoglobin
3. Infectious mononucleosis
4. Congenital absence (ahaptoglobinemia), which occurs in approximately 3 percent of the black race, rare in other races

Patient Preparation. No special preparation is necessary.

13.4 TESTS FOR HEMOLYTIC DISEASE

13.4.1 Coombs' Test—Direct, Indirect, and Quantitative (Non-maternity)

Synonyms

Direct	Direct antiglobulin test, DAGT
Indirect	Indirect antiglobulin test, IAGT, antibody screening test
Coombs' test	Antiglobulin test, AGT
Quantitative test	RBC antibody, quantitative; RBC antibody assay

Reactions Reported

Direct	Normal/negative
Indirect	Normal/negative
Quantitative	Normal range: 0–35 molecules/RBC

Explanation of the Tests. This antiglobulin testing (AGT) is known as the Coombs' test to honor one of the men who produced the first anti-human serum antibody used as a laboratory reagent for the test. AGT is based on the principle that anti-human globulin antibodies will cause agglutination of RBCs that have been coated with globulin antibodies (sensitized). Globulin antibodies often attach themselves to RBCs without causing RBC agglutination. Complement-activating antibodies will also attach a complement component to an RBC at times without adhering to the RBC themselves. Because RBC-attached globulin, or complement fragments, are difficult to visualize and their presence indicates unexpected or abnormal antibodies, AGT is used for visualization by causing agglutination of previously dispersed RBCs. The anti-human serum antibody reagents (or Coombs' serum) used for testing vary in makeup depending on what is suspected or what is to be identified. There is a broad-spectrum antiserum globulin (ASG) used for screening as well as single antibody serums or various combinations (e.g., anti-IgG, anti-Rh_0 (D), anti-Ig plus anti-C_3d). The tests then can be used to diagnose causes of hemolytic disease, determine blood types, or investigate causes of transfusion reactions.

The *direct test* is so called because it is a one-step process done directly on the patient's cells. Anti-human serum antibody is mixed with the patient's washed RBCs. (The washing is an important step because the Coombs' serum will react, and even reacts preferentially, with any unbound globulin present.) If agglutination of the patient's RBCs occurs, this indicates the presence of an antibody on the cells but does not identify the antibody.

The *indirect test,* or antibody screening test, is a two-step process in which RBCs with known antigenic makeup are exposed to the patient's serum. The outcomes of that combination are then visualized by the second stage of the test in which Coombs' serum is added to the known antigen RBCs and patient's serum mixture after careful washing of the RBCs to remove free globulin. If the patient's serum contains the antibody to the RBCs' specific antigen, agglutination takes place, and the antibody is identified. The first stage of the indirect test can also be done by using a known specific antibody serum that is exposed to washed RBCs from the patient. The indirect test can then detect and identify either the free antibody in a patient's serum or specific red cell antigens (Ravel, 1984; Widmann, 1983).

It is estimated that 100 to 500 IgG molecules bound on RBCs are required for detection by the routine (direct–indirect) Coombs' tests. Any smaller number will produce a negative reaction. When immunohemolytic anemia is suspected and routine Coombs' testing produces negative results, a *quantitative test* may be done. It is also useful for following the response to treatment in immunohemolytic anemias as the amount of antibody decreases. The quantitative test can be done as a complement fixation assay of the patient's serum incubated with antihuman antibody from rabbits (Coombs' serum) in which the amount of lysis is compared with a control.

INDICATIONS FOR USE (Expected Positive Reactions):*

1. Direct test
   a. Diagnosis of hemolytic disease of the newborn
   b. Diagnosis of acquired autoimmune hemolytic anemias, both idiopathic and secondary (e.g., erythroblastosis fetalis)
   c. Investigation of hemolytic transfusion reaction, incompatibility, within the first hour after a reaction
2. Indirect test (Used in transplant preparation)
   a. Detection and identification of antibodies to the antigenic blood systems such as Duffy (Fy), Kidd (jk), Kell (K), or Rh (e.g., in the pregnant woman)
   b. Detection of immunoglobulin antibodies for which IgG antibodies are available against platelets and leukocytes
   c. Demonstration of autoantibodies in patients with autoimmune hemolytic anemia
3. *Findings:*
   a. *Positive direct test*
      (1) hemolytic disease of newborns
      (2) autoimmune hemolytic anemia
      (3) hemolytic transfusion reactions
   b. *Positive Indirect Coombs*
      (1) detection of: IgG antibodies;
      (2) blood factors for which IgG antibodies are available
      (3) demonstrating autoantibodies in patients with autoimmune hemolytic anemia
(Laboratory of Pathology, 1991)

Patient Preparation. No special preparation is necessary.

---

*Now referred to as "Mother-Baby Studies" and include Rh.

13.4.2 Glucose-6-Phosphate Dehydrogenase

Synonym: G-6-PD screen

Reaction Reported: Normal or abnormal

Normal Findings: 8–8.6 U/g hemoglobin

Explanation of the Test. G-6-PD is a red cell enzyme. It controls one of the glucose metabolic pathways in the RBC. Deficiency of G-6-PD is the most common of the rather uncommon RBC enzyme defects (Miale, 1972). The defect is a sex-linked genetic one that is determined by a gene on the X chromosome. The disease is most severe in males, although some females who have abnormal genes on both X chromosomes are equally affected. Females with only one abnormal gene are carriers and may be asymptomatic or moderately affected. The G-6-PD defect is found mainly in blacks and to a lesser degree in other Mediterranean races (e.g., Italian, Greek, Sephardic Jews).

When the defective RBCs are exposed to certain chemicals in sufficient concentrations, they are destroyed, which causes a drug-induced hemolysis. The older RBCs are destroyed preferentially, because they have lost much of their G-6-PD activity in the process of aging. If treatment with the chemical (drug) is discontinued, hemolysis will stop within 48 to 72 hours. The few whites affected are likely to have a more intense hemolysis and thus are more likely to be anemic. Hemolytic anemia does not develop in all persons with the defect, and there are many molecular variants of the disease.

The test is specific to G-6-PD and is used as a screening test for the enzyme defect. It is based on the length of time needed for an oxidative reduction to occur. The greater the time required, the less G-6-PD present. Other tests such as the Heinz body preparations (stain)—an old test rarely used—have been used to detect this defect but are less specific. For example, Heinz bodies appear in some normal newborns and postsplenectomy patients as well as in thalassemia major patients (Luckmann & Sorensen, 1987).

EPISODES OF HEMOLYSIS OCCUR IN:

1. Individuals with G-6-PD defect after exposure to certain drugs such as antimalarials (primaquine, quinacrine), sulfonamides and sulfones (many but not all varieties), analgesics (acetanilid, phenacetin [not in all variants]), nonsulfa antibacterials agents (chloramphenicol [not in all variants], nitrofurantoin)
2. Individuals with a G-6-PD defect after ingestion of fava beans (favism) and may be seen in patients with the defect who are being treated for parkinsonism with L-dopa. L-dopa may be the precursor of the active hemolytic principle in fava beans

FALSE NORMAL REACTIONS MAY OCCUR IN:

1. Individuals with very elevated reticulocyte counts, as in a patient with the G-6-PD defect 3 to 10 days after a severe hemolysis. Because reticulocytes are young cells, their enzyme levels are proportionately greater
2. Heterozygote females (only one X chromosomal defect)

Patient Preparation. No special preparation is necessary.

13.4.3 Pyruvate Kinase Deficiency

Synonyms: PKD, PK

Fluorescence test (qualitative test)

Reaction Reported

Normal	Decreased or no fluorescence
Abnormal	Persistence of fluorescence

Serum assay (quantitative test)
Routine assay
Normal Range: 2.0–8.8 U/g

Low substrate assay
Normal Range: 0.9–3.0 U/g hemaglobin

Explanation of the Test. Pyruvate kinase deficiency (PKD), a rare condition, is an autosomal recessive trait causing severe, chronic, nonspherocytic hemolysis and is brought on or made worse by stresses such as infection. Despite the rarity, PKD is the second most frequent deficiency in RBC enzymes.

The fluorescence test is based on the known activity of PK in the RBC. It catalyzes the reaction producing adenosine triphosphate (ATP) from adenosine diphosphate (ADP) and forming pyruvate. Pyruvate is required to oxidize nicotinamide adenine dinucleotide (NADH) to (reduced) nicotinamide adenine dinucleotide (NAD) and form lactate. NADH fluoresces; NAD and lactate do not. Therefore, the loss of fluorescence indicates the presence of active PK and vice versa. The quantitative assay measures the level of PK in the hemoglobin. For these tests any WBCs must be carefully removed from the blood sample because they normally contain about 300 times as much PK as do RBCs and do not share the defect when it is present (Hamilton, 1986; Miale, 1972).

Patient Preparation. No special preparation is necessary.

13.4.4 Pyruvic Acid

Synonym: Pyruvate

Purpose of the Test. This test is principally used to calculate the lactate pyruvate ratio, which, along with lactate and glucose determinations, diagnose malignant hypothermia (Tietz, 1990, pp. 484–485).

Explanation of the Test. Pyruvate is found in the metabolic pathways of carbohydrates, fats, and amino acids. Any inborn error of pyruvate metabolism can, therefore, cause a wide variety of disturbances. For example, an increase in blood lactate levels can be caused by an alteration of pyruvate concentration (Laboratory of Pathology, 1991).

Administration of IV glucose causes a rise in pyruvate levels. The blood lactate levels rise in response to increased pyruvate. The increased blood lactate levels must then be distinguished from lactate produced from tissue hypoxia (McCance & Huether, p. 18).

Pyruvate acid is very unstable and must be treated if not examined immediately (precipitated and refrigerated).

Patient Preparation. In some laboratories, the patient is required to be fasting and at rest (Laboratory of Pathology). Check the procedure required by the laboratory doing the test.

Implications for Nursing
1. Any increase in pyruvic level found through the test should be brought to the immediate attention of the physician managing the medical care of the individual.
2. Question the use of IV glucose prior to the test for the hospitalized patient. Be sure the laboratory doing the test is aware of the glucose administration.

13.5 BLOOD TYPING AND CROSSMATCHING

13.5.1 Type and Rh Factor

Synonyms: ABO and Rh, Rh factor and type, blood groups

Reactions Reported:

ABO blood group: A, B, AB, O (no abnormals)
Rh = normal = positive or negative

Explanation of the Tests. Blood typing tests are required to determine compatibility before any whole blood or most blood components can be given. A, B, AB, O, and Rh are designations of red cell antigens, chemical structures that cause the surface of the RBCs to have differing properties, depending on the antigen. Blood typing to determine the blood group is the identification of the antigen present on an individual's RBC surface. Antigens are identified by their agglutination properties. Within the body they cause antibody production. The blood types serve as antigens. The O phenotype is a very weak antigen, so for all practical purposes it can be considered nonantigenic. Each blood type produces antibodies to the other blood types but not to its own. Type O therefore has antibodies to both types A and B (Table 13–4). Type A has the strongest antigenic properties.

Blood typing is also used to corroborate parentage and for definition of medicolegal problems such as inheritance (Miale, 1972).

Patients needing transfusions are given blood of their own type whenever possible. In cases of real emergency the secondarily acceptable blood types can be given, but only in dire need and only until truly compatible blood is available. Whole-blood transfusions are rarely given. Blood components are given instead—a specific part of the blood to treat a specific deficiency. This approach has been found safer and more effective. It also allows better utilization of available blood stores (McGowan, 1980) (see Table 13–5 for a quick overview of the blood components and their uses).

TABLE 13–4. ABO BLOOD TYPES AND COMPATIBILITY

Blood Group and Phenotype	Can Accept from	Can Donate to	Antigen Present on RBC	Antibodies Present in Serum	Frequency of Occurrence (%) in U.S., Rank-Ordered	
O		A, B	None	Anti-A	1	46
OO	O	AB and O[a]		Anti-B		
A	A	A	A	Anti-B	2	42
AA	O	AB	Has strongest			
AO			antigenic activity			
B	B	B				
BB	O	AB	B	Anti-A	3	9
BO						
AB	AB	AB	A and B	None	4	2
AB	A, B, O[b]					

[a]Known as the universal donor, depending on antibody titer. If more than 1:100, it is not used for replacement.
[b]Known as the universal recipient. This is not necessarily true; it depends on the titers of anti-A or anti-B in the donor's blood (Miale, 1972).
Data from Miale, 1972; Whaley & Wong, 1983; Watson, 1979; and Widmann, 1983.

Rh Factor. Many blood groups or systems exist, which makes the process of crossmatching essential whenever blood or blood components are given. The best known blood group after ABO is the Rh system. There are eight subgroups of agglutinogens in the Rh system. The factors produced are known by two classifications and generally identified by both. One, the American or Wiener classification, uses hr', hr'', rh', rh'', RH_0, and various combinations of the designations.

TABLE 13–5. BLOOD COMPONENTS AND THEIR USES

Component	Indicated in	Comments
Whole blood	Hypovolemia, hypovolemic shock because of acute hemorrhage	
RBCs (packed cells)	Nonhypovolemic deficits of RBC mass, symptomatic hypoxia in acute or chronic anemia	Use of cells without serum reduces the possibility of antigen–antibody reactions to plasma constituents and volume overload
RBC with crystalloids	In patients with whole-blood needs other than serum proteins Prophylactic transfusions for pre-renal–transplant patients	Cause of anemia should be known before use. Nutritional replacement best if feasible for deficiency anemias
Frozen-thawed-washed RBCs	As for RBCs plus in the presence of leukocyte antibodies (multiple transfusions or pregnancies); history of febrile transfusion reactions; hemodialysis patients; possible candidates for organ transplantation	Makes available rare blood by storing it; can be used as a mechanism for storage in advance when autogenous (self) transfusion is necessary (transplantation); washing removes any unbound globulin—a potential antigen; most expensive RBC replacement
Fresh-washed RBCs		Outdated in 24 hr

TABLE 13–5. (Continued)

Component	Indicated in	Comments
Platelet concentrate	Thrombocytopenia, aplastic anemia	Most effective with thrombocytopenia due to decreased platelet production or increased platelet loss; least effective with platelet destruction. Transfuse as rarely as possible because of increased risk of human lymphocyte antigen (HLA) antibody formation. HLA-matched platelets from single donor used in high-risk patients—marrow transplant
Leukocyte concentrate (buffy coat/buffy poor RBC) (granulocyte concentrate)	Severe granulocytopenia; infection refractory to intensive antibiotic treatment Only those who have had a transfusion reaction or have received leukofiltered RBC's before are given this component (Lab. of Pathology, 1991).	Usually given daily until clinical evidence of improvement; concentrate collected and given as closely together as possible. Its use prophylactically is controversial
Fresh-frozen plasma (FFP)	Multiple or single coagulation deficiencies (e.g., severe liver disease, massive transfusion reaction treatment)	Can be stored for a year, thus immediately available; provides coagulation factors; not used as a volume expander
Normal serum albumin (25% solution)	Treatment of conditions causing protein loss (nephrosis) or hypoproteinemia Both used in conditions requiring blood volume expansion	Prepared from pooled plasma and treated to inactive hepatitis virus; a purified preparation of albumin only
Plasma protein fraction	Initial treatment of shock resulting from hemorrhage, plasma loss (burns), or dehydration	Contains albumin and alpha and beta globulins; long storage life even without refrigeration
Cryoprecipitate	Hemophilia, severe burns, hemorrhagic shock	Prepared from frozen plasma. Contains factor VIII concentrated 15 to 40 times normal; also rich in factors VII and I (fibrinogen); must be kept frozen. Was a frequent source of AIDS transmission prior to extensive donor testing
Factor VIII	Severe hemophilia; heated factor VIII used when factor level <5%	Can be stored at home and self-administered. Heated factor VIII decreases risk of AIDS and hepatitis transmission
Immune serum globulin (human)	Conditions with reduced naturally occurring antibody content: hypogammaglobulinemia, agammaglobulinemia; prophylaxis or attenuation of certain infectious diseases: hepatitis B, tetanus, pertussis, mumps, vaccinia, etc. Provides passive immunity for non-A, non-B hepatitis	Prepared from pooled plasma Specific immune globulin solutions can be prepared from individuals with high titers of specific antibodies

Data from Lenes, 1987; McGowan, 1980; and Phipps et al., 1983.

The English, or Fisher-Race, classification is based on a theory of three genes per chromosome and has, therefore, three major designations, in both capital and lowercase letters (i.e., Cc, Dd, and Ee). Each gene contains one of each letter in combinations of lowercase and capital letters (e.g., Cde, cdE, CDe).

The most important of the Rh antigens is Rh_0 (D). When it is present, the person is considered Rh-positive; 20 percent of the white population lack Rh_0 (D) and are therefore Rh-negative. (The percentage of Rh-negative persons is much less in the black race [5 to 7 percent] as well as in the Native American or Mongoloid races [1 percent].) Rh_0 (D) is often the only subtype tested for, but further testing is done if Rh_0 (D) is not present. Frequently, Rh_0 variant (D^u), will be tested for, as it often fails to give a strong positive reaction in general screening tests and a false Rh-negative reaction can occur. The other subtypes are checked when necessary.

All blood groups (antigens) are present on each person's RBCs, and the need to screen for the presence of antibodies to groups other than ABO and Rh increases as the number of persons in the population who have been transfused increases. Usually, these systems produce reaction only with prior sensitization, as is true with the Rh group. These other groups include the Kell system (K), Duffy system (Fy), the Kidd system (jk), the MN, P, Lewis (Le), and Lutheran (Lu) systems as well as subgroups of A (A_1, A_2, A_i, etc.) (Miale, 1982; Ravel, 1989).

13.5.2 Blood Crossmatch

Synonym: Compatibility testing

Reactions Reported

Compatible	No agglutination or hemolysis
Incompatible	Clumping (agglutination) and/or hemolysis occur

Explanation of the Test. Not only must the ABO and the Rh blood types of patient and donor blood or constituents be known before introducing alien blood into a body system, but also a pretest for match is done between the two supposedly compatible sets of blood to eliminate the chance of any other blood group incompatibility. The recipient's serum is also screened routinely for the presence of antibodies. Transfusion reactions occur with incompatible blood and can be fatal. A transfusion reaction is the body's response to alien antigens by way of antibody production, with subsequent agglutination and hemolysis. The ABO blood types react immediately. The others usually require presensitization.

Crossmatching can be done by mixing the transfusion recipient's serum (which would contain antibodies if sensitized) with the donor's cells and examining the mixture for agglutination. It is possible that antibodies in the donor serum could cause problems with specific antigens on the recipient's cells, but this is not ordinarily a major concern, as the donor blood component will be greatly diluted when in the recipient's plasma.

There are three techniques used to detect as many incompatibilities as possible: antiglobulin, albumin media, and enzyme-treated cells. At least one procedure is done at room temperature in serum or saline to detect any cold agglutinins (antigens). The use of indirect AGT is done at 37°C to detect nonagglutinating antibodies.

Antibodies do not appear spontaneously to antigens except to the ABO system. A transfusion of Rh-positive blood in an Rh-negative person will cause antibodies to form slowly. Only with a second transfusion, again with Rh-positive blood, will agglutination and hemolysis of RBCs occur. The same principle applies when an Rh-negative mother carries an Rh-positive fetus. The first child has usually no ill effects unless the mother has been previously sensitized by an Rh-positive transfusion. Subsequent pregnancies with Rh-positive fetuses will be threatened, however. In the instance of an Rh-positive mother or recipient and an Rh-negative child or donor, there is usually no difficulty for the pregnant mother or the transfused individual.

HLA typing (see Section 12.4) has become useful in parentage studies because the antigens are fully developed at birth and there is great diversity among unrelated persons. Phenotypes of one parent and the child are all that are necessary to determine whether a given man or woman is the other parent (Widmann, 1983). HLA typing is rarely if ever done with a "routine" type and crossmatch of blood for transfusion.

Types of Transfusion Reactions

Hemolytic/Immunologic. The hemolytic/immunologic transfusion reaction is most important because it is the most life-threatening. It is *caused* by incompatability between donor and blood recipient or a mismatch between ABO groups. It is also found with mismatches of other blood groups in previously sensitized individuals (previous tranfusion or pregnancy). *Signs and symptoms* are variable but classically include pain in the lumbar region, a rapid increase in temperature and pulse, chills, flushing of the skin, nausea and vomiting, precordial pain, and possible blood pressure decrease (Table 13–6). *Nursing action* entails stopping the transfusion (see "Implications for Nursing: Urinary Hemoglobin," item 4 in Section 4.10). Save the remainder of the blood and all equipment for examination. Check the blood against patient data for a possible clerical error. Report event.

Pyrogenic. Not seen as much with the use of disposable intravenous equipment, a pyrogenic reaction will most likely occur in components stored at room temperature but can occur with refrigerated products. Devastating effects can occur in response to the bacterial endotoxins produced (fever, shock, hemoglobinuria, disseminated intravascular coagulation [DIC], and renal failure). *Causes* include contamination of transfusion substances, usually bacterial, or contamination in the process of the intravenous puncture. *Signs and symptoms* are fever shortly after the transfusion begins, which may be accompanied by chills, mild or severe. *Nursing action* entails stopping the transfusion. Save the remainder of the blood and all equipment for examination. Treat symptomatically. Report event.

Allergic. An allergic reaction is usually caused by the presence of an allergen—often derived from food—in the blood to which the recipient is sensitive. *Signs and symptoms* may only be urticaria, or there may be acute bronchial asthma, angioneurotic edema, or anaphylactic shock. *Nursing action* entails giving antihistamines. Report event. Depending on the severity,

TABLE 13–6. SIGNS AND SYMPTOMS OF SPECIFIC TRANSFUSION REACTIONS

Reaction Type	Cause	Specific Signs and Symptoms
Allergic reaction	Sensitivity of the *donor* to allergens (eggs, pollens, etc.)	Hives, rash, itching
Anaphylactic reaction	Antibodies against IgA immunoglobulins usually because of previous transfusion or pregnancy	Generalized flushing, bronchospasm, dyspnea, substernal pain, laryngeal edema, or collapse
Febrile nonhemolytic reaction	Sensitization to WBCs, platelets, and plasma antigens that is related to multiple transfusions	Initial chill followed by fever (within I hr of tranfusion start), may also have headache, nausea, and vomiting, or back and leg pain
Hemolytic reaction		
Acute (intravascular)	ABO incompatibility; RBC exposure to hypertonic solutions; improper storage of blood (freezing, storage >35 days; warming above 40°C)	Multiple: anxiety, restlessness; nausea and vomiting; flushing; chest and lumbar pain; rapid respiration and heart rate; chills followed by fever; hemoglobinuria
Delayed (extravascular)	Antibodies of Rh system (anti-D, anti-c, anti-E)	Occur a week or more after transfusion; milder forms of malaise, fever, decreased Hgb count; positive Coombs' test response, hyperbilirubinemia
Nonimmunologic reactions		
Circulatory overload	Large quantity of blood tranfused in short period of time; blood transfused more rapidly than can be tolerated by person with cardiac or renal insufficiency	Dyspnea, shortness of breath; labored breathing, dry cough, rales at base of lungs
Air embolism	Air introduced into IV line	Cyanosis, dyspnea, signs and symptoms of shock, cardiac arrest

Data from Lewis & Collier, 1983; and Luckmann & Sorensen, 1987.

blood administration may be stopped. To prevent an allergic transfusion reaction, all donors should be fasting, all donors with active allergies should be eliminated, and premedication with antihistamine should be instituted in patients with a history of an allergic reaction to transfusion.

Hemoclastic—Reaction to Unidentified Plasma Component. Occurring with plasma transfusions, its *cause* is unknown but may be nonspecific or a leukoagglutinin reaction. *Signs and symptoms* include chills, fever, backache, and leg pain. *Nursing action* indicates stopping the transfusion and reporting the event.

Circulatory Overload. Seen most often in children, the elderly, and persons with heart disease, a circulatory overload may be *caused* by too large a quantity of blood given, or blood given at too rapid a rate. *Signs and symptoms* are those of heart failure: dyspnea, cough, cyanosis. *Nursing actions* include discontinuing the blood transfusion immediately, changing tubing of the blood line, and switching to hydrating fluid to a "keep-open" (TKO) rate, procuring medical orders for rapid diuresis, and, with pulmonary edema, taking appropriate steps to decrease cardiac return (e.g., rotating tourniquets, sitting position—legs dependent).

Hemorrhagic Reaction. An infrequent occurrence, a hemorrhagic reaction may be *caused* by DIC or washing out of platelets and other coagulation factors in exchange transfusions with inadequate replacement. *Signs and symptoms* include petechial hemorrhages, ecchymoses, hematuria, gastrointestinal hemorrhage (tarry stool), and uncontrollable bleeding from an operative site. *Nursing actions* include reporting the event after stopping the transfusion and maintaining an open access to the vein with hydrating fluids at a TKO rate.

Patient Preparation. No special preparation is necessary.

IMPLICATIONS FOR NURSING: BLOOD TYPING AND CROSSMATCHING

1. Before the administration of blood
   a. Check for completion of type and crossmatch tests and the compatibility between patient and donor blood
   b. Check the blood to be given, and validate with another nurse or a physician. See that the label is correct in *all* details. *Any* discrepancy on the label means that the blood is not to be given
2. Start the infusion slowly, not to exceed 20 drops/min, run the infusion at that rate for the first 50 ml, and stay with the patient for that time. The usual rate in the adult, depending on the person's condition, is 30 drops/min, or 500 ml over a span of 4 hours. If the person should receive more than 100 ml of incompatible blood, irreversible shock, total renal shutdown, and death can occur
3. Check vital signs every 15 minutes to one-half hour, depending on the general condition of the patient getting the blood. Particularly close surveillance is suggested if the individual's mobility or awareness is impaired
4. Observe for or inquire after any sign or symptom of reaction, (e.g., chills, fever, low back pain). Occasionally, early signs may be urticaria or flushing, a sense of uneasiness, and/or mild air hunger. Should a person receiving blood complain about feeling "funny," this vague complaint should be given immediate attention. A *minimal* response on the part of the nurse is to decrease the rate of blood flow to a (TKO) (keep vein open [KVO]) rate and report the situation to the physician. In some hospitals it is required that the transfusion be discontinued at this point. The nurse should also stay with the patient until the situation is resolved. Should slightly more overt signs or symptoms of a reaction occur, the steps listed in item 5 should be followed
5. With any confirmed sign of reaction
   a. Discontinue the blood transfusion, but do not discard it
   b. Change the intravenous tubing, and maintain vascular access with normal saline, or one-fourth normal saline. Glucose in water is not recommended for administration immediately after blood because the absence of electrolytes can precipitate hemolysis and clotting in the needle or in the tubing if it has not been changed
   c. Notify the physician. Epinephrine HCl, 1:1000, and sodium lactate (1/6 mol/L) may be ordered to reduce the precipitation of Hgb globin in the kidney

d. If the reaction is a hemolytic one, an immediate laboratory test is imperative. Two tubes of blood are drawn from the patient and sent to the laboratory

e. Evaluate renal function by using strict intake and output measurement. If the reaction is severe, a catheter may be required. Frequent urine specimens may be examined for hemolysis. Do not discard the urine until it is known that a test will not be done. Maintain hydration through an intravenous line, but check for evidence of an overload. Check for other bleeding (hemolysis may be severe enough to cause massive platelet loss and defibrination due to consumptive coagulopathy—DIC)

13.6 LEUKEMIA DIFFERENTIATION

13.6.1 Leukocyte Alkaline Phosphatase Stain

Synonyms: None (LAP is not used because of probable confusion with leukocyte acid stain or leucine aminopeptidase)

Normal Range: 60–140 points (see process, specific to test laboratory)

Explanation of the Test. Staining indicates leukocyte alkaline phosphatase (LAP) activity in neutrophils, which in turn indicates intercellular metabolic activity. Visible pigment is formed at the site of phosphatase activity. The test helps differentiate chronic granulocytic leukemia from neutrophilic leukemoid reactions (see "Decreased Scores in," item 1). Because this is a difficult test, it is generally used to support a diagnosis rather than as a definitive diagnostic test.

Process. A stained slide (whole blood) is examined, and 100 neutrophils are graded 0 to 4+, depending on the amount of alkaline phosphatase stain present in each cell. The total count for the 100 cells is added. The grading is based on a scale developed by each laboratory. An example is: 0 count/neutrophil, no granules, no staining; 4 count/neutrophil, medium-sized granules filling the entire cell, no protoplasm visible (SHMC, 1984).

DECREASED SCORES IN:

1. Chronic myelocytic (granulocytic) leukemia, irrespective of the total leukocyte count. (Therefore, useful in differentiating a nonleukemic myeloid reaction [increased granulocytes] from a chronic myeloid reaction, especially with a WBC count greater than 30,000/mm³, and a score of less than 30)
2. Paroxysmal nocturnal hemoglobinuria
3. Hereditary hypophosphatasia
4. Aplastic anemia

INCREASED SCORES IN:

1. Polycythemia vera
2. Myelofibrosis
3. Neutrophilia secondary to infection due to an increase in the total number of leukocytes
4. Active Hodgkin's disease

PHYSIOLOGICAL INCREASED SCORES IN:

- Pregnancy

Patient Preparation. No special preparation is required.

13.6.2 Leukocyte Acid Phosphatase Stain (Bone Marrow or Whole Blood)

Synonym: Stain for tartrate-resistant acid phosphatase (LAP is not used because of probable confusion with leukocyte alkaline phosphatase or leucine aminopeptidase)

Normal Range: None—an interpretation of findings is given

Explanation of the Test. When granular cytoplasm is placed on a slide and treated with tartaric acid, a visible pigment is formed at the site of phosphatase activity. This indicates the presence of tartrate-resistant acid phosphatase. Such staining is found to occur primarily in the cytoplasm of leukemic reticuloendothelial cells (so-called hairy cells). The test is used to diagnose hairy cell leukemia:

1. Positive staining in most cases of hairy cell (reticuloendothelial) leukemia
2. Weak staining possible in some non-hairy cell lymphoproliferative processes
3. Negative staining in all other leukemias. (Some cases of non-hairy cell lymphoproliferative processes do not stain)

Patient Preparation. No special preparation is necessary.

RELATED NURSING DIAGNOSES (NOT PRIORITIZED): HEMATOLOGIC SYSTEM

Almost any catabolic disorder in humans ultimately leads to some degree of anemia. Therefore, almost all nursing diagnoses *could* apply to the individual with anemic, leukopenic, or thrombocytopenic problems. The selection of diagnoses for this section was based on those found to most consistently occur with such problems, no matter what the medical diagnosis.

Comfort and learning needs are assumed to be important nursing diagnoses in *any* illness, but they are so variable in the focus of nursing for almost all the illnesses included in the category of hematologic problems that they are not addressed here.

The primary physiological cause of dysfunction in anemias is related to an impairment in gas exchange. At the level of implementation of nursing care, this diagnosis might be most usefully addressed as it relates to the individual's level of function, not as "gas exchange" per se. For example, if the lack of oxygen-carrying power is due to a nutritional deficit or a potential or actual injury (e.g., bleeding, trauma, falls) is present, there are independent nursing measures that may be taken to assist the client to at least maintain his or her present level of wellness. Nursing also has an active and independent role in the assessment and management of such areas as impaired activity and safety, in teaching the client and family, and in fostering self-care.

Potential Injury, Physiological*

Falls, Cuts, and Thermal Injuries Related to

1. Cerebral hypoxia secondary to decreased gas exchange causing confusion, dizziness, altered thought processes, slowed physical and mental response to stimuli, decreased attention span, and visual impairment (see diagnosis for Impaired Physical Mobility)
2. Potential dysrrhythmias secondary to cardiac muscle hypoxia
3. Muscle weakness secondary to peripheral hypoxia
4. Decreased healing power of skin and mucous membranes secondary to peripheral hypoxia and/or nutritional deficiencies
5. Impaired mobility (see diagnosis for Activity Intolerance)

Bleeding Related to

1. Decreased production or increased destruction of clotting factors
2. Increased risk of injury (see "Falls, Cuts, and Thermal Injuries")

Potential for Infection Related to

1. Poor wound healing (see "Falls, Cuts, and Thermal Injuries")
2. Decreased leukocyte production (pernicious anemia, leukemias)
3. Ineffective leukocytes in circulation (leukemias)

Alteration in Nutrition (Less Than Body Requirements) Related to

1. Deficient intake or utilization of nutrients for adequate production of blood cellular products (deficiency of iron, vitamin B_{12}, folic acid)
2. Deficient caloric intake secondary to physical discomfort associated with some blood dyscrasias (glossitis, stomatitis, dyspepsia, nausea, anorexia)
3. Deficient intake secondary to fatigue/weakness. (See Diagnosis above)

Impaired Physical Mobility Related to

1. Weakness and fatigue secondary to nutritional deficits and hypoxia
2. Balance and gait disturbance (B_{12} deficiency)
3. Prescribed activity restrictions
4. Pain (sickle cell crisis)
5. Decreased visual acuity (retinal hemorrhage in leukemia, aplastic anemia, pernicious anemia)

Activity Intolerance Related to

1. Rapid onset of fatigue with activity secondary to tissue hypoxia and/or decreased muscle mass (see diagnosis for Alteration in Nutrition)
2. Pain (joint pain in acute sickle cell anemia, anginal pain with cardiac hypoxia)
3. Decreased cardiac output (arrythmias secondary to cardiac hypoxia)
4. Dyspnea on exertion (decreased gas exchange with decreased hemotocrit)
5. Fear of falling or injury (see diagnosis for Potential Injury: Physiological)
6. Apathy secondary to chronic illness

---

*Medical diagnoses, given in parentheses, are examples only and do not reflect all possible causes for the sign or symptom given.

F O U R T E E N

THE NEUROLOGIC SYSTEM

RECOGNITION OF NEUROLOGIC DYSFUNCTION

Individuals who suffer from neurologic problems often have minor, perhaps transitory signs and symptoms that are ignored because they *are* transitory, are adapted to without awareness of the adaptations, or are erroneously credited to the aging process. Neural disorders of such subtle onset are one of the greatest diagnostic challenges. Much hope is placed in the diagnostic use of new technology such as positron emission tomography (PET) for earlier diagnosis (see Section 17.8.1).

14.1 LABORATORY AND CLINICAL INDICATIONS OF NEUROLOGIC SYSTEM DYSFUNCTION

Laboratory Findings. Findings may be specific for an infectious causative disorder or indicative of the general physical state of the individual. In general, laboratory findings from screening tests are nonspecific and not useful as clues to neurologic problems.

Clinical Findings. Indication of risk groups include a history of vascular disease (arteriosclerosis), any condition that significantly reduces cardiac output and blood pressure, and age over 40 (increased risk for transient ischemic attack [TIA] with potential for stroke); a history of persistent headache longer than 1 year in previously uncomplaining person warrants a neurologic consultation, as should a history of head injury plus any of the following signs or symptoms. In children (exclusive to or more frequent in), projectile vomiting, an increase in head circumference, tight or bulging fontanels with history of upper respiratory infection (URI) or otitis media, poor feeding, increased restlessness, and irritability are indications. In adults, signs and symptoms include alterations in level of consciousness (LOC); impaired mentation (orientation, cognition, memory); muscular changes: weakness (palsy), spasticity, rigidity, particularly nuchal (inability to press chin on chest), tremors (intention and nonintention), and changes in handwriting; changes in reflex response: presence of pathological reflexes (e.g., Babinski), increased deep tendon reflexes, absence of reflexes, hyperreflexia, clonus; changes in gait, movement, and posture; changes in sensation: numbness, hyperesthesia (increased or altered response to superficial sensation), paresthesias ("funny feelings"), "trigger points" for pain sensation; visual changes: acuity/blurring, photophobia, diminution of vision, total vision loss, field or visual cuts (contralateral to muscular changes indicate stroke), diplopia; dizziness, lightheadedness, dizziness with postural change; changes in personality or behavior (inappropriate); changes in speech: slurring, dysphasia, aphasia; and abnormal sleep patterns (Conn & Conn, 1985; Conway-Rutkowski, 1982).

14.2 LUMBAR PUNCTURE

Synonyms: LP, spinal tap, examination of cerebrospinal fluid (CSF)

Normal Ranges: See Table 14–1

Explanation of the Test. Examination of the aspirated CSF is composed of many separate tests, not all having to do with visualizing fluid contents (e.g., measurement of CSF pressure). Some observations or tests are not done routinely, but for the "routine" spinal or lumbar puncture (LP), if such a thing exists, the tests include measurement of pressure, examination of gross appearance (consistency, turbidity, viscosity, tendency to clot), measurement of protein and glucose concentrations, and a cell count including a differential count when indicated. (Serum protein levels must be normal to interpret any CSF protein values, therefore are done concurrently. [Wallach, 1992, p. 220].)

Brief Physiology Review. CSF is formed in the ventricles of the brain; circulates over and bathes the surface of the brain, spinal cord, and nerve roots; and is reabsorbed by the arachnoid villa (the arachnoid is the delicate membrane between the dura and the pia mater that covers the brain and spinal cord). There is no direct communication between the CSF and the cerebral blood supply (the blood–brain barrier) in the normal healthy person. Substances can cross these barriers by way of active transport (chemical ions such as K^+, H^+, Mg^+, Ca^+), and in some instances, substances will diffuse rather rapidly across the barrier (e.g., water, chloride). Several pathological mechanisms open the barrier (e.g., acute hypertension, hypercapnia) as do nonpathological, but intrusive procedures, such as the injection of radiographic dyes. The LP is carried out at the L3–4 space or lower in adults to avoid the spinal cord. The cord persists lower in children, and the tap must be done at L4–5 space or lower (Henry, 1991).

Indications for LP

1. Suspected meningitis, encephalitis, brain abscess, subarachnoid hemorrhage, leukemia involving the CNS, multiple sclerosis (MS), Guillain-Barré syndrome, and spinal cord tumor (*not* intracranial tumors)
2. To document impairment of CSF flow
3. Differential diagnosis of hemorrhagic versus ischemic syndromes in cerebral-vascular disease (TIA, stroke) or the differential diagnosis of cerebral infarct versus intracerebral hemorrhage

TABLE 14–1. REFERENCE VALUES FOR LUMBAR CSF

Constituent	CNS	Serum	SI Units
Protein (total)	15–45 mg/dl	6.0–7.8 g/dl	0.150–0.450 g/L
Pediatric			
Neonatal	20–170 mg/dl		up to 0.7 g/L
Infant	10–30 mg/dl		
Children and senior adult	30–60 mg/dl		
Senior adult			up to 0.7 g/L
Prealbumin	2–5%	—	
Albumin	56–76%	52–67%	
Alpha$_1$-globulin	2–7%	2–5%	
Alpha$_2$-globulin	4–12%	6–14%	
Beta globulin	8–18%	8–16%	
Gamma globulin	3–12%	10–22%	
Electrolytes			
Sodium	136–150 mEq/L	136–150 mEq/L	
Potassium			
Lumbar CSF	2.6–3.0 mEq/L	3.0–4.5 mEq/L	
Cisternal CSF	2.3–2.7 mEq/L	—	
Chloride	118–130 mEq/L	96–104 mEq/L	120–130 mmol/L
Bicarbonate	20–25 mEq/L	21–26 mEq/L	
Calcium	2.1–2.7 mEq/L	4.6–5.4 mEq/L	
Magnesium	2.4–3.0 mEq/L	1.5–2.4 mEq/L	
Lactate	10–22 mg/dl	3–7 mg/dl	
Osmolality	280–295 mosm/L	280–295 mosm/L	
Acid Base			
pH			
Lumbar CSF	7.28–7.32	7.38–7.42	
Cisternal CSF	7.32–7.34	(arterial)	
Pco_2			
Lumbar CSF	44–50 mm Hg	36–40 mm Hg	
Cisternal CSF	40–44 mm Hg	(arterial)	
Pco_2	40–44 mm Hg	45–100 mm Hg	
Special chemistry			
Ammonia	0.5–1.0 mg/ml	1.0–2.0 µg/ml	
		(arterial)	
Creatinine	0.5–1.2 µg/dl	0.5–1.2 mg/dl	
Glucose	50–80 mg/dl	70–100 mg/dl	2.8–4.2 mmol/L
Iron	1–2 µg/dl	50–150 µg/dl	
Phosphorus	1.2–2.0 mg/dl	3.0–4.5 mg/dl	
Urea	6–16 mg/dl	8–20 mg/dl	
Uric acid	0.5–3.0 mg/dl	2.0–8.0 mg/dl	
Zinc	2.0–6.0 µg/dl	50–150 µg/dl	
Pressure	50–180 mm of CSF lateral recumbent position		

Adapted from Kreig, A. (1979). Cerebral spinal fluid and other body fluids. In J. B. Henry (Ed.), *Clinical diagnosis and management by laboratory methods* (16th ed.). Philadelphia: Saunders, with permission; Data from Conn, 1987.

4. Introduction of anesthetics, radiographic contrast media, or certain medication (e.g., methotrexate [meningeal leukemia], amphotericin [fungal meningitis])
5. Removal of blood from CSF after subarachnoid hemorrhage (McCormick, 1986, p. 648)

Contraindications for LP

1. Presence of or suspected presence of intracranial tumors because of the potential for tentorial herniation with pressure shifts
2. In most cases when increased intracranial pressure (IICP) and papilledema (edema and hyperemia of the optic disk—choked disk) are present, for the reason given with item 1. The criteria necessary for a physician to proceed with an LP when the foregoing situation is present include
   a. Necessary information is not available by any other means
   b. The probability is high that the CSF findings will have a significant impact on *both* treatment and outcome
   c. Neurosurgical consultation is available (Henry, 1991)
3. In most patients with primary clotting defects (thrombocytopenia) or those defects secondary to anticoagulant drug use because of the possibility of the formation of extradural or subdural hematoma and resultant paralysis
4. In the presence of systemic sepsis as well as infection or severe dermatologic disease in the lumbar area because of the potential for meningitis
5. Some spinal deformities and in extreme age in some cases because of the difficulty in the procedure
6. In some cases of severe personality problems in the patient because the trauma can become the basis of further personality disruption

Routine Tests with LP. See Tables 14–2 to 14–8.

Patient Preparation

1. If an accurate determination of CNS glucose levels is particularly important, the test should be done in the fasting patient (n.p.o. except for water for 8 to 12 hours before the test). All "routine" lumbar taps—as opposed to emergency taps—are best done on a fasting patient.
2. Lumbar tap is one of the more fear-producing diagnostic tests. Any measures that will reduce patient anxiety and increase cooperation during the procedure should be undertaken. Infants and children are usually restrained.
3. Inform the laboratory of any suspected infective organisms when requesting a stain and/or culture on the CSF.

Postprocedural Care

1. A postprocedural headache may occur within a few hours or several days after the lumbar puncture. It is believed to occur because of the leakage of spinal fluid at the puncture site into surrounding tissues, which is finally absorbed by the lymphatics. The loss of fluid, if large enough, allows the brain to settle when the client sits upright, thereby causing tension or traction on the venous sinuses, which causes pain.   (*cont'd.* p. 459)

TABLE 14–2. GROSS APPEARANCE OF CSF IN ADULTS

Normal	Variations from Normal and Significance
Clear	Changes causing turbidity may be due to increased presence of leukocytes—at least 200 cells/µl of CSF necessary to cause slight turbidity (see also Table 12–1, for a numerical identification of degree of turbidity); increase in turbidity also due to increased erythrocytes—at 400 cells/µl CSF; presence of microorganisms (bacteria, fungi, ammoebas) or contrast media; also due to aspiration of epidural fat with spinal puncture
No clot formation	Clots often due to increased protein in CSF; always occurs when protein levels are 1000 mg/dl or greater; very fine clotting occurring with lower levels can be seen if specimen is refrigerated 12–24 hr; occurs with increased fibrinogen levels resulting from traumatic tap and certain types of meningitis or neurosyphilis
Viscosity of water	Increased viscosity reported with metastatic mucinous adenocarcinoma of the meninges
Colorless	White or cloudy because of high WBC count (over 500 WBC/µl) or increased protein levels
	Xanthochromia: yellowish discoloration, can actually range from pale pink to orange and yellow; change in color indicates presence of RBCs, usually, and their age—the younger the cell, the pinker the color; specimen must be examined within l hr after tap to prevent false-positive result because of lysis; RBC increase and presence of xanthochromia most often due to subarachnoid hemorrhage; color change can also be due to presence of bilirubin with increased serum bilirubin, presence of carotenoids with increased serum carotene, or presence of melanin due to meningeal melanosarcoma; xanthochromia expected in premature infants because of increased bilirubin, increased CSF protein, and immaturity of blood–brain barrier

Data from Henry, 1984, and Ravel, 1984.

TABLE 14–3. CSF PRESSURE

Normal and Comments	Increased in	Decreased in
50–180 mm of CSF (lateral recumbent position)	Anxiety: if over 180 at start of tap, check for breath holding, muscle tightening, jugular compression	Actually a rare occurrence
Minor variations occur with respiration	Infections: high with bacteria or TBc lesser increase with encephalitis, neurosyphilis	Circulatory collapse
		Severe dehydration
		Acute hyperosmolality
If initial pressure is over 200 mm Hg, only 1–2 ml CSF should be removed	Meningeal inflammation	Loss of CSF with leakage (dural tear, CSF rhinorrhea, previous puncture)
	Congestive heart failure	
A 25–50% drop in ICP after removal of 1–2 ml CSF indicates cerebral herniation or spinal cord compression	Acute obstruction of the superior vena cava—early	Complete spinal subarachnoid block (noncommunication)
	Thrombosis and obstruction of IC venous sinuses	With no initial increase in pressure, CSF pressure should not drop more than 5–10 mm for each ml CSF fluid removed
Normal pressure, sitting position: over 300 mm H_2O	Acute hypoosmolality due to hemodialysis	If final pressure drop is less than the 5–10 mm/ml after fluid is removed, an increased CSF pool is indicated (e.g., hydrocephalus)
	Increased CSF protein concentration or hemorrhage (subarachnoid) impairing CSF reabsorption	

(continued)

TABLE 14–3. (Continued)

Normal and Comments	Increased in	Decreased in
	Mass lesions (tumor, abscess, IC hemorrhage), cerebral edema	If final pressure drop is greater than the norm, a decreased CSF pool is indicated (e.g., tumor, spinal block)

Abbreviations: TBc, tuberculosis; ICP, intracranial pressure; IC, intracranial
Data from Henry, 1984, and Widmann, 1983.

TABLE 14–4. QUECKENSTEDT TEST

Procedure	Normal Response and Comments	Variations from Normal
Bilateral jugular compression for 10 sec Indications for use: suspicion of subarachnoid block or spinal cord tumor *Not* a routine test	CSF pressure increases rapidly to 300 mm and rapidly returns to normal when compression ceases Principle: CSF space is a closed system; pressure exerted in one part of a closed system should be reflected in all other parts	CSF pressure decreased or delayed (more than 20 sec) = a "positive" test; occurs in: sinus thrombosis; obstruction at foramen magnum; mass spinal canal lesion With abnormal or positive test result, the normal variations of pressure with respiration are absent

Data from Clark, 1975, and Henry, 1984.

TABLE 14–5. CSF GLUCOSE[a]

Increased in	Decreased in	Comments
Some cases of aseptic or viral meningitis False increase with serum hyperglycemia	50% of patients with bacterial meningitis 25% of patients with mumps meningoencephalitis Variable decrease in meningitis (due to TB, fungus, virus) Subarachnoid hemorrhage (4–8 days after onset) Some cases of neurosyphilis; false decrease secondary to hypoglycemia	Normal level is usually about half to one third that of serum glucose Must be compared with serum concentration to detect false increase or decrease (CSF glucose level rises or falls approximately 2 hr after plasma levels change) Major pathological significance found in decreased levels Decrease usually due to impairment of active transport or increased use

[a]See Table 14–1 for normal range.
Data from Conn, 1985, and Henry, 1984.

TABLE 14–6. CSF TOTAL PROTEIN[a]

Increased in	Decreased in	Comments
Normally in neonate and older adult	CSF loss from leakage as in dural tear with trauma; rhinorrhea; otorrhea; increased intracranial pressure because of increased filtration through the arachnoid	Increased CSF protein level is roughly proportional to the degree of leukocytosis; thus cell count usually increases as well
Presence of blood (traumatic tap) 1 ml blood can increase protein to 400 mg/dl	Hyperthydroidism, mechanism unknown	Protein from plasma diffuses into CSF
Increased permeability of blood–CSF barrier; common cause of pathological increases, as in bacterial, fungal, TB, meningitis; subarachnoid hemorrhage; cerebral thrombosis; IC hemorrhage		Concentration varies slightly with age
		Protein can also be fractionated by electrophoresis (see Table 14–1 for normals); increases in gammaglobulin level most important in detection of multiple sclerosis
Obstruction of CSF circulation as in tumor; herniated disk		
Increased CNS synthesis of IgG as in Guillain-Barré syndrome; collagen diseases; multiple sclerosis		
Tissue degeneration as in amyotrophic lateral sclerosis (ALS)		

[a]See Table 14–1 for normal range.
Data from Henry, 1984, and Ravel, 1994.

TABLE 14–7. CSF LACTATE (LACTIC ACID)

Increased in	Decreased in	Comments
Any condition with a decreased cerebral blood flow, decreased oxygenation of the brain, or IICP, as in traumatic brain injury; seizures; respiratory alkalosis; IC hemorrhage; hydrocephalus; TIA; multiple sclerosis; bacterial meningitis	Decreases are of little clinical importance	Lactate concentrations may be of assistance in the differential diagnosis between bacterial meningitis (lactate level increased to over 25 mg/dl) and aseptic meningitis (most cases have no increase in lactate levels)
		Also may be useful as a screening test to detect CNS disease; becoming a more routine test because of this

See Table 14–1 for normal range.
Data from Henry, 1984.

TABLE 14–8. CELL COUNT (CSF CELL COUNT; SPINAL FLUID CELL COUNT)[a]

| Cell Type (Normal Cells) | Normal Range (%) | | Increased in |
	Adults	*Neonates*	
Lymphocytes	62 ± 34	20 ± 18	Increased in many infectious and in partially treated bacterial meningitis; in parasitic disease (toxoplasmosis), subacute sclerosis panencephalitis (SSPE) secondary to measles virus, multiple sclerosis, drug abuse encephalitis, Guillain-Barré syndrome, polyneuritis, periarteritis
Pia–arachnoid mesothelial (PAM) cells and monocytes	36 ± 20	72 ± 22	Increased in mixed reactions, with many other cell counts increased, such as in TB and fungal, chronic bacterial, and leptospiral meningitis; amoebic encephalomyelitis; rupture of brain abcess
Neutrophils	2 ± 5	3 ± 5	When increased with monocytes, may indicate TB meningitis; some authorities consider even one neutrophil abnormal; numbers increase with traumatic tap, bacterial infections, early in viral infections, and other infectious processes; also increased in CNS hemorrhage, injections of foreign materials into subarachnoid space, in metastatic tumor, and in infarct
Histiocytes	Rare	5 ± 4	
Ependymal cells	Rare	Rare	Ependymal cells are cells from the ventricular and central canal of the spinal membrane lining; increased after pneumoencephalograms, with hydrocephalus, after cisternal or ventricular puncture, or after administration of chemotherapeutic agents intrathecally
Eosinophils	Rare	Rare	Increased over 5% in some cases of pneumococcal meningitis, TB meningitis, fungal meningitis (coccidioidomycosis), and syphilis meningoencephalitis; in parasitic infection and after foreign protein injections (radioactive serum albumin); after rabies vaccination, intracranial shunts; with allergic or hypersensitive reactions to food or drugs; in allergic asthma; in CNS lymphocytic leukemia
			Found in
Plasma cells	0	0	Often associated with lymphocytic reactions; may be the only abnormality in multiple sclerosis; lymphocytes may undergo transformation to plasma cells in CNS
Basophils	0	0	Found with CNS granulocytic leukemia
Macrophages (includes giant cells)	0	0	Found in TB mycotic meningitis, after brain surgery, after trauma, after subarachnoid hemorrhage
Leukemic cells	0	0	Uncommon initially in leukemias; occur with long-established disease after severe illness, usually during remissions; most common in lymphoblastic leukemia and acute myeloblastic leukemia
Tumor cells	0	0	From primary or metastatic cancer

[a]*Normal Range:* Just what cells can appear normally and in what amount is somewhat controversial. Each laboratory provides its "normal," which is usually given as a count of cells rather than a percentage. When more than the accepted normal number are seen, a WBC differential is performed, and all cells noted are identified. The counts are percentages of total cells usually seen, including some rather controversial "usuals."
Data from Henry, 1984.

2. Keep the client flat for several hours (6 to 12 hours is still recommended in many settings), and provide him or her with a liberal fluid intake (unless contraindicated). Replenishing lost fluid prevents the brain from settling in the base of the skull.

3. If the headache persists, an epidural blood patch may be done. A small amount of blood is removed from the client's vein and is injected into the same site as the spinal puncture. The rationale is that blood will clot and close off the leak.

Other Tests Done on CSF

1. Organism stain—slide stain (see Section 5.1.1 for more detailed information). Gram's stain, Wright's stain, and India ink stains are used to assist in the identification of infective organisms or the presence of malignant cells

2. Organism culture is usually done to help isolate an infective organism (see Sections 5.1.2 and 5.1.3)

3. Serology—specifically the Venereal Disease Research Laboratory Test (VDRL) and/or the fluorescent treponemal antibody absorption test (FTA-ABS) can be done on both blood and CSF when syphilis is suspected or must be ruled out (see Section 6.3.2.D)

4. See also "Diagnostic Tests," Chapter 17: 17.3.5.C, "Carotid Arteriogram; 17.3.5.E, "Cerebral Arteriogram"; 17.4.1.B, "Brain Scan"; 17.4.1.D, "Cisternogram"; 17.6.B, "Brain Sonography" (encephalogram); and "Drug level testing," Chapter 18, Table 18–3 "Anticonvulsive Drugs: Therapeutic and Toxic Levels."

RELATED NURSING DIAGNOSES (NOT PRIORITIZED)

The diagnoses selected here can reflect only a few of the possible diagnoses that may be involved in neurologic dysfunction. The neural system is intrinsically involved with all body functions. Anything that interferes with the function of a given part of the neurologic network will involve nursing diagnoses related specifically to that function. For that reason the diagnoses here are an attempt to select those of particular importance in neurologic dysfunction.

There are some major overlaps, such as alteration in comfort or pain because of the unique meaning headache has in intracranial injury. Self-care deficit is included because of the overwhelming impact permanent paralysis, or paresis has on *all* aspects of life, not just tissue perfusion, skin integrity, elimination, and gas exchange, which are usually the major concerns with temporary mobility impairment.

With a few exceptions (such as pain or headache) the focus of the nursing diagnoses here is on the neurologically stable individual in a rehabilitative or chronic but progressive stage of illness. Knowledge deficit is assumed; necessary teaching is considered an integral part of all administration of nursing care under all nursing diagnoses.

Alteration in Comfort—Pain, Related to

1. Headache secondary to increased intercranial pressure (cerebrovascular accident [CVA], brain injury related to surgical or accidental trauma, space-occupying lesions of the brain)
2. Irritation or compression of nerves (herniated intervertebral disk, vascular spasm, inflammation of surrounding tissues)
3. Muscle spasm cramping
4. Paresthesias
5. Dysfunctional body temperature control due to damage of regulatory centers of the brain (subarachnoid hemorrhage, spinal cord lesions)

Potential for Injury
Trauma, Related to

1. Muscle atrophy secondary to decreased physical mobility (bed rest, paralysis or paresis, restricted movement secondary to pain, fear of injury, and prescribed rest)
2. Loss of muscular control or consciousness secondary to seizure activity
3. Alteration in somatic sensation (touch, pressure, pain, temperature):
   a. Neglect syndrome secondary to lack of awareness of the existence of a body part (CVA), e.g., one-sided neglect of affected side
   b. Tactile agnosia—inability to recognize things touched such as the keen edge of a knife
   c. Lack of awareness of body's position or specific body parts in space (loss of proprioceptive sense) secondary to brain injury
4. Potential for violence (against self or others) due to brain injury
5. Potential for aspiration secondary to muscle weakness (or function loss) or loss of sensation in the oropharynx (CVA)
6. Loss of reflex activity (eye blink, withdrawal from pain) with paresis, paralysis
7. Balance and gait problems secondary to neurochemical imbalance (Parkinson's disease)
8. Incomplete reception of environmental stimuli due to unilateral brain damage with ischemia or actual neuron destruction (CVA, neurosurgery)
9. Alterations in blood pressure secondary to changes in intracranial pressure (increased) or lack of peripheral vasoconstriction secondary to decreased skeletal muscle activity
10. Alteration in thought processes due to sensory/perceptual deprivation such as:
    a. Poor judgment (right-sided CVA, Alzheimer's disease)
    b. Poor memory for recent information (CVA)
    c. Wandering secondary to memory loss, inability to maintain orientation to physical environment
    d. Decreased attention span, increased distractibility
    e. Decreased level of awareness or consciousness secondary to ICCP
    f. Anxiety

Bleeding Related to

Predisposition to gastritis/peptic ulcer secondary to prolonged stress

Complications

1. Autonomic hyperreflexia secondary to spinal injury above T7
2. Infection secondary to decreased immune response due to decreased mobility and decreased nutritional status; need for catheterization with loss of bladder control; and increased risk of injury

Impaired Verbal Communication, Related to

1. Dysarthria (slurred speech) secondary to loss of motor function for speech articulation
2. Dysphasia (also known as aphasia) secondary to damage of speech centers of the brain (e.g., Wernicke's or Broca's areas); can include loss of ability to speak (use language), loss of ability to understand verbal language, loss of ability to understand written language, and/or loss of ability to write
3. Inadequate respiratory function (breathlessness or labored breathing) to power speech (Guillain–Barré syndrome, trauma to neck/cervical spine)
4. Agnosia (loss of ability to understand the meaning or significance of what is seen [visual agnosia], what is heard [verbal agnosia], or what is felt [tactile agnosia] or the loss of ability to recognize familiar things/people)
5. Decreased phonation (whispering speech) secondary to damage to innervation of vocal cords or incoordination of muscles controlling respiration, phonation, articulation, and prosody (rate, rhythm, intonation of speech) (Parkinson's disease) (Ozuna, 1986)

Alteration in Nutrition (Less than Body Requirements), Related to

1. Impaired swallowing secondary to sensory and perceptual deficits of both the mucous membrane of the affected side of the mouth (food pocketing) and control of muscles necessary to chewing and swallowing (CVA, damage to cranial nerves or brain stem)

2. Alteration or loss of senses of taste and smell
3. Decreased appetite and intake secondary to decreased activity, emotional lability, or depression

Self-Care Deficits, Related to

Differential diagnosis between self-care deficits, self-concept, and home maintenance management, depending on level of recovery

1. See the first four diagnoses
2. Decreased mobility secondary to paralysis, paresis, lack of equilibrium, increased pain on activity, muscular spasm on activity, disuse atrophy of skeletal muscles
3. Lack of motivation for self-care secondary to slow or no progress over time and lack of ability to concentrate and recall instructions, increased discomfort with self-care activities
4. Dressing apraxia (inability to recall how to do a once-learned activity)
5. Use apraxia (inability to use once-familiar objects appropriately, e.g., eat with fork, knife, spoon; drink from a cup)
6. Fear of injury

Sexual Dysfunction, Related to

1. Decrease or loss of libido secondary to neural damage (cerebral lesions) or decreased self-concept
2. Decrease or loss of ability to attain or maintain erection (both neural and psychological causes)
3. Physical inability to manage sex act without assistance (quadraplegia)
4. Rejection by partner (actual or assumed) due to change in body image
5. Involuntary unacceptable or undesirable behavior on part of the patient (Alzheimer's disease, right-sided CVA)
6. Cultural and societal strictures on acceptability of sexuality in persons with major handicaps
7. Lack of knowledge of alternative methods for obtaining sexual satisfaction

Disturbance in Self-concept, All Areas, Related to

1. Loss of physical control of body functions, total or partial (e.g., bowel or bladder incontinence or retention; locomotion)
2. Loss of emotional control (lability of emotional response)
3. Increased dependency in all areas (e.g., inability to perform activities of daily living without assistance, inability to provide for own economic needs)
4. Impaired memory
5. Loss of work role, family role, social role, and relationships sustained by these roles
6. Negatively perceived change in physical appearance (facial muscle weakness, contractures or spasticity of extremities)

Alteration in Family Process, Related to

Differential diagnosis with anticipatory or dysfunctional grieving, depending on the process in each family

1. Change in family dynamics with loss of patient's usual group role
2. Burden of care on member(s) of family group
3. Feelings of anger, blame toward patient because of perceived lack of prevention of problems
4. Grief, anticipatory or active
5. Economic problems secondary to loss of income from patient's usual work role and secondary to cost of care
6. Inability to effectively communicate with patient
7. Loss of control over physical care and well-being of patient to health professionals
8. Unacceptable behavioral or personality changes on the part of the patient (temporary acting out, permanent deterioration)

FIFTEEN

THE REPRODUCTIVE SYSTEM

15.1 PREGNANCY

Introduction. The very first screening test in pregnancy is usually the test that validates the fact that the woman is indeed pregnant. Table 15–2, "Tests of Gonadal Function," in Section 15.2 describes those used most often by the physician in the office, women's health clinics, and hospitals in order to confirm signs and symptoms of pregnancy and to follow the progress of a possibly threatened pregnancy. The basis of such tests is the change in the levels of human chorionic gonadatropin (hCG) produced almost immediately on implantation of a fertilized ovum in the uterus. The most specific tests, therefore the most accurate, are done on the blood.

15.1.1 Pregnancy Testing

A. *Home Tests for Pregnancy*

Almost all home test kits reactions are now based on a very sensitive (100%) monoclonal antibody–antigen (immunologic) process that detects the presence of hCG in urine or more recently a radioimmunoassay (RIA) for B subunit of hCG. The later test process is very sensitive and can detect pregnancy before a woman misses her menstrual period.

Self-testing has become the standard first test for pregnancy. Since the inception of home testing, the process has become easier and more accurate. Depending on the test selected, home tests can detect pregnancy before menses are expected; from the first day after an expected, but nonoccurring, menstrual period; or up to 9 days after. The only instruction that is almost universal in the testing is the importance of using first-voided urine because of the increased concentration of hCG.

Results are available immediately or in a matter of minutes, depending on the test. The most recent method to be marketed is the simplest—a matter of placing the small paper strip in the urine stream; others include catching a first-void, midstream urine sample from which drops are placed on specific areas of the test paper, in specific amounts, and waiting a variable amount of time for a color change (usually to blue) caused by an antigen–antibody reaction.

If the test is negative, most self-testing methods recommend a second test if menses do not occur within 1 week.

IMPLICATIONS FOR NURSING

Because of the potential for error in the use of home tests, the woman should be counseled at the earliest possible time to have the pregnancy confirmed officially by a physician. This will provide opportunity not only to affirm the diagnosis but also to review medications in use, some of which could have caused invalid testing, some of which could be dangerous to the fetus.

B. Serum Pregnancy Test

Synonyms: Early pregnancy detection test (EPT); pregnancy test immunoassay

Normal Range (mIU/ml)

Negative (nonpregnant female)	0–4.9
Positive (pregnant female)	26 or above
Borderline	5–25

Serum concentrations of hCG (a glycoprotein) are secreted (produced) on implantation of a fertilized ovum (blastocyst) into the endometrium of the uterus. Detectable in serum as early as 6 days after implantation, it continues to increase during the first trimester of pregnancy. Serum hCG testing is more sensitive than urine pregnancy tests and is, therefore, useful to assess ectopic pregnancy or other aberrant pregnancies in which hCG levels are elevated. (See also Section 16.6, "hCG-Beta Subunit, Quantitative")

INCREASED IN:

1. Pregnancy
2. Ectopic pregnancy (hCG levels are low for gestational age)
3. Any hCG-producing tumors
4. Inflammatory bowel disease
5. Ulcers (gastric)
6. Cirrhosis

IMPLICATIONS FOR NURSING

1. Urine specimens should be delivered to the laboratory without delay as the constituents are stable for a maximum of 12 hours at room temperature. Refrigerate if the specimen cannot be delivered promptly.
2. Urine specimen pH levels less than 5 or greater than 9 can produce false-positive reactions, as can specific gravity outside the ranges of 1.005 to 1.035.

C. Urine: Pregnancy Test

Synonyms: None

Normal Range

Negative for nonpregnant females

---

hCG's main function is to maintain the corpus luteum during the first trimester of pregnancy. An important function of the corpus luteum is to ensure adequate production of progestins, which are necessary for the growth (proliferation) and integrity of the endometrium (Laboratory of Pathology, 1991).

Urine testing of hCG has the advantage of being noninvasive, but it is somewhat less reliable than serum testing. Therefore, the test is frequently useful as a follow-up test of pregnancy initially confirmed by serum testing.

Specimens can be positive as early as 7 to 10 days postconception.

POSITIVE IN:

1. Pregnancy (usually 10 days postconception)
2. Postpartum (specimens taken up to 1 week after delivery)

FALSE POSITIVE IN:

- Individuals with choriocarcinoma, hydatidiform mole, or testicular tumor

FALSE NEGATIVE (OR LOW TITER) IN:

- Threatened abortion or ectopic pregnancies

15.1.2 Pregnancy Norms for Laboratory Tests

Introduction. Pregnancy causes some structural and functional changes in almost all body systems. Because of these changes, laboratory findings will differ from standard reference ranges, yet are not intrinsically abnormal. Unless the pregnant woman's tests are evaluated by reference ranges or norms relative to pregnancy function, much unnecessary concern can occur, and treatment of a nonexisting pathology could also occur. Specialists in the maternal–child area of nursing are unlikely to be confused by this. But neophytes or experienced medical-surgical nurses who suddenly find themselves confronted with the care of a pregnant woman for a medical or surgical problem—which may be totally unrelated to the pregnancy—can be readily led astray or thoroughly confused by these "normal abnormal" findings.

The most commonly checked laboratory tests whose results are altered by pregnancy are listed in Table 15–1. The physiological alteration causing the change in values is given when known. Possible, but not proven, causes for change are also given and identified as such.

TABLE 15–1. PREGNANCY REFERENCE RANGES (NORMS) FOR LABORATORY TESTS

Test Name	Pregnancy Reference Range
Chemistry	
Serum glucose, fasting	Usually decreased; mean, 65 mg/dl (standard mean, 75–80 mg/dl)
2-hr postprandial	145 mg/dl, upper limit of normal (standard upper limit, 110–120 mg/dl)
Plasma bicarbonate	Decreased by 10–15% to approximately 24–25.3 to 31.9–33.4 mEq/L arterial (standard norm [S norm], 22–29 mEq/L)
Serum albumin	As low as 2.7 g/dl (S norm, 3.5–5 g/dl)
Total protein	Variable
Serum IgG and IgA	Decreased
Serum amylase	Variable—increased or normal (S norm, 20–30 IU/L)
Serum alkaline phosphatase	Massive increases, 2,400–18,900 IU/L (S norm, 12–63 IU/L)
Serum cholesterol	Increased 30–40% over standard norms; levels vary with age (see Section 1.11)
Serum free fatty acids	Increased 50–60% (S norm, 239–843 UEq/L)

Underlying Physiological Mechanisms	Comments and Nursing Implications
Increased cortisol, increased progesterone levels cause decreased entry of glucose into the cells In healthy women insulin level will increase, thereby leading to normal or slightly decreased serum glucose content In pregnant women with impaired glucose tolerance (IGT) the pancreas may be unable to respond adequately	Gestational diabetes is defined as an abnormal insulin metabolism (decrease) occurring only during pregnancy and reverting with termination of pregnancy Individuals at risk: family history of diabetes mellitus (DM), 20% overweight, over 40 yr old Increased index of suspicion: previous history of (1) large-for-gestational-age baby (400 g or more), (2) previous delivery of child with congenital anomalies, (3) previous unexplained intrauterine or neonatal death, (4) repeated late abortions, (5) infertility Done as a screening test at 26–30 wk, will be done at first visit, given aforementioned risk factors
Decreased in compensation for chronic hyperventilation due to decreased ventilation capacity	The gravid woman is more susceptible to rapid changes in blood gases and hypoxia because of respiratory system changes, especially with a history of respiratory disease
Partially due to hemodilution plus increased albumin breakdown with no increase in synthesis Decreases can be due to increased degradation	Protein requirements for gravid women are at least 30+ g/day over nonpregnant needs for maintenance and growth of tissue Decreased albumin level is progressive throughout pregnancy and does not return to normal until approximately 8 wk postpartum
May be decreased because of increased fluid volume, renal protein loss, or increased degradation (?) May be increased because of increased levels of transport proteins and fibrinogen	
Increased degradation (?)	Potential for decreased resistence to infection due to decreased IgG levels
May be increased because of increases in estrogen/progesterone levels Increase is due to increase in placental fraction	Increase related to growth and tissue building rather than dysfunction
Increase is due to effect of placental hormone Placenta synthesizes cholesterol for fetal use and hormone production	The increase is temporary unless other factors are involved and returns to normal when pregnancy terminates
Increase is due to combined effect of increased levels of cortisol, estrogen, progesterone, and placental lactogen, all of which are due to decreased insulin activity	Increases can also be related to emotional stress

(continued)

TABLE 15–1. (Continued)

Test Name	Pregnancy Reference Range
Serum creatinine	Decreased to *less* than 0.7–1.5 mg/dl (S norm, 0.7–1.5 mg/dl)
Serum urea nitrogen	Decreased to less than 4–22 mg/dl (S norm, 4–22 mg/dl)
Plasma sodium	Variable; increased *total body sodium content*; plasma sodium level may be within normal limits (WNL) or decreased (S norm, 136–145 mEq/L)
Plasma cortisol, total	Increased over S norm of 8–24 µg/dl (8 AM); 4–12 µg/dl (4 PM); 2–12 µg/dl (8 PM)
Plasma adrenocorticotropic hormone (ACTH) Serum thyroid 1. Total T$_4$ (thyroxine) 2. Thyroxine-binding globulin (TBG) 3. Total T$_3$ 4. Resin T$_3$ uptake 5. Thyroid-stimulating hormone (TSH)	Markedly increased in early months (S norm, 20–100 pg/ml, 8 AM fasting) 1. Increased (S norm, 4.5–12.5 µg/dl), 2. Markedly increased (levels higher than 12 µg/dl, probable *true* hyperthyroidism [S norm varies with lab]) 3. Increased (S norm, 80–200 ng/dl) 4. Decreased to hypothyroid range of (S norm varies with lab) 5. Within normal (S norm, 2–10 µIU/ml) All related to increased estrogen levels
Plasma renin-angiotensin	Increased in second half of pregnancy (S norm, 75–275 ng liberated/ml/hr angiotension; renin, 0.6 × 10 GU/dl) (GU: Goldbatt units)
Hematology Hemoglobin (Hgb)	Slight decrease midpregnancy with a mean level of 11.5 g/dl; late pregnancy, mean level of 12.3 g/dl (S norm, 12–15/g/dl)

Underlying Physiological Mechanisms	Comments and Nursing Implications
Decrease is due to increased cardiac output plus increased plasma volume causing increased renal plasma flow (RPF) and increased glomerular filtration rate (GFR) of 20–50% Perhaps due to effect of human placental lactogen (hPl) in 1st and 2nd trimester	GFR drops to near normal in 3rd trimester. Serum creatinine determination provides an accurate test of renal function during pregnancy Levels at or below 1.5 mg/dl must be considered abnormal and must be reported
Mechanism very similar to that of serum creatinine	Findings in high-normal standard range should be considered abnormal
Decreases occur because of dilution with increased plasma volume and/or increased losses in renal filtration Total body sodium concentration increased because of increased aldosterone levels throughout pregnancy	Kidney compensation for sodium loss is often inadequate during pregnancy, thus leading to inappropriate sodium loss before retention readjusts. Increased filtration because of increased blood volume and renal blood flow causes a small constant drop in sodium; thus, an increased serum sodium level above normal should be reported ASAP. Accurate input and output (I & O) monitoring imperative at this time
Increased level of binding proteins (protein transport) occurs with increased estrogen level, which allows increased cortisol levels	Until adjusted to the increased levels, the pregnant woman may be at increased risk for infection and may have trouble sleeping
Increase is due to increased circulating cortisol levels (?) 1. Increased along with TBG, but not quite so high. Only bound fraction increases 2. Increase starts at fertilization and plateaus at 12 weeks' gestation 3. —— 4. Increased because of increased TBG available in excess of hormone 5. WNL because of increased demand for thyroid despite increased levels All related to increased levels	Overt signs of hyperthyroidism should not occur with pregnancy-caused increases in the hormone. Failure of the TBG to rise suggests either actual hypothyroidism or inadequate estrogen level, which reduces the chance of successful pregnancy, i.e., increased rate of spontaneous abortion Many of these changes can be seen in women who take estrogen. (To validate, check serum cholesterol level, which does not necessarily increase with estrogen but will do so in pregnancy)
Increased ovarian synthesis (?)	After 18–20 wk, there is normally a decreased response to vasoconstrictors except in those with preeclampsia, who continue to respond
A dilutional decrease because of increased plasma volume; total blood volume increases 30–50%	Less than 11 g/dl should be reported; Hgb/Hct routinely checked at initial visit and around wk 30

(continued)

TABLE 15–1. (Continued)

Test Name	Pregnancy Reference Range
Hematocrit 36–45%	Slight decrease to 32–34 (S norm, 36–45%)
Reticulocyte count	Slight increase over norm of $50–75 \times 10^3 mm^3$
White blood count	Increased to $5–15 \times 10^3 \ mm^3$ occasional myelocyte or metamyelocyte (S norm, $4–10 \times 10^3/\mu l$)
Leukocyte alkaline phosphatase stain (differs with each laboratory)	Increased (S norm approximately 5–100 based on arbitrary scale)
Leukocyte stain	Positive for Döhle's bodies (may be normal in pregnancy)
Serum iron	Slight decrease or normal (S norm, 60–175 µg/dl)
Iron-binding capacity, total (TIBC)	Increased, greater than 20–45% saturation (S norm, 250–450 µg/dl)
Serum folate	Decreased serum levels in pregnancy; levels in red blood cells (RBCs) same as S norm (S norm, serum: more than 1.5 ng/ml; RBC level: more than 100 ng/ml)
Erythrocyte sedimentation rate (ESR; sed. rate)	Increased markedly over S norm of 1–10 mm/hr

Coagulation tests: All coagulation factors increase at least a little during pregnancy except

Fibrinogen	Large increase, up to 50% (S norm, 160–300 ng/dl); 3rd trimester levels, 400–600 ng/dl

Underlying Physiological Mechanisms	Comments and Nursing Implications
As for HgB	Less than 32% is to be considered anemia; usually iron supplement started (oral). If no clinical improvement, Hct rechecked before 30 wk (fetal need increases). Fetus always receives priority for iron, so fetus is rarely anemic, but iron stores may be low
The degree of reticulocytosis is proportional to erythropoietic activity; greatest increase is found in the 2nd trimester	
Increase is due to increase in neutrophils (no increase in lymphocytes). Further rise during labor and immediately postpartum; very similar to stress response	Can mask infection response; therefore nurse needs to check for clinical signs and symptoms of infection, especially urinary tract infection (UTI)
Increased with total leukocyte increase of increased intracellular metabolism; no relationship to serum alkaline phosphatase	Indicative only of increased leukocyte count and stress response in pregnancy; can be mistaken for or mask infection (see white blood cells [WBCs])
Reflects some metabolic alteration such as those stimulating rapid neutrophil generation	
Decrease is due to rapid increase in maternal RBC production and fetal needs. Transferrin levels are increased also, but with low saturation	Iron deficiency anemia is the most common anemia in pregnancy. Increased index of suspicion with history of heavy menses, inadequate iron in diet
Increase is due to increased estrogen production, which causes increased protein synthesis, primarily transferrin	See total protein
Fetal needs for folate are substantial and maternal tissues absorb more folate than usual	Serum folate levels can be falsely increased after ingestion of ordinary diet
Increase occurs after 3rd or 4th mo of pregnancy and is related to the increase in fibrinogen levels	Most types of anemia will falsely increase the ESR

XI [plasma thromboplastin] and XIII [fibrin-stabilizing factor])

Increase is due to release of thromboplastin-like substance from the placenta and amniotic fluid into the maternal circulation; also related to presence of increased levels of estrogen (see Section 3.6)	Venous thrombosis occurs more often in pregnant than nonpregnant women. The risk is even greater during the postpartum period. (Disseminated intravascular clotting [DIC] also can occur but is not common.) Besides the increased levels of clotting factors, venous stasis is due to enlargement of the uterus and possible decreased activity, which decreases the use of the somatic pump to return blood from the lower extremities; all add to the risk

(continued)

TABLE 15–1. (Continued)

Test Name	Pregnancy Reference Range
Platelets	Usually normal count during pregnancy but increased markedly at delivery (S norm, 250,000–500,000/mm^3)
Prothrombin (PT) and partial thromboplastin times (PTT)	Normal or slightly shortened (S norms, PT: 11–18 s, PTT: 35–45 s/APTT)
Antithrombin III	Markedly decreased (S norms not available for antithrombin III, fibrin split products, and plasminogen)
Fibrin split products	Increased slightly
Plasminogen	Increased
Urine Tests	
Urine glucose	Negative or 1 + (S norm, negative)
Urine protein	Negative except at the time of labor when a trace (less than 100 mg/dl) normally occurs (S norm, negative)
Creatinine clearance	Results somewhat increased in first two trimesters (S norm 70–130 ml/min)
Urine concentration tests	Rather unreliable
Urine bacteria screen	Negative for organisms in freshly voided, clean-catch specimen

Underlying Physiological Mechanisms	Comments and Nursing Implications
Mechanism very similar to the stress response	
Cause for change unclear; most marked post delivery. Stress (?)	Physiological changes tend to support clotting and prevent clot lysis
A decreased renal threshold exists in most pregnancies as well as an increased GRF, which presents more glucose for filtration	There is no consensus on whether a 1+ urinary glucose result is normal in pregnancy. Given the presence of other risk factors (see serum glucose), even a 1+ should be carefully monitored. Glucosuria is more common in the last trimester in any case
Physiological changes in glomerular filtration occur with strenuous activity and allow traces of protein to be eliminated in the urine. Protein may also occur because of the breakdown of bacteria secondary to a silent UTI	Any proteinuria is generally considered an ominous sign in pregnancy (see Fig. 15–2)
Increases are due to increased cardiac output with increased plasma volume, which causes increased RPF and GFR	GFR decreases markedly with pregnancy-induced hypertension (PIH), and clearance of creatinine will decrease (see Section 16.4)
Related to edema fluid excretion that occurs during sleep	Maintain careful check of I & O as well as weight changes if any question of fluid imbalance
Dilation and hypokinesis (decreased function) of pelves and ureters favor development of UTI during pregnancy because of resultant fairly static urine in upper port of tract	UTI in pregnancy can lead to acute pyelonephritis (25% incidence), which in turn can cause chronic pyelonephritis and renal failure. The infant will be predisposed to sepsis, and acute pyelonephritis is associated with premature labor and low birth weight. Asymptomatic bacteriuria occurs in 2–12% of pregnant women. At risk: Black women with sickle cell trait and women with diabetes mellitus (DM)

Data from Olds, London, & Ladewig, 1984; Ravel, 1984; Schneider, 1978; Wheeler, 1984; and Widmann, 1983.

15.1.3 Hematology

A. Hemoglobin and Hematocrit

Reason for Checking

1. Pregnant women are susceptible to iron deficiency anemia. Because of the increased red cell volume (approximately 33 percent in pregnancy), increased amounts of iron are required. Although gastrointestinal absorption does increase, it is rarely sufficient, and supplemental iron is needed
2. Physiological anemia or pseudoanemia of pregnancy (due to hemodilution) is an expectation
3. A slight hypercoaguability exists because of increased clotting factors. Should hemodilution decrease for whatever reason (evident usually by an increased Hct), measures can be taken to decrease the chance of thrombosis and treat the fluid imbalance

See also Figure 15–1 and Table 15–1.

B. White Blood Count and Differential

Reason for Checking

1. Prolonged increases in the estrogen level cause increases in the serum cortisol concentration, which in turn tends to increase the number of circulating neutrophils. Establishment of a baseline for the individual is important for later assessment
2. Pregnant women are at increased risk for UTIs; thus, the baseline WBC count is necessary to determine the presence of the body's response to infection

C. Blood Typing

Reason for Checking. Any disparity in the gravid female's blood type and that of the fetus poses the potential of significant harm to the fetus or early termination of pregnancy by spontaneous abortion (Olds et al., 1988, p. 329). The result is either a high-risk pregnancy, or a high-risk infant. Clinically significant hemolytic disease (isoimmune hemolytic disease or erythroblastosis fetalis) is associated with D factor in the Rh blood group and with ABO blood types. ABO incompatibility occurs more frequently than does RhD but rarely results in as severe a hemolytic disease. The most common incompatibility with the ABO group is that of a type O mother and a type A or B infant (type A produces the strongest response) and usually presents as jaundice in the infant (Olds et al., 1988, p. 84). (See also Section 13.5, "Blood Typing and Crossmatching.")

D. Antibody Screen

Reason for Checking. As for blood typing, the presence of antibodies to other blood factors (such as antibodies to type A in the type O mother) indicates previous sensitization, perhaps by an earlier pregnancy or a blood transfusion. Antibody levels are reported as "titers." The presence of such antibodies in significant concentrations, as determined by the local laboratories,

(Decision points in heavy outline)

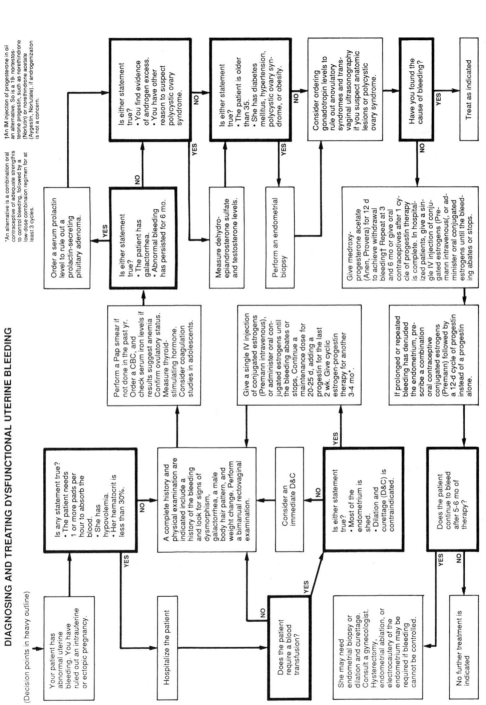

Figure 15–1. Diagnosing and treating dysfunctional uterine bleeding. (Reproduced with permission from *Patient Care*, May 15, 1992. Copyright © Medical Economics Publishing, Montvale, NJ. All rights reserved.)

indicates the need for further assessment. (See also Section 1.10 "Total Serum Bilirubin Levels Increased In"; and "Implications for Nursing," care of the neonate with hyperbilirubinemia.)

E. Serology for Syphilis

Reason for Checking. If the gravid female does have syphilis, treatment started before the 16th to 18th weeks should prevent the effects of syphilis in the infant. If treatment is not started until after that time, the infant may die in utero or will require treatment for prenatal (congenital) syphilis after birth and will be likely to have some congenital defects. See also VDRL or rapid plasma reagin (RPR) tests in Section 6.3.2.D.

F. Rubella Titer

Hemagglutination Inhibition Test, HAI: Titers greater than 1:16 indicate immunity. Titers less than 1:8 indicate susceptibility.

Reason for Checking. The gravid woman in whom an immunity to rubella (German measles) has not developed and who contracts the disease during pregnancy will suffer no greater effects from the infection than if it is contracted at any other time; however, the risk to the fetus is great. Possible teratogenic effects on the fetus, and the percentage of risk are as follows:

1. First trimester
   a. Third to seventh week, death of fetus
   b. Second month, 25 percent will have serious defects
   c. Third month, 15 percent will have serious defects
2. Second trimester—early, permanent hearing impairment
3. Possible defects
   a. Congenital heart disease (patent ductus arteriosus, narrowing of peripheral pulmonary arteries)
   b. Cataracts (can be present both at birth or develop in neonatal period; unilateral or bilateral)
   c. Petechial rash
   d. Hepatosplenomegaly, hyperbilirubinemia
   e. Mental retardation
   f. Cerebral palsy

The infant may also be born with an active rubella infection.

G. Two-Hour Postprandial Blood Glucose

Reason for Checking. Impaired glucose tolerance (IGT), previously called latent DM, is often triggered during pregnancy and produces the probability of recurrence with future pregnancies at best, or lifelong diabetes at worst (Table 15–1).

15.1.4 Urine Tests

A. Assessment of Proteinuria

Reason for Checking. Because of the increase in size of the uterus, the distensibility of the bladder and the ability of the kidneys and ureters to drain, especially on the right side of the body, are hampered. These changes, along with an increased GFR that changes to nearer the usual flow in the third trimester, all increase the risk of UTI in the gravid female.

B. Urine for Glucose and Protein Determinations

Reason for Checking. To detect and manage impaired glucose tolerance, UTI (see Fig. 15–2), and early warning signs of preeclampsia.

15.1.5 Tests for Risk Populations
See also Section 15.1.6 "Newborn Screening Tests."

A. Culture for Gonorrhea*

Reason for Checking

1. Many practitioners routinely do a culture for gonorrhea; others do so only when there seems to be indication of need; however, many women are asymptomatic but will present with positive smears and cultures. There is an increased incidence of sexually transmitted disease in the adolescent age group
2. If gonorrhea is present, it presents risks for the gravid female and for the fetus. At the time of membrane rupture the infection can spread upward in the mother and lead to endometritis, salpingitis, oophoritis, and even pelvic peritonitis. Sterility can be an outcome
3. The fetus is at risk for prematurity because of premature labor. If delivered through the infected canal, the infant is at particular risk for eye infection. Other areas such as the ear, the oropharynx, the stomach, and even the anus can also become infected. (See also Section 6.3 "Diagnosis of Common Sexually Transmitted Organisms")

B. Sickle Cell Screen
See also Table 13–3, "Clinical Syndromes of Hemoglobinopathies."

Reason for Checking

1. If the mother has sickle cell disease rather than only the trait, she will be at risk for experiencing more frequent crises during the course of the pregnancy and has a one-in-three chance of developing preeclampsia
2. There is a 50-percent risk of perinatal death, usually with spontaneous abortion, prematurity, or intrauterine growth retardation
3. If the mother is a carrier of the trait, then both parents must be tested so that genetic counseling can be undertaken. Sickle cell anemia is an autosomal recessive disease
4. Prepregnancy screening is often done in susceptible individuals. The disease afflicts only those of African-American descent (Brookoff, 1992, p. 138)

C. Tay-Sachs Screen

Reason for Checking

1. As sickle cell anemia, Tay-Sachs is an autosomal recessive disease that, although less common than sickle cell anemia, is perhaps even more devastating because the child seldom lives beyond 4 years of age

---

*Other tests for gonorrhea, for herpes virus hominis, type 2, and for AIDS will be found in Chapter 6.

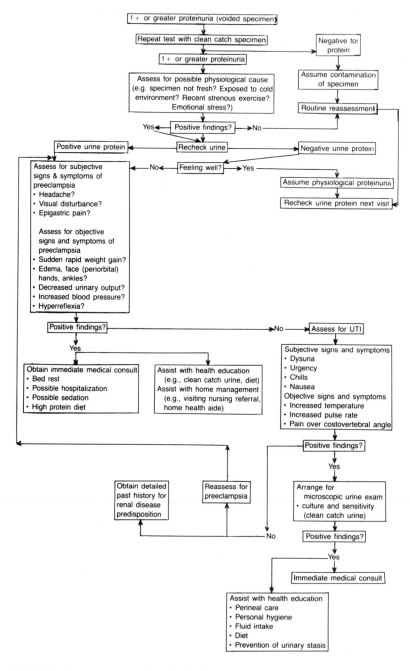

Figure 15–2. Nursing assessment of proteinuria in the pregnant woman. *(Data from Wheeler, 1984.)*

2. Prepregnancy screening is often done in susceptible individuals (e.g., those of eastern or central European Jewish ancestry)

D. Chorionic Villus Sampling (CVS)

Purpose of the Test. CVS is used to diagnose chromosomal and genetic abnormalities in the fetus during the first 12 weeks of pregnancy. Amniocentesis is not done before 16 to 18 menstrual weeks of pregnancy, and results can rarely be reported before 3 weeks. A 5-month fetus may be viable, which makes the decision for abortion much more difficult as well as distasteful to many people. The procedure is medically more difficult in later pregnancy, thus a greater risk as well. CVS may replace amniocentesis when its use becomes more commonplace.

Process. With the patient under topical anesthesia, a very thin, flexible, hollow tube is inserted into the uterus and guided by ultrasonography. A few cells are taken with gentle suction from a site on the placenta that contains fetal cells. The procedure takes only about 20 minutes to perform. The fetal cells are examined for chromosomal or biochemical defects after about 2 days of preparation. A cell culture is usually done to confirm the diagnosis but is not required. All chromosomal abnormalities (e.g., cri du chat, trisomy 13, 18, and 21) can be identified by this method.* Given an adequate family history, many genetic abnormalities can also be identified (Tay-Sachs, cystinosis [Fanconi's syndrome], cystic fibrosis, hemophilia, sickle cell anemia).

Time Required. Results of the culture—depending on what is being tested for, or whether a direct preparation of the sample cells can be made, and on the viability of the cells or their ability to reproduce well—may be from 2 to 3 days to 2 to 3 weeks.

E. Alpha-fetoprotein, Serum, Amniotic Fluid

Synonyms: AFP, A-fetoprotein, alpha-1-fetoprotein; alpha-fetoglobulin

Normal Range: Nonpregnant adult: 0–25 IU/ml

Serum Reference Values		*Amniotic Fluid Reference Values*	
Gestation Week	*Range (0.025–2.5 × median) (IU/ml)*	*Gestation Week*	*Range[a] (Mean ± 3SD) (KIU/ml)*
15	5.7–57	16	6.0–27
15½	6.2–62	17	5.8–25
16	7.1–71	18	4.5–22
16½	7.9–79	19	4.0–17
17	8.6–86	20	3.0–15
17½	9.3–93		
18	10.1–101		
18½	10.7–107		
19	11.6–116		

[a]Assume log-normal distribution (SHMC Laboratory, 1984).

Definition. Alpha fetoprotein (AFP) is a serum protein (globulin) that is normally produced during fetal development. The testing of AFP levels is presently the only screening test using the

---

*An HCG-beta subunit quantitative test is also frequently used; which can detect very low levels of human chorionic gonadotropin (β-subunit). (See tests to monitor cancer, Section 16.6.)

mother's blood to screen for genetic defects. The defects (neural tube defects [NTD]—see "Pathophysiology") it identifies, through increased levels of AFP in the mother's blood or amniotic fluid, are presently incurable. It should be born in mind, however, that the overall incidence of NTDs is only about 1 in every 1000 births and that false positives can and do occur.

Should the AFP levels be low, there is the possibility of a Down's syndrome baby.

Unfortunately the mother or parents are left with rather limited options should the test(s) indicate an increased level. One option would be to deliver a baby who may not survive, or who may be severely physically or mentally handicapped. The other option would be to terminate the pregnancy, which conflicts with many individuals' ethical and religious beliefs. With decreased levels the dilemma is perhaps not so acute. The test is not considered highly accurate. "About 20% of Down's cases may be detected by AFP screening & follow-up evaluation. . . . The vast majority of these cases [with low AFP levels] will, nevertheless, prove to be normal" (Harvard Medical School Letter, 1987, p. 7).

Physiology. AFP is synthesized by the embryonal yolk sac, the liver, and the gastrointestinal tract. It is normally present only in the fetal circulation but is found in minute amounts in the mother's circulation during pregnancy. AFP has a high affinity for oxygen and composes approximately 80 percent of fetal hemoglobin. Its persistence into adult life is abnormal.

Pathophysiology. If the neural tube of the embryo fails to close properly, usually at the end of the first month of gestation, large amounts of AFP leak into the amniotic fluid, and some transfers to the mother's circulation. If the neural tube's failure to close occurs at its upper portion, skull and brain development is arrested. Anencephaly (absence of a brain) can occur and is always fatal, sometimes in utero, sometimes shortly after birth. If the neural tube's failure to close occurs at the lower end, spina bifida (split spine) is the result. This is a malformation of the spine and the spinal cord that frequently (90 percent of cases) is also associated with hydrocephalus, a block in the drainage of fluid circulating in the brain, which can cause learning disabilities or severe retardation. Spina bifida is also associated with meningocele or myelomeningocele, conditions in which the neural tissue of the spinal cord is directly visible or covered only with a thin membrane. In only 29% of the cases is the area covered by skin or a thick layer of membrane. The results of this deformity can include bilateral paralysis of the legs, alterations in bowel and bladder control, and ultimately severe contractures of the lower extremities.

NTDs occur in approximately 2 of 1000 births in the United States. The occurrence of Down's syndrome with some decreases in AFP levels is an unexpected and as yet unexplained occurrence.

AFP LEVELS INCREASED IN:*

1. NTDs of the spinal cord because of an abnormal opening in the fetal body that leaks AFP into the amniotic fluid. (This is assumed to be the reason for increased AFP levels in the maternal circulation as well [Harvard Medical School Letter, 1987, p. 7])

---

*AFP is also increased in a number of disorders unrelated to fetal-maternal interaction. For example, increases are found in primary cancer of the liver, some types of testicular cancer, aplastic anemia, leukemia, and some cases of Hodgkin's disease and lymphoma. The theory as to their cause is that neoplastic disease arises from so-called germ cells, very primitive cells that may involve continued production of fetal hemoglobin. Congenital nephrosis and thalassemia also tend to show increased AFP levels, probably because of a hereditary or genetic defect.

2. Congenital protrusion of the intestines (omphalocele)—rationale as for item 1 (very rare)
3. Fetal deaths in utero, possibly because of increased permeability of membranes related to stress
4. Fetal distress (see "Pathophysiology")

FALSE AFP LEVELS INCREASED IN:

1. Incorrect estimation of fetal age (levels of AFP increase with age of the fetus—see normal ranges)
2. Presence of more than one fetus (e.g., twins), which increases AFP release in utero
3. Fetal hemorrhage, which causes blood contamination of the amniotic fluid

FALSE AFP NORMAL VALUES IN:

• Cases where the gestational age of the fetus has been underestimated

AFP LEVELS DECREASED IN:

• Down's syndrome, in some cases

IMPLICATIONS FOR NURSING: ALPHA-FETOPROTEIN, SERUM, AMNIOTIC FLUID

1. Active nursing diagnosis. A lack of knowledge related to the purpose for testing, process of testing, implications of any findings from the testing, risks involved in choices made on basis of testing—due to the genetic nature of the problem and no previous knowledge
2. Nursing actions
   a. Ensure that the client is fully counseled, either by the physician or a geneticist, as to the purpose, process, risks, and possible outcomes of the testing. Ensure that a significant other is included in the counseling
   b. Recall or gather as much updated information as possible to be able to accurately clarify the client's recall of counseling and to be able to provide knowledgeable support. At this point the test is done as a *routine* screening test only in some prenatal settings. Requirement by law has been mandated in a few areas. It has been endorsed, with reservations, by both the American College of Obstetrics and Gynecology and the American Society of Human Genetics. The reservations are that it be done only as a part of a "comprehensive program that includes patient education, qualified laboratories capable of measuring and interpreting AFP levels, and medical back-up, including ultrasound and amniocentesis" (Harvard Medical School Letter, 1987, p. 8)
   c. When the client expresses interest in or a need for the information, explain what the usual sequence is for testing, what the procedure is for each step, and what will be expected of the client
3. Sequence for tests
   a. The usual procedure is for the maternal blood sample to be drawn first at 16 to 20 weeks' gestation (AFP is measurable in the blood then)
      (1) This involves a simple venipuncture or a fingerstick if necessary
      (2) The laboratory performing the test may require the following information for a more accurate interpretation of its findings
         (a) Mother's age and fetal gestational age
         (b) Maternal weight
         (c) Race
         (d) History of diabetes, blood disorders, or Down's syndrome in the family

       (3) Results are usually ready in 2 to 4 days

       (4) If both serum and amniotic samples are to be taken at the same time, the serum sample should be drawn first because amniocentesis may cause an increase in circulating AFP levels

    b. If the serum sample has elevated AFP levels, a second blood test is done to confirm the finding

    c. If the second blood test also shows elevated AFP levels, an ultrasound test is done to check fetal development. (See Obstetric Sonogram, 17.5.1.F)

    d. If the ultrasound examination indicates a problem in development, an amniocentesis will be suggested

  4. Procedure for amniocentesis

    a. A signed informed consent is required

    b. The test must be done in a setting that allows access to ultrasound to assist with placement of the sampling needle

    c. The client should void before the procedure to reduce the risk of puncturing the bladder and to increase comfort during the procedure

    d. Fetal heart tones are assessed and recorded before and after the test, to ensure the health of the fetus

    e. The client may experience some mild cramping during the procedure that often can be lessened with relaxation techniques

    f. The client will be asked to lie on her back with hands behind her head. This helps to remind her to keep her arms and body still and her hands away from the sterile field

    g. The abdomen will be cleansed and draped with sterile linen, and the ultrasound machine will be used to locate the position of the placenta, the fetus, and the pool of amniotic fluid. It may also indicate a multiple birth, which can make the amniocentesis unnecessary (see "False AFP Level Increased in")

    h. Amniotic fluid is removed with a syringe attached to a long needle that has a stylet. No more than two attempts to obtain an amniotic sample are usually made

    i. Amniotic fluid is withdrawn (15 to 20 ml) after the stylet is removed from the needle. The needle is removed and the puncture site dressed—often with just a Band-Aid

    j. The syringe with the amniotic fluid is placed in a container to protect it from light and sent *immediately* to the laboratory.

    k. Time needed for the test, usually less than one-half hour

F. Prenatal Risk Profile

Synonym: PRP

Definition. Factors other than findings from tests for patients at risk (e.g., AFP or CVS) are included in a risk profile. Maternal data include age, weight, diabetic status, gestational age in weeks and days (determined by date of last menstrual period and ultrasound); laboratory test outcomes of hCG b-subunit, and estrogen in the form of estradiol (see Table 15–2, estriol range by gestational week, in Section 15.2). Maternal and paternal family history of importance includes previous history of neural tube defects or Down's syndrome and race. All data are factored in to determine risks for the infant.

Patient Preparation. The test must be performed between 15 and 20 weeks of gestation.

Process. A computer program is available to laboratories to calculate risk factors for neural tube defect and Down's syndrome based on maternal age, serum AFP, hCG, and U-estriol (uE3/urine estriol in MOM units).

Prior to computer use, 60 percent of Down's affected infants could be identified using maternal age, AFP, uE3, and hCG levels with a 5-percent false-positive rate. Screening, using maternal age alone or with AFP levels, results in a detection rate of 20 to 35 percent; screening by amniocentesis detects only 5 percent of cases (Laboratory of Pathology, 1991).

G. Fetal Cell Analysis for Embryonic Defects

Definition. This promising, but still investigational, test is expected to ultimately replace many of the testing techniques currently in use. Fetal cell analysis uses monoclonal antibodies to test surface proteins from early blood cells (usually erythroblasts or trophoblasts) shed by the fetus and carried in maternal blood. Only recently has it been possible to separate fetal cells from maternal cells by identifying surface proteins that are present on fetal cells but absent from maternal cells.

Purpose. At present, the studies have focused on finding fetal cells with an extra chromosome. Other genetic defects cannot as yet be analyzed because the fetal cells are still "contaminated" with the maternal cells and, if the mother is a carrier of the genetic defect, the test will not identify the defect as hers or that of the fetus.

Because the test is done on a blood sample from the mother, the fetus is not at risk for injury as with an amniocentesis or chorionic villus sampling (CVS).

The expectation is that within a year the techniques will be refined so that *all* the mother's cells will be removed from the testing process, allowing identification of many other genetic defects by this risk-free process (Hall, 1993).

H. Bilirubin Amniocentesis

Synonym: Amniotic bilirubin

Normal Range[a]

Not affected–mildly affected
Moderately affected
Severely affected

[a]The significance of the concentration of bilirubin present in the amniotic fluid is based on the week of gestation (length of pregnancy). Findings are often reported in a graph form rather than by numbers (Liley's prediction graph).

Definition. Amniotic fluid bilirubin is believed to result from fetal hemoglobin in Rh isoimmunization disease. Hemolysis of fetal erythrocytes occurs when maternal antibodies (IgG) to the fetal erythrocyte Rh antigens cross the placenta into the amniotic fluid.

Purpose. The values determined by the test are used to characterize the significance of the bilirubin concentration during that relatively short time.

Normal Values. Amniotic fluid bilirubin is measured as "optical density" (OD). Peak elevation occurs before the 20th week of gestation, decreasing at a constant rate thereafter. Rather than being reported in numbers, findings are entered on a "prediction graph" plotting the logarithm of OD versus the week of gestation. These predictive values are valid only for 1 week after the amniocentesis sample is taken.

FINDINGS:

1. Less than 0.220 OD: Fetus nonaffected to mildly affected
2. 0.220–0.340: Fetus moderately affected; usually requires one or more transfusions; usually survive if transfused
3. 0.340 or greater: Fetus severely affected; most often delivered stillborn or dies in the neonatal period despite exchange transfusion

FALSE FINDINGS PRESENT IN:

1. Fetal bleeding into the amniotic fluid (can be corrected by extraction)
2. Meconium in the amniotic fluid—an indicator of some kind of fetal distress (Laboratory of Pathology, 1991)

I. b-hCG Pregnancy Test

Synonym: b-subunit human chorionic gonadotropin (hCG) assay

Normal Range

Mean doubling time in normal pregnancy: 1.98 days (approximately every 2 days up to the 10th wk of gestation)
Precipitous drop first 6 days postoperation
Normal clearance time postoperation: 2–28 days

Abnormal Range

Increase in hCG or progesterone 6 days after tissue removal (persistent ectopic gestation?)

Definition. Quantitative measures of b-hCG can be detected in maternal serum as early as 7 days after conception. b-hCG measures can be used to confirm both ectopic pregnancy and spontaneous abortion by comparing values with those for similar-age intrauterine pregnancies. However its use requires that the last menstrual period *be known* for accurate comparison, an uncertain fact in almost one third of women with ectopic pregnancy.

Purpose. In clinically stable patients known to have an ectopic pregnancy, serial hCG determinations can be followed to determine if spontaneous resorption is occurring. Spontaneous resorption is rare but does occur. However, the most frequent approach is to try to make the diagnosis as early as possible so as to allow prompt intervention, avoiding rupture, hemorrhage, and destruction of the fallopian tube. Only one third of women who have sustained an ectopic pregnancy will go on to deliver a live born infant in the future (Henry, 1991, p. 478; Leach, pp. 31–46).

J. Toxoplasmosis

Explanation of the Disease. Toxoplasmosis is the most frequently occurring parasital disease (Tietz, 1990, p. 809). It occurs world wide in humans and mammals. Birds act as intermediate hosts. Congenital toxoplasmosis is a grave danger to the fetus.

Transmission. While there is no *direct* transmission of the disease, it can be transmitted via the placenta if the expectant mother has an active infection (McFarland et al., 1993, pp. 1078–81). Fifty percent of women infected during pregnancy have a congenitally infected infant. The later the mother is infected during pregnancy, the greater is the chance of transmission to the fetus. However, the earlier in gestation that the mother is infected, the greater the chance of the infant being *severely* infected (Berkow, 1992, p. 2041).

Clinical Manifestations in the Newborn. The infected fetus with clinical manifestations is usually born prematurely and may demonstrate interuterine growth retardation, jaundice, enlarged spleen, and rashes. Neurological involvement can include chorioretinitis, hydrocephalus, intracranial calcification, microcephaly, and seizures. The fetal outcome of infection varies from early death to long-term neurologic problems and can include mental retardation, deafness, seizures, or other neurological manifestations. Even the infant that appears normal at birth can display one or more of these manifestations thereafter.

Tests for Toxoplasmosis
The most reliable, therefore most used tests to determine the presence of toxoplasmosis are immunoglobulin tests.

A. Toxoplasmosis IgM

Synonym: None

Normal Range: Outcomes are reported by written interpretation

Patient Preparation (Physical): None

Explanation and Findings of the Test. This is a whole blood test (plasma is not accepted) primarily used to detect current infection. IgM titers rise before IgG, usually 5 to 14 days from the time of infection and peak within 2 to 4 weeks, though this can occur as early as the first week. Usually the titer becomes negative within 3 weeks. In rare cases, the titer elevation can persist for more than a year.

Diagnosis of recently acquired, acute or reactivated infection is made on the basis of a single high titer drawn within 2 weeks of symptom onset, or a serial rise in titer in two tubes run in parallel.

Time Required (for test results). Variable, depending on the length of time from infection. (Laboratory of Pathology, 1991)

B. Toxoplasmosis IgG (Both IgM [see above] and IgG tests can be run at the same time)

Synonym: None

Normal Range: Outcomes are reported by written interpretation

---

Patient Preparation. No physical preparation. The purpose, meaning, and preparation for testing should be clearly explained to the person being tested.

Explanation of the Test. A sample of the patient's whole blood (plasma cannot be used) is exposed to an appropriate dried antigen. If the blood contains antibody, the antibody binds to the antigen, which is then treated with fluorescein-tagged antihuman IgG (a dried antigen). When the antihuman IgG binds positively with the patient's antibody, indicating a positive response, the combination fluoresces and is detected by a fluorometer.

Time Required (for test results). Usually 2 to 5 days.

Findings. (High titers decrease slowly, may be detectable for years)

- A titer greater than 1:1000 is highly suggestive of recent infection
- Rising titer: active infection is indicated
- Titer < than 1:16 indicates no infection
- Stable titer indicates infection at some time
- Titer of 1:16 to 1:24 needs to be retested—equivocal
- Titer of 1:201 to 1:1000 indicates possibility of recent infection or reflection of past exposure.

Acute specimens must be drawn within 2 weeks of symptom onset; convalescent serum is drawn at least 3 weeks after the acute specimen (Laboratory of Pathology, 1991).

15.1.6 Newborn Screening Tests

A. Test for Phenylketonuria

Synonyms: Phenylpyruvic acid, Guthrie test

Normal Ranges

Less than 4 mg/dl phenylalanine, reported as negative
Levels of 4–8 mg/dl, reported as presumptively positive

Generalized systemic screening of all newborn infants for phenylketonuria (PKU) is mandatory in 43 states of the United States. The remaining states offer voluntary screening. PKU causes a hereditary type of mental and physical retardation but is one of the few hereditary diseases in which the negative effects can be prevented by early recognition and treatment (Ravel, 1989), thus the widespread and even mandatory screening of newborns.

The Guthrie test is the most widely used screening test. It is sensitive and accurate enough to detect definitely abnormal blood levels (4 mg/dl or greater) and is the most reliable test available for screening purposes as well as being relatively inexpensive. It is a bacterial inhibition test. Fresh capillary blood is obtained by a heelstick, and three areas of blood are placed on a special filter paper, which in turn is placed on a special culture medium containing *Bacillus subtilis.* The bacterium's growth is inhibited by the special culture medium but is stimulated by the presence of sufficient concentrations of phenylalanine—greater than the normal plasma level of 2 mg/dl or less. Therefore, a growth of bacteria indicates a positive reaction and the presence of PKU. With a positive response, further tests are done to confirm and investigate further to rule out false positives. A typical PKU plasma concentration of phenylalanine is usually greater than 15 mg/dl, and tyrosine levels are lower than 5 mg/dl (Ravel, 1989).

Urine screening tests are available but are not usually of value until the infant is over 2 weeks of age, because the serum level of phenylalanine must exceed 10 to 15 mg/dl for phenylpyruvic acid to present in the urine (Whaley & Wong, 1991). By that time irreversible mental deficiencies may have already occurred. Therefore, a more sensitive test that is responsive to lower plasma concentrations such as the Guthrie test is necessary for early diagnosis. Carriers can be identified by a phenylalanine loading or tolerance test, which is similar to a glucose tolerance test (Harvey et al., 1991).

Physiology. The metabolism of the essential amino acid phenylalanine and, subsequently, that of the amino acid tyrosine is extremely complex and not yet fully understood. Phenylalanine cannot be synthesized by the body but is required by it to function. Usually, dietary phenylalanine, which is found in all protein, is acted on by the hepatic enzyme phenylalanine hydroxylase, which converts it to yet another amino acid, tyrosine. Tyrosine is needed for the formation of the pigment melanin and the hormones epinephrine and thyroxin (Howard & Herbold, 1982).

Pathophysiology. The primary defect in PKU is the absence or deficiency of the enzyme phenylalanine hydroxylase. In its absence, phenylalanine cannot be converted to tyrosine, nor can the subsequent conversions take place. This defect can be noted only after the infant has ingested foods (usually milk) containing protein because the amino acid is not synthesized by the body. With the administration of protein phenylalanine, the plasma concentration rises and "alternate catabolites" accumulate in the blood to be excreted in urine once the plasma levels reach the renal threshold (greater than 4 mg/dl, usually 10 mg/dl or more). In infants or children with still-maturing central nervous system (CNS) structures, mental development is retarded, either because of the increased levels of plasma phenylalanine and its increased levels in the spinal fluid or because of the presence of various phenylketones in the blood. Brain development is abnormal, nerve sheath myelinization is defective, cystic degeneration of the gray and white matter occurs, and cortical lamination is disturbed. CNS destruction and, therefore, possible mental retardation occurs before the abnormal metabolites (the phenylketones) begin to be excreted in the urine (Whaley & Wong, 1991).

The decreased production of melanin is thought to be responsible for the phenotypic appearance of PKU victims. They routinely have blond hair, fair skin, and blue eyes (Ravel, 1989).

Because the excess presence of phenylalanine is the single defect, and because it occurs in the body only by exogenous administration, the disease can be successfully treated by extremely strict diet manipulation. If begun in the first month of life and continued faithfully, it can prevent mental or physical retardation. It has not been established with any certainty just how long the diet must be maintained. Some authorities believe that it can be terminated at school age—the rationale being that the brain has achieved maximum growth by then. Others recommend dietary management indefinitely (Howard & Herbold, 1982). Most authorities recommend the former course, continuing treatment until the age of 6 or 8.

PKU FALSE-POSITIVE RESPONSES IN:

1. Liver disease because of defective metabolism, which results in increased levels of precursors
2. Galactosemia because of secondary liver disease
3. Transient states of hyperphenylalaninemia or variants of PKU that do not require dietary treatment

PKU FALSE-NEGATIVE RESPONSES IN:

1. Testing done before 4 days postbirth*
2. Testing done in premature infants because of delayed maturation of enzymes required for phenylalanine catabolism (Harper et al., 1979)
3. Testing done before the infant has ingested sufficient quantities of protein. This may be due to insufficient feedings secondary to the infant's refusal to eat because of anorexia or vomiting. Infants with PKU tend to vomit and refuse to eat more often than do normal infants

---

IMPLICATIONS FOR NURSING: TEST FOR PHENYLKETONURIA

1. Before having the Guthrie test done, it is important that the infant ingest at least two high-protein feedings. Because normal plasma values of phenylalanine are related to both age and protein intake, the test is usually done approximately 4 days after birth. False negatives can occur if the test is done before 4 days or before enough protein has been ingested. The testing should be done on all such infants within 1 to 2 weeks (Lab. of Pathology, 1991)
2. Case finding is a shared responsibility among all health care workers. The nurse can assist in the process by
   a. Validating that all newborns in the nurse's care are tested before leaving the hospital
   b. Being alert for any "mousey, musty, horsey" odor in urine from any infant or child in the nurse's care and immediately doing a urine or diaper test for PKU
   c. Reinforcing the need for a recheck test, usually within a month of birth, with the parents. This can be done by
      (1) Being sure that the parents fully understand the purpose of the test
      (2) Informing the parents of the correctable nature of the defect and the essential role that only the parents can play in the future well-being of the infant
      (3) Helping the parents deal with feelings of blame and guilt that often occur in reaction to a positive test. Because there is a number of false positives with the initial Guthrie test (some reports state that the majority of initially positive Guthrie test results are not due to PKU [Ravel, 1989]), this possibility can be mentioned, but should not be stressed in helping encourage the return for the second test and in dealing with feelings
3. Follow-up support and guidance in management of the child as he or she grows is an important area for nursing intervention, especially in a clinic or home setting
   a. Although complete dietary control is possible with the infant, the older child is likely to rebel, particularly as children become more independent and can find their own food or as the attitude of their peer group becomes important
   b. The philosophy of the approach to a handicapped child applies in this instance. Helping the child to be as well-socialized as possible given the restrictions necessary, placing the responsibility of dietary control increasingly with the child as he or she matures, and understanding and dealing realistically with the child's negative feelings are all concepts to be applied to the child with PKU

---

*In premature infants the serum phenylalanine level is usually low at birth and rises to levels of 9 mg/dl or higher in 1 to 2 weeks.

    c. Helping the family to deal with other possible effects of the illness in the child is equally important. These can include failure to thrive, frequent vomiting, irritability, hyperactivity, unpredictable or erratic behavior, fright reactions, bizarre behavior, screaming episodes, unusual posturing, and eczema or other dermatologic problems. Any of these would require major adaptation and coping on the part of the parents. The nurse might assist the parents to

       (1) Arrange and accept relief time from child care without guilt feelings

       (2) Reinforce the knowledge that the behavior is due to the disease and may be temporary and reversible. Consult with the physician about this

    d. The need for careful and systematic follow-up must be reinforced at frequent intervals and the parents assisted with the process. Changes will be necessary in the diet to cope with growth spurts and developmental changes in the child. The nurse can help with the necessary teaching and support to provide for

       (1) Monitoring changes in behavior that indicate inadequate phenylalanine intake (e.g., anorexia, rash, listlessness, failure to grow)

       (2) Monitoring growth by keeping daily (infant) or weekly (child) records of height and weight, which can provide positive reinforcement for the child and the parents

       (3) Using an exchange equivalent list to provide for more flexible, less cumbersome diet planning. If the parent does not have such a list, consult with the dietician to provide one or to update it to make it more suitable to the age of the child. Free access to a dietician is a high-priority need for parents of PKU children

       (4) Establishing a schedule for blood phenylalanine determinations (Guthrie test) usually twice weekly during the initial diet stabilization period, weekly for infants, at 2- to 3-week intervals for toddlers, and monthly thereafter as long as the diet is continued

       (5) Routinely testing urine, especially if the child has not been adhering closely to the diet

         (a) Diaper test using 10 percent ferric chloride solution in drops, which is inexpensive and easy to do

         (b) Phenistix text—more accurate but more expensive than the diaper test. It is not useful until the child is 6 weeks old or older

         (c) Dinitrophenyl hydrazine (DNPH)—a more complex process but the least expensive and very accurate. It might be suggested for use if a parent or health care worker is accustomed to dealing with testing

4. Special counseling is indicated for adult carriers who plan to marry and for the female adult with PKU who plans pregnancy

    a. Refer those planning marriage or motherhood for genetic counseling if necessary or possible

    b. Acquire sufficient knowledge and understanding of the genetic pattern to be able to reinforce and elaborate on the genetic counseling given or, in the absence of such a service, to provide accurate and necessary counseling

    c. Women with PKU who wish to bear children should receive a phenylalanine-restricted diet regardless of their serum levels at the time. The outcomes of such pregnancies are as yet unknown

B. Test for Galactosemia

Synonym: UDP—galactose transferase utilization test

Normal Range: 2.5–9 IU enzyme activity/g hemoglobin

Definition. Testing for galactosemia is a semiquantitative measurement of the amount of enzyme activity that is deficient or totally absent in the inherited disease of galactosemia. The enzyme measured is one of the three needed for the conversion of galactose to glucose in the body and is the one deficient or absent in this disease (galactose-1-phosphate uridyl transferase) (Henry, 1991). This blood test is considered to be a better screening test for the condition than is the older approach of urine testing (e.g., Clinitest) because it will yield a positive result whether or not the child has been eating, whereas the urine test depends on the ingestion of lactose. As in PKU, the infant with galactosemia may refuse milk or may be vomiting.

Not all infants are tested routinely. Usually, those that are suspected of having the disease (e.g., both parents are known carriers) have the cord blood tested at birth. Others are often picked up by a combination of physical findings and urine testing. Such a case finding is confirmed by further testing using the red cell utilization test or blood galactose determination. Galactosemia is of sufficient importance, although rare, to be included among the general screening tests in that finding it can be lifesaving or markedly increase the future quality of life. The disease is sufficiently treatable to eliminate the negative consequences and is often "outgrown" (Ravel, 1989).

Physiology. Figure 15–3 illustrates the metabolism of galactose.

Pathophysiology. Galactosemia is a hereditary autosomal recessive disease. At birth the child appears normal. After feeding the infant usually vomits, and weight loss ensues. There is an absence or deficiency of the final enzyme in the metabolism of galactose (see "Physiology"). Increased amounts of galactose-1-phosphate accumulate in the plasma; at the same time, a state of hypoglycemia exists because galactose is not processed to glucose. The hypoglycemic state can lead to convulsions and mental deficiency. Proteinuria and aminoaciduria also occur.

By an unknown mechanism the accumulation of galactose-1-phosphate causes cerebral damage, aminoaciduria, and liver damage in the form of a cirrhotic process and enlargement. Jaundice can occur by the second week of life. Splenomegaly follows the liver damage, which is

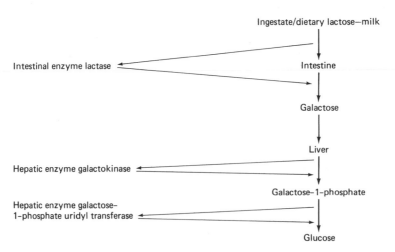

Figure 15–3. Galactose metabolism.

secondary to portal hypertension. Recognizable cataracts appear by the end of the first or second month if untreated. The excessive galactose is excreted in the urine.

Carriers are asymoptomatic but may show a spontaneous dislike for or avoidance of galactose-containing food, primarily milk, milk products, and legumes (Howard & Herbold, 1982; Whaley & Wong, 1991).

IMPLICATIONS FOR NURSING: TEST FOR GALACTOSEMIA

1. No special preparation is necessary for the test
2. Because galactosemia is a genetic and treatable disease, genetic counseling is encouraged
3. Because not all children are routinely screened for the disease, the nurse needs to be alert for signs and symptoms of its presence. Many of these signs and symptoms are similar to those of PKU, and the nurse must be able to recognize differences if they occur
    a. Initial signs and symptoms are vomiting and a failure to gain or an actual loss of weight below birthweight. Drowsiness, failure to feed well, failure to thrive, and diarrhea often follow. None of these symptoms differs substantially from those of infants with PKU
    b. An enlarged liver or spleen frequently develops in the child with galactosemia, and such a child frequently has aminoaciduria and proteinuria. None of these problems is normally found in children with PKU
    c. Independent testing of urine (positive Clinitest versus negative strip or dipstick test results indicate galactosemia) and urinalysis results should be checked
4. Dietary teaching is of major importance because dietary manipulation is the primary treatment
    a. A diet totally free of all milk and milk products (e.g., cream, cream soups, butter, cheese, ice cream, sherbet, yogurt) is prescribed
    b. The family or patient needs to be especially aware of the inclusion of lactose in many prepared foods and needs to be advised to read the labels of such foods very carefully
    c. The family should also be instructed to read labels on patent medicines with care. Many contain lactose as a filler. They also need to consult with their pharmacist when obtaining prescription drugs so as to eliminate drugs containing lactose as a filler
5. It is generally easier to get compliance with the therapeutic regimen for galactosemia than for PKU. The substitution of soybean formula is usually well accepted by the child, although the odor may be objectionable to the parent, and the probability of being able to include milk and milk products some day adds to the ease with which the diet is accepted by the growing child. Such compliance does not eliminate the need to stress the importance of compliance and the potentially harmful effects, as well as irreversible effects of noncompliance. Follow-up should be consistent and supportive

---

C. Sickledex

Synonyms: Sickle cell solubility, sickle-turbidity test, sickle cell test

Normal Range: Negative

Definition. The Sickledex is a highly specific screening test because it is used to screen for only one form of bleeding disorder, hemoglobin S (Hb-S). This variant form of hemoglobin produces sickle cell anemia or sickle cell trait, which occurs almost exclusively in blacks. It will detect both homozygous (sickle cell anemia) and heterozygous (sickle cell trait) states but does not differentiate between them (Laboratory of Pathology, 1991). Hemoglobin electrophoresis is used to differentiate between the trait and the disease (Whaley & Wong, 1991).

The principle underlying the test is that deoxygenated Hb-S is virtually insoluble in certain media (e.g., high-phosphate buffer solution) and will form a cloudy or turbid mixture when mixed in the solution. All other forms of hemoglobin (A, A$_2$, F, C, D) produce a clear suspension (Ravel, 1989). The test is felt to be reliable as a screening test despite some false-positive and/or false-negative results (listed later), and it can be quickly done using blood obtained from a fingerstick. Hemoglobin electrophoresis is often necessary after a positive Sickledex result to differentiate between trait, disease, or a false-positive result that is due to other hemoglobinopathies (Whaley & Wong, 1991). It is included as a routine screening test for newborn blacks in many hospitals.

Physiology. See "Physiology" in Section 2.1.2.

Pathophysiology. Sickle cell anemia (or trait) is a recessive, hereditary blood dyscrasia that is characterized by the presence of Hb-S in place of hemoglobin A (Hb-A) in the RBCs. This variant hemoglobin differs from normal hemoglobin only in that one of the 574 amino acids making up its structure is different (valine instead of glutamine). Such a small alteration in the hemoglobin molecule causes remarkable changes in the characteristics of the RBCs containing it. The hemoglobin is markedly decreased in its solubility. When it is exposed to decreased environmental pH or decreased oxygen, the hemoglobin forms long slender crystals that deform the RBC into a crescent, or sickle, shape. This causes the blood to become more viscous because the cells tend to become sticky and adhere to one another. Sickling will also occur when there is inadequate fluid—dehydration states—which enhances the viscosity. The situation readily progresses to thrombosis after venous stasis. Thrombosis further decreases oxygenation locally, hypoxia is increased, and more sickling results. Cells with Hb-S are more fragile and hemolyze readily, their life span is 26 to 35 days compared with a normal of 120 days, and anemia results despite increased production of RBCs. The defective Hb-S also has a greatly reduced ability to transport oxygen, which increases the body's hypoxia.

The disease is characterized by symptom-free periods interspersed with episodes of acute crises that are most frequently related to vascular occlusion, which is accompanied by excruciating pain in the area or organ affected. The severity and site of the crisis episodes are not predictable (Groer & Shekleton, 1983).

The person afflicted with the trait (genetic inheritance from only one parent) rather than the disease (genetic inheritance from both parents) does not usually have symptoms unless severely stressed, because the majority of his or her blood has normal hemoglobin.

The disease is not evident in infants until they are approximately 6 months of age because of the high percentage of hemoglobin F (Hb-F) found in the newborn. Once the infant replaces the Hb-F with the defective hemoglobin, symptoms will appear. Pathological changes throughout the body can include changes in the following tissues:

1. Spleen: Enlargement, ultimately fibrotic changes ("autosplenectomy")
2. Blood: Hemolysis, anemia (normocytic, normochromic), hyperplastic bone marrow, decreased hemoglobin (7 to 10 percent), bilirubinemia, reticulocytosis

3. Kidney: Ischemia (causing an inability to concentrate urine), enuresis, hematuria
4. Skin: Chronic leg ulcers because of decreased peripheral circulation and thrombosis
5. Liver: Enlargement secondary to circulatory stasis; cirrhosis may occur secondary to capillary obstruction, necrosis, and scarring, Hemosiderosis (increased storage of iron) secondary to hemolysis and may also occur in the spleen, bone marrow, kidney, and lymph nodes
6. CNS: Possible cerebrovascular accident (CVA) secondary to thrombosis, signs and symptoms of minor brain hypoxia—headache, weakness, convulsions, and visual disturbances including a loss of vision from progressive retinopathy and retinal detachment
7. Heart: Potential congestive heart disease secondary to chronic anemia
8. Bones: Osteoporosis secondary to bone marrow hyperplasia and congestion, skeletal deformities secondary to the weakening of bone (especially lumbar and thoracic regions), arthralgia secondary to erythrostasis in joints, hand-foot syndrome secondary to infarction of the short tubular bones (swelling and pain), aseptic necrosis of the femoral head secondary to chronic ischemia (Whaley & Wong, 1991)

SICKLEDEX FALSE-NEGATIVE RESULTS OCCUR IN:

1. Persons with a hemoglobin concentration of 10 g/dl or less
2. Infants less than 6 months of age because of the presence of Hb-F (Lab. of Pathology, 1990)

SICKLEDEX FALSE-POSITIVE RESULTS OCCUR IN:

1. Non–S-sickling hemoglobinopathies (rare occurrence) (e.g., hemoglobin C [Harlem, Georgetown, and perhaps Alexandria]) (SHMC, 1984)
2. Dysglobulinemias such as Waldenström's disease, myeloma, cryoglobulinemia

---

IMPLICATIONS FOR NURSING: SICKLEDEX

1. No special patient preparation is necessary
2. Not all people agree with the use of screening tests for the identification, in particular, of sickle cell trait. One criterion for the use of screening tests is not met in the use of the Sickledex for identification of the trait, which helps provide a rationale for opposing its use. The unmet criterion is that the test be used for the purpose of uncovering a serious or common disease that *is treatable* (see the introduction to Part I). Hb-S trait is treatable only through selective reproduction, which can easily be viewed as racial genocide by the most affected race, the blacks. The nurse needs to be aware of this point of view to understand and deal tactfully and effectively with negative responses to "routine" screening tests
3. The nurse will need to acquire knowledge in the area of genetic transmission so as to correctly reinforce genetic counseling or to provide such when necessary. For example, it is well to know that each child born to parents both carrying the sickle trait has a 25 percent chance of having the disease
4. Implications for nursing applicable for hyperbilirubinemia may also apply in this instance. Monitor the blood levels of bilirubin as well as urinary bilirubin and urobilinogen
5. Assess gently for enlargement of the liver or spleen. If a physician is doing this on a routine basis, there is no need to subject the patient to a second palpation. A decrease in size is, of course, a favorable sign and vice versa

6. By following the list of potential pathological changes (see pathophysiology), do an initial assessment of each area as a baseline for future comparisons to determine the effectiveness of therapy or progress of the disease

7. The major nursing goal in the care of the individual with sickle cell disease, not in crisis, is to prevent sickling by preventing hypoxia and providing adequate hydration. This is done not only by implementing a well-conceived plan of care but also by teaching that plan of care to the patient, family, home caretaker with an adequate and compelling rationale to increase compliance. Some possible interventions are as follows

  a. Provision of adequate hydration for hemodilution by

    (1) Calculating the child's intake based on a minimum of 100 to 125 ml/kg/day

    (2) Providing highly specific instructions for intake in terms of numbers of glasses, bottles, or cups per day rather than in ml/day

    (3) Listing and using high-fluid content foods particularly enjoyed by the patient (e.g., fruit with a high water content, popsicles, soups)

    (4) Arranging patient or family access to a variety of fluids for "self-service"

    (5) Offering a small amount of a different fluid on each contact with the patient—encouraging the family to do the same

  b. Evaluation for adequate hydration by

    (1) Observing the absence of physical signs and symptoms of sickling (e.g., complaints of severe pain, evidence of increased hemolysis [jaundice, hematuria])

    (2) Checking for moist mucous membranes

    (3) Ascertaining that the intake and output are balanced when corrected for insensible losses

    (4) Seeing that infant fontanelles are full, not sunken

    (5) Checking that weight is either increased or at baseline

    (6) Knowing that the urine will be dilute because of the kidney's inability to concentrate; therefore, urine specific gravity is not a good criterion for measurement

  c. Prevention of fluid loss by

    (1) Preventing perspiration by control of ambient temperature

      (a) Avoid undue exposure to the sun

      (b) Avoid excessive clothing/bedding

      (c) Look at or check with the patient rather than assuming that the room temperature is correct

    (2) Knowing that enuresis frequently occurs, even in adults, because of the kidney defect

      (a) If dehydration threatens, weigh the bedding dry and then wet for a better calculation of loss

      (b) Use diapers when appropriate—weigh them

      (c) Arrange ready access to a toilet during day and night; instruct in urine measurement

      (d) Take to the toilet during the night if sleep patterns will not be disturbed

      (e) Adapt toilet training in youngsters to allow for a blameless lack of success. Psychological problems occur readily with enuresis

    (3) Monitoring lab reports and signs and symptoms for electrolyte loss. The loss of potassium in urine can precipitate acidosis, which enhances sickling

  d. Prevention of hypoxia by preventing increased cellular oxygen demand through

    (1) Preventing infection (see "Implications for Nursing" in Section 1.9.2 and items 2c, 3a, and 3c in Section 2.2.3)

    (2) Monitoring laboratory reports for evidence of acidosis (see Appendix A) (e.g., decreased venous CO_2 concentration)

    (3) Preventing overheating; see item c (1)

    (4) Monitoring the RBC count, hematocrit, and hemoglobin for changes in oxygen-carrying capacity

    (5) Limiting physical activity on the basis of the results of item (4) plus evidence of fatigue, complaints of dyspnea on exertion, and the acceptance of the limitations by the patient without emotional stress

    (6) Identifying and preventing, if possible, emotional stressors. Work independently with the patient or family in positively managing stressors

(7) Providing analgesia promptly after a report of pain (other than aspirin, which promotes bleeding) and giving oxygen if the pain is due to sickling, but with judicious restraint, because a prolonged use of oxygen will decrease the stimulus for erythropoietin production, thus increasing the anemia and hypoxia

(8) Providing passive range of motion (ROM) exercises to prevent thrombus formation as well as maintain muscle mass for later active exercise while decreasing the immediate oxygen demand

(9) Providing a diet with adequate nutrients to replace lost blood cells and provide energy (see "Implications for Nursing" in Section 1.8 items #5 and 6).

(10) Preventing infection due, in part, to impaired ability of the reticuloendotheilial system to clear bacteria from the blood. Salmonella and pneumococcal infections are prevalent (Henry, 1991, pp. 651–652).

Infants (starting at 6 weeks of age) and children at risk, (with their parents' consent) are often placed on a preventative treatment program of oral penicillin (125U); twice daily. Dosage is increased at intervals to a maximum of 250 units, and given to the child through age six (Personal Interviews. B. Horton RN and D. Martin MD, October 1992).

15.1.7 Tests Related to Preeclampsia

Definition. Preeclampsia or pregnancy-induced hypertension (PIH) is defined as a blood pressure of 140/90 mm Hg during the second half of pregnancy in a previously normotensive woman or an increase of 30 mm Hg systolic and an increase of 15 mm Hg diastolic in a previously hypertensive woman. It is also defined as a "chronic disease, confined to pregnancy" (Worley, 1984, pp. 821–822).

Rationale for Use

1. With careful attention to warning signs (clinical signs and symptoms and laboratory data), convulsions (eclampsia) can be prevented, and a live infant delivered

2. Hypertensive diseases are the most common medical complication of pregnancy; PIH is the most common hypertensive disease in pregnancy

3. Even if convulsions are prevented, there may be serious consequences for the fetus because of decreased placental blood flow during the pregnancy, and early delivery by cesarean section may be indicated

4. PIH does not always present with classic signs and symptoms (see Fig. 15–4). Even though eclampsia is now a rare occurrence, when it does occur it is seen most frequently in the atypical presentation, which can easily be misdiagnosed as obstructive cholecystitis, pancreatitis, or another abdominal dysfunction

A. Urine Tests

1. Protein test results will be positive with a 24-hour urine sample; random sampling may be negative

2. Creatinine clearance test responses will be at or above normal clearance levels during pregnancy (pregnancy norm, 120 to 150 ml/min; the standard norm is approximately 100 ml/min in the nonpregnant state). The 24-hour creatinine clearance test depends on many variables that must be taken into account, such as fluid intake, physical position during collection. Some feel that the lateral recumbent position best reflects renal function and sodium intake

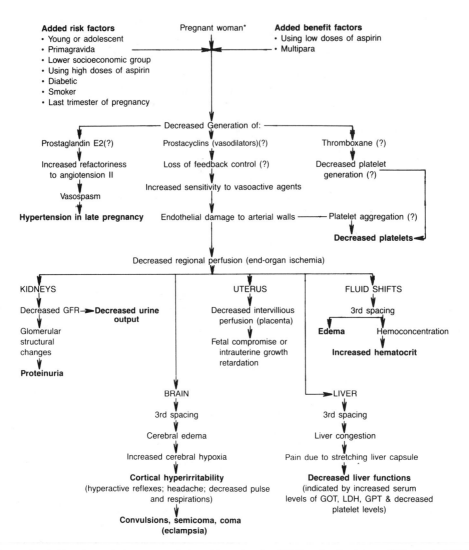

Figure 15–4. Preeclampsia (pregnancy-induced hypertension [PIH]) pathophysiology. With atypical PIH, those patients presenting without evidence of hypertension, or without proteinuria perhaps, the presence of right upper quadrant pain and elevated low-density lipoprotein levels with a decreased platelet count and increased hematocrit should cause the practitioner to develop a high level of suspicion of the presence of PIH. In patients who have a superimposed chronic hypertension, the symptoms of PIH will occur earlier and be more severe. *(Data from DeVoe & O'Shaughnessy, 1984; Wolfe, 1985; and Worley, 1985.)*

B. Blood Chemistry

1. Serum uric acid: Markedly increased in severe PIH, in part because of a decreased GFR and in part because of an alteration in reabsorption in the proximal convoluted tubules
2. Serum iron: Striking elevations to a mean of 135.3 μg/dl in pregnant women with diagnosed preeclampsia as compared with a mean of 61.6 μg/dl in normotensive gravidas and

a mean of 72.5 µg/dl in gravidas with hypertensive disease (Entman & Richardson, 1983, pp. 196, 568)

3. Hepatic function tests: Used to confirm rather than diagnose PIH; generally used only when the pregnant woman complains of right upper quadrant (RUQ) pain
   a. Serum bilirubin, increased
   b. Serum aspartate transaminase (SAST), increased
   c. Alkaline phosphatase, increased
   d. Total lactic dehydrogenase, increased
   e. Serum glutamic pyruvic transaminase (GPT), increased

C. Coagulation Studies

1. Thrombin time: Prolonged because of an alteration in liver function (?) greater than the standard norm, which is within 3 seconds of the control (usually 10 to 15 seconds)
2. Platelet count: Decreased to less than 150,000 platelets/mm³. The decrease appears to correlate with the severity and duration of hypertension. A decrease is found in 18 percent of preeclamptics and 39 percent of eclamptics
   a. Can be lower in more severe cases
   b. Decreased platelet count is much more common than changes in any other clotting factors in PIH. Some researchers believe the decrease to be the *first* sign of preeclampsia
   c. Decrease may be related to platelet aggregation secondary to endothelial injury in the microcirculation (DeVoe & O'Shaughnessy, 1984, p. 845)

D. Hematology

Only the hematocrit (Hct) change is useful in the diagnosis of PIH. Because of the third spacing that occurs secondarily to the increase in blood pressure and increased capillary permeability, intravascular fluid is decreased, which causes a fluid-related increase in the Hct (relative increase).

E. Critical Indices in the Nontypical Pregnancy Induced Hypertension (PIH) Case

Given a pregnant woman in the last trimester who is complaining of RUQ pain, if the Hct is increased, the platelet count decreased, and the liver enzyme levels, specifically AST and GPT, increased, the chances are excellent that she is suffering from PIH whether she is showing protein in the urine, or whether or not her blood pressure is notably increased (Wolfe, 1985).

15.2 REPRODUCTIVE HORMONES: GONADAL FUNCTION

Introduction. The term *gonad* refers to a sex gland: the ovary in the female, the testes in the male. The ovary produces ova, and the testes produce spermatozoa. Gonadal function is not limited to reproduction. Both sex glands produce hormones that control sexual maturation, pubertal reproductive organ development, and physical traits that define femininity and masculinity (e.g., voice pitch, body form, muscular development, hair growth patterns). The principal hormones produced are estrogen and progesterone by the ovary and testosterone by the testes.

Gonadal function is under the control of the pituitary (luteinizing hormone [LH] and follicle stimulating hormone [FSH]), and there is evidence to suggest that the hypothalamus secretes a single peptide-releasing hormone that controls the secretion of both gonadotropins. This factor is known by several names (e.g., luteinizing releasing hormone [LRH], LH/FSH-releasing hormone [RH], or gonadotropin-releasing hormone [GnRH]). LH is sometimes called interstitial cell stimulating hormone (ICSH) in males (see Fig. 15–5).

Another hormone of importance in reproduction is human gonadotropin (hCG), a so-called hormone of pregnancy, which is produced by the placenta. The placenta also produces estrogen and progesterone and increases those serum levels during pregnancy.

A. Laboratory and Clinical Indications of Gonadal Dysfunction

Laboratory Findings. Screening tests do not provide indicators of congenital gonadal dysfunction other than a marked increase in urinary 17-KS levels, a test that is rarely done in screening. In acquired dysfunction the screening tests reflect the primary disorder without specific clues to gonadal dysfunction.

Clinical Findings. Findings include adolescent failure to develop appropriate or any secondary sex characteristics; the presence in the infant or young child of intersex genitalia, hypospadias, clitoral enlargement, webbing of the neck, lymphedema; in adult women, menstrual disorders, such as abnormal uterine bleeding, absence of menarche, amenorrhea, painful menses, signs of pregnancy; hirsutism; virilization; in men or women, evidence of infertility; and in adult males, hypogonadism, change in body hair patterns, impotence.

B. Tests of Gonadal Function
Table 15–2 lists the normal ranges, uses, and characteristics of major gonadal function tests.

C. Associated Tests

C.1 Buccal Smear

Synonyms: Barr test, sex chromatin test, S-chromatin study

Reported Results (normal)

Female	Barr body–positive, single (20–40% of cells)
Male	Barr body–negative

Indications for Use. The buccal smear test is indicated for ambiguous or abnormal genitalia, male or female infertility without other known cause, and symptoms suggestive of Turner's or Klinefelter's syndromes.

Explanation of the Test. The buccal smear test is primarily a screening test for the purpose of visualizing Barr bodies. The Barr body is normally found in the nuclei of various body cells and is produced by inactivation of one of the X chromosomes in female cells. (Females carry XX chromosomes; males carry XY). This occurs at the time of embryonic implantation in the uterus. Only one X chromosome is needed to transfer genetic information. The X chromosome inacti-

(*continued p. 506*)

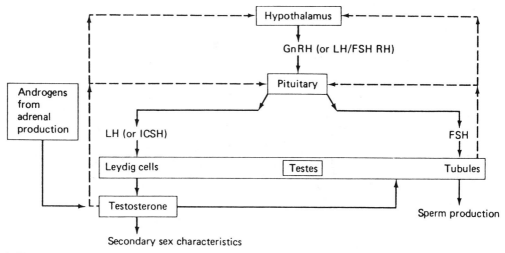

A. Male gonadal function

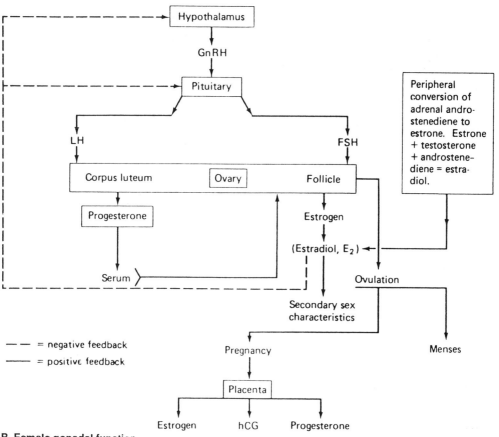

B. Female gonadal function

Figure 15–5. Gonadal Function

TABLE 15–2. TESTS OF GONADAL FUNCTION

Name of Test	Normal Ranges		Comments	Purpose, Increases, Decreases
Estrogen Tests	Adult Female	pg/ml	Estradiol is the predominant estrogen in human serum. Produced in small amounts in the male testes and large quantities in the adult female ovary, the product of maturing ovarian follicle and corpus luteum	**Detects** secondary ovarian failure (decreases pituitary production of gonadotrophins), primary ovary failure due to ovarian dysgenesis or menopause causing amenorrhea and infertility
Estradiol, serum (E₂, Beta 17 estradiol)	Follicular phase	30–120		
	Preovulation	150–350		**Evaluates** abnormal uterine bleeding and proliferative endometrium (see Fig. 15–1)
	Luteal phase	100–210		
	Postmenopausal	10–35		**Monitors** treatment to induce ovulation in subfertile women
	Pregnancy	Up to 35,000		**Evaluates** estrogen-producing tumors; estrogen hypersecretion in males
	Human Menopausal gonadotrophin (HMG) treatment	350–750		
				Assesses gynecomastia
	Adult Male (over 12 years)	10–35		
	Prepubertal Children	2–10		
Estriol, serum (E₃; Free estriol)	Estriol Range (ng/ml)		Free Estriol arises from the placenta primarily and depends on precursors from the fetal adrenal. First detected at 9 weeks gestation	A useful index of fetal and placental function as its continued production depends on a live fetus and functioning placenta
	Gestation (Weeks)			
	30	3.3–8.7	If serial samples are to be collected (which is recommended), they should be gathered at the same time each day because of diurnal variation. The estimated date of confinement (EDC) should be noted on the order form	**Decreased in:**
	31	3.3–10.8		• Fetal death with a sharp drop within 1–2 hours
	32	3.3–14.5		• Low levels with fetal adrenal hypoplasia and hydatidiform moles
	33	3.8–14.0		• Sudden decreases occur with maternal diabetes and hypertension
	34	5.0–15.0		• Drops of 4 mg/ml in last 6 mo of pregnancy strongly suggest fetal distress
	35	5.0–18.3		
	36	5.3–19.8		**Increased in:**
	37	5.7–24.1		• Twin gestation
	38	5.0–28.0		
	39	5.4–29.0		
	40	6.4–31.8		

500

Test	Reference Values	Patient Preparation	Clinical Significance
Estriol, urine (pregnancy urine for Estriol [E₃])	Depends on # of weeks of gestation Weeks mg/specimen 32–34 5–27 35–37 8–39 38–40 11–44 (Concentration of total estriol in the unknown [patient] sample is determined on a standard curve)	Note week of gestation and diabetes status on the order form. A 24-hr urine collection is required No other special patient preparation is necessary This is a competitive binding test using anti-estriol antibody Drugs interfering with the test include ampicillin and exogenous corticosteroids	Estriol is the primary urinary estrogen compound excreted during pregnancy **Decreased in:** • Fetal distress • Placental insufficiency • Fetal adrenal atrophy related to anencephaly with very low levels • Conditions of anemia, malnutrition, pylonephritis, intestinal disease or hemoglobinopathies of the mother **Increased in:** • Erythroblastosis fetalis, with the fetus in no apparent distress • Twin gestation
Estrogen fractionation (Estrogen by Brown's fractionation)	Total Estrogen (µg/24 specimen) Female 4–60 Male 4–24 Female only E¹ (Estrone) 2–25 E² (Estradiol) 0–10 E³ (Estriol) 2–30	A 24-hr urine collection No special patient preparation A quantitative test by spectrophotometric process	Levels rise and fall in conjunction with the menstrual cycle Estriol excretion is always equal to or greater than estrone. Estrodial always has the lowest excretion rate **Increased in:** • Pregnancy • Some ovarian and andrenocortical tumors **Decreased in:** • Menopause • End-organ failure

(continued)

TABLE 15–2. (Continued)

Name of Test	Normal Range		Comments	Purpose, Increases, Decreases
Serum progesterone (No synonyms)	Females	ng/ml	A direct assay of radio-labeled antibody binding and inhibition by an unlabeled antigen, counted by gamma counter	Used primarily to evaluate subfertile or infertile women (e.g., ovulation, oligoovulation, luteal phase defect)
	Prepubertal	0.10–0.34		Useful in first 12 weeks of pregnancy to detect and manage patients threatened with abortion, or those with a history of habitual spontaneous first trimester abortion
	Follicular	0.20–0.90	No special patient preparation	
	Luteal	3.0–36.0	Progesterone serves to maintain the female endometrium. It is produced by the ovary, placenta, and adrenals in the female and by the adrenals and testes in males	
	Pregnant	Up to 300		
	Postmenopausal	0.3–30.0		**Decreased levels occur in:**
	Males			• The absence of fertilization as the luteal phase ends
	Prepubertal	0.4–0.26	In women, progesterone has a cyclic pattern (see normal ranges) in conjunction with the luteinizing hormone cycle peaking half way through the luteal phase	• In many cases of adrenogenital syndrome
	Adult	0.12–0.31		
Testosterone Serum testosterone	Females	ng/dl	An RIA test with no special patient preparation	**Used to evaluate:**
	Males	25–100	Testosterone is produced by the testes in the male, controlled by pituitary FSH and LH, and by the ovary and adrenal gland in the female	• Premature and delayed puberty in males (e.g., Klinefelter's syndrome)
	Prepubertal males	300–800		• Differentiation of testicular tumors of males
		>100		• Hirsutism and virilization syndromes in females
				Increased in:
				• Polycystic ovary
				• Adrenogenital syndrome
				• Precocious maturity in males
				Decreased in:
				• Delayed puberty in males
				• Male hypogonadism due to primary pituitary failure in males (LH levels also decrease)
				• Some patients with cirrhosis

Testosterone battery (Total testosterone; free Testosterone and Testosterone binding protein ([TeBG])	Testosterone	ng/dl	Age and sex should be noted on the order form
	Male	350–1030	Specimen, if not immediately tested, should be frozen within 1 hr of collection
	Female	10–55	
	Free testosterone	(pg/ml)	Serum testosterone *may* be normal in hirsute females, probably because of elevated clearance rates and therefore can be misleading when measured alone
	Male	52–280	
	Female	1.1–6.3	
	TeBG	(ug/dl)	
	Male	0.9–1.9	
	Female	1.0–3.0	

The battery is used to evaluate androgenizing disorders causing virilization syndromes in women

Free testosterone:
- Decreased in patients receiving estrogen or glucocorticoid therapy
- Increased in androgenizing disorders

TeBG:
- Decreased in androgenizing disorders and adrenal problems
- Increased in hyperthyroid women and patients receiving estrogen

FSH, serum (follicle stimulating hormone)	Male	mIU/mll	An RIA test with no special patient preparation
		3–20	May be used with a hormonal stimulator (e.g., Clomiphene or gonadotropin-releasing factor)
	Female		This will increase FSH secretion in normal subjects, but not those with pituitary failure. Indicate on the request slip if stimulators have been given
	Follicular phase	3–20	
	Ovulatory peak	0–40	
	Luteal phase	2–40	FSH, with LH, stimulates Leydig cell production of testosterone and spermatogenesis in males. In females, FSH stimulates ovarian follicle maturation; LH supports the corpus luteum. FSH is produced by the ovaries and adrenal glands in females. Estrogen has a positive feedback effect on FSH and LH, and progesterone has a negative feedback
	Postmenopausal	40–200	
	Pediatric	Up to 12	

Helpful in diagnosis of pituitary failure and diagnosis of delayed puberty, testicular failure, primary precocious puberty due to disorders of the pituitary—gonadal axis

Increased in:
- Primary gonadal failure

Decreased in:
- Hypothalamic or pituitary failure

(continued)

TABLE 15–2. (Continued)

Name of Test	Normal Range		Comments	Purpose, Increases, Decreases
FSH, urine			FSH and LH are secreted in bursts so that single measurements vary widely (50% above or below the mean), therefore 3 samples are usually drawn 30 minutes apart and the samples pooled	This test is rarely, if ever, used and thought to be much inferior to the serum FSH test
Serum LH (luteinizing hormone)		mIU/mll	An RIA test with no special preparation necessary	Helpful in the diagnosis of pituitary failure
	Children (prepubertal)	0–4	Indicate on order form when high levels might be expected (as with stimulation tests such as clomiphene, a gonadotropin, or in the presence of a gonadotropin-producing neoplasm). Clomiphene increases secretion of FSH and LH in normal individuals, but not in pituitary failure	Increased, along with FSH in primary gonadal failure
	Adult			False increase occurs when high levels of HCG are present
	Male	0–12		Decreased, along with FSH, in hypothalamic or pituitary failure
	Female		Results of the test are equivocal when done on a person with increased HCG	
	Follicular	0–15		
	Ovulatory	0–17		
	Luteal	0–15		
	Postmenopausal	0–75		
Serum prolactin (PRL; lactogenic hormone; mammotropin)		ng/ml	An RIA test with no special preparation necessary	Helpful in diagnosis of hypothalamic tumors
	Adult		Prolactin production and release can be controlled by a hypothalamic inhibitory factor	**Increased in:**
	Female	1–15.8		• One third of pituitary tumors
	Male	0–12.2	There is a diurnal variation in prolactin levels with a 50% rise during sleep over levels while awake	• Some patients with amenorrhea (approximately 10%)
				• The majority of patients with amenorrhea and galactorrhea
				• Physiological conditions occurring in stress, pregnancy, and lactation
				• False elevations occur with the administration of estrogens, phenothiazines, and reserpine

Test	Normal range	Description	Clinical significance
hCG-beta subunit, quantitative (human chorionic gonadotropin assay; hCG assay; "pregnancy test")	Males and nonpregnant females: 0–5 mIU/ml	An RIA test using monoclonal antibody, in this case reporting the presence but not the amount of hCG in the blood. It is very sensitive, reporting levels as low as 1.5 mIU/ml of hCG, beta subunit. This test is not useful as a screening test for neoplasms, nor does it supply any information about tumor location, or specific tumor type. It does not cross-react with LH	Used primarily now as a "tumor marker" in sequential checks on hCG secretion from gestational neoplasms (e.g., hydatidiform moles, choriocarcinoma) as well as testicular and other types of neoplasms. Increase or decrease of serum levels are used as an indicator of patient response to treatment and evidence of residual hCG secreting tumor. **Increased in:** • Gestational trophoblastic neoplasms (see above) • Slight amounts in a small percentage of patients with gastric or duodenal ulcers; inflammatory bowel disease; and cirrhosis
Serum pregnancy test (early pregnancy detection test [EPT]; qualitative hCG-beta subunit; Biocept Pregnancy test; test for ectopic pregnancy; pregnancy test—RIA)	Normal Range: Negative (nonpregnant female) 0–5 mIU/ml; Positive (pregnant female) 26 or greater; Borderline Between 6 and 25	A qualitative monoclonal antibody test that provides measurement of intact hCG specific for the beta receptors. Because it is so specific, it does not cross react with other hormones (i.e., FSH, LH, TSH). It can be performed in approximately 2 hr and requires no special patient preparation. Neither hemolysis nor marked jaundice interfere with the test results. High serum lipids will require a careful interpretation of the test results. hCG is secreted by the trophoblast when the fertilized ovum is implanted and can be detected as early as 6 days after conception using this test. Levels continue to increase during the first trimester of pregnancy	This is the most frequently used test for pregnancy in laboratory settings. It is much more sensitive than the urine pregnancy tests based on the same general principle (see Section 15.1.1.A). Because of the high sensitivity it is used in the workup of ectopic and other aberrant pregnancies. **Increased in:** • Normal pregnancy • Trophoblastic disorders • hCG-producing tumors • Inflammatory bowel disease • Peptic and duodenal ulcer • Cirrhosis. Low elevations (less than expected for gestational stage) in ectopic pregnancy

Data from Lab. of Pathology, 1990; Henry, 1984; and Raven, 1984.

vated can be either of maternal or paternal origin, and all cells descending from that specific cell will have the same X inactivated. The presence of a Barr body is characteristic of the nuclei of cells in normal females; its lack is characteristic in normal males. The Barr body appears in certain sex chromosomal abnormalities. Presumptive diagnosis of these abnormalities can be made by comparison of the results of the buccal smear test with the individual's genitalia and secondary sex characteristics. The buccal smear test does not indicate true genetic sex; it only shows the number of female (X) chromosomes present. Confirmation of presumptive diagnoses can be done by chromosome karyotyping.

Special staining techniques of buccal cells are necessary to use the smear in defining gonosomal intersexuality (mixed gonadal dysgenesis) or Y chromosome abnormalities such as the XYY or "supermale" condition. Karyotyping is preferable and usually necessary in any case.

The Barr test can also be done on epithelial cells of vaginal smears, urinary sediment, or amniotic fluid. Any sex chromosomal abnormality can be diagnosed by amniocentesis at 15 to 16 weeks' gestation and karyotyping.

Note: Inaccurate reports of the Barr test can occur. Poor slide preparation or degenerating cells can cause false-negative reports. Artifacts such as bacteria can cause false-positive reports. Only 40 to 60 percent of normal female cells contain identifiable Barr bodies, so a sufficient number, usually at least 100, must be examined.

Patient Preparation

1. Buccal smears should not be done during the first week of life or during adrenal corticosteroid or estrogen treatment. False decreases in the incidence of Barr bodies occur
2. The outermost layer of epithelium does not demonstrate Barr bodies and must be removed before collecting the specimen. Specimen collection is probably best done by a cytotechnologist
3. Several slides should be prepared and must be immersed immediately after collection in fixative (Pap test fixative) because the Barr bodies fade rapidly when exposed to air

C.2 Semen Analysis

Synonym: Semen examination

Normal Ranges (complete test)

pH	7–8.5 (less than 7 abnormal)
Volume	1.5–5.0 ml (infertile males tend to have increased volume)
Count	60–150 million/ml (less than 20 million is abnormal)
Motility	60% motile at 3 hr 50% motile at 6 hr
Morphology	At least 70% of sperm normally formed
Microscopic	No RBC; none to occasional WBC; occasional to few cells; no crystals

Explanation of the Test. Usually a semen test is part of a thorough workup of both partners to investigate fertility, or it may be done to check the outcome of a vasectomy.

Patient Preparation

1. Varying periods of continence are suggested before sample collection (3 days or a period equal to the usual frequency of coitus for the couple)
2. Collection is most satisfactory if done as near as possible to the facility where it will be examined
3. Specimens must be kept at a constant body temperature after collection, with no extreme changes, until examined
4. The time of collection must be known and be accurate. After 2 hours the sample should not be used for full examination. Postvasectomy examinations (microscopic only) can be done on 2-hr specimens, but the fresher the sample, the more accurate the test result

C.3 Serum Alkaline Phosphatase

See Section 1.12.1 for more detailed information on this test. Marked elevations of heat-stable alkaline phosphatase occur in the third trimester of pregnancy. Used as a placental function test in the past, it is no longer used as a test in pregnancy. Plasma and urinary estriol measurements have replaced it. It may be found to be a useful tumor "marker" in the future.

C.4 Pregnancy-Associated Plasma Proteins, Serum

Alpha- and beta-globulins appearing with a specificity comparable to hCG are now called pregnancy-associated plasma proteins (PAPP). Clinical values have not yet been established, but in time it might be expected that these proteins will be used to diagnose first-trimester pregnancy and evaluate placental function (Henry, 1984).

RELATED NURSING DIAGNOSES

Despite the disparity of body functions linked to the various endocrine glands, patients with endocrine dysfunctions share a remarkable number of actual or potential nursing diagnoses in common.

The following listing is submitted as a tool for primary nursing assessment of the patient with suspected or diagnosed endocrine dysfunction. Representative data from five of the most common endocrine disorders are presented with each of the nursing diagnoses selected as being the most likely to be common problems with all endocrine patients.

Activity Intolerance Related to Inadequate Rest, Sleep, or Exercise

1. Hyperthyroidism secondary to decreased metabolic and arousal rate, anemia, and hypotonia of muscles (hypothyroidism)
2. Hyperthyroidism secondary to physical exhaustion due to increased metabolic rate and inability to replace nutritional stores by ordinary food intake, which is accompanied by weight loss, loss of muscle mass, weakness, rapid fatigue, and an increased response to sensory stimuli.
3. Hypercortisolism—Cushing's disease or syndrome—secondary to protein tissue wasting, loss of muscle mass, hypokalemia, and a disturbance in sleep patterns related to the elevated concentration of circulating cortisol
4. Hypocortisolism and hypoaldosteronism—Addison's Disease—secondary to hyponatremia, hyperkalemia, dehydration, and hypoglycemia
5. (Hyperglycemia—diabetes mellitus—Secondary to potential or actual fluid and electrolyte imbalances, e.g., hyperkalemia, hypovolemia due to osmotic diuresis; acid-base imbalance, (i.e., metabolic acidosis (noncarbonic acidosis); and intracellular hypoglycemia due to lack of insulin

Potential or Actual Disturbance in Self-Concept Related to Alterations in Body Image/Self-esteem and Role Performance Secondary to

1. Hypothyroidism: Mucosaccharide deposits causing thickening or dulling of facial characteristics; dry brittle hair, male hair pattern in females, premature greying; presence of goiter (rare); decreased mental acuity, weight gain due to decreased metabolic activity and poor food selection (high caloric, easily digested foods); decreased or absent libido
2. Hyperthyroidism: Awareness of decreased emotional control due to increased sensitivity to environmental and physical stimuli; negative body changes, e.g., severe weight loss, exophthalmos (limited), increased oil production of hair follicles and skin with acne; inability to concentrate
3. Hypocortisolism: Physical weakness and lethargy; pigmentation changes
4. Hypercortisolism: Alterations in fat and water distribution, effects of virilism (skin and hair changes), and mood swings
5. Hyperglycemia: Adaptation to chronic illness as change in self-image, alteration in daily schedule for self-care and body monitoring, consideration of possible complications and their effects on quality of life

Potential for Injury (Falls, Trauma, Infection, or Bleeding) Related to

1. Hypothyroidism: Decreased nutritional status with weakness and hypotension (see diagnosis, decreased skin integrity due to dry skin and decreased peripheral circulation, decreased phagocytic activity of leukocytes (cause?), potential for arrhythmias because of potassium imbalance
2. Hyperthyroidism: Physical weakness (see first Diagnosis, Activity, Intolerance), elevated blood pressure, potential for cardiac arrhythmias because of potassium imbalance, decreased attention span and hyperactivity
3. Hypocortisolism: Postural hypotension due to hyponatremia/fluid loss; potential for addisonian crisis
4. Hypercortisolism: Weakness due to loss of muscle mass and potential for fractures due to decreased calcium storage in bones and demineralization, potential for cardiac arrhythmias because of potassium imbalance, potential for bleeding due to stress/ulcer formation, decreased effectiveness of leukocytes, decreased effectiveness of skin barrier due to thinning
5. Hyperglycemia: Blood pressure instability due to possible sudden fluid loss with hyperglycemia, decreased sensation (balance, pain, pressure) in lower extremities due to diabetic neuropathy, possible visual impairment (blurring with hyperglycemia, retinal damage long term or cataracts), decreased effective bacterial resistence due to high blood glucose levels

Lack of Knowledge Related to

1. Hypothyroidism: Reversibility of physical changes with treatment over time; time frame for changes; lifelong hormone replacement, expected effects, side effects to be monitored or reported
2. Hyperthyroidism: Disease process, e.g., reversibility of physical changes with treatment over time; time frame for changes; medication; antithyroid, side effects to be noted or reported; preparation for surgical treatment if needed, risks versus benefits; self-care postsurgery (hormone replacement)
3. Hypocortisolism: Purpose and effect of support or replacement hormones, how administered, monitoring or reporting changes and/or side effects
4. Hypercortisolism: Treatment options (depending on cause); monitoring and reporting possible secondary or side effects of decreasing hormone levels as well as signs and symptoms of complications due to increased levels (e.g., hypertension, peptic ulcer disease, bone fractures)
5. Diabetes: Disease process, complications, prevention of complications, self-care procedures (body monitoring, foot care, insulin or hypoglycemic medication administration, testing for glucose, diet and exercise management)

SIXTEEN

TESTS TO MONITOR CANCER
TUMOR MARKERS

INTRODUCTION

This chapter focuses on the use of "tumor markers" primarily in use at present to monitor therapy in some cancers. Other body substances alter in the presence of cancer but are not referred to as tumor markers. For example, lactate dehydrogenase (LD/LDH) is always found in human serum at a given level. Isoenzyme $LD_{2,3}$ will increase in malignancy, but the increase is believed to be secondary to the disorganized cancer growth rate and perhaps oxygen-supply imbalance, not as an element of malignant transformation. Its rise is highly nonspecific (Henry, 1991, p. 293; McCance & Huether, 1990, pp. 298-9,).

Tumor markers, or potential tumor markers, can be defined as a broad category of substances produced by both malignant and benign cells, the benign cells responding to the presence of malignant cells. The markers include hormones, enzymes, and antigens found in body fluids and tissue specimens (or tissue extracts). Tissue section staining (histochemical stains) for tumor markers may provide information about the origin of the tumor, the cell type from which it is derived, from which it is different, and/or the degree of that difference. In short, markers offer data on where the tumor started, which cell type at that site is involved, whether it differs from the original cell, and how much. Other markers indicate the presence and/or amount of antibody (Henry, 1991, p. 285). Only those tests fairly frequently used at present are included here.

There are multiple uses for tumor markers, and not all markers do the same thing. They can detect, identify, monitor, radiolocalize (define), and even treat malignancy. They are extremely useful in laboratory work, primarily for detection, identification, and monitoring. Laboratory testing with tumor markers can help confirm the presence of suspected malignancy and identify what kind of malignancy it is so that appropriate, optimum treatment can be given. This identification can include information about the prognosis and whether the cancer is at a treatable stage. Tumor markers are also used to monitor the disease course of confirmed malignancies (Henry, 1991).

To date, none of the identified tumor markers have been found suitable for malignancy screening in the general population. They have not been sensitive enough in *early* disease to allow detection when the course of the malignancy might be altered (McCance & Huether, 1990, pp. 298–301). Most tumor markers identified to date lack specificity for cancer, showing elevations in more common benign disorders as well. Both sensitivity and specificity do tend to increase in later cancer stages, providing accurate diagnosis. Unfortunately, at present, detection at that time rarely favorably alters the course of the disease (Henry, 1991, p. 285).

TABLE 16–1. AMERICAN CANCER SOCIETY RECOMMENDATIONS FOR THE EARLY DETECTION OF CANCER IN ASYMPTOMATIC PEOPLE.

Test or Procedure	Sex	Age	Frequency
Sigmoidoscopy, preferably flexible	M & F	50 and over	Every 3–5 yr
Fecal occult blood test	M & F	50 and over	Every yr
Digital rectal examination	M & F	40 and over	Every yr
Prostate exam[a]	M	50 and over	Every yr
Pap test	F	All women who are or who have been sexually active, or have reached age 18, should have an annual Pap test and pelvic examination. After a woman has had three or more consecutive satisfactory normal annual examinations, the Pap test may be performed less frequently at the discretion of her physician.	
Pelvic examination	F	18–40 Over 40	Every 1–3 yr with Pap test every yr
Endometrial tissue sample	F	All menopause, if at high risk[b]	At menopause and thereafter at the discretion of the physician
Breast self-examination	F	20 and over	Every month
Breast clinical examination	F	20–40 Over 40	Every 3 yr Every yr
Mammography[c]	F	40–49 50 and over	Every 1–2 yr Every yr
Health counseling and cancer checkup[d]	M & F M & F	Over 20 Over 40	Every 3 yr Every yr

[a]Annual digital rectal examination and prostate specific antigen testing should be performed on men age 50 and older. If either is abnormal, further evaluation should be considered.
[b]History of infertility, obesity, failure to ovulate, abnormal uterine bleeding, or unopposed estrogen or tamoxifen therapy.
[c]Screening mammography should begin by age 40.
[d]To include examination for cancers of the thyroid, testicles, ovaries, lymph nodes, oral region, and skin.

Table 16–1 provides a more overall view of tests useful in *early* detection of cancer in the asymptomatic patient. Some overlap with tests indicated as tumor markers in this chapter is evident and usually relates to their use in different stages of the malignancy, underscoring the need for constant review and updating of tests and their uses (Mettlin et al., 1993, p. 42).

16.1 CARCINOEMBRYONIC ANTIGEN TEST

Synonym: CEA, plasma

Normal Ranges (ng/dl)[a]

Nonsmoker	0–3
Smoker	0–5

[a]Levels suggestive of tumor: greater than upper normal range (Laboratory of Pathology, 1991) or 25.3 ng/ml (Torosian, 1992, p. 26)—varies among laboratories.

Definition. Carcinoembryonic antigen test (CEA), a venous plasma test, is based on the presence of tumor-specific antigens (glycoproteins) on the surface of tumor cells. The test is a radioimmunoassay (RIA) using antibodies that have been developed to react with extracted CEA (embryonic tissue). It is no longer used as a screening test for cancer per se, nor is it specific for one type of cancer. Furthermore, it is not considered to be the sole criterion for cancer diagnosis because the findings in CEA levels overlap in both cancerous and noncancerous conditions (Laboratory of Pathology, 1991). It has been found useful as a tumor marker for metastatic meningeal cancer (Henry, 1991, p. 455). Its primary present use is in testing for recurrence of treated cancers.

Physiology. CEA usually appears during the first or second trimester of fetal life, decreasing before birth (embryonic tissue is fast growing). It may normally be present throughout life in very small amounts (see normal ranges), circulated by the lymphatic and vascular systems. CEA is a glycoprotein polysaccharide secreted by surface mucosal cells, primarily those lining the gastrointestinal (GI) tract but also from other sites such as the pancreas and liver.

Benign conditions causing transient CEA elevations include (in decreasing order of occurrence): benign prostatic hypertrophy; bronchitis; colonic polyps; diverticulitis; gastritis; hepatocellular obstructive biliary disease; inflammatory bowel disease; and renal disease (Torosian, 1992, p. 26).

Pathophysiology. The most frequent (though not only) morbid pathology causing increased CEA levels is cancer of any one of several organs (see "Physiology") secondary to disruption of mucosal cells by cellular proliferation, causing basement membrane damage. CEA is released into underlying connective tissue and absorbed by the lymphatic or vascular system. Patients with small or early tumors often test negative. Tumors testing at levels greater than 10 ng/ml are felt to imply a worse prognosis. A normal CEA does *not* exclude even far advanced tumors, nor do high CEA titers mean a cancer is so far advanced that it cannot be resected successfully (Laboratory of Pathology, 1991). High titers can be considered reasonable, if not conclusive evidence, against *early* stage tumors.

A negative response is possible in the presence of cancer, as well as a positive response in the absence of cancer (McIntosh, 1992, p. 49). Combination monitoring of colorectal cancer with CEA *and* a tumor-associated glycoprotein called TAG72 that has been able to pick up as much as 91 percent of *recurrent* disease is under study at this time. The combination of the two tests appears most important. CEA alone detected only 20%; TAG72 alone detected only 42 percent of primary and recurrent disease. Combined they picked up over 56 percent (Fry et al., 1989, p. 31).

CEA INCREASED TITERS IN:

1. Many types of cancer: 70 percent of colon (colorectal) cancer—those cancers that have penetrated the bowel wall; 90 percent of pancreatic cancer; 30 percent of breast cancer
2. Many tumor recurrences
3. Presence of metastasis
4. Pregnant women
5. Some benign disorders, usually those with tissue inflammation or obstruction (Ravel, 1989, p. 588):
   a. Heavy cigarette smokers (McCance & Huether, 1990, p. 339)
   b. Benign liver disease (Conn, 1991, p. 713)
6. Pleural effusion fluid secondary to various malignancies (not a consistent finding) (Ravel, 1989, p. 588)

CEA DECREASED OR ABSENT TITERS IN:

1. Healthy individuals
2. Newborns
3. Early stage tumor (one that has not penetrated the bowel wall) (Fry et al., 1989, p. 16)

IMPLICATIONS FOR NURSING

1. No patient preparation is required for the test itself, other than the usual preparation of the patient for venipuncture. The test can be done on blood serum or plasma, but plasma is preferred (Fry et al., 1989, p. 16)
2. Inform the patient about when to expect test results, usually 3 to 5 days
3. Because the test is frequently used to monitor the level of CEA of known cancer patients before and after therapy, the nurse will need to validate the meaning of the outcomes prior to answering the client's questions related to those findings
4. Assess the patient's anxiety level, and reinforce information about the test findings based on her or his ability to understand or accept the meaning of the results
5. Understanding the meaning of the "staging" often done with the initial test will be helpful in support-ing the client. Unlike other solid tumors, the *size* of the primary cancer does not seem to be an indi-cator of prognosis in colon cancer, rather staging is based on:
   a. Extent of penetration into the bowel wall
   b. Regional lymph node involvement
   c. Presence of distant metastases
      Dukes's Classification System (Modified)
      Stage A   Tumor confined to bowel wall
      Stage B   Tumor penetrates bowel; invades pericolonic or perirectal tissue; no lymph node metastases
      Stage C   Metastases in regional lymph nodes
      Stage D   Peritoneal "seeding," omental implant, or liver metastases beyond the limits of sur-gical resection (Fry et al., 1989, p. 16)

16.2 SERUM ACID PHOSPHOTASE (BIOCHEMICAL)

Synonyms: SAP; prostatic acid phosphotase (ACP/PAP)

Normal Range

Males   1.4–4.8 u/L[a]

---

[a]Only normal values for males are listed here as the test is used almost exclusively for evaluation of changes in *prostatic* acid phosphotase.

Definition. The acid phosphotase (SAP or PAP) test is primarily used to monitor levels of acid phosphotase in the serum of men having been diagnosed with and under treatment for prostatic cancer in order to evaluate response to therapy. This biochemical assay produces an estimated level of acid phosphotase rather than directly measuring it. The level is determined by the amount of change occurring in a specific measurement of substrate (a substance that can be changed by the action of the enzyme) (Ravel, 1989).

Physiology. Acid phosphotase consists of a group of closely related enzymes sharing certain bio-chemical characteristics (Ravel, 1989), specifically the ability to hydrolyze phosphate esters in an acid pH environment (Lab. of Pathology, 1991). These enzymes are found in all body tissues

TABLE 16–2. PROSTATE CANCER STAGING

Stage A_0	Normal rectal examination. Surgery for presumed benign disease
A_1	Three or fewer cancer positive chips after transurethral resection of prostate for presumed benign disease and:
	• Involvement of <5% of total prostate volume
	• Tumor is well differentiated
A_2	Involves >5% of total prostrate volume
	• Any grade of tumor other than well differentiated
	• Can be associated with lymph node metastases
Stage B	Detectable by rectal exam
B_1	From 1.5 to 2 cm in diameter
B_2	Larger than 2 cm in diameter
Stage C_0	Extension outside prostate gland, but no distant metastases
C_1	Minimal extension
C_2	Extension may involve the seminal vesicle or ureters
Stage D	Associated with distant metastases
D_0	Tumor clinically located with normal bone scan
D_1	Involvement of local lymph nodes
D_2	Distant nodal involvement (outside the pelvis). May be visceral or in bone
D_3	Disease progresses after appropriate hormonal therapy

Data from Conn, 1991.

and fluids but with much higher, more concentrated amounts in prostatic tissues, erythrocytes (erythrocyte phosphotase), platelets, and leukocytes (Laboratory of Pathology, 1991). Lesser amounts are found in the liver and spleen. Females as a group, because of the lack of the prostatic enzyme, also have lower levels. The two major enzyme producers in humans are the prostate and red blood cells (RBCs) (Diagnostics, pp. 116–117, 1986).

Pathophysiology. In carcinoma of the prostate, prostatic tissue cells multiply. When cellular metastasis occurs, the level of PAP increases in the serum. Rarely is the alkaline phosphotase level increased when the cancer is contained within the prostate. The more widespread the metastasis, the greater the likelihood of high SAP levels (Diagnostics, 1986) because the tumor cells retain the ability to produce the enzyme.

POSITIVE INCREASES IN:

• Five to ten percent of tests on men with known prostatic cancer

FALSE-POSITIVE INCREASES IN:

1. Infarcts—temporary increase
2. Benign prostatic hyperplasia (BPH) without evidence of cancer (0–19 percent)
3. Nonprostatic cancer with metastasis to the bone
4. Certain metabolic disease (e.g., Paget's disease; primary hyperthyroidism)
5. Gaucher's disease
6. Some platelet disorders; thrombocytosis; platelet destruction (Ravel, 1989)
7. Rarely with increased alkaline phosphotase activity (Lab. of Pathology, 1991)
8. Samples collected following rectal examination (Ravel, 1986)

FALSE-NEGATIVE REACTIONS IN:

- Tests done on serum left at room temperature for as little as 1 hour after exposure to air

---

IMPLICATIONS FOR NURSING

1. Make sure that the blood sample taken for this test is not exposed to air. In many labs the sample will also be frozen as soon as possible. Check out the protocol operating in the facility doing the test
2. Only serum is used for testing. Plasma cannot be used because of false positives occurring related to the presence of RBCs (RBC acid phosphotase)
3. See also Implications for Nursing with serum acid phosphotase (Multisystem Screening Tests, Chapter 1, Section 1.12.1)

16.3 PROSTATE SPECIFIC ANTIGEN (SERUM)

Synonyms: PSA; PA; PSA-RIA

Normal Ranges

Males	0–2.5 ng/ml (Laboratory of Pathology, 1991)
	<4 ng/dl (Fracchia, 1992, p. 28)
Range for detection of local disease	4–10 ng/mL (Crawford, 1992, p. 57)
Poor prognostic sign	>10 µg/L (Catalona, Nov. 1991, p. 139)[a]

[a]Upper limits of normal vary with specific testing material: monoclonal PSA (m-PSA) = 4.0 ng/ml; polyclonal PSA (p-PSA) = 2.5 ng/ml (Littrup, June 1992, p. 38).

Definition. Prostate specific antigen (PSA) is glycoprotein used as a serum and tissue marker of prostatic adenocarcinoma. The test is an immunoassay that has great specificity for prostatic tissue (Henry, 1991, p. 292). Prostate cancer is the second most prevalent cancer and the third most common cause of cancer deaths of men in the United States. PSA has been found to be significantly related to disease progression risk after treatment and closely related to length of patient survival after treatment (Lab. of Pathology, 1991).

Physiology. PSA is a highly immunogenic glycoprotein (a serine protease) produced exclusively in the prostate glands' tissues (the epithelial cells of the prostate acini and ducts) and found in its fluid and seminal plasma. It is present normally in low concentrations in the sera of well males. Because it is found exclusively in the one tissue and very sensitive to testing, it is a useful biological "marker" specific to the prostate (Catalona, 1991, p. 139; Crawford, 1992, pp. 57–58; McIntosh, 1992, pp. 49–50). It is, therefore, a very valuable instrument for monitoring results of therapy as well as for indicating disease recurrence (McIntosh, 1992, p. 49).

Pathophysiology. PSA testing is presently used to follow up on treatment of prostatic cancer and to support its diagnosis, rather than as a screening test. Its presence is not unique to cancer. For example, it can be found in many instances of benign prostatic hypertrophy (10–20 percent) (Crawford, 1992, p. 57). PSA levels elevate approximately 0.3 ng/ml per gram of benign prostatic hypertrophy tissue compared to 3.0 ng/ml per gram of cancer (Littrup, 1992, p. 38). However, the combination of digital rectal examination (DRE) and PSA is believed by some to offer the best detection rate for prostatic cancer at present (Crawford, 1992, p. 58). Others see promise of increased positive, predictive/detective rates of prostatic cancer when PSA is combined with transrectal ultrasound (TRUS) (Littrup, 1992, p. 38). The PSA test alone does not distinguish between indolent and fast-growing cancer (Kritz, 1992, p. 28), and some researchers believe that PSA testing in men over 50 is questionable for this reason (Crawford, 1992, p. 57). The test has been found to be twice as accurate as DRE alone. It is very useful and therefore widely used as a detector of residual or recurrent disease in patients after a radical prostatic resection (Crawford, 1992, p. 57).

At least one group of researchers suggests PSA testing over a period of 5 to 10 years showing an average rate of increase of 0.75 ug/1 or greater per year as a criterion for detecting prostate cancer. In their research only 10 percent of the group studied were misclassified, a specificity of 90 percent. Those misclassified had BPH (Carter et al., 1992, pp. 105–06).

PSA LEVELS INCREASED (MODERATE TO HIGH CONCENTRATIONS) IN:

1. Prostatic cancer (to include individuals in stage A disease) (Laboratory of Pathology, 1991). (See Table 16–2, "Prostate Cancer Staging")
2. Benign prostatic hypertrophy
3. Following DRE
4. Persistent elevation after radical prostatectomy indicates residual tumor (Fracchia, 1992, p. 28)

PSA ABSENT IN:

- All females (normal finding)

PSA LEVELS DECREASED OR ABSENT IN:

- After successful radical prostatectomy (near or to 0 ng/ml or dl)

IMPLICATIONS FOR NURSING

Patient/family teaching:
1. Provide information about prostatic cancer as needed and applicable to the case:
   a. Nineteen percent of all cancers in men are found in prostate
   b. Eighty percent or more of diagnosed prostatic cancers are already metastastatic (perhaps because testing had not been done routinely)
   c. Prostatic cancer is slow growing
   d. U.S. incidence: Approximately 86,000 new cases diagnosed each year with a higher incidence in married and black men. Rarely found in men under 60 years of age
   e. Approximately 25,000 deaths due to prostate cancer occur yearly (Lewis & Collier, 1992, p. 1458)
2. Explain as needed:
   a. The importance of preventative actions that can and should be taken for early discovery, when treatment is more readily effective
   b. Awareness of symptoms that may indicate the disease, such as changes in urinary flow: frequency, hematuria, hesitancy, nocturia, retention, urgency
   c. Yearly checkups to include direct rectal examination (DRE) with PSA and prostatic acid phosphotase (PAP) testing and/or ultrasonography with a needle biopsy to better examine prostatic cell status
   d. Explain briefly what each of the tests accomplish to help in early diagnosis of both prostatic cancer or benign prostatic hypertrophy

16.4 ALPHA-FETOPROTEIN (SERUM) TEST: TUMOR MARKER RADIOIMMUNOASSAY

Synonyms: AFP; A-fetoprotein; alpha-1-fetoprotein

Normal Range

Nonpregnant adult	0–25 IU/ml (Lab. of Pathology, 1991)
	<25/ng/ml (Burrell, 1992, p. 1758)

Definition. Alpha-fetoprotein (AFP), an oncofetal antigen, is normally produced by the fetal liver, and low levels continue to be produced up until age 1 year (see 15.1.5.E). A similar protein is produced in the adult primarily as a result of the development of specific carcinomas (Ravel, 1989, p. 309) The test is used to (not in order of use):

1. Assist in making a diagnosis of cancer by the amount of tumor marker present. (Most common tumor sites include: liver, ovaries, testes) (McCance & Huether, 1990, p. 300)
2. Determine metastatic spread of tumors
3. Monitor the effectiveness of treatment (primary test use)
4. Stage tumor (Burrell, 1992, p. 1758)
5. Check for recurrence after surgical removal

Pathophysiology. Both testicular cancer and hepatoma are believed to produce AFP (Burrell, 1992, p. 50). Cancer cells contain proteins not present in normal cells. These proteins are called *tumor-specific antigens* (TSA). When inserted into the cell membrane of a normal cell a cytotoxic immune response occurs. Because cancer cells reproduce so rapidly, this immune response is inadequate to deal with tumor growth. AFP enters the vascular system when a malignancy occurs. The amount of AFP is regulated by genes in the tumor cells (Burrell, 1992, p. 1758).

AFP LEVELS INCREASED IN:

1. Liver cancer: May be a marked increase (>400 ng/ml) in primary liver cancer) (McCance & Huether, 1990, p. 1260)
2. Testicular cancer (gonadal cancer)
3. Hepatitis (Burrell, 1992, p. 1738), one of the few nonneoplastic disorders to cause AFP increases (McCance & Huether, 1990, p. 339). (Excessively high levels have been correlated with Hepatitis B antigen, rapid tumor growth, and poor tumor differentiation) (ibid, 1260)
4. Liver cirrhosis, alcohol related (small transient increases)
5. Pancreatic cancer (McCance & Huether, 1990)

IMPLICATIONS FOR NURSING: TESTICULAR CANCER

1. The nurse needs to be as completely informed as possible about the best estimate of prognosis; the type of tumor involved; treatment planned or already carried out; what the tumor stage is; the

meaning the diagnosis and planned or completed treatment has to the individual and his wife or significant other in order to intelligently respond to questions and concerns

2. The most frequent treatment is surgical; preferably a radical inguinal orchiectomy regardless of cell type or staging. The nurse needs to know the rationale for radical surgery, which can be any of or a combination of the following:
   a. Virtual 100 percent effective control of local disease
   b. A necessary approach when histologic diagnosis and extent of the disease are difficult or impossible to determine prior to surgery
   c. If the cancer is confined to the testes, the treatment affords a cure
   d. Risk of complications or side effects is minimal
   e. Surgical mortality is virtually nil
3. If cancer is only suspected, treatment may be confined to a radical inguinal orchiectomy plus a high ligation of the spermatic cord. (A bilateral orchiectomy may be done in these cases because of the great incidence of cancer appearing in the presently unaffected testis)
4. Radiation or chemotherapy may be the procedure of choice when surgery is not feasible or if intraabdominal masses are present and inoperable. Its use as an adjunct to surgery has become less desirable over time.
5. With the removal of only one testis and a desire to maintain fertility, the client and wife or significant other need to know that removal of lymph nodes in the area (iliac and lumbar) can cause sympathetic nerve damage, which, in turn, can cause retrograde ejaculation (due to failure of the bladder opening to close) with semen backflow into the bladder. This precludes seminal ejaculation during intercourse. If conception is the goal, artificial insemination is possible, but results are poor
6. Periodic follow-ups with CT scans or other tests to check for recurrence and/or metastasis are extremely important
7. Testicular biopsy is contraindicated because of the expected risk of tumor spread
8. Adjuncts to surgical treatment include radiation or chemotherapy. The chemotherapy cure is believed to exceed 70 percent (Burrell, 1972, pp. 1780–81)

16.5 PAPANICOLAOU SMEAR

Synonyms: Pap smear; cervical smear; gynecological smear; vaginal smear

Normal Findings

Normal appearing cells; no malignant or abnormal cells

Definition. A study of the structure and function of cells from the cervical or vaginal lining, the test is done to detect cells that are undergoing change (Burrell, 1992, p. 1681) or to monitor possible pathology indicated in previous testing.

Findings. If a Pap smear is suggestive of a malignancy, a biopsy is usually done to confirm the diagnosis and to determine the extent and characteristics of the malignancy (Ravel, 1989, p. 577). The findings are reported in several different ways, two of which are given here:

Grading	Grade I	Normal appearing cells
	Grade II	Atypical cytology with evidence of malignancy
	Grade III	Inconclusive with suggestion of malignancy
	Grade IV	Strongly suggestive of malignancy
	Grade V	Conclusive of malignancy

Or   Normal
            Inflammatory
            Mild cervical intraepithelial neoplasm (CIN)
            Severe CIN cancer (Burrell, 1992)

Process. A Pap smear, done during a vaginal examination, can be performed in a multitude of ways, and the detection ability of the processes vary considerably, as do the reports of those abilities in the literature. According to Ravel (1989, pp. 576–77), the detective abilities of the different methods are:

Test	Device	Detection (%)
Biopsy	Vibra aspiratory	80–100%
	Novak suction curette	77–94
Cytology	Isaac's cell sampler	98–100
Lavage	Gravlee cell wash	78–100
Mechanical Cell	Mimark endopap	less than 90
Dislodgement	Endometrial brush	57–92
Smears from vaginal pool		18–90
Specimens from the cervix		25–55

Cervical cancer is uncommon in women who have never been sexually active. Cancer incidence rises markedly with a history of early sexual intercourse, multiple sexual partners, frequent sexually transmitted diseases and, most recently determined, with sexual transmission of human papillomavirus (HPV). HPV subtypes (determined by DNA typing) most likely to progress to dysplastic or invasive carcinomas are:

1. HPV types 6 and 11: Causing condylomas and low-grade dysplasias
2. HPV types 16 and 18: Commonly associated with lesions that evolve to high-grade dysplasias and invasive cervical malignancy

HPV produces morphological changes that may be interpreted on the Pap smear (Larson et al., 1992, p. 31).

IMPLICATIONS FOR NURSING:

1. History gathering is essential and usually includes:
   a. Whether the patient is pregnant (if so, use of the "brush" is contraindicated)
   b. Date of last menstrual period (cellular change can be anticipated); if the patient is menstruating, the test is not usually performed
   c. Use of intravaginal device (IVD)
   d. History of clinical cancer, especially of reproductive organs
   e. History or present use of hormone treatment
   f. History of menstruation: regularity, duration, degree of discomfort
   g. History of vaginal pain, itching, exudate
   h. Personal and/or family history of gynecological disorders
   i. Medical history (Laboratory of Pathology, 1991)

2. Client instruction (may or may not be nursing duty, but essential that it be done):
   a. No intercourse, douches, or vaginally inserted medications for at least 24 hours prior to the test because of loss of cellular deposits and changes in vaginal pH that will affect test outcomes
   b. A lubricant will not be used with the vaginal speculum, but it may be dipped in sterile water before use. Review relaxation techniques with client prior to the speculum insertion
   c. The procedure is not unlike a routine vaginal examination
   d. Probable maximum time for the procedure 20 minutes to 1/2 hour, assuming inclusion of a bimanual examination as well as visual examination and sample collection
   e. Have the client empty her bladder just prior to the examination
3. All samples collected must be labeled correctly, depending on the requirements of the laboratory doing the study. Labels usually require the patient's name, age, date of last menstrual period, collection site(s), and method. Any slides must be preserved *immediately*. Check the technique for the institution in which the test is being done. (Usually the slides are either sprayed with a commercial fixative or placed in a fixative solution)
4. There are usually no posttest restrictions (Kayes, 1986, pp. 696–99; Laboratory of Pathology, 1991)

16.6 hCG-BETA SUBUNIT, QUANTITATIVE (SERUM)

Synonym: Human chorionic gonadotropin B-subunit, quantitative

Normal Findings

Males, nonpregnant females	0–5 mIU/ml
Pregnant females	2–25 IU/L (1–2 wk postconception)

Definition. This is a very sensitive test (a fluorometric enzyme immunoassay) that is highly specific for hCG, having almost no cross-reactivity with luteinizing hormone. It is particularly useful as it can detect low quantities of hCG in serum. It is used as a tumor marker in following up on the status of certain kinds of cancer (choriocarcinoma; testicular neoplasm). In testing for these cancers, hCG increases or decreases indicate response—or lack of response—to therapy (Laboratory of Pathology, 1991). It is also useful in determining abortions, missed abortions, and ectopic pregnancies (Henry, 1991, pp. 478–479). (See also 15.2.3 Tests for Risk Populations; hCG Pregnancy Test.)

Physiology. Being a glycoprotein hormone, hCG has two subunits (A and B) that differ in composition, although they are structurally similar. hCG's biological and immunologic specificity is conferred by the beta unit.

Some tumors produce "ectopic hormones," a term used to describe the production of hormones by tumors of nonendocrine origin (McCance & Huether, 1990, p. 299). hCG is one of these hormones, acting as an indicator of cancer activity. Ectopic pregnancy and abortion may cause an increase in hCG levels at the same rate as in normal pregnancy, up to a certain point.

In ectopic pregnancy that point is usually less than 4 to 6 weeks, at which time the hCG levels plateau or begin to decrease (Tietz, 1990, pp. 126, 130–131). With abortion of the fetus, hCG usually decreases, or the expected increase slows considerably.

These patterns are not absolutes and may vary considerably. Findings in this test are not useful to screen for cancer in the absence of known disease, nor does the test inform about tumor location or tumor type (Laboratory of Pathology, 1991).

LEVELS INCREASED IN:

Normal pregnancy
Gestational trophoblastic neoplasms
   a. Choriocarcinoma
   b. Hydatidiform moles
   c. Testicular neoplasms

LEVELS STATIC OR DECREASED IN:

   1. Ectopic pregnancy
   2. Threatened, incomplete, or complete abortion

IMPLICATIONS FOR NURSING:

Because the conditions that will exist to require the use of this test tend to focus on the potential of death for the patient or fetus, nursing actions are best centered on providing psychological support, while also focusing on physical comfort.

   Some suggestions for maintaining both kinds of comfort—other than providing medication for pain in a timely manner—include:
1. Be honest in answering questions or giving information. Do not provide answers using unexplained medical terminology.
2. Provide factual information about the fetus, or patient's status openly and honestly and at a time when he or she needs or wants to know.
3. Help the patient or family to deal with the impact of the situation by helping them to determine those things with which they are able to cope and those with which they are not.
4. Make continued human contact available and rewarding (e.g., arrange for the presence of family or friends the patient expresses a desire to see, and tactfully deter the presence of those who look to the patient for their support.)
5. Assist the patient to get adequate comfort and rest by administering pain medication and physical care in a timely and understanding way
6. Encourage, rather than discourage, joking and laughter with the patient

---

Part

IV

DIAGNOSTIC IMAGING

The term *diagnostic modalities* in this text is meant to exclude those diagnostic tests that are performed in the clinical laboratory on *samples* from the patient. Instead, diagnostic modalities refer to tests requiring the presence of the person being examined during the testing procedure. The testing modalities discussed in this section are not totally inclusive of all such tests. In particular, electrocardiography, endoscopy, and pulmonary function testing are excluded. They were seen to require more extensive detail for clarity and adequate understanding than did the other testing modalities. To include the topics and exclude the detail would be a great disservice to the reader. To include the detail would require almost a book in itself. Because there are excellent texts available on each subject, the categories are not included here.

INTRODUCTION

This section of the book begins with one of the oldest and best known diagnostic tools, the x-ray, and ends with the newer modalities, such as magnetic resonance imaging (MR or MRI), computerized positron emission tomography (PET), and single photon emission computed tomography (SPECT).

The focus of this section is on understanding the purpose and process of testing using imaging modalities, and on conveying that information to the client (teaching and learning). Less stress is placed on cellular physiology and pathophysiology as specific structural or functional change is the major focus for most diagnostic testing, with the probable exception of MRI, PET, and SPECT testing.

Test findings generally provide a medical diagnosis rather than a nursing diagnosis. Therefore, nursing implications focus on how to prepare the client for a successful and safe test, with a minimum of anxiety and a maximum of knowledge about the purpose and process of the test itself.

The nursing role related to diagnostic testing is that of information giver and expeditor. The aims of these roles are to allay apprehension and increase the ability and willingness of the patient to cooperate in what may be a frightening or uncomfortable experience. If this goal is accomplished, then the goal of expediting the process is partially met because the chance for a satisfactory test being completed the first time are greatly increased.

To help the nurse fill these roles adequately, the diagnostic test information given in this section focuses strongly on meeting the learning needs of both the novice nurse and the client to help ensure a successful test through adequate physical and mental preparation and aftercare. The nurse would do well to check the process and procedures in use at the facility where he or she works. There is seldom *one* right way, and given the relative newness of this area of testing, changes are to be expected and looked for.

S E V E N T E E N

DIAGNOSTIC MODALITIES

SEQUENCING OF IMAGING EXAMINATIONS

In order to prevent interference in other testing due to the use of contrast agents in many tests, thereby causing delays in subsequent studies, the following sequence is recommended (Montgomery & Lieckti, 1991, p. D):

1. All noncontrast studies should be done before any type of contrast study
2. All ultrasound (US) studies should be done before barium studies
3. All nuclear medicine studies should be done before barium studies
4. All computerized tomography (CT) scans requiring oral or rectal contrast should be done before barium studies (unless time allows for reprepping of the patient)
5. All iodine contrast examinations should precede all barium studies
6. All gastrointestinal (GI) tract studies should be done before any upper GI tract procedures
7. Oral cholecystograms *must* precede GI, small-bowel or large-bowel studies
8. Intravenous pyelogram (IVP) and bladder studies should be done before barium studies

17.1 X-RAY

17.1.1 Explanation of the Process

X-ray is one of the oldest diagnostic modalities; discovered in 1895 and made clinically safe by 1900, x-ray was initially called roentgenography after the discoverer, W. C. Roentgen, a German physicist. (See Appendix E for more detailed information.) The main disadvantage in the use of x-ray for diagnosis is that the rays can damage living tissue, kill cells, or alter them so that they cannot reproduce. The basis for the use of x-ray (i.e., radiation) as a treatment for malignancy [cancer] is that radiation readily destroys rapidly reproducing cells. Exposure to x-ray is also cumulative, so repeated exposure at less than cell-destroying levels can still pose serious risks. X-ray exposure is measured in roentgen equivalents for man (REMS). In practice, x-ray exposure is most frequently measured in RADs, an acronym for radiation absorbed dose. (See also Appendix E.)

Certain populations such as pregnant women should not be exposed to *any* x-ray. Except in emergencies, women of childbearing age should have x-rays only up to 14 days after the first day of their menstrual period to protect the fetus (if one exists) from radiation damage (Corbett, 1987, p. 6).

17.1.2 Types of X-Rays

A. Diagnostic Radiography

Synonyms: Roentgenograms, x-ray films, x-ray pictures

X-ray films are used for the initial screening diagnosis of body structures.

B. Tomography

Synonyms: Laminogram/graphy; planigrams/graphy; polytome; stratiogram/graphy. (See also 17.7.2 Tomography; A. Computerized Tomography; B. Angiograms; C. 3-D Reconstruction; D. PET; and E. PET-FDG

Tomography is any one of several noninvasive techniques of roentgenography (x-ray). It is especially designed to show detailed images of body structures in a preselected plane (layer) of tissue in a two-dimensional view. It produces a film that represents a detailed cross section of tissue structure. This is done by blurring images of all structures in other planes, and by elimination of super-imposed dense structures, which can hide defects in standard x-ray. This feature is particularly useful in the identification of space occupying lesions. The imaging is more detailed than standard x-ray and can eliminate the need for many other tests.

Tomography is more costly than x-ray. Multiple settings may be necessary for tomography to discover a lesion within tissue. It also requires a special radiographic apparatus that moves in a linear or polydirectional fashion while filming. The films must move in the opposite direction.

C. Contrast Studies, Definitions

Synonym: Radiopaque studies

The x-ray contrast between body structures that occurs naturally in some areas such as the chest which contains air, blood, fat, and bone is not found in some sites (e.g., the extremities). To visualize these areas, a solid, liquid, or gaseous substance is given that either absorbs more or less radiation than the surrounding tissue. Contrast material can be given either orally, rectally, intravenously, by urinary catheter, by inhalation, or percutaneously.

Contrast substances that absorb more x-rays than do most body tissues are those with high atomic numbers (e.g., barium). Others, such as air, have the same atomic number as body tissue but are less dense, thereby absorbing fewer x-rays. Contrast agents are introduced into a hollow viscus, which allows the area to be visualized. (See Sections 17.2.3 through 17.2.11, and 17.3, 1 through 6, for examples.)

IMPLICATIONS FOR NURSING: REACTION TO CONTRAST MEDIA

Any foreign material has the potential to cause a reaction, an allergic response, when placed in the body. The reaction can be immediate—which is the most common type—or it can be delayed. Although most centers do not use reaction assessment (Cyr, 1986), it remains good nursing practice to be aware of signs and symptoms and preventative measures.

1. Prevent reactions by assessing for sensitivity to the material to be used. A common ingredient in contrast media is iodine, which is also a fairly common allergen. Check for a past history of an allergy to saltwater fish or a reaction to previous diagnostic testing with any contrast material. Be sure to record any positive responses, no matter how vague, and call the response(s) to the attention of the radiology department and the physician.

2. Identify reactions early by awareness of probable early signs and symptoms (e.g., pallor, sweating, increased heart rate, feelings of anxiety [something "not right"], headache, dizziness, nausea or vomiting, flushing, complaints of warmth, shortness of breath, dyspnea, and at times, coughing or sneezing). Early identification is also in part based on a knowledge of the person's pretest status, which should be assessed and recorded. *Always* check the blood pressure (BP), pulse, and respiration before and after diagnostic tests using contrast media.

3. Immediate hypersensitivity, also called anaphylactic shock, occurs almost immediately. Parenteral epinephrine, 1:1000 (or a like drug), should be readily at hand wherever a contrast test is being done for immediate administration should a reaction occur. (It counteracts the primary signs and symptoms by increasing the BP, heart rate, and cardiac output; relaxing bronchial musculature; constricting bronchial arterioles; and inhibiting histamine release, thereby reducing pulmonary congestion.) It can be given subcutaneously, intramuscularly, or intravenously, with intravenous the route of choice. Intramuscular injections should not be given in the buttocks. If the drug is given intravenously, a cardiac monitor should be attached to the patient before administration. The BP should be taken repeatedly for the first 5 minutes, and it should be checked every 2 or 3 minutes thereafter until stable. A full crash cart should also be immediately available for defibrillation or cardioversion if needed. The incidence of severe hypersensitivity is very low, but should it occur, it is essential to be ready to treat it immediately

4. Be prepared to deal with allergic responses immediately in a susceptible person by obtaining an order for an antihistamine or corticosteroid as occasion requires (p.r.n.) before the test. If the contrast medium is to be given intravenously, check for a local reaction after the test. Report and record the reaction. Treat any subsequent phlebitis at the injection site with warm compresses.

5. Assist with elimination of the contrast media used
   a. Intravenous material is excreted in the urine and usually acts as an osmotic diuretic. The client will need extra fluids to help dilute and eliminate the material unless this is contraindicated. Extra fluid will also help prevent the bladder and urethral irritation that is often caused by the contrast media.
   b. Barium, used in visualizing the GI tract, is eliminated through the rectum. Obtain an order for bowel care if none has been written. Removal of barium almost always requires assistance such as cathartics, enemas, and so on. If barium is not fully excreted, an obstruction of the bowel can occur. Provision of extra fluids, if not contraindicated, is also helpful for the elimination of barium.

6. Prepare the patient for what to expect (i.e., the usual response to an intravenous injection of contrast media [often called dye] or its absorption). Usually intravenous contrast material causes a flushed and warm sensation. There may also be a taste sensation, a metallic/salty taste, with iodine injection. An aching sensation at the point of injection also can occur. Check with the radiology department if information is not available to you otherwise.

Fluoroscopy. This use of x-ray is based on the x-ray's ability to cause objects to fluoresce on the x-ray plate. In this case the fluorescence is projected onto a screen held over or in front of the part of the patient's body to be examined. The visualization of the organ's structure can be seen as on an x-ray film, but the movement of the body parts visualized can also be continuously observed. Often a contrast substance will be given (e.g., a barium swallow). The major disadvantage of fluoroscopy is that it exposes the patient (and the operator to a lesser degree because of protective clothing) to more radiation than does a standard x-ray.

Cineradiography. Often used with fluoroscopy, cineradiography is the recording of the visualized body parts' movement on either videotape or motion picture film. This provides for a review of the process, in slow motion if needed, to determine abnormal function. Fluoroscopy and cineradiology have been used most extensively with cardiac catheterizations but are also used with transhepatic cholangiograms, barium swallows, and chest films (to detect phrenic nerve paralysis).

Xerography (Xeroradiography). Xerography uses a photoelectric developing process (much like that of an office copier), as opposed to diagnostic radiology, which is a photochemical process. It provides a "positive" picture, one in bas-relief, rather than the "negative" picture produced by an x-ray. The process provides accuracy because of greater image resolution; greater contrast helps identify small areas of increased density, and xerography involves less exposure to radiation than does an x-ray. It is used primarily for soft tissue and extremity visualization.

17.2 COMMONLY USED X-RAY STUDIES

17.2.1 Chest Film

Synonym: Chest x-ray

Explanation of the Test. A chest film is the most commonly used x-ray study. It can be done in the radiology department or, as a "portable" x-ray, taken to the client in a hospital room or to a community setting in a van. For some time the chest film was used routinely as a screening test each year with a physical examination or on admission to the hospital. Because of the risk of additional, unnecessary radiation, this is no longer the case. Presently it is used to determine lung ventilation; heart position and size; vascular patterns in chronic respiratory disease; and the presence of atelectasis, hydrothorax, pneumothorax, infection, tuberculosis, lung tumors, and infiltrate. A comparison with previous chest films for change often provides the most valuable information.

IMPLICATIONS FOR NURSING: CHEST FILM

1. No permit is needed
2. No physical preparation of the patient is necessary
3. Patient education: It is important to stand as straight and "tall" as possible; a front and side view (called an anterior/posterior [A&P] and lateral) are usually the minimum number of views. Clothing must be removed to the waist. No jewelry such as necklaces may be worn, nor should cardiac monitor patches be left in place. The patient will be required to take two deep breaths and hold the second one for approximately 15 seconds
4. Length of time needed: Usually only a few minutes

17.2.2 Plain Film of the Abdomen

Synonyms: Scout film, KUB (kidneys, ureter, bladder), flat plate of the abdomen

Explanation of the Test. A plain film of the abdomen is usually done as first step in the diagnosis of abdominal pain/discomfort, trauma, enlargement of the abdomen, or with any examination of the GI system. The presence of excessive gas in the bowel (bowel distention), ascites, or the position of the liver, spleen, and kidneys can be determined, as can the location of abdominal trauma. Bile stones can also be visualized at times, depending on their composition, and a viscous perforation can be detected by the presence of air under the diaphragm, which will elevate it.

IMPLICATIONS FOR NURSING: PLAIN FILM OF THE ABDOMEN

1. No permit is needed for this procedure
2. Physical preparation: Bowel preparation is sometimes required, but most often the abdominal plain film is done without preparation because of insufficient knowledge as to the cause of the abdominal problems. Check with the physician. In the absence of specific instructions, no preparation should be done. Unless otherwise specified, the bladder should be emptied before the test
3. Patient education. The person will need to know that there should be little or no discomfort associated with the test other than lying briefly on a hard surface. If it is possible, one view at least will be taken with the individual standing (or sitting). If that is not possible, a view will be taken with the patient on his or her left side
4. Length of time needed: Usually only a few minutes

17.2.3 Arthrogram

Synonym: Joint film

Explanation of the Test. An arthrogram is an x-ray of a joint space after injection of a contrast medium. The contrast medium can either be a positive substance (as an iodine solution) or a negative substance (such as air). This test is usually done on an outpatient basis in a hospital or in the doctor's office. The purpose is to help explain the presence of joint pain or discomfort that is persistent and without demonstrable cause. The knee is the joint most often studied because it is most often injured, but any encapsulated joint can be so studied. Vertebrae are also examined with this method.

The test is done using a sterile procedure with a local anesthetic. If there is fluid in the joint, it is aspirated before the contrast media is introduced (see Synovial Fluid Analysis, Section 12.2.2.D.2). Several x-ray views of the joint are taken (e.g., at rest, at full extension, and at full flexion). Findings from the test can help diagnose synovial abnormality, ligamental tears, arthritis, or dislocation.

IMPLICATIONS FOR NURSING: ARTHROGRAM

1. A permit is needed for this procedure in some hospitals, and the patient may need to be assessed for an allergy to iodine
2. Physical preparation: Because this is a sterile procedure, the area that is to be perforated to introduce contrast media will need sterile preparation, usually just before the process. Shaving is considered necessary only if there is abundant hair at the site
3. Patient education: There may be an increase in pain during the procedure because of the position changes of the joint that are necessary for the multiple x-ray views. The person needs to be reassured that a mild analgesic will be available for this pain if necessary. If it is an outpatient procedure, patients should be advised to plan to rest for a while afterward to help decrease the discomfort until they are able to walk out
4. Postdischarge teaching: Information concerning the management of subsequent discomfort (which is usually due to a mild to severe local reaction to the contrast media that causes redness, heat, and pain in and around the joint for several days) should be given (e.g., ice packs help reduce acute swelling). The joint should be rested for at least 12 hours after the procedure; an elastic bandage or support may be useful for several days, especially if the knee joint is involved. Pain may be due to muscle fatigue as well, in which case *warm* compresses are useful. The individual should also be alerted to the possibility of joint "noise" on movement for 1 or 2 days after the procedure, which is to be expected. If it lasts longer than this, the doctor should be informed
5. Length of time needed: Variable with a minimum of one-half hour*

---

*Arthroscopy is *not* the same thing as an arthrogram. Arthroscopy is the fiberoptic, direct visual examination of the interior of a joint by an optical instrument and is a surgical examination. The knee joint is the most commonly examined joint, although any encapsulated joint interior can be fully visualized and damage to parts of the joint identified. It is a minor surgical procedure, usually done under local anesthesia. A general anesthetic is used when minor repairs of the joint are done through the arthroscope. Possible minor repairs include the removal of calcium deposits, scar tissue, cartilage, the meniscus, or bone spurs from within the joint.

17.2.4 Bronchoscopy and Bronchogram

Explanation of the Test

1. Bronchoscopy is an endoscopic,* direct lighted visualization of the larynx, trachea, and bronchi. The use of a flexible fiber-optic bronchoscope has for the most part replaced the use of the rigid bronchoscope, which was more uncomfortable for patients, often requiring general anesthesia. The scope can be inserted by way of either the nose or mouth (most common) and can be passed into the trachea and the main stem bronchi. Bronchoscopy can be either diagnostic or therapeutic

   a. Diagnostic: Visualization for the identification of strictures, tumors, or inflammation; biopsy; aspiration of deep sputum specimens for culture, sensitivity, and cytology examinations; brushings of tissue for cytological examination; and determination as to whether a lesion is resectable

---

Endoscopy is a general term referring to visual inspection of any body cavity (end/endo = within, inner; scope/scopy = watcher/examination of). It implies the use of an instrument, here a "scope."

b. Therapeutic: Removal of foreign objects, deep suctioning of retained secretions (as with airway obstruction and postoperative atelectasis), location and control of bleeding/hemorrhage

2. A bronchogram is an x-ray examination of the bronchial tree by using a contrast medium. A radioopaque iodine contrast solution, usually with an oil base, is injected into the tracheobronchial area through a catheter. It is a diagnostic measure, helpful in detecting deep bronchial obstructions (e.g., foreign bodies, cysts, cavities, or bronchiectasis). This procedure is less frequently done now with the increased availability of tomography. When done, it usually accompanies a bronchoscopy

Bronchoscopy is contraindicated for pregnant women and for patients with severe shortness of breath who cannot tolerate any impediment to high oxygen flow.

IMPLICATIONS FOR NURSING: BRONCHOSCOPY AND BRONCHOGRAM

1. Most in-hospital bronchoscopies and bronchograms require that a permit be signed. Check with the regulations of the facility where the procedure is to be done
2. Physical preparation: The patient should be kept n.p.o. at least 6 to 8 hours before the test(s), usually after midnight, or if an afternoon test, the meal before the test is omitted. Check with the physician for special orders for patients with chronic respiratory congestion. An expectorant or respiratory treatment measures may be ordered. Report any occurrence of fever. Provide thorough mouth care to decrease the chance of introducing any bacteria into the lungs during the procedure. Dentures *must* be removed before the procedure, and any oral lesions or loose teeth must be reported to the physician and radiology department or surgical department, depending on where the procedure is scheduled. Preprocedure medications are usually given: sedation or tranquilizers to relax the patient (diazepam [Valium] is frequently used because it also helps to relax the musculature, which will help with the passage of the scope) and ephedrine or atropine to dry up secretions. A narcotic may also be given. Because the throat is usually sprayed or swabbed with a topical anesthetic, the patient must be assessed for sensitivity to such agents as well as sensitivity to iodine (see also Implications for Nursing: Reaction to Contrast Media, Section 17.1.2.C)
3. Patient education
   a. Determine what the patient and family already know or believe about the procedure and correct any misconceptions. Determine what their immediate learning needs are, and start there
   b. The patient and family will need to know what to expect and what will be expected of them (see "Physical preparation," item 2) and the rationale for each expectation (e.g., n.p.o. to decrease the chance of vomiting and aspiration during the procedure)
   c. The patient will need to know the importance of restraining any cough during the procedure and that the spray or swabbing of the throat will help decrease the urge to cough and the ability to swallow. Rapid, shallow breathing will help to restrain the urge
   d. Explain the need to breathe through the nose during the test even though the mouth will be kept open (the patient may need or want to practice this) and to communicate by nonverbal means (e.g., hand signals)
   e. Inform the patient that the swallow reflex will be absent for a while after the procedure is over and that no fluid or food can be taken until it returns
   f. Assure the patient that oxygen can be and often is routinely given during the test and that she or he *can* breathe despite the tube in the air passages
   g. Inform the patient that she or he will need to change position several times when the contrast media is given to reach the maximal area of the bronchial tree
4. Posttest care and teaching

a. The patient will usually cough up most of the contrast media

b. To assist in expectoration of the contrast media after the test, the patient may be asked to do postural drainage (explain this only if probable) or may be placed prone in Trendelenburg's position for 15 to 20 minutes three times a day. Describe or demonstrate either of the procedures that are followed in the facility where the test is being done

c. Inform the patient that an expectorant is often given to help remove secretions and contrast medium. Forcing fluids, unless contraindicated, is also helpful for this

d. The patient should also know that she or he will have a slight sore throat for a while after the test

e. Given time and a receptive patient, teaching relaxation exercises can be helpful to the patient

5. Length of time needed: Approximately 1 hour for a bronchogram

17.2.5 Barium Enema

Synonyms: Double-contrast study of the colon, air contrast study of the colon, lower GI study

Explanation of the Test. The barium enema is a study of the large bowel by using barium as a contrast medium; barium is introduced through the rectum by a tube retrograde flow and retained as the radiologist observes the bowel filling under fluoroscopy. X-rays are taken as well during the filling process and again after the patient has eliminated as much barium as is possible.

A double-contrast, or air contrast study, is the introduction of a thicker barium solution that is expelled and air introduced to "push" the barium against the colon walls, thereby outlining them.

This process is particularly useful in the identification of wall lesions such as polyps or bleeding sites. The double-contrast study can only be done with a patient who is mobile because many position changes are necessary, and it requires a well-prepared bowel. Fecal deposits can mimic lesions.

Barium enemas are indicated in any suspected lower intestinal disease or problem such as tumors, polyps, diverticula, occult bleeding, the presence of mucus or pus in the stool, complaints of lower abdominal pain, changes in bowel habits or stool formation, positional anomalies, or any form of obstruction.

Individuals at risk with barium enemas are the elderly (over 72 years old) and nonfunctional individuals. The elderly have shown a tendency toward fluid imbalances after barium enemas that lead to changes in mental status. The threat occurs because of the preparation for the test (laxatives, enemas, restriction of fluid) plus the diarrhea that often follows use of laxatives in the aged and a decrease with age in the ability to return to normal homeostatic fluid balance (Robinson & Demuth, 1985, pp. 7–9).

Barium enemas are contraindicated when a perforated viscus is suspected (severe abdominal pain/cramping).

IMPLICATIONS FOR NURSING: BARIUM ENEMA

1. Permits are not usually required

2. Physical preparation: Notify the physician if the patient has severe abdominal cramping or pain before the test. Check the intake and output (I&O) and blood pressure on the elderly patient, the non-

functional person in his or her 70s. Inform the radiology department if the patient is unable to retain enema fluid so that a special tube can be used during the test itself. What is done in preparation of the bowel depends, in part, on what the usual procedures are for the facility in which the test is done and, in part, on what the problem is suspected or known to be. One possible set of preparation schedules is given here

    a. Preparation: a completely clean colon (use: examination for small polyps, early inflammatory, or infiltrating lesions)

        (1) Liquid diet for 3 days before the test if possible

        (2) Two ounces of castor oil (or an acceptable substitute such as GoLYTELY) on the third day at noon

        (3) Provide an increased fluid intake until midnight of the third day

        (4) Enemas until clear (maximum of three) in the morning of the day of the examination

    b. Preparation for varying degrees of obstruction (anular tumors, diverticulitis, intussusception, volvulus)

        (1) Two ounces of castor oil at 4:00 PM the day before the test (substitute as for 2a(2) above). The castor oil is omitted if the patient is partially or totally obstructed

        (2) Light liquid dinner. Provide increased fluids until midnight

        (3) n.p.o. after midnight

        (4) Enema (tap water or Fleet) until clear or three times starting at 6:00 AM on the day of the examination

    c. Preparation for acute inflammatory bowel disease determining the source of more gross bleeding only (e.g., ulcerative colitis, granulomatous colitis, acute diverticulitis). This preparation is not standardized. It is done on an individual basis determined by the physician and the diagnostic department (Laboratory of Pathology, 1992)

3. Patient education

    a. The elderly will need more thorough, repeated instruction as to their responsibility regarding fluid intake after the procedure. If the test is done on an outpatient basis, it is most important to involve a home caretaker in these instructions as well

    b. List the steps in the test preparation, and give a rationale for each. Provide the patient with a preparation slip if available. Such a slip is vital for the outpatient. Stress the importance of adequate preparation to prevent having to redo the test. Determine and inform the patient whether the administration of routine oral medications is to be held and whether they should be taken later in the day

    c. Explain the procedure and the need to change the position of the table and his or her own position to facilitate passage of the barium into the colon; the maximum amount of barium to be instilled will be no more than 1½ qt, usually much less, which most people can retain without problems. The patient will be asked to first hold the barium and then expel it while still in the x-ray department—which can take up to 30 minutes. A final x-ray film will be taken after the barium is expelled

4. Posttest care

    a. The patient will also need to know the importance of removing *all* the barium after the test. She or he can recognize the presence of barium in the stool by the unusually light color of the stool or by streaks of white in the stool

    b. Inform him or her that there is usually a need for enemas or cathartics (e.g., Milk of Magnesia) to complete the removal of barium and that the doctor will order this. Include the reason for this process, the possibility of obstruction because of retained barium

    c. Include the need to replace lost fluids, especially for the elderly; a minimum of 2000 ml is needed each day unless contraindicated

    d. Inform the patient that the test is often very fatiguing and that she or he should plan to rest at least the remainder of the day of the test

5. Length of time needed: Approximately 1 hour

17.2.6 Cholecystograms and Cholangiograms

A. *Oral Cholecystograms*

Synonyms: OCG, gallbladder series, GB series, oral cholecystography, gallbladder radiography

Explanation of the Test. Oral cholecystography is an x-ray test, rarely done with the advent of ultrasound, using an oral contrast medium in capsule form to visualize the internal anatomy of the gallbladder in order to evaluate its function (filling, concentration, contraction, and empty-ing) and the patency of the cystic duct, as well as to determine the presence of nonradiopaque gallstones. Radiopaque gallstones, composed of calcium carbonate, are the least commonly oc-curring stones. The more common gallstones are composed of cholesterol and bile pigments and require the use of contrast medium to be seen. The contrast medium, taken orally, is iodine based (e.g., iopanoic acid [Telepaque], iodoalphionic acid [Priodox], sodium ipodate [Oragrafin]), absorbed by the liver, and excreted by the biliary tree to end in the gallbladder where it is concentrated. If the gallbladder is not visualized after the contrast medium is given, which indicates that the dye has not entered the gallbladder to be concentrated, the test may be rescheduled for the following day with a double dose of the contrast medium used. If there is still no visualization, the cause can be an obstruction of the cystic duct by stones, a chronic in-flammation, inadequate preparation, or an unknown cause (see "Intravenous Cholangiogram," B. in this section).

Ultrasound is now considered the gold standard for the diagnosis of cholelithiasis and has largely replaced OCG for the diagnosis of gallstones.

THIS TEST IS CONTRAINDICATED IN:

1. Any liver dysfunction (e.g., serum bilirubin level greater than 3 to 4 mg/dl)
2. Patients allergic to the contrast medium. The intravenous cholangiogram can be substi-tuted, but if the purpose is to determine concentration ability of the gallbladder, the in-travenous test will not show this
3. Early pregnancy (first trimester). The contrast medium may have teratogenic effects on the fetus at this time, and x-ray itself is a hazard

---

IMPLICATIONS FOR NURSING: ORAL CHOLECYSTOGRAM

1. No permit is needed
2. Physical preparation
   a. Scans involving iodine (e.g., thyroid uptake, protein-bound iodine [PBI]) must be done before a gallbladder study
   b. Cholecystograms should precede any barium studies because barium will interfere with visual-ization of the gallbladder
   c. Cholecystograms can be scheduled with—*to precede*—upper GI, small bowel, and colon (bari-um enema) studies

    d. Fat-free meals, at least the evening meal before the test. In some facilities all meals of the preceding day are fat free. In others a high-fat noon meal is given to empty the gallbladder

    e. Radiopaque tablets or capsules are given 2 hours after the evening meal; directions on the packet should be followed. Usually the "dye" is taken in six capsules 5 minutes apart. At least 250 ml of water should be taken with the capsules to ensure their absorption

    f. Patient should be kept n.p.o. thereafter. Most radiology departments prohibit smoking and gum chewing as well to prevent stimulation of gallbladder contraction

    g. No laxatives until after the test. (Some facilities schedule bowel preparation [enemas or suppositories] the morning of the test to clear possible obscuring feces in the lower colon)

    h. Check the patient for iodine sensitivity. The dye can cause nausea, vomiting, and/or diarrhea. Only if vomiting occurs will the contrast medium be lost and the test need to be cancelled

    i. Check for signs, symptoms, and a history of liver disease. Report *any* positive findings

    j. Inform the radiology department if the patient receives any morphine before the test because it can cause a spasm of the spincter of Oddi

3. Patient education

    a. Explain the purpose of the test and the process of the physical preparation necessary for it along with an adequate rationale for the test and preparation

    b. Especially if the test is done on an outpatient basis, a written list of the steps in the procedure and expectations of the patient is helpful

    c. Provide explanations in terms the patient can understand

    d. Inform the patient that the test often needs to be repeated. This is not cause for alarm because it is usually due to a lack of dye, not disease. The patient should remain on a low-fat diet if the test is to be repeated the next day

    e. Reinforce the need to drink large amounts of water (unless contraindicated) with the dye capsules or tablets

    f. The patient will be asked to change positions several times during the test for the radiologist to differentiate between gallstones and air bubbles (air bubbles will rise with position changes)

    g. If the ability of the gallbladder to contract and empty is to be evaluated, the patient will be given a fatty meal after the first series of films are taken, and more x-ray films will be taken at intervals until all the dye has been expelled

    h. The contrast medium is excreted in the urine, therefore fluid intake is important. Some patients report slight dysuria with dye excretion. This will be minimized by dilution of the urine

4. Length of time needed: Approximately 1 hour, depending on whether the emptying time is being evaluated and the speed with which the contrast medium is eliminated

B. Cholangiograms

Explanation of the Test. Cholangiograms differ from cholecystograms in the way the dye, or contrast medium, is given and in the purpose for which they are done. Cholangiograms are done to visualize the cystic, hepatic, and common bile ducts, primarily to assess their patency. The contrast medium, rather than given orally, can be administered in four different ways, depending on the situation:

1. Intravenous Cholangiograms (IVC): Done to study the hepatic and common biliary ducts, or the biliary "tree." It demonstrates stones in the ducts, strictures, or space-occupying lesions. IVC is done in patients with symptoms of gallstones but after they have already had a cholecystectomy, in those in whom the gallbladder cannot be visualized

with an oral cholecystogram (in patients with acute abdominal imflammatory processes not related to the biliary system, such as pancreatitis, the gallbladder is often not visualized for unknown reasons), to visualize suspected ductal stones, and for those patients who cannot tolerate oral contrast medium. Indications for use of this test have decreased since endoscopic retrograde cholangiopancreatography (ERCP) and percutaneous transhepatic cholangiography (PTC/PTHC) have been introduced

2. T tube cholangiogram: Done during surgical procedures to check for obscure gallstones in the common duct or done several days postoperatively to check the patency of the biliary tree. This usually is a fluoroscopic examination

3. Percutaneous transhepatic cholangiogram (PTHC): Also a fluoroscopic examination, but one in which a cannula is inserted percutaneously into an intrahepatic duct, often the common bile duct, to inject a contrast medium. This method is used when jaundice or another hepatic disorder is present that indicates a lack of liver function; and it provides direct visualization of the ducts

4. Operative cholangiogram: The cystic or common bile duct is cannulated after surgical exposure, and contrast medium is introduced to provide immediate information to the surgeon

---

IMPLICATIONS FOR NURSING: CHOLANGIOGRAMS

1. A permit is required for any of the aforementioned methods of testing
2. Patient preparation: (Only preparation for the IVC is covered here because it is the most commonly used test)
   a. The patient is kept n.p.o. 6 to 8 hours before the test. If the test is done in the afternoon, the meal before the test is withheld
   b. A bowel preparation (laxative, suppository, Fleet enema) is usually ordered
   c. The contrast medium is administered in the radiology department
   d. Determine any history of allergic response to iodinated contrast medium, and inform the radiologist prior to the procedure. An antihistamine or steriod may be ordered to be given before testing
3. Patient education
   a. Determine what the patient/family knows and what they want to know and start there
   b. Explain the procedural steps and the rationale for them
   c. The patient and family need to know that this is a long procedure, up to 8 hours. It will require that the patient make several position changes. It is not a particularly uncomfortable test except for the need to remain on the hard x-ray table for prolonged periods of time and the "flush" sensation of the contrast medium administration
   d. Films are taken every 15 to 30 minutes until the "dye" reaches the common bile duct and that duct can be visualized. Tomography may be used for better visualization of the duct system
   e. Encourage the patient to inform the doctor or technician of any nausea or other uncomfortable or unusual responses during the test
4. Posttest care
   a. Provide fluids to help flush the contrast medium from the body
   b. Food should be made available. Usually these patients will be on a low-fat diet
5. Length of time needed: 2 to 4 or, rarely, 8 hours

C. Endoscopic Retrograde Cholangiopancreatography (ERCP)

Synonym: ERCP—biliary and pancreatic ducts

Normal Findings: Normal biliary and pancreatic ducts

Explanation of the Test. Usually performed following abdominal ultrasound, CT, liver scan, or biliary tract x-ray, primarily to confirm diagnosis. Only ERCP and percutaneous transhepatic cholangiography (PTHC) (see item 3 in B.) provide radiographic visualization of either biliary or pancreatic ducts. Such visualization, in turn, provides information related to the presence and kind of obstruction of these ducts. Although ERCP is the more difficult of the two tests, requiring an experienced endoscopist, the morbidity outcome is much less than that of PTHC. ERCP is able to visualize the biliary tree in the presence of high bilirubin levels, which is not possible with oral cholecystograms, or IV cholangiograms. Fiber-optic endoscopy visualizes the pancreatic ducts, identifying the cause and degree of obstruction.

Purpose of the Test. ERCP is performed to identify the cause of biliary obstruction (e.g., stricture, cyst, stones, or tumor).

IMPLICATIONS FOR NURSING

1. Informed consent must be obtained before the test
2. Patient preparation: The process should be explained at the level and felt need of the patient. Some fairly uniform preparatory steps include:
    a. The patient is kept n.p.o. from midnight before the test
    b. Some form of sedation is usually provided (sedative, narcotic, or hypnotic) to allow easier passage of the scope
    c. Prior to inserting the endoscope through the nose or mouth, the gag reflex is usually suppressed or obliterated by spraying the pharynx with a local anesthetic (check for sensitivity to local anesthetics before its use)
    d. The fiber-optic duodenoscope is inserted through the mouth and will initially cause some gagging
    e. Glucagon may be given IV at this time to decrease duodenal spasm and to facilitate visualization of the ampulla of vater
    f. A small catheter is inserted via the scope, through the ampulla, and into the pancretic, or common vile ducts
    g. Radiographic dye is then inserted via catheter, and x-ray films are done
3. Contraindications: ERCP cannot be used in the presence of:
    a. Acute or recent (less than 6 weeks) pancreatitis
    b. Barium in the bowel
    c. Pregnancy (potential harm of ionizing radiation to the fetus)
4. Posttest care
    a. Assess for respiratory depression. Have equipment for resuscitation immediately available
    b. Nothing by mouth until gag reflex is present
    c. Assess for signs and symptoms of ERCP-induced pancreatitis (e.g., abdominal pain, nausea, vomiting), septicemia (e.g., fever, shaking chills, nausea, vomiting, diarrhea)
    d. Maintain safety while the patient is sedated (e.g., bed rails up, frequent slight position changes, airway unobstructed)
5. Length of time needed: Minimum of 1 hour

17.2.7 Bladder Examinations

A. Cystograms

A cystogram (cystography, voiding cystogram, cystourethrogram) is an x-ray of the bladder that uses contrast medium inserted through a Foley catheter. The filling is observed under fluoroscopy by the radiologist to assess for filling defects or shadows within the bladder that may indicate bladder tumors (usually primary); distortions or compression of the bladder that indicates the location and size of pelvic tumors or hematomas; extravasation of the contrast medium out of the bladder into the peritoneum to indicate bladder rupture, which may be secondary to trauma; or backflow of urine from the bladder to the ureters (vesicoureteral reflux) or a neurogenic bladder. This is a useful test when cystoscopy or retrograde pyelography are contraindicated.

B. Cystoscopy

Cystoscopy is the direct, lighted visualization of the bladder and urethra by use of a cystoscope. Usually performed by a urologist, it is used not only for direct inspection of possible defects of the bladder (listed under cystogram, in A.) but also for biopsy, collection of separate urine specimens from each kidney (using ureteral catheters passed through the scope), identification of calculi, and measurement of bladder capacity. As with other endoscopic examinations, cystoscopy has therapeutic as well as diagnostic uses. Cystoscopy is used for coagulation of bleeding areas in the bladder; implantation of radium seed into a bladder tumor; drainage of blocked kidney pelves; and removal of small stones, tumors, or other bodies.

C. Cystometry

Cystometry, a study of intravesical pressures during filling and emptying of the bladder (detrusor muscle function), can be done at the same time as a voiding cystogram or done with cystoscopy, but it is usually done as a separate study because it does not require the use of contrast media other than air or water. Cystometry helps determine whether the malfunction of the bladder is due to neurogenic, obstructive, or infectious causes. Signs and symptoms indicating a need to measure bladder pressures include dysuria, enuresis, stress (overflow) incontinence, weak urinary stream, and/or frequency of urination. Medical diagnoses indicating a need for this test include neurological problems such as myelomeningocele, spina bifida, and tabes dorsalis. Neural trauma such as cord injury may also be an indication. During cystometry sensation related to neural stimulation of the bladder is checked (e.g., sensations of heat and cold, fullness, urge to void, flushing, sweating, nausea, pain, or discomfort), and response to the administration of cholinergic and anticholinergic drugs can be assessed.

D. Retrograde Pyelography

Retrograde pyelography (retrograde pyelogram) is a radiographic visualization of the kidney pelves, as well as the rest of the lower urinary tract. It is done with cystoscopy. Ureteral catheters are placed and a contrast medium injected into the ureters and renal pelves. This test is indicated when an intravenous pyelogram (IVP) does not visualize a kidney, when an IVP is contraindicated because of an allergy to the contrast medium (there is much less absorption of the contrast medium with this test than with an IVP, thus much lower risk of allergic response), when there is severely decreased renal plasma flow (RPF), or when there is need to rule out unilateral ureteral obstruction. It also provides excellent visualization of the total urinary tract, which is not possible with an IVP.

IMPLICATIONS FOR NURSING: BLADDER EXAMINATIONS

(For all teaching, always determine what the client and family know, what they believe to be true, and what they want to find out about first, and start teaching from there.)

1. No permit is needed for a cystogram or for cystometry. A permit is necessary for cystoscopy or a retrograde pyelogram when done in a hospital. Both can be done on an outpatient basis in a urologist's office
2. Physical preparation
    a. Cystogram
        (1) A Foley catheter is inserted before going to the radiology department
        (2) In some facilities only clear liquids are given for breakfast on the day of the examination
        (3) Assess for a history of allergy to iodine
        (4) Assess for signs and symptoms of urinary tract infection (UTI), and report immediately if present
    b. Cystoscopy
        (1) Fluids are pushed for several hours before the test, if not contraindicated, to maintain a continuous flow of urine during the test. A full liquid diet is given the morning of the test. (If a general anesthesia is to be used, the patient should be kept n.p.o. with an intravenous line. General anesthesia can be used for children and highly anxious or uncooperative adults)
        (2) Baseline vital signs should be taken
        (3) Topical preparation (scrub and topical spray with antiseptic solutions) will be done in the cystoscopy room—part of most surgical departments of hospitals—or in the urologist's office
        (4) A tranquilizer with a narcotic analgesic is usually given an hour before the examination for sedation and comfort
        (5) Assess for an allergy to local anesthetics (unless general anesthesia is planned)
    c. Cystometry: No physical preparation is necessary unless the test is done in conjunction with cystoscopy or a cystogram, in which case the preparation is as given for those tests
    d. Retrograde pyleography: Preparation is as for cystoscopy with the addition of an assessment for a history of an allergic response to iodine, shellfish, or past contrast studies. A bowel preparation may also be ordered
3. Patient education
    a. Cystogram
        (1) Explain the steps in the procedure and the rationale for each
        (2) Spell out diet restrictions, if any
        (3) Explain the purpose and procedure for catheterization with a Foley catheter
        (4) Make understood the need for at least 2400 ml of fluid for 24 hours after the test, unless contraindicated, to ensure elimination of all contrast material
    b. Cystoscopy
        (1) Explain the steps of the procedure and the rationale for each
        (2) Reassure the patient that, although there will be discomfort, it is not usually severe because of the use of local anesthesia through the catheter before insertion of the cystoscope and that she or he may experience a strong urge to void

(3) If a general anesthesia is planned, instruct the patient in routine pre- and postoperative measures (e.g., deep breathing, coughing, the presence of an intravenous line)

(4) Stress the importance of fluid intake both before the test and afterward to maintain good urine flow and to help eliminate any dye or possible contaminant

(5) Tell the patient that the test is usually done in the lithotomy position, with his or her legs in stirrups and suitably covered

(6) Postprocedure care

   (a) Explain that some hematuria is not uncommon

   (b) I&O should be monitored for a minimum of 24 hours. Adults should take in a minimum of 2500 ml over those 24 hours. Any decrease in output, less than the intake, may be the result of retention, as would small, frequent voidings. Alterations in voiding should be reported. Medications can be given to stimulate voiding if necessary

   (c) The chance of a UTI is increased after this test because of trauma to the urinary tract with instrumentation. This trauma also increases the chance of transient bacteremia. A prophylactic antibacterial is often ordered to prevent the problem, but the patient will need to be aware of signs and symptoms of both UTI and bacteremia so that they can be reported immediately and treatment started. Dysuria and changes in color or odor of the urine would be early infection indicators. A urinalysis is usually done routinely a day or so after the test

     • Dysuria can also occur because of the physical trauma to sensitive tissues of the urinary tract as well as excretion of the contrast medium

     • Increased fluid intake when not contraindicated, administration of medication for bladder spasm or mild analgesics, and application of heat to the abdomen (by warm tub baths if allowed) usually manage the discomfort

     • Check for the presence of a ureteral catheter. If one is present, ensure that no tension is applied to the catheter

c. Cystometry

  (1) Explain the steps of the procedure and rationale for each step

  (2) Inform the patient that there should be minimal discomfort with this test, and stress the importance of telling the urologist when discomfort does occur

d. Retrograde pyleography

  (1) All items given under cystoscopy apply here, plus the following

  (2) It is important that the patient not be dehydrated before the test. Inform the patient of signs and symptoms of dehydration and ask that she or he report any that occur. Make clear the importance of taking in the amount of fluids allowed before and after the test

  (3) Laxatives or cleansing enemas may be ordered before the test

  (4) X-rays are taken once the contrast medium has been injected and again after the ureteral catheters have been removed

  (5) List signs and symptoms the patient should report after the test (e.g., itching, rash, hives, flush, shortness of breath, increased heart rate) because these may indicate the beginning of an allergic response to the contrast medium and can be best controlled early by the administration of antihistamines or cortisone if necessary

4. Length of time needed

  a. Cystogram: 15 to 30 minutes

  b. Cystoscopy: Under local anesthesia, from 25 minutes to 1 hour

  c. Cystometry: 30 minutes to 1 hour

  d. Retrograde pyelogram: 1 to 1½ hours

17.2.8 Intravenous Pyelogram

Synonyms: IVP, excretory urogram

Explanation of the Test. An IVP is a frequently used x-ray study of the kidney that delineates the calyx, pelvis, and lower part of the urinary tract through the use of an intravenous, iodinated contrast medium that is excreted by the urinary system. For the contrast medium to appear on the x-ray film after intravenous injection and, thus, dilution by the blood, the contrast medium must be secreted and then concentrated by the kidney, two tubular functions. The IVP, therefore, can provide some information about those functions as well as the renal structure. This test is done by a radiologist. After injection of the contrast medium, x-ray films are taken at timed intervals (e.g., every minute for 5 minutes; at 2, 5, and 7 minutes; or at 7- to 12-minute intervals) during which the cortex of the kidney is visualized. In approximately 15 minutes the x-rays will define the renal calyx and pelvis. In approximately 45 minutes the bladder should be visualized. At this point the patient is asked to empty his or her bladder, and a final x-ray film is taken to check for any urinary retention. This test helps the diagnosis by making structural defects evident; by outlining tumors or indicating their presence by structural distortion; by indicating the status of renal function by the length of time taken for the contrast medium to appear in the kidney cortex and be excreted by each kidney; by identifying a lack of arterial blood flow or the presence of calculi in the kidney, ureters, or bladder; and by assessing the effects of trauma. *Retrograde pyelography* was frequently used in the past, particularly if a patient was allergic to the contrast media of an IVP or if the results of an IVP were equivocal (e.g., congenital absence of the kidney or decreased renal perfusion). It is done less frequently at present, probably because of the availability of better options such as a renogram, which is the test of choice when an allergy to contrast medium is suspected. Tomography (see Section 17.7.2) is often used as a follow-up test to localize and better visualize the pathology indicated by the IVP.

An IVP is contraindicated:

1. If the blood urea nitrogen (BUN) concentration is greater than 50 mg/dl
2. With a history of sensitivity to the contrast medium
3. In states of severe dehydration or oliguria
4. In patients being medicated for chronic respiratory conditions such as emphysema, asthma, or bronchitis

---

IMPLICATIONS FOR NURSING: INTRAVENOUS PYELOGRAM

1. No permit is required in many facilities; others do require one. Check with the radiology department of the facility doing the test
2. Patient preparation
   a. Assess for any history of allergic response to shellfish or previous contrast material. Skin testing may be done. Antihistamines or a steroid may be given before the test for susceptible persons
   b. Schedule any barium studies to follow this test
   c. Some bowel preparation is usually done the evening before the test in the adult. Bowel preparations vary with the status of the patient (e.g., unlikely to be done with a diagnosis of ulcerative colitis or in the very elderly or the very young)
   d. Fluid restriction may apply because maximum concentration of urine by the kidney helps visualization of the dye. Some facilities provide a clear liquid dinner and breakfast before the test; others require a strict 12-hour n.p.o. period before the test. Keeping an I&O record and taking vital signs provide useful baseline data for all patients

3. Patient education
   a. Explain the steps of the preparation and procedure with rationale for each
      (1) Generally the contrast medium is given by intravenous drip, but it may be given by a bolus injection
      (2) There will be several position changes: supine, Trendelenburg (to retain the contrast medium in the kidneys for a longer interval, heavy pressure may be applied externally as well for this purpose and can be very uncomfortable), and upright (to check the stability of the kidneys and to help drain them)
      (3) Patients will be asked to empty their bladders and then have another film taken. If unable to void, they may be returned to the nursing unit until able to void—at which time they must return to the x-ray department immediately
   b. Remind the patient of the sensations to be expected with injection of contrast medium. (See "Contrast Studies," Section 17.1.2.C)
   c. Stress the importance of letting the radiologist or technician know of any sensations such as itching, shortness of breath, or any other discomfort. (The risks of the test, such as minimal radiation and allergic reaction to the contrast medium, should be discussed by the patient's physician or the radiologist before the test. Check to ensure that this has been done)
4. Posttest care
   a. Fluids should be taken to tolerance, if not contraindicated, to help with the elimination of contrast medium and to overcome dehydration
   b. Usually the patient will return to the previous diet immediately, unless other tests are scheduled
   c. Bed rest should be encouraged if any posttest weakness is present
   d. Teach the signs and symptoms of delayed sensitivity and that they should be reported as soon as possible to obtain rapid treatment as prescribed by the physician
5. Length of time needed: Approximately 45 minutes to 1 hour

17.2.9 Upper Gastrointestinal Series

Synonyms: Barium swallow, esophagram, upper GI series and small-bowel series, enteroclysis study, hypotonic duodenography

Explanation of the Tests. These tests make up what is generally referred to as the GI series and can be used to study one or all parts of the upper GI tract. Because of this, the series is variously titled to indicate the focus or the scope of the examination to be done. Visualization of the esophagus—position, patency, and contour—is called an *esophagram* and is often done to diagnose a hiatal hernia; examination of the motor function of the esophagus (peristalsis) is usually called a *barium swallow*. If the total upper GI tract is to be observed, the test is referred to as an *upper* GI series; a *small-bowel series* implies that the focus is on or includes examination of the jejunum and ileum. To study the small bowel requires ingestion of additional barium by the patient. An *enteroclysis study* is one form of small-bowel study that uses double-contrast media and also differs in the method of approach. All of the other aforementioned tests are done by having the patient drink a barium mixture. A series of x-rays or fluoroscopy shows this radiopaque material filling the esophagus, stomach, and small bowel. (The farther down the GI tract the x-rays are to be taken, the more time it takes to be visualized.) The enteroclysis study involves an enema using a methylcellulose solution and barium, much like a barium enema. It is, however, introduced to reach the small bowel. Because it does visualize the small bowel, it is considered to be part of the study of the upper GI tract and, thus, fits with the other tests given here.

The procedure used is similar to that used in doing a cardiac series (see Section 17.4.1.C). Barium sulfate is the most commonly used contrast medium, but if a leak (e.g., a fistula) or an obstruction—which would cause regurgitation and aspiration—is present, the radiologist will use a water-soluble solution such as methylglucamine diatrizoate (Gastrografin).

As indicated before, the purpose of these tests is to detect structural abnormalities (e.g., esophageal varices, hiatal hernia, gastric diverticuli), anatomic malposition of organs, pathology (e.g., tumors, gastritis, ulcers, polyps), and disorders of function (e.g., hyperperistalsis, uncoordinated peristalsis, or hypoperistalsis; incompetent or spastic cardiac or pyloric valves) causing an increased or decreased transit time of the contrast medium.

Certain drugs may be given in conjunction with any of these tests. To decrease bowel spasm, glucagon can be given. Metoclopramide (Reglan) helps decrease the transit time of the barium through the pyloric valve, which aids in visualization of the small bowel.

A *hypotonic duodenoscopy* is a term applied to slowing the action of the small intestine by the use of propantheline bromide (Pro-Banthine), an anticholinergic.

Upper GI tests are contraindicated for any patient with suspected or known total bowel obstruction or those with a perforated viscus.

IMPLICATIONS FOR NURSING: UPPER GASTROINTESTINAL SERIES

1. A permit is not required
2. Physical preparation
   a. If a barium enema is also to be done and there is no preference stated by the physician, schedule it to be done the day after the GI series rather than the same day
   b. A light meal is given the evening before the test. A low-residue diet for 2 to 3 days before the test is suggested by some radiologists. To decrease gastric secretion and GI motility, smoking and gum chewing are restricted in some facilities
   c. Patients should be kept n.p.o. after midnight. Oral medications should be withheld or new orders for injectable medications obtained. In some cases medications will be given up to 2 hours before the test. Regular insulin is usually withheld, but long-acting insulin may be given if the procedure is not expected to last more than 4 to 5 hours. Check for orders
   d. Notify the radiology department if any narcotics or anticholinergic drugs have been given. They slow the motility of the GI tract
   e. Use of the small-bowel series prolongs the test by hours. Suggest that the patient take along something to help pass the time. The very ill or the elderly will need special preparation to keep them comfortable (e.g., use of a stretcher instead of a wheelchair and ample pillows, blankets, footlets, etc., to keep the patient warm)
3. Patient education: Explain the steps in preparation and procedure along with the rationale for each step
   a. All barium given the patient must be swallowed to provide adequate contrast
   b. The test should not cause significant discomfort other than that of lying on the hard x-ray table, being n.p.o., and taking the barium, which most people find somewhat unpleasant
   c. Usually an x-ray film will be taken before the contrast medium is given
   d. If a barium swallow is being done, the process of swallowing will be observed by fluoroscopy with the patient upright
   e. As the stomach fills, the radiologist may palpate it (using a lead-lined glove) to visualize all parts of the stomach and duodenum while x-ray films are taken
   f. The table will be tilted to help move the barium or hold it in place
   g. The small-bowel series prolongs the study by hours (see item 2e). The patient usually waits in the radiology department while films are taken every 15 to 20 minutes. Only when the contrast

medium has reached the terminal ileum will the patient be free to return to the nursing unit or home

h. If the patient is to wait in the x-ray department for the small-bowel series, suggest that she or he take something with them to help pass the time. The very ill or elderly patient should be monitored every 15 minutes at a minimum

4. Posttest care

a. Return to the usual diet unless other tests are scheduled

b. Fluids are given to tolerance to treat any dehydration because of the n.p.o. status and to assist in softening the stool to help in eliminating the barium or other contrast medium

c. The stool will be light or streaked with white if barium was used, and a laxative or enema may be ordered to help prevent constipation. Inform the patient of the importance of eliminating *all* of the barium to prevent obstruction

d. If the patient has an ulcer or ulcer symptoms, he or she should take an antacid or food as soon as possible on return from the test

5. Length of time needed

a. Barium swallow: 15 to 20 minutes

b. Upper GI series: 1 hour

c. Upper GI series with small-bowel series: 1 to 3 hours or longer (can be up to 5 hours), depending on how rapidly the barium moves

d. Enteroclysis: 1 hour

17.2.10 Mammogram

Synonyms: Breast radiography, breast xerography

Explanation of the Test. A mammogram is an x-ray examination of the breast on x-ray film. Xerography, a form of x-ray using paper rather than film, is frequently used for breast examination (see Section 17.1.2.F, "Xerography") because it exposes the person to less radiation than a regular x-ray.

Mammograms are used primarily to detect early breast cancers that are not palpable. Breast masses are usually not palpable until they are 1 cm in size. Mammograms are also taken to follow up after breast cancer surgery or treatment and for those patients at high risk for breast cancer. Cysts are also demonstrated by mammograms, but because they are often larger, they are usually palpable fairly early. The mammogram is considered much more diagnostic than conventional x-rays because the dense breast parts are sharply defined.

Persons at risk for breast cancer (family history in grandmother, mother, or sister) and those treated for other types of cancer may be asked to have yearly mammograms. Guidelines from the American Cancer Society, modified in 1983 and not updated since, recommend:

1. Age 20: Monthly breast self-examination
2. Ages 20 to 40: Physical examination of the breast at 3-year intervals
3. Ages 35 to 40: Annual baseline mammogram and/or breast physical exam
4. Ages 40 to 49: Annual or biennial mammograms or check with physician for individual assessment as to need
5. Age 50 on: Annual mammograms

(Dodd, G. p. 178, 1992)

Women who have had breast cancer resection should have yearly mammograms, regardless of age. Because a low-energy beam is used and because the mass of tissue exposed is small, the benefits of yearly mammograms are felt to outweigh the risk of radiation exposure.

Two or more views are taken by an x-ray technician (craniocaudal, lateral, and oblique) while the patient is seated or standing.

There are no contraindications to this test.

Ultrasound is often used to define characteristics of a mass suspected or seen on mammography. In many centers ultrasound localization, aspiration, and fine-needle biopsy is preferred to mammography.

IMPLICATIONS FOR NURSING: MAMMOGRAM

1. A permit is not required
2. Physical preparation: No physical preparation is required. In many facilities the use of deodorant, perfume, and powder are discouraged on the day of the test because the chemicals can interfere with the imaging. Dressing in a blouse, and slacks or skirt with a half-slip will facilitate clothing removal for the test
3. Patient education
   a. Because this test is known to be done primarily to diagnose or rule out cancer, the anxiety level is frequently quite high. The patient may benefit from knowing that approximately eight out of ten breast lumps are benign
   b. The patient should expect some discomfort, which is related to having the breasts exposed and held firmly in position against the film holder to eliminate skin folds and spread the breast tissue out as much as possible. The presence of chronic cystic breast disease or pendulous breasts will increase the discomfort. Pressure is only necessary for short periods at any one time, however
   c. This is a good time to assess whether the patient knows how to do a self-examination of the breasts and to provide written directions, as well as verbal instruction and demonstration, if needed. Make clear the advantages of early detection of any changes in breast tissue
4. Length of time needed: 45 minutes

17.2.11 Myelogram

Synonym: Myelography

Explanation of the Test. A myelogram is a fluoroscopic and radiological examination of the spinal canal, specifically the arachnoid space. Approximately 15 ml (from 5 to 15) of cerebral spinal fluid (CSF) is aspirated, and contrast medium (radiopaque material or air) is injected into the lumbar area by lumbar puncture. This test is done in the x-ray department by a radiologist, a neurologist, a neurosurgeon, or an orthopedic surgeon.

The radiopaque material can either be water soluble or have an oil base. If an oil-based material is used, it must be removed from the canal after the test because it cannot be absorbed and eliminated by the body. (It can be left in place, with special precautions for the patient's comfort and well-being, if the test is to be repeated, to spare the patient a second lumbar puncture.) Usually after removal of the CSF and injection of an oil-based material, the lumbar puncture needle is left in place for aspiration of the contrast medium after the test.

The contrast medium outlines the spinal cord and nerve roots to show any distortion. It is used when compression of spinal nerve roots or posterior fossa neural structures is suspected. The best known cause for its use is the suspicion of a ruptured intravertebral disk.

Oil contrast medium is heavier than spinal fluid and does not mix with the water-based spinal fluid, so the x-ray table must be tilted down at the head to allow the material to flow in that direction and visualize the upper portion of the spinal cord. Usually the patient is placed in a prone position on the table. The flow of the contrast material, and the outlining of structures is observed under fluoroscopy, and x-ray films are taken. Several different positions of the table may be necessary to adequately visualize the full spinal canal. The contrast material is not allowed to flow up into CSF circulation.

IMPLICATIONS FOR NURSING: MYELOGRAM

1. A permit is required
2. Physical preparation
   a. Check for iodine allergy (shellfish, previous contrast medium)
   b. The patient should be kept n.p.o. from 4 to 8 hours before the test. If the test is scheduled for the afternoon, usually a light or liquid lunch is given
   c. A bowel preparation (cleansing enema, suppository) may be ordered for the evening before or in the early morning of the day of the test
   d. Some premedication for anxiety and comfort may also be ordered. If none is and the patient is anxious, request such an order
   e. If metrizamide (a water-soluble iodine contrast medium) is used, the physician may give a loading dose of phenytoin (Dilantin) before the procedure because metrizamide may cause generalized seizures if it enters the cranial subarachnoid space
3. Patient education
   a. Determine the client's/family's previous knowledge and beliefs about the procedure. Help clarify misconceptions. Determine what information is wanted first, and start teaching with it
   b. Explain the steps in the preparation and procedure, and provide a rationale for each
   c. Be sure to explain the need for the multiple strap restraints while the patient is on the x-ray table, which are used more to keep the patient safe from falling as the table is tilted than to keep the patient "down." She or he will not be restrained, except by physical support, during the lumbar puncture
4. Posttest care
   a. If the dye is to be left in place, the head of the bed must be slightly elevated to prevent meningeal irritation, which causes severe headache. This is true whether the contrast medium is being left there to be absorbed (with water-soluble contrast media or air) or whether the material is left in place for further study at a later time. Oil-based dyes are ordinarily removed with the injecting syringe
   b. Bed rest is usually necessary for several hours after the test. When oil-based dyes are used and removed, the patient will be kept flat, often in a prone position, for 6 to 8 hours. At times the patient must be kept flat for 24 hours or longer if the dye could not be removed because of an obstruction. Turning from side to side is permitted, but the spinal column may not be bent
   c. Free fluids, to 2400 ml, are important in helping replace the CSF, to help the dye be absorbed, and to prevent a headache. Explain this, and have fluids easily accessible (unless contraindicated)

d. Neural and sensory function of the lower extremities will be assessed after the test to ensure that there has been no nerve damage during the test

e. It is important for the urine output to be recorded. Because of possible meningeal irritation or arachnoiditis, myleography can temporarily interrupt neural function. Urine retention is not an uncommon side effect because of this

f. Vital signs will be recorded every 4 hours for the 24 hours after the test to check for hemodynamic changes (e.g., drop in BP) related to a late hypersensitivity response

g. Because of possible irritation of the meninges by the contrast medium, the patient may have a headache. Because of the need to lie quietly on the x-ray table plus understandable tension, as well as possible muscle pain from the underlying problem for which the test was done, analgesics will be made available and should be taken to allow rest

h. Nausea and vomiting occur in a small percentage of those tested. Very rarely seizure activity occurs because of the meningeal irritation. Antiemetics and antiseizure drugs may be ordered on a p.r.n. basis; if not, they can be requested

5. Length of time needed: Usually about 1 hour

17.3 ANGIOGRAMS

An angiogram is literally a picture (gram) of a vessel or the vasculature (angio). In practice, it is a method of x-ray used to examine the transportation systems of the body, the arteries, the veins, and the lymphatic channels. The angiographic examination of each transport system can be and usually is designated specifically by using the system's name (i.e., lymphogram, venogram, and arteriogram). The general term *angiogram* is often used interchangeably with arteriogram.

An angiogram involves the injection of a contrast medium into a vessel through a catheter selectively placed to visualize a specific part of the system under review. The catheter placement is done under fluoroscopy by a radiologist. Cineradiography (see Section 17.1.2.E) is frequently used as well. Angiograms, especially arteriograms, are often given names that coincide with the vessels to be studied or the vessel used for access. The most common site for contrast medium injection for arteriograms is the femoral artery.

Angiograms are invasive studies (i.e., a substance is introduced into the body by an orifice other than a natural one) and as such, they carry a higher risk of harm than noninvasive studies. They also tend to cause the patient more apprehension and may have more discomfort associated with them.

17.3.1 Lymphangiograms

Synonym: Lymphograms

Explanation of the Test. A lymphangiogram is an x-ray examination using a special contrast medium to visualize lymph vessels and nodes in the legs, pelvis, abdomen, and less commonly, the chest (axillary and supraclavicular nodes). The contrast medium used is an iodine contrast oil (Ethiodol). The lymph system is a very fine network that is not palpable, as are the venous and arterial systems. This is overcome by first injecting a dye (Evans blue) into peripheral tissues (webs of toes or rarely fingers). The blue dye is picked up by the lymph system in about one-half hour. A lymph vessel can then be dissected (similar to a vein "cutdown") under local anesthesia and a small cannula and catheter (no. 126 or smaller) inserted under fluoroscopy to carry the iodine contrast medium. The iodine is infused very slowly, over at least 1 1/2 hours, using a pump. Once the contrast material has been injected, x-ray films are taken. X-ray films are again taken in 24 hours. By that time the contrast medium should have reached the area's lymphatic nodes. The lymphatic system retains the contrast medium for a matter of weeks, months, or even up to a year. One advantage to this long retention is that follow-up x-ray films can be taken over long periods without the need to inject more contrast material. However, the retained dye is rarely visible for more than 48 hours.

Purpose. Lymphangiograms are done to determine the presence of retroperitoneal lymphomas in patients with Hodgkin's disease, for staging of malignant lymphomas, to identify lymph node involvement in malignancies, to detect abnormal lymphatic structure, and to check on the effects of therapy.

IMPLICATIONS FOR NURSING: LYMPHANGIOGRAMS

1. A permit is required
2. Physical preparation
   a. Check for a history of iodine allergy (shellfish, previous contrast medium) and allergies to local anesthetics. Inform the physician and radiologist of any positive findings
   b. There is no restriction of food or fluids
   c. A sedative is frequently ordered because the procedure is prolonged and rather uncomfortable at times and requires that the patient remain still while the lymph vessel is isolated and the contrast medium injected
   d. An oral antihistamine preparation is usually ordered for patients at risk for an allergic response. For a severe allergy a noniodine dye can be used or the test cancelled
   e. The part to be injected, usually the foot, will need to be thoroughly cleaned
3. Patient education
   a. Explain the procedure and pretest preparation simply and completely, and give a rationale for each step. The entire examination is done lying down. After the area is sterilized a blue tracer dye is injected into a cannulated vein at the top of a foot to visualize lymph channels. This takes from 2 to 3 hours
   b. Be sure the patient is aware of how much time is to be spent in the x-ray department (e.g., all morning) and that she or he will have to return to the x-ray department the following day for a short session of follow-up x-rays when the contrast medium gets to the nodes. There will be no further injections of contrast material the second day, however
   c. Analgesics will be available for comfort
   d. The affected limb is often elevated to facilitate lymphatic drainage and prevent edema
4. Posttest care
   a. Inform the patient that the blue dye used to locate lymph vessels will stain the skin for up to 48 hours and then should disappear. Also inform the patient that the blue dye is excreted in both the urine and the stool and can be expected to stain them for several days after the test
   b. The patient will be on bed rest for about 24 hours posttest as ordered by the physician. She or he can expect to be quite tired after the test as well. The patient's feet should remain dry for 3 days because of possible contamination of the stitches
   c. If the lymph channels of the upper part of the body are visualized, the chest will be carefully assessed after the test because it is possible for the contrast medium to enter the lungs through the thoracic duct, which can cause an upper respiratory irritation and possible infection. It will be

important then to change position every 2 hours, deep breathe, and cough to keep the lungs expanded and clear. The health team will also observe carefully for respiratory complications
  d. There will be small stitches at the point of the injection that should not be allowed to get wet for a day or two. The stitches are usually removed by 7 to 10 days
  e. Any discomfort or numbness distal to the incision in the affected extremity should be reported. Discomfort could be related to inflammation or infection at the injection site. Numbness could indicate some peripheral nerve trauma
5. Length of time needed
  a. Three to 5 hours for initial test
  b. Fifteen to 30 minutes the second day

17.3.2 Venograms

Synonyms: Venography, phlebography, vascular evaluation

Explanation of the Test. A venogram is a fluoroscopic and x-ray examination of the venous system of a particular organ or body structure by using a contrast medium injected into a vein. It is used primarily to study the deep leg veins because it is the definitive test for deep vein thrombosis (DVT), which occurs primarily in the lower extremities. The test is also used to study the right side of the heart (see "Cardiac Catheterization," Section 17.3.6) to identify congenital venous abnormalities (e.g., arteriovenous fistula) and to identify a vein for cardiac arterial bypass grafting (CABG) before the surgery. As in a lymphogram or an arteriogram, a venogram shows only structure and flow. In cases of suspected DVT, a duplex ultrasound, if available, is usually done first as a screening procedure (See Section 17.6.1 "Impedence Plethysomography" [IPG]). A venogram is an invasive test, whereas duplex ultrasound is not; thus, the risks and discomfort associated with a venogram are greater.

Procedure. To do the test on a lower extremity, contrast medium (usually iodine based) is injected into either the ankle or the dorsum of the foot. The contrast material is preceded by a normal saline solution drip. A tourniquet may be placed above the ankle to retard the upward flow of the contrast material into superficial veins. The x-ray table is tilted, foot down, at a 40° to 60° angle to keep the dye in the distal veins longer, and no weight bearing is allowed on the leg being tested because this would cause a decreased vascular flow. The contrast material is injected slowly, and this is followed by fluoroscopy and x-ray films at intervals. After the test the injected vein is flushed with normal saline to help dilute and remove the dye. The patient will need to hold the leg absolutely still to prevent blurring of the films during the test.

IMPLICATIONS FOR NURSING: VENOGRAMS

1. A permit is required. In some facilities the permit will be obtained by the radiologist after she or he explains the test to the patient. The permit must be signed before any sedation is given
2. Physical preparation
  a. Assess for a history of iodine allergy (shellfish, previous contrast dye), and report any positive findings

b. Fluid and food restriction vary. In some facilities the patient will be n.p.o. after midnight; others require an n.p.o. status for only 4 hours before the test; still others restrict only food for 4 hours before the test, with clear fluids allowed up to the time of the test

c. A sedative may be ordered to decrease the patient anxiety

d. A skin test, antihistamines, or steroids may be ordered for those at risk for an allergic reaction

3. Patient education

a. Explain in simple-to-understand terms the steps of the procedure and preparation. Provide a rationale for each one step

b. The patient will need to know the signs and symptoms of a sensitivity response and should be requested to report any such occurrence. (See "Patient Education"—"Arteriogram")

4. Posttest care

a. Pulses in the affected leg should be checked on a routine basis

b. The injection site will be covered with a small bandage and should be checked for bleeding

c. The extremity may be elevated

d. Fluids will be offered to tolerance, if not contraindicated, to help in the elimination of contrast material

5. Length of time needed: 30 minutes to 1 hour

17.3.3 Digital Radiography: Digital Subtraction Angiography

Synonyms: DSA, transverse digital subtraction, digital fluorography

Explanation of the Test. A refinement of angiography, this process is a hybrid test—an examination of the arteries by using a venogram.

Digital radiography has similarities to computerized tomography in that it uses a computer to remove distracting superimposed images (a process called *high spatial resolution*). Ordinary x-ray imaging loses information because it must present three-dimensional pictures in two-dimensional form. DSA provides "depth" by removing everything from an image except that which the doctor wants to see. (See Appendix E for more information.)

Procedure. As in the procedure for a venogram, in DSA the solutions are injected through a peripherally inserted catheter, introduced into a vein, and threaded through to the superior vena cava where the contrast medium is injected and follows the cardiac/pulmonary circulation. The contrast medium is administered by a mechanized injector at 14 ml/s, but at intervals to allow the pulmonary distribution to clear so that other vessel outlines are distinct. The process is observed by fluoroscopy and imaged by the computer after converting the image to a digital form.

Purpose. DSA is used for the evaluation of almost all soft-tissue structures of the body. It is invaluable for balloon angioplasty, visualizing abnormalities, as well as improving function after treatment (e.g., the kidney [renal vascular hypertension, renal tumors]); identification of persons at risk for cerebral vascular accident (stroke); preoperative evaluation of coronary arteries and aortofemoral occlusive disease, aneurysm, and vascular mapping of suspected hypervascular abdominal tumors; postoperative evaluation of coronary artery bypass graft (CABG) patency and left ventricular wall motion (gated-wall study—see Section 17.4.1.C) patency of arterial grafts and endarterectomies; and cranial evaluation of suspected aneurysm/vascular malformations.

IMPLICATIONS FOR NURSING: DIGITAL RADIOGRAPHY: DIGITAL SUBTRACTION ANGIOGRAPHY

1. A permit is required
2. Physical preparation
   a. Assess for iodine allergy (shellfish or previous contrast dye)
   b. Restriction of food and fluid is variable. Check with the facility in which the test is to be done
   c. Sedation may be ordered to decrease anxiety and to help the patient remain still during the test. Movement will blur the picture
3. Patient education
   a. Explain the steps of the preparation and procedure, and give a rationale for each
   b. Caution the patient about the need to remain still during the test
   c. Inform the patient of early signs of an allergic response, and impress the need to report these to the radiologist or technician
   d. As with other central injection of contrast material, the patient may experience brief moments of nausea, a metallic/salty taste, and/or flushing. These are transitory and normal
   e. Glucagon may be given orally to decrease GI movement, which can also blur the picture
4. Length of time needed: From 30 to 45 minutes

17.3.4 Arteriograms

Synonym: Arteriography

Explanation of the Test. An arteriogram is a fluoroscopic and x-ray study of selected arteries. An arteriogram involves greater risks than does a venogram or a lymphangiogram in that arterial puncture involves the risk of hemorrhage and embolus formation. An arterial catheter is radiopaque, so its insertion can be checked under fluoroscopy. Usually, the catheter will be inserted into the femoral, brachial, or carotid artery, depending on what part of the arterial system is to be visualized. It will be advanced into position with a guide wire. (The carotid artery is rarely directly entered for tests because of the risk of disrupting athrosclerotic plaques and causing embolization into the cerebral circulation. Other arteries are used instead, or DSA is done. See the preceding section.) Ultrasound doppler may be used to determine the need for an arteriogram, depending on the vessels to be evaluated. Carotid duplex scanning, in conjunction with an MRI scan of the carotid vessels, has replaced carotid arteriograms in some centers. These tests are less invasive and less costly to perform, yet provide all necessary information for vascular surgery.

Purposes. Arteriograms are useful in determining the patency of arterial vessels, in indentifying abnormal vascularization (as with neoplasms), and in detecting lesions amenable to surgery.

GENERAL IMPLICATIONS FOR NURSING: ARTERIOGRAMS

1. A permit is required
2. Physical preparation
   a. The patient should be assessed for sensitivity to iodine (shellfish or previous contrast studies)
   b. Antihistamines or steroids may by ordered for administration before the injection of contrast material in allergy-susceptible individuals
   c. The patient will be n.p.o. 6 to 8 hours before the test. (In some facilities clear liquids are allowed up to the time of the test)
   d. Depending on the site for injection, an area may need to be shaved, although this is usually done in the radiology department
3. Patient education
   a. Steps in the preparation and procedures need to be explained clearly, yet simply, with an adequate rationale for each
   b. The patient will need to know the expected and nonthreatening sensations she or he may have in response to the contrast medium used (flushed, warm sensation, brassy or salty taste, transient nausea)
   c. Early signs of allergic response should be explained (nausea, vomiting, palpitations, dizziness, dyspnea), and the need should be stressed for the patient to tell the radiologist or technologist of these signs and symptoms as soon as they occur
4. Posttest care
   a. Extra fluid is important, if not contraindicated, to help replace fluids lost in the urine (a contrast medium acts as an osmotic diuretic) as well as help flush the contrast medium from the body
   b. Elimination of contrast medium may cause some slight dysuria, extra fluids will help prevent this as well
   c. Urine specific gravity will be higher than normal and therefore should not be used for assessment purposes until all the contrast material has been passed
   d. Food and fluid intake will be resumed as soon as all x-ray films have been taken. Some tests require a "post film"
   e. The site of arterial puncture will have a pressure dressing in place that should not be removed for at least 6 hours
   f. An ice bag may be placed on the puncture site to help constrict vessels and prevent bleeding
   g. Pulses distal to the puncture site will be checked at regular intervals of decreasing frequency
   h. Some discomfort may occur, and analgesics are usually ordered for this purpose. The patient should be instructed to report any pain distal to the puncture site because it may be related to clot formation or embolization
5. Length of time needed: Variable with the area being examined—from 30 minutes to 3 hours

17.3.5 Specific Arteriograms (Arteriography, Angiograms, Angiography)

See also "Arteriograms," Section 17.3.4.

A. Adrenal Arteriograms

1. Purpose: For detection of benign or malignant tumors that interfere with adrenal function (pheochromocytoma, adrenal adenomas, adrenal carcinomas) or the presence of bilateral adrenal hyperplasia
2. Possible complications include
   a. Allergic response to the contrast medium (dye)

    b. Hemorrhage secondary to arterial puncture

    c. Embolization because of dislodgement of an atherosclerotic plaque. (Complications a to c are true for all types of arteriograms)

    d. Severe, even fatal hypertension with pheochromocytoma. Usually alpha-adrenergic blockers (e.g., phenoxybenzamine [Dibenzyline]) and beta-adrenergic blockers (e.g., propranolol [Inderal]) will be given for several days before the test to prevent this complication from occurring

3. Contraindications (as for arteriograms in general plus items that follow)

    a. Severe sensitivity/allergic response to the contrast medium

    b. Physiologically or psychologically unstable patients

4. Procedure (see also "Arteriograms"): In this test a branch of the renal artery, the inferior adrenal artery, is cannulated to visualize the adrenal gland

5. Specific nursing implications

    a. Baseline vital signs are especially important, BP being of greatest import

    b. With a diagnosis of pheochromocytoma, check to be sure that alpha- and beta-adrenergic blockers have been ordered and administered for several days before the test. If not, consult with the physician

B. Brachial Arteriogram

1. Purpose: To observe structure, patency, and flow to an upper extremity

2. Possible complications: As for "Adrenal Arteriograms"

3. Contraindications: As for "Adrenal Arteriograms"

4. Procedure: The brachial artery is cannulated directly

5. Specific nursing implications

    a. BP must not be taken on the examined arm after the test because the distal circulation would be compromised

    b. Any distal pain or numbness should be reported immediately

C. Carotid Arteriograms

1. Purpose: Although usually preceded by a Doppler and/or duplex ultrasound scan, the arteriogram is used to determine the patency of the carotid artery or the reason for any abnormality. It is rarely done directly into the carotid artery because of an increased potential for transient ischemic attacks (TIA) and stroke

2. Possible complications: As for "Adrenal Arteriograms"

3. Contraindications: As for "Adrenal Arteriograms"

4. Procedure: This examination is not done directly into the carotid if that can be avoided because of the danger of dislodging atherosclerotic plaques into the cerebral circulation. The femoral artery is usually the site for cannulation. If that is not feasible, the axillary artery can be used

5. Specific nursing implications posttest

    a. With a femoral approach

        (1) The patient should be kept flat in bed for 6 hours. To prevent meningeal irritation the person's head should be raised slightly

        (2) With groin injection, the leg on the affected side should not be bent for 6 hours

  (3) Check vital signs and pedal pulses every 30 minutes for 4 hours

  (4) Check the site every 15 to 30 minutes for 4 hours for bleeding

  (5) If bleeding occurs, apply pressure directly on the puncture site, and notify the x-ray department

  (6) Resume the usual diet and fluids immediately after the test

 b. With an axillary approach

  (1) The patient may be up and about, but the affected arm should be immobilized for 6 hours. The use of a sling and binding to the chest is suggested

  (2) Vital signs and radial pulses should be checked every 15 minutes for 4 hours. BP is not taken in the affected arm

  (3) Check the arm for bleeding and swelling every 15 minutes for 4 hours. If bleeding occurs, apply pressure on the puncture site, and notify the x-ray department

 c. If the carotid has been directly cannulated (rare)

  (1) Have a tracheostomy set at the bedside

  (2) Check both temporal pulses with other vital signs, and compare one side with the other

  (3) Assess for signs and symptoms of transient ischemic attacks (TIA) (facial weakness, visual disturbance, or slurred speech) as well as evidence of difficulty in breathing or swallowing

D. Celiac Arteriogram; Hepatic Arteriogram

1. Purpose: To visualize one branch of the visceral arterial circulation, (e.g., the celiac trunk), to detect vascular and structural abnormalities. Many visceral organs and areas can be visualized (e.g., the upper part of the stomach, lower portion of the esophagus, pancreas, duodenum, gallbladder, and liver)
2. Possible complications: As for "Adrenal Arteriograms"
3. Contraindications: As for "Adrenal Arteriograms"
4. Procedure: Usually the femoral artery is cannulated and the catheter threaded into the desired area. If it is not feasible to use the femoral artery, the axillary artery can be used
5. Specific nursing implications (See also "Specific Arteriograms", Section 17.3.5): As for "Carotid Arteriogram"

E. Cerebral Arteriograms

Similar to the carotid test; the terms are often used interchangeably. A noninvasive approach, that is, a transcranial doppler, used in conjunction with a carotid duplex scan, yields information about cerebral circulation in a noninvasive way. Availability and cost are factors to be considered however.

1. Purpose: To detect abnormalities in cerebral circulation (aneurysm, occlusion, spasm, arteriovenous malformations, tumors, abscesses, and hematomas)
2. Possible complications: As for "Adrenal Arteriograms"
3. Contraindications: As for "Adrenal Arteriograms"
4. Procedure: The vertebral, subclavian, brachial, femoral, or common carotid arteries can be used for this study. Cerebral scans have almost replaced the use of cerebral or carotid arteriography as screening tests because of the decreased risks with a scan
5. Specific nursing implications

a. As for "Carotid Arteriograms" and

b. After the test: Neurological evaluation every 15 minutes for 4 hours; then every 30 minutes for 4 hours; then every hour for 4 hours; and every 4 hours thereafter, if still indicated

c. If access was through any arteries in or near the neck, assessment for swelling is especially important (hoarseness, difficulty in breathing). A tracheostomy set should be kept in the room and any abnormalities reported immediately

F. Femoral Arteriograms

1. Purpose: The femoral artery is often cannulated as an access to other, smaller arteries in both the upper and lower parts of the body. Therefore, all information under these other arteriograms applies here, depending on the site ultimately to be visualized

2. Possible complications: As for "Adrenal Arteriograms"

3. Contraindications: As for "Adrenal Arteriograms"

4. Procedure: See "Celiac Arteriograms" or "Carotid Arteriograms"

5. Specific nursing implications

   a. As for "Celiac Arteriograms"

   b. Pedal pulses should be checked. The use of a Doppler instrument may be necessary for this. Compare with the pretest baseline values

   c. Compare the warmth and sensation between the right and left legs and feet. Also compare the findings in the affected leg or foot with pretest baseline values

   d. Any increase in pain in the affected leg after the test should be reported immediately

G. Pulmonary Arteriograms

1. Purpose: This test is especially useful in examination of the pulmonary vessels, usually to support a diagnosis of pulmonary embolism after a positive lung scan result. It can also detect a variety of congenital abnormalities or acquired pulmonary lesions

2. Possible complications: As for "Adrenal Arteriograms" plus the patient should be monitored for cardiac arrhythmias during the arteriogram. The most frequently occurring arrhythmia is a premature ventricular contraction (PVC)

3. Contraindications: As for "Adrenal Arteriograms"

4. Procedure: Usually access to the pulmonary artery is through the femoral *vein*. The catheter is threaded through the vein to the inferior vena cava, through the right atrium and ventricle, and into the main pulmonary artery where the contrast medium is injected

5. Specific nursing implications: As for "Celiac Arteriograms" or "Femoral Arteriograms" plus the patient should be on a cardiac monitor if any arrhythmias occurred during the course of the examination

H. Renal Arteriograms (See also Renal Artery Doppler/Renal Sonogram)

1. Purpose: This test has been less frequently used as the first diagnostic study when the renal artery Doppler ultrasound test is available. Doppler may be done on both native and transplanted kidneys. When color doppler is added, renal artery stenosis can also be detected and renal perfusion qualitatively evaluated. Also, duplex scanning of a transplanted kidney can be used to evaluate rejection.

Renal arteriograms are still used, especially when ultrasound imaging is not available or when cost is a major problem. They provide information related to arthrosclerotic narrowing (stenosis) of the renal artery and can also be used to detect increased renal vascularization secondary to tumor growth.

2. Possible complications: As for "Adrenal Arteriograms"
3. Contraindications: As for "Adrenal Arteriograms"
4. Procedure: Again, the femoral artery is the insertion site of choice, and the catheter is threaded into the renal artery under the direction of fluoroscopy
5. Specific nursing implications
    a. As for all previous femoral cannulations
    b. BP should be carefully watched and compared with baseline findings. The procedure can cause a temporary decrease in renin production, which will cause the decrease in BP
6. Alternative scanning: If available and affordable, renal artery Doppler of both native and transplanted kidneys is often recommended as the first probable study, as is use of color Doppler for detection of renal artery stenosis and qualitative evaluation of renal perfusion. Duplex scanning of a transplanted kidney for possible rejection of the kidney is also recommended.

17.3.6 Cardiac Catheterization

Synonyms: Coronary arteriogram, angiocardiography, right and/or left heart catheterization

Results of echocardiography (17.5.C)—particularly Doppler—use before catheterization, to correlate findings about valve area pressure gradients in certain diseases, for example, stenosis/regurgitation, may eliminate need for cardiac catheterization.

Explanation of the Test. Cardiac catheterization is a very sophisticated test that requires a team of highly trained and skilled professionals to perform. Cardiac catheterization is performed by a cardiologist, usually in a special "cath lab." It is used when less invasive tests have not provided enough information to determine a course of treatment (often whether heart surgery is indicated). It involves an arteriogram of the coronary circulation and left heart chambers as well as a venogram of the right side of the heart and pulmonary circulation. The test

1. Visualizes coronary circulation and any deficits and pinpoints area(s) of obstruction
2. Checks BPs in the heart chambers
3. Measures the cardiac output and ejection fractions through each valve
4. Identifies congenital malformations and cardiac enlargement

Results of echocardiography, and Doppler in particular, are often used to correlate with cardiac catheterization. They are especially useful with regard to valve areas and pressure gradients in certain defects (e.g., stenosis and regurgitation). The echocardiogram is done before the catheterization, and if the findings warrant it, cardiac catheterization may not need to be done.*

---

*Thanks are due to Susan Adams, B.S., R.D.M.S., R.D.C.S., and Andrea Skelley, B.S., R.D.M.S., R.D.C.S., for revisions to this section.

Procedure. A long catheter is passed into a peripheral artery, usually the brachial or the femoral artery, and/or a vein, often the antecubital or femoral vein, and threaded by means of a guide wire into the heart by way of the aorta (arterial line) or the vena cava (venous line). The catheter has sensors at the tip to read chamber pressures, and flow rates can also be measured. The full process is followed with fluoroscopy. An arterial catheterization is also referred to as a left heart catheterization because the catheter enters the left heart in a retrograde fashion. The venous approach can be called a right heart catheterization in which the catheter enters the right atrium through the vena cava. It is then "floated" into the right ventricle and into the pulmonary artery. Pulmonary artery pressure and pulmonary wedge pressure (a reflection of left heart pressure in the pulmonary arterioles) can be checked by this catheter, as can be heart chamber pressures. It is also possible to check the left side of the heart with a venous catheter. When the catheter enters the right atrium, it can be maneuvered transeptally through a potential opening in the atrial septum, a remnant of fetal development, which can sometimes be opened by forcing the catheter through, or a needle puncture of the septum can be done. The increased BP of the left heart seals the septum, thus preventing backflow. Cardiac catheterization also checks the blood flow rate on both sides of the heart and actual coronary perfusion with the use of a radiopaque contrast medium introduced through the catheter, observed with fluoroscopy, and recorded with cineradiography (see Section 17.1.2.E). Blood samples are tested in the various chambers to check oxygen saturation. The patient is placed on a cardiac monitor for the full procedure because catheter irritation of heart muscle might cause an arrhythmia. The test is contraindicated for patients with gross cardiomegaly and those physiologically unstable enough to require intense nursing care at all times.

Results of echocardiography and Doppler in particular (see "Ultrasound Diagnostic Tests," Section 17.5.1.C, "Echocardiograms") are often used to correlate with cardiac catheterization, especially with regard to valve area and pressure gradients in certain diseases (e.g., stenosis and regurgitation). In these instances, the echocardiogram is done before the cardiac catheterization, and, if the data obtained are good enough, the catheterization is not done (Adams & Skelley, 1993).

IMPLICATIONS FOR NURSING: CARDIAC CATHETERIZATION

1. A permit is necessary. The physician is responsible for discussing the procedure, the risk factors, and the possible complications versus benefits with the patient and family before the consent is signed

2. Physical preparation

   a. Usually the patient will be kept n.p.o. for 6 to 8 hours before the test. There is a danger of aspiration in emergency situations

   b. Check for sensitivity to local anesthetics (used with arterial catheter insertion) and iodine (shellfish or previous contrast studies), and report any positive findings. Give any ordered antihistamines or steroids

   c. The dosage of any oral anticoagulants may be decreased, or use of the drug discontinued, to prevent excess bleeding. Heparin may be ordered, however, as a short-acting anticoagulant to prevent thrombosis. Other routine medications may be withheld but are usually given

   d. Usually no bowel preparation is ordered, but the patient should void and empty his or her bowel, if possible before the test

   e. Check baseline vital signs, with special attention to BP and peripheral pulses. Check radial, apical, and pedal pulses, at a minimum
   f. The skin preparation is usually done in the "cath lab," but shaving the groin may be requested before the test
   g. Check the patient's height and weight, and record. These measurements are used to calculate the amount of contrast medium necessary
   h. Premedications (often merperidine [Demerol] with diazepam [Valium] or hydroxyzine pamoate [Vistaril]) are given to decrease anxiety and provide comfort through the long test
   i. The patient will be awake, and most facilities allow patients to keep dentures in place and wear a watch and glasses if they wish
3. Patient education
   a. Explain the procedure and pretest preparation as needed after the physician's explanation, and give rationales
   b. The patient will need to be prepared for the physical reaction to the contrast medium. Central delivery of contrast medium tends to cause a more severe and prolonged "rush" of heat to the patient's head along with a metallic taste for a minute or so
   c. An intravenous line will be started in the cath lab to provide access for medication as needed
   d. The patient may be given nitroglycerin sublingually to help dilate the coronary arteries for contrast media filling, not necessarily for angina
   e. The arterial puncture, even with local anesthesia, is usually somewhat uncomfortable
   f. As the catheter enters the ventricle, the patient may feel a "flutter," a "missed beat," or a "racing" pulse. Assure the patient that this is transitory and due to the irritation of the heart by the catheter and that the heart is monitored constantly by an electrocardiograph (ECG) visible to the cardiologist
   g. The patient will have to lie still for a protracted period of time on the hard x-ray table. The patient needs to know that the table position will change from time to time, even though she or he does not move on it
4. Posttest care
   a. Vital signs, particularly pedal, apical, and radial pulses, will be taken at lengthening intervals for at least 4 hours
   b. The patient may be placed on a cardiac monitor
   c. The intravenous line will remain in place for at least 12 hours
   d. Bed rest is usually required. With arterial puncture, bed rest for 6 to 12 hours is usual. (See "Posttest Nursing Implications for Arteriograms," Section 17.3.4)
   e. The patient should report any dyspnea, and the nurse will check for or ask about changes in pulses and BP (dyspnea, narrowing of pulse pressure, paradoxical pulse, and distended neck veins when the patient sits forward are signs of cardiac tamponade, a rare but possible complication)
5. Length of time needed: 1 to 3 hours

17.4 NUCLEAR DIAGNOSTIC TESTS: SCANS AND IMAGING

Synonyms: Radionuclide imaging studies, scans; scintiscan; scintiphotography; radioisotope scans

Explanation of the Process. Radionuclide studies are usually done in a department of nuclear medicine within a hospital or other medical facility. This department is concerned with both therapeutic and diagnostic uses of radioactive materials. (See Appendix E for a discussion of radionuclides/radioisotopes and radiopharmaceuticals.) Radionuclides used in nuclear medicine *or nuclear diagnostic testing* generally have half-lives of 24 hours or less. Radionuclides can be used for both in vitro *and* in vivo testing. For in vitro testing samples from the body are collected after a radionuclide has been given orally or intravenously, depending on what is to be imaged, and the sample is tested for the degree of radioactivity uptake. Examples of in vitro tests include blood volume, red cell mass, red cell survival and the Schilling Test. The in vivo tests measure the amount of radionuclide uptake in a specific area or organ within the body. This section deals only with in vivo tests (i.e., radionuclide scans).

Still, the most common type of imaging device presently used for radionuclide scans is the gamma scintillation camera. It detects gamma rays emitted by the radionuclide the patient has inhaled, ingested, or had injected, similar to the action of a Geiger counter. The rays are converted into two-dimensional images on an oscilloscope screen. The results are then transferred to x-ray film. A computer can be used to enhance the statistical difference of radionuclide concentrations in normal versus abnormal tissues, hence the term *computer-enhanced nuclear scans.*

The scanning may be done immediately after the radionuclide has been given, or it may be done hours later. The delay time before scanning depends on the length of time it takes the specific tissue being scanned to take up the radionuclide and localize it. The scan can be produced as a black-and-white dot matrix or more usefully in shades of gray where better definition is possible. Color imaging is a more recent technique that requires computer assistance and is, perhaps, the more easily read. The shades of gray or color vary with the relative distribution of the radionuclide in different parts of the tissue or organ.

Diagnostic scanning is based on an understanding of:

TABLE 17–1. RADIOPHARMACEUTICAL SPECIFICITY

Tissue or Organ	Radionuclide
Bone	Technetium tagged to phosphate (Tc-99m)
Brain	Radioiodinated human serum albumin (RISHA)
	Diethylene triamine pentaacetic acid (DTPA)
	Technetium 99m (Tc-99m) pertechnetate or glucohaptanate—for perfusion study
Gallbladder	Tc-99m + EHIDA
	Tc-99m + PIPIDA
	Tc-99m + DISIDA (hepatolite)
Heart	Thallium 201 (^{201}T, Th-201)—for perfusion scan
	Tc-99m pyrophosphate
	Albumin or red blood cells (RBCs) tagged with Tc-99m—for ejection fraction studies
Kidneys (renal)	I-131-Hippuran (iodohippurate sodium)
	Tc-99m + DTPA, DSMA (Glucohapatanate)—for static view
	I-131 or I-123 tagged to orthoiodohippurate
Liver	Tc-99m tagged to sulfur colloid
Lung	Tc-99m with albumin—for perfusion study
	Krypton 91 (Kr-91)—for lung ventilation scan
	Xenon 133 (Xe-133)—for lung ventilation scan
Thyroid	Tc-99m pertechnetate—for screening
	Iodine 123 (I-123)—for screening and/or uptake
	Iodine 131 (I-131)—for uptake
Total-body scans	Gallium citrate (Ga-67)—for inflammatory lesions and neoplasms
	Tagged leukocytes with In-111—for inflammatory lesions only

Data from Corbett, 1983; Fischbach, 1984; and SHMC, 1985.

1. The specificity of a particular radiopharmaceutical for the organ or tissue being examined (See Table 17–1)
2. The expected distribution ("hot spots" indicate an increased uptake of the radionuclide that images very darkly; "cold spots" indicate a decreased uptake of the radionuclide that images lighter) of the radiopharmaceutical in the organ or tissue under "normal" versus diseased conditions

The most commonly used radionuclide for diagnostic testing is technetium (Tc-99m). It may be combined with organ-specific compounds, such as phosphorus for bone, or given alone. A non-radioactive blocking agent such as potassium chloride used with technetium in brain scans helps to prevent excessive uptake of the radioactive substance by tissues other than those to be studied.

Timing of the scan after administration of the radionuclide depends on the speed with which the material is taken up by the part to be scanned. The time can vary from an immediate uptake to a period of 24 to 72 hours, as in total-body gallium scans for infectious disease or tumor.

Generally, radionuclide scans are contraindicated for pregnant women and growing children unless no other diagnostic measure will suffice. (With new techniques now under study this stricture may not apply. Check with the nuclear medicine department doing the test.) The 14-day rule (see "Explanation of the Process" under "X-ray," Section 17.1) for women of childbearing age applies here. Mothers should be cautioned not to nurse their infants while having nuclear tests performed.

17.4.1 Commonly Used Nuclear Tests

A. Bone Scans

Synonym: Three-stage bone scan

Purpose. Bone scans are used to check for metastatic lesions of primary cancers, particularly breast and prostatic cancer. They are also used to detect early bone disease, such as osteoporosis, osteomyelitis, osteoarthritis, stress fractures, as well as bone response to antineoplastic agents. A three-stage bone scan is used to evaluate inflammatory joint disease, bony infection (e.g., osteomyelitis), and/or injury.

Procedure. The patient is injected intravenously 1½ to 3 hours before to the scan. She or he will have to lie supine or prone for the entire study, approximately 1 hour. One and one half to 3 hours after the injection the patient is taken to the nuclear medicine department for the scan to be done. In the three-stage bone scan the patient goes to the nuclear medicine department for the intravenous injection. Blood flow and blood pool images are taken at that time and bone images later.

IMPLICATIONS FOR NURSING: BONE SCANS

1. Usually a specific permit is not required
2. Physical preparation: Except for having the patient empty his or her bladder to decrease bladder activity and to increase visibility, there is no physical preparation. A sedative may be ordered if the

patient has difficulty remaining in one position for long periods. When technetium is used, water intake is forced to at least six glasses, unless contraindicated, to help in the distribution of the radionuclide

3. Patient education
   a. Explain the steps of the procedure, especially the purpose of the waiting period after the injection, and the preparation, providing adequate rationales
   b. There is no restriction in activity before the test
   c. Explain the limited dose of radiation involved with the scan, its short half-life, and the lack of radiation danger to the patient or any visitors
   d. In a whole-body bone scan, the camera and/or the scanning bed will move as the picture is being taken. Static images of a specific area are often also required. The image is similar to a time exposure of regular film. There is no radiation from the scanner. It simply identifies the concentration of the radioisotope in the patient's body and records it
   e. Explain the importance of moving only when and as instructed to prevent blurring the image
   f. Any jewelry or other metallic material that might obscure the area of study should be removed
   g. Assess female clients for possible pregnancy and inform the department doing the test if possible, or diagnosed. The fetus will need protection from ionizing rays

4. Posttest care
   a. The patient can return to his or her usual activities of daily living as soon as the test is completed
   b. The radiopharmaceutical used for bone scanning is excreted by the kidneys, so urine should be handled with appropriate precautions. Urine samples should not be taken for analysis for 24 hours, and nurses should wear gloves when emptying catheter bags in this period

5. Length of time needed
   a. Total of 2 to 4½ hours from the time of the intravenous injection
   b. Approximately 1 hour for the scan itself

B. Brain Scans

Synonyms: Cerebral flow scan, brain circulation scan, isotope brain scan, radionuclide brain scan

Purpose. A scan is done primarily to evaluate the distribution of the radiopharmaceutical carried in the vessels and tissues of the brain. Brain scans are useful in detecting intracranial masses but do not differentiate the type of mass or lesion located. They can be used to establish brain death as well as evaluate herpes simplex encephalitis, dementia, and seizures (Detmer, 1992, p. 24). They are helpful in locating areas of cerebral ischemia, infarction, or hemorrhage, and they are used to evaluate a lesion's response to therapy or status postoperatively. The timing of a brain scan is important in its use. For example, in cases of CVA there will be no pathology evident on a brain scan for about a week or more than a month after the event. A cerebral thrombosis without infarction may never produce an abnormal brain scan result.

Two types of brain scans are usually done—a circulation or perfusion study (cerebral flow, brain circulation) and a static image study, which is used to help determine the site of the pathological tissue. If a lesion has damaged the blood–brain barrier, more of the radionuclide will enter the cerebral circulation, diffuse into and localize in the area of the lesion, thereby causing a "hot spot."

Procedure. Agitated patients may be sedated prior to the test. The patient may receive a blocking agent (e.g., potassium chloride or perchlorate) in the form of a tasteless capsule or a rather flat tasting liquid about one-half hour before an intravenous injection of the radionuclide. If a circulation or flow scan is to be done, images will be taken immediately after the radionuclide injection. Flow dynamics are compared between the two sides of the brain, and images are stored for later study. One and one half to 4 hours later the static brain scan views are done, the isotope having become localized in the brain tissues. Each picture takes up to 5 to 10 minutes. Isotopes preferentially localize in abnormal regions of the brain such as within tumors, subdural hematomas, and abscesses (only the outer rim of the abscess takes up the isotope).

IMPLICATIONS FOR NURSING: BRAIN SCAN

1. A permit is not required
2. Physical preparation: As for "Bone Scan" (see Section 17.4.1.A)
3. Patient education
   a. As for "Bone Scan" to include caution in pregnancy due to potential for fetal harm from ionizing radiation
   b. For cerebral blood flow (circulation) studies, the patient is placed in a supine position for the isotope injection, and the scanner will be placed over her or his head immediately
   c. To maintain the position of the head during each image, the technologist may use masking tape across the patient's forehead
4. Posttest care: The patient's urine should not be used for urine testing for at least 24 hours after the radionuclide injection. (The half-life of Technetium 99 is 6 hours)
5. Length of time needed
   a. For cerebral circulation/flow study, 15 minutes
   b. For static brain scan, maximum of 1 hour
   c. Total time including the administration of a blocking agent and radionuclide plus both scans, 4 hours

---

C. Cardiac Nuclear Scans (Radioisotope scans/radionuclide imaging; scintiscans/scintigram/scintigraphy)

Definition of Terms. *Nuclear scans* are those that make use of radioactive isotopes, used for diagnosis. Radioactive isotopes are those that emit radiation as they disintegrate. Each isotope tends to concentrate in specific body areas and tends to do so at a higher rate if the area is diseased.

Scintiscan* refers to the use of camera detection of the isotopes. Cameras are used for imaging the body reaction; that is, hypofunction (light areas on the film = hypofunction; dark areas = hyperfunction; also called "cold spots" and "hot spots").

---

*Scintigrams or scintiscans are defined as those in vivo tests utilizing a scintillation camera that are displayed using the gray scale, that is, shades of gray rather than black and white as in x-rays. Scintigrams can be used to localize the area and assess the status of the infarct in myocardial infarction and to evaluate the response to pharmacological therapy and the effects of cardiotoxic drugs (Miller & Keane, p. 477). (See 17.4, "Explanation of the Process.")

This section of tests is made up of a number of separate tests that can be divided into two broad categories: (1) perfusion studies (studies of blood delivery throughout the heart/presence of infarcts); (2) ventriculography (evaluation of ventricular wall motion; ventricular function; hypertrophy).

Cardiac Nuclear Test Uses (General)

1. Evaluation of chest pain and/or ECG changes and determination of cause
2. Pre- and post–operative follow-up on effectiveness of coronary artery bypass surgery (e.g., increased myocardial perfusion)
3. Myocardial dysfunction: Primary disease and/or follow-up evaluation of cardiac function
4. Screening for infarction (suspected or previously diagnosed)

Contraindications for Cardiac Nuclear Scans

1. Pregnancy (usually)
2. Recent nuclear scans may interfere

Explanation of the Process. Although the tests in this section can be done individually, generally more than one is done, especially in the process of diagnosis rather than follow-up. Individual tests often have multiple names applied to them such as "radionuclide ventriculography," that refers primarily to gated-wall (or pool) ejection fractions.

Multigated Acquisition Scans

Synonyms: MUGA; gated equilibrium heart scan

Explanation of the Process. MUGA is an additive to scanning that involves synchronized monitoring of cardiac function by electrocardiograph (ECG) and scintillation camera (a gallium scan). The ECG activity triggers the scintillation camera that then images cardiac blood flow as well as cardiac muscle (wall motion) function at specific, predetermined points through several cardiac cycles. From one to 64 points in a *single* cardiac cycle can be recorded and up to 1000 cardiac cycles may be imaged. The data recorded are compiled by a computer, indicating, for example, the time interval (fractions of a second) between one R wave peak to the next (these time intervals are referred to as *gates*, hence the test name) or whatever cardiac activity is to be examined. The data are then compared by computer to a norm for cardiac function, and a printout is done of the ECG as well as of sequential heart images. The later provide a "moving picture" of the heart. As indicated, several testing approaches can be assisted with the addition of MUGA.

Purpose. MUGA (or gated) studies are used to evaluate myocardial health and cardiac blood pool/wall function in persons with suspected or known cardiomyopathies (e.g., ischemic heart disease secondary to bundle branch block, myocardial infarct [MI]), to localize the area and assess the status of the dysfunction, and to evaluate response to pharmacological therapy or effects of cardiotoxic drugs.

Patient Preparation for Nuclear or Scintillation Scans. Red blood cells (RBCs) may be "harvested" from the patient prior to the test. These cells are labeled with a radionuclide (usually Tc-99m/technetium, a very unstable form with a half-life of only 6 hours) and reinjected. Or the cells may remain in the bloodstream and be labeled by IV injection. In this case, the process of labeling first consists of an injection of a nonradioactive substance to which RBCs bind in the plasma such as HiSnPyrophosphate. One-half hour later an IV injection of Tc-99m/technetium is done to provide the radioactive substance for imaging.

1. First Pass Imaging

Synonym: First transit studies

Procedure. With the gamma ray scanner over the supine patient's chest (precordium), the labeled cells, pumped by myocardial contraction, pass through the valves for the first time. If further tests are to be done, the patient is repositioned a total of four times (lateral, right and left oblique) as the scanner images the complete heart and its activity. MUGA is rarely used if only the first pass test is to be done. No patient preparation is usually necessary other than that of providing the patient with an overview of what the testing will be and how long it can be expected to last. The test duration will depend on how many of the tests in this sequence will be done at one session. Check with the department doing the study or studies.

Purpose. The test provides a rapid and relatively easy way to evaluate ventricular function, at rest or after exercise. Often used as an early, singular screening test for heart valve function, it also shows the shape or structure of the ventricles (which, when recorded on film, are also called ventriculograms).

Time Required. Immediate. The first pass study can be done as a separate test or as the first step of a total gated-wall motion study. It is especially useful in *right* ventricle evaluation. Right heart findings are not included in the selective computerized program of gated imaging. Contrary to left heart studies, which are preprogrammed, computer regions of interest for right heart study must be individually selected (e.g., function of the right heart valve; amount of tracer left in the ventricle; shape and structure of the ventricles; presence of any atrial ventricular (AV) shunts usually from right to left heart).

2. Ejection Fraction

Synonyms: EF; gated EF, gated pool/wall imaging ejection fraction

Explanation of the Test. Ejection fraction (EF) is defined as the percentage of total ventricular volume ejected during each heart contraction, (i.e., stroke volume divided by end-diastolic volume).

Procedure. This test is almost always combined with MUGA testing, i.e., gated, and is rarely done in a single test. Cardiac atrial and diastolic function is imaged using a contrast agent.

Technetium-99m pertechnate or technetium-labeled albumin is often used as the radioactive substance for computer measurement of ejection fractions (EFs). Computers calculate the cardiac output of both ventricles and printouts are done to show both resting and stressed ejection fractions (see also Thallium scan stress test) as well as any abnormalities. The ejection fraction is reliable for ventricles of any size, even ones with aneurysm.

Patient Preparation. The patient, after having IV lines inserted for the contrast agent, is asked to lie as quietly as possible and not to talk during the actual imaging, so that it need not be repeated. The scanning can be interrupted, if necessary, but will prolong the imaging time. No other patient preparation is required.

Time Required. Scanning to pick up cardiac output (ejection fraction) alone usually takes a total of 1/2 hr. or less. If the full MUGA test is done, the time is greatly extended.

Purpose. This test is a frequently used index of ventricular, especially right ventricular (RV), function.

NORMAL EF FINDING (RESTING):

1. Sixty-five to 75 percent of normal end-diastolic volume right ventricle
2. Over 55 to 65 percent left ventricle
3. Lesser values indicate decreased cardiac contractility

EF INCREASED BY:

1. Increased contractility (e.g., increased sympathetic nervous system activity)
2. Decreased contractility (e.g., heart failure; MI)
3. Increased afterload (e.g., arterial hypertension)
4. Decreased afterload (e.g., decreased peripheral resistance) (McCance & Huether, p. 883).

Imaging agents used. Tc-99 (pyrophosphate) or technetium pertechnetate

Time Required. Immediate; both ventricles are studied.

ABNORMAL FINDINGS IN:

• Decreased output with myocardial damage (e.g., infarction, decreased perfusion)

3. Gated Blood Pool Imaging

Synonym: Gated wall motion study

Purpose. To provide information on left ventricular muscle function or coronary blood distribution by computerized photography (motion picture images) of the myocardial wall while in motion (wall motion study) through several cardiac cycles. It is especially useful in *right* ventricle evaluation.

1. Imaging agent: Tc-99 (pyrophosphate) or technetium pertechnetate (used in four different projections of the heart) are employed.
2. Time required: Immediate imaging is obtained, followed by 1 or 2 hours of continuous imaging.
3. Findings:
    a. information on both left and right ventricular function and on cardiac output
    b. detecting LV aneurysms (sensitivity and specificity: >90%).

4. Thallium Scans: Stress and Resting Tests

Synonyms: Myocardial perfusion scan, exercise thallium profusion imaging test, thallium stress test

---

Explanation of the Test. Thallium scans are noninvasive, radionuclear cardiac scans. Several different imaging materials can be used, the most common being thallium-201, technetium-99m pertechnate, or technetium-99m pyrophosphate.

Purpose. All normal myocardial cells take up thallium, thus ischemic or infarcted cells appear as "cold spots" on scanning. Tc-99m pyrophosphate is taken up only by ischemic cells. Thus, poorly perfused or ischemic areas such as infarcts, will appear as "hot spots" with this test. That is, normal myocardium will show greater thallium activity than poorly perfused myocardium.

Indication for Use of Stress Test. In borderline situations there may be no evidence of myocardial ischemia in the resting state. Testing while stressing the cardiovascular system (i.e., stress testing) may be done. The patient must be closely monitored throughout stress testing.

Procedure. Usually, and preferably, the patient is in a fasting state for perfusion scans. Thallium 201 is given IV while the patient exercises, usually on a treadmill. Close monitoring throughout the test is imperative, preferably by a cardiologist.

Thallium will accumulate in the myocardium directly in proportion to the regional blood flow. There can be five stages of testing, depending on the individual's tolerance of the process. Each stage is made up of a 3 percent increase in the speed of the treadmill as well as in the treadmill incline. Testing is preceded by a baseline evaluation of the individual's heart action with an electrocardiograph (ECG). The electrodes are left in place to monitor heart action throughout the test. Indicators for stopping the test before its usual time span (30 minutes) include:

1. Maximum pulse rate
2. Severe angina
3. Second- or third-degree heart block
4. Reported or evident severe fatigue, dyspnea, any chest pain
5. Rapid increase in pulse or blood pressure

6. Evidence of life-threatening arrhythmias (e.g., ventricular tachycardia; more than 10 premature ventricular contractions (PVC) in 1 minute)
7. Flat or down-sloping ECG stress testing segment depression (suggestive of a 3.5 percent greater risk of multivessel disease)

The findings from the stress test are compared to the resting thallium scan.

Time Involved. Preliminary assessment and exercise segment take over approximately 10 to 15 minutes each. See the following two tests for alternative tests.

5. Dipyridamole-Thallium Scans

Synonym: Persantine-thallium scan

Explanation of the Test. Dipyridamole-thallium scans are in order when exercise stress testing is not advisable or the individual is unable to exercise enough to stress the heart. Dipyridamole is a coronary vasodilator that increases myocardial coronary artery blood flow, except for flow distal to stenosed areas, simulating the exercise portion of the preceding test, leading to an increased thallium 201 uptake in "normal" coronary arteries and relatively decreased distal to stenotic areas.

Procedure. With the patient lying on an examination table or in bed, thallium 201 is injected IV 3 to 5 minutes after dipyridamole. Imaging of thallium 201 distribution can be done with a conventional scintillation camera. The patient should be told to expect the "camera" to rotate about him or her and that it will produce a sound such as a 'click' when actually scanning (See also Implications for Nursing, this section)

Purpose. The test is useful in the:

1. Initial evaluation of chest pain of uncertain origin
2. Determination of the functional significance of coronary artery stenosis (as determined by angiography)
3. Follow-up on bypass surgery, transluminal angioplasty, or thrombolysis
4. Estimation of prognosis after an acute myocardial infarction
5. Estimation of the extent of scarring after an infarct

The test's sensitivity for significant coronary artery disease is similar to exercise testing (80 to 85%), and its specificity is over 90 percent.

6. Exercise Gated-Wall Motion Studies

Purpose. Exercised gated-wall motion studies are another alternative to thallium scans and enable the visualization of any abnormalities of cardiac wall motion and the extent of mitral valve regurgitation under stress for the patient known to be at greater risk in exercise testing.

Time required. 2 to 2-1/2 hours

Procedure. After administration of a radionuclide (see patient preparation for scintilation scans), the heart is scanned from four different projections. The patient pedals a specially adapted exercise bicycle while supine and the heart action is again scanned during the activity.

Preparation for the Test. The patient should be kept n.p.o. 4 hours prior to testing, and a resting 12-lead ECG is done before the test, usually in the morning. A cardiologist must be present. The test lasts from 2 to 2½ hours.

IMPLICATIONS FOR NURSING: CARDIAC NUCLEAR SCANS

1. Consent of the patient or his/her guardian is usually required for all cardiac scans. Ensure that the physician has or will be informing the patient of the risks and benefits of the proposed scan
2. Physical preparation: Usually minimal to none. Alcohol and caffeine should be omitted prior to the test
3. Patient education
   a. Determine the patient's understanding of the test(s) to be done, and provide additional information or reinforcement of previous knowledge, as indicated. Bear in mind the fatigue level of the cardiac patient as well as the effects of psychological stress. Retention of information may be low, as may be tolerance of stress. Teaching must be highly individualized and well coordinated with the medical staff
   b. Activity is not usually restricted. However, rest after the scan should be encouraged
   c. Reassure the patient that, except for the minor discomfort of the intravenous injection, testing is painless and fairly uncomplicated
   d. If postimaging is to be done, be sure that the patient is aware of this and of when it is to be done (often 4 to 6 hours after the injection of the imaging agent)
4. Some scans can be done at the bedside. If the patient's condition is likely to deteriorate with transfer or if transfer would cause undo hardship, determine whether the scan could be done at the bedside
5. Explain the purpose of and process used for radioactive labeling of the client's blood prior to the test. Emphasize the low level of reactivity and its short half-life and explain terminology (i.e., half-life) as needed
6. The patient may be reassured to know that a physician will be present during cardiac stress testing
7. An electrocardiogram is usually done before cardiac scans and may be repeated after the test is completed. An ECG is done throughout MUGA testing
8. Delayed redistribution scans (such as the dipyridamole-thallium scan) require a return to the imaging area in 4 to 24 hours for further scanning. This can take up to 1 hour
9. Length of time needed:
   a. First pass imaging (only): 1 to 2 minutes after the injection when other tests are to follow. If only the first pass test is done, more images are taken. Time: 15 to 30 minutes
   b. Ejection fraction: as for first pass imaging
   c. Gated-wall motion study (alone): 1 to 1½ hours
   d. Stress test(s) with MUGA: 2 to 2½ hours
   e. Dipyridamole thallium scan: 30 minutes (possible return for imaging after 4 to 24 hours for a 1-hour scan)

D. *Cisternograms*

Synonyms: Cisternography, cerebral spinal fluid flow scan, CSF flow scan

Purpose. A cisternogram is done when there is a need to assess normal and abnormal pathways as well as the hydrodynamics of the CSF. The test is helpful in detecting obstruction to CSF flow and therefore in determining the cause for hydrocephalus as well as helping determining the feasibility of and plans for treatment such as the type of and location for shunt formation.

  Other pathology that can be detected by this procedure includes third-ventricle tumors, subdural hematomas, cysts of the posterior fossa or subarachnoid space, and spinal lesions.

Procedure. Although a cisternal puncture can be done when a lumbar deformity or some other condition that precludes a lumbar approach exist, the hazards of such a puncture so close to the brain stem make the lumbar approach the method of choice.

  A sterile lumbar puncture is performed, usually by a neurologist, and a radionuclide is injected into the CSF. Delayed images of the brain (and spinal canal if important) are then taken at prolonged intervals, for example, at 2, 6, 24, and 48 hours. The timing and number of delayed images taken are determined by the physician.

IMPLICATIONS FOR NURSING: CISTERNOGRAM

1. A permit is usually required for the lumbar puncture
2. Physical preparation
   a. As for any lumbar puncture, the patient is positioned (side-lying in full flexion, or sitting while leaning over a chair back). Sedation is given if overly anxious; moral support is always given. Sterile preparation of the puncture site and sterile draping as well as injection of local anesthesia at the site of the puncture are usually done by the physician. The skin preparation is generally done in the nuclear medicine department
   b. The nurse should assess for sensitivity to local anesthetics. Positive findings should be reported to the nuclear medicine department before the time of the test
   c. If a *CSF leak test* is also to be done, instructions will be given the nurse about placing small sterile cotton balls or pledgets in each nostril. These are replaced and deposited in specially marked vials when they become saturated. It is best if the nurse wears clean gloves to do this or scrubs her or his hands thoroughly beforehand
3. Patient education
   a. Explain the steps in the procedure and physical preparation, to include the lumbar puncture, clearly, concisely, and with adequate rationale
   b. The patient will be expected to lie flat for a period of time after the puncture, e.g., ½ to 6 hours (check with the physician for the specific time interval). If there is a CSF leak, however, the head of the bed might be raised slightly to prevent retrograde flow of the CSF. The nurse should treat the area about the nares as a clean field and not introduce any contaminants through contact
   c. Given a CSF leak or if the physician orders a "Leak Test" the patient will need to be protected against cross-contamination. The pledgets should be removed when saturated to prevent ascending infection; the patient should be instructed to
      (1) Not touch the nose or upper lip with the hands

(2) Not sniff secretions back into the throat because this can cause contaminated secretions to enter the cranial vault

(3) Avoid, if possible, coughing and sneezing for the same reason

(4) Always have the head of the bed elevated *slightly* to prevent retrograde drainage

4. Length of time needed

- Each set of images requires 30 to 60 minutes. As with a brain scan, the technologist will use tape to immobilize the patient's head during each imaging

E. Gallium Scans

Synonyms: Total-body scan, whole-body scan

Purpose. Gallium citrate (Ga-67) is taken up by a number of body tissues (e.g., liver, spleen, bone, breast, large bowel). It also localizes in most inflammatory lesions and in certain neoplasms. Because it does have an affinity for both benign and malignant neoplasms, further tests are required to determine malignancy, such as the use of CT scans or ultrasound imaging. The gallium scan is used to locate hidden abscesses and metastatic nodules and localize infections within organs or elsewhere in the body. Gallium scanning is also useful in evaluation of malignant lymphomas, focal liver defects, the tumors as well as the staging of Hodgkin's disease, and bronchogenic cancer. It can be used to evaluate tumor response to therapy.

Procedure. Gallium is injected 24 to 48 hours before the scan. For the scan, the patient may be positioned standing or supine. The uptake probe and the detector head of the gamma scintillation camera may touch the skin in the process of scanning. The length of time each scan takes depends on how much of the body is to be scanned. Delayed image scans may be done 42, 72, 96, and/or 120 hours post injection. The number of delayed image scans done depends, in part, on the kind of disease process being studied. Two scanning heads may be used, one above and one below the body. This gives pictures of several tissues layers, somewhat like a tomograph scan. (For a yet more sophisticated type of scan that is based on this principle as well as on the principle of tomography, see Section 17.7.2.D, "Positron Emission Tomography.")

IMPLICATIONS FOR NURSING: GALLIUM SCAN

1. A permit is not required
2. Physical preparation
   a. As for "Bone Scans," Section 17.4.1.A
   b. Bowel preparation: Necessary for scans of the abdomen. This will usually be clarified by the nuclear medicine technologist at the time of the injection
      (1) Regular diet with bran products and fresh fruit
      (2) Laxative the afternoon before a scheduled scan (4 tablespoons milk of magnesia or two ounces castor oil)
      (3) Warm water or Fleet's enema, until clear the morning of the scan, early enough to produce results before imaging time (usually 1 to 2 hours before the scan)

(4) Repeat preparation and diet changes may be requested for delayed images on subsequent days. (Gallium collects in the bowel, which causes an abnormal concentration that confuses diagnosis and obscures visualization)

   c. If bowel preparation is contraindicated (presence of colostomy, allergies, hemorrhoids, acute phase of colitis), the nuclear medicine department must be notified

   d. If possible, schedule any barium studies after the gallium scan or at least 1 week before

3. Patient education
   a. As for a bone scan, plus
   b. Explain the steps of the procedure and preparation clearly, concisely, and with adequate rationale
   c. The patient will be expected to remain still for the duration of the scan

4. Posttest: If the initial scan is suggestive of bowel disease, a cleansing enema may be ordered before any of the delayed image scans to prevent inadequate visualization

5. Length of time needed
   a. Initial scan: 1½ to 2 hours
   b. Delayed scans: usually 45 to 60 mins each. Some delayed imaging can be scheduled at 48, 72, 96, and 120 hours after gallium injection (A total-body scan, head to toe, can vary from 6 to 30 minutes) (Dudley & Searle, 1992, pp. 14–15)

F. GI Bleeding Scans

Synonym: Gastrointestinal bleeding scan

Purpose. A bleeding scan is used to localize the site of active GI hemorrhage of labeled red cells, particularly in the lower tract. Although angiography will identify the presence of blood in the tract, it will only do so when active bleeding is occurring. Because most GI bleeds are intermittent, this test is the more likely to be successful.

Procedure. In some laboratories a blood sample is taken from the patient; the RBCs are separated and labeled with Tc-99m. The RBCs are then reinjected intravenously into the patient, and the abdomen is imaged continuously for the first hour. If necessary, further images are taken at several-hour intervals—up to 24 hours, although these later images are less accurate because they cannot be continuous and free blood moves rapidly in the bowel (Dudley & Searle, 1992, p. 19).

More recently the patient is initially injected (IV) with 3cc of HiSnPyrophosphate and a second smaller injection 20–30 minutes later. At the same time as this injection, blood image of the lower abdomen are taken (usually using tomography). Images are then taken every minute for 1 and ½ hours. Delayed images are also often done. (Dudley & Searle, 1992, p. 19)

IMPLICATIONS FOR NURSING: GI BLEEDING SCAN

1. A permit is usually not required
2. Patient preparation: None
3. Patient teaching: Explain the purpose and procedure of the test clearly with an adequate rationale on the basis of the patient and the family's learning needs as well as readiness and ability to learn.

> Stress the relative noninvasiveness of the test and its ability to pinpoint the bleeding site, which will speed treatment and make it more specific and therefore effective
> 4. Length of time needed: Variable, from 1 hour up to 24 hours, discontinuously

G. Indium-WBC Scans

Synonyms: Indium scan, Indium 111 autologous white blood cell scan, In-111

Purpose. The indium-WBC scan is a noninvasive test that is used to detect or localize inflammation, infections or abscesses deep within body cavities that have been suspected or known for 7 days or less. It can locate the infected site and determine whether it is a localized, walled-off abscess that may or should be drained. It replaces the use of the gallium scan because the In-111 is not taken up by neoplastic lesions or noninfected healing wounds as gallium is. It also has better imaging capability in the abdominal area than does gallium because it is not excreted into the colon.

Procedure. A sample of the patient's own blood (60 cc) is obtained. Granulocytes are isolated, separated, and labeled with the In-111 isotope; this process takes 3–4 hrs. The tagged cells are then reinjected intravenously, and whole-body imaging is done 18 to 24 hours post injection for suspected infections. If Crohn's disease is suspected, imaging will also be done 2 to 3 hours after the injection (Dudley & Searle, 1992, p. 24). Persons with low white cell counts, such as leukemics, can be transfused with tagged donor white cells. With ambiguous findings, ultrasound or CT scans can be used (Alport & Havron, 1980, p. 18).

IMPLICATIONS FOR NURSING: INDIUM-WBC SCAN

1. A permit is usually not required
2. Patient preparation: None. The patient must have a WBC of 300 or more for effective testing
3. Patient teaching: Explain the purpose and the procedure of the test clearly, and give adequate rationale for them. Base your information on both the patient and the family's identified learning needs and on their readiness and ability to learn. Stress the relative noninvasive characteristics of the test and its ability to help the physician determine the most appropriate treatment regimen
4. Delay views may be done as well in 36–48 hrs
5. Length of time needed: 18 to 24 hours to complete all scans. Preparation of tagged white cells before reinfusion takes from 1 to 1¾ hours

---

H. Liver/Spleen Scans

Synonyms: Blood vessel structural scan, hepatobiliary scan

Purpose. Hepatobiliary scans have been used to primarily evaluate biliary function, but because any agent used to outline the biliary tree will pass through the spleen and be excreted by the liver, their function is assessed as well. Liver scans are used to locate space-occupying lesions, as with suspected cancer metastasis, and to determine the severity of disease of the parenchymal liver cells as in cirrhosis. It is useful in the differential diagnosis of jaundice and in identifying hematomas secondary to trauma. Liver scans also image the spleen and therefore are used to demonstrate splenomegaly and to evaluate the distribution of radioactive colloid particles in the reticuloendothelial cells of the liver and spleen (Dudley & Searle, 1992, May, p. 26B). Liver and spleen scans frequently require further tests such as CT scans, ultrasonography, or gallium scan to confirm the findings.

Procedure. A radionuclide, often Tc-99m, is given intravenously, and 15 to 30 minutes later the abdomen is scanned as the patient is asked to change position on the table. The position change provides maximum visualization of all areas of the liver or spleen.

Patient Position	Liver Visualization
Supine	Ability to descend with inspiration
Left anterior oblique	Anterior portion of liver
Prone	Right area of liver; best view of the spleen
Right anterior oblique	Left area of the liver

IMPLICATIONS FOR NURSING: LIVER SCAN

1. A permit is usually not required
2. Physical preparation
   a. Neither food nor fluid is restricted before the test
   b. Scanning is usually contraindicated in pregnant women, during lactation, and for children
3. Patient teaching
   a. Explain the purpose and procedure for the test on the basis of the patient's and family's previous knowledge and understanding of the test, and gear it to their identified learning needs as well as their readiness and ability to learn
   b. Inform the patient that she or he will be asked to assume many different positions for the test, and even though the prone and or supine positions may be uncomfortable because of ascites, assure him or her that the time will be short and that it is important that she or he stay still to have a successful test
4. Length of time needed: 45 minutes to 1 hr

I. Lung Scans

Synonyms: Lung perfusion scan/lung scintiscan, ventilation/perfusion scan (VPS), ventilation quantification (VQ), quantitation lung scan

---

Purpose. The VPS evaluates the blood and air supply to the lungs, primarily to rule out or diagnose a pulmonary embolism (PE). It is thought to be the most accurate, noninvasive modality for diagnosing PE. It detects the percentage of the lung that has normal function, and by using a quantitative process, it provides an assessment of pulmonary vascular function. The chief drawback in using perfusion scans alone for the diagnosis of a PE is that the abnormalities of flow in various regions are highly nonspecific as to cause because these defects can be due to congestive heart failure (CHF), chronic obstructive pulmonary disease (COPD), pneumonia, or cancer. Using ventilation scans with perfusion scans increases the specificity of the process. Although a normal VPS result virtually rules out PE, the error factor is great enough to indicate further workup when PE is highly likely on a clinical basis.

The tests are also used preoperatively to evaluate pulmonary function in the patient with marginal lung reserves. It is, however, inappropriate for use in checking for pulmonary tumors unless these tumors have invaded the pulmonary vasculature. Other less time-consuming and less expensive tests such as a chest film are best used for preliminary screening. Pulmonary function tests are frequently done along with the lung scan.

Procedure

Perfusion Scans (usually performed first). A radiopharmaceutical is injected (e.g., human serum microspheres or macroaggregated albumin labeled with technetium). The patient lies supine for the injection. Abnormal images occur if the total dose is given while the patient is upright because particles of the tracer dose settle in the lung bases. Once at least half of the tracer has been injected, the patient is placed upright if at all possible for the scan. Several projections are imaged: anterior, posterior, and both lateral views at a minimum; therefore the patient should expect to change position. Perfusion scans can be done on a portable basis if necessary.

Ventilation Scans. A ventilation scan requires patient cooperation as well as the ability to breathe without assistance; therefore the patient with a decreased level of consciousness or any mental incapacity and the patient breathing on a respirator cannot be scanned except under extreme conditions.

The patient is given an inert radioactive gas (e.g., xenon [Xe-133], krypton [Kr-83], or an aerosolized solution such as TcDTPA) to breathe by mask or mouthpiece. If using a mouthpiece, the patient is instructed not to breathe through the nose, or she or he may wear a nose clip. The patient will be asked to take deep breaths on command and hold them as scanning is done. The patient then breathes normally through the mask for approximately 5 minutes. The scan focuses on three phases: the "wash-in" phase as the patient builds up the tracer gas in the lungs, the "equilibrium" phase while the patient rebreathes from a breathing bag and the radioactivity in the lung becomes fairly steady, and the "wash-out" phase as the tracer is fully expelled.

Quantitative Lung Scan. This combines both of the aforementioned tests; however, the ventilation scan is performed first while images are acquired on a computer. A perfusion scan follows, also collected on computer images. An analysis (quantitative) of the data collected is then done by the computer.

IMPLICATIONS FOR NURSING: LUNG SCAN

1. A permit is not usually required. Check with the department doing the test
2. Physical preparation
   a. A recent chest x-ray film should be made available, if possible
   b. There are no food or fluid restrictions before the test
   c. All jewelry or metal around the chest area should be removed before the test
3. Patient education
   a. Explain the steps in the preparation and procedure clearly and concisely, with an adequate rationale for each
   b. Except for the injection of the intravenous radionuclide, there is little, if any, discomfort with these tests. Some patients have difficulty accepting the use of the mask or nose clip, especially those who have any degree of anxiety or dyspnea. Stress that "normal" air is present through the mask or tube in the usual amounts and that the tracer gas makes up only a minute amount of the air taken in. A practice session might be useful
   c. Scans will be taken on inspiration, while breath holding, and after expiration. The patient will have to remain still during the scan
4. Length of time needed:
   a. Perfusion scan: Approximately 30 minutes
   b. Ventilation scan: Approximately 10 to 15 minutes
   c. Quantitative perfusion and ventilation scans, 1 hour

J. Renal Scans

Synonyms: Kidney scan, radionuclide renal imaging, renogram/renography/renocystogram, DMSA[a] renal scan/DTPA[b] renal scan

[a]Dimercaptosuccinic acid
[b]Diethylenetriaminepentaacetic acid

Purpose. Renal scans can look at renal tissue (parenchyma), renal structure, renal plasma flow, and renal function. These objectives can be met by individual scans for each objective, or through the use of two intravenous injections of different tracer materials, perfusion, structure, and urinary excretion can be studied at one imaging session. A third type of renal scan uses Tc-DSMA and is used to evaluate tumors, cysts, and other space-occupying lesions. Tc-DMSA binds to the renal cortex and is stable over several hours. The IV injection is usually done 2 hours before images are taken.

Renal scans evaluate renovascular hypertension, acute or chronic renal disease, renal trauma, obstruction (such as space-occupying lesions or vascular occlusion), and the status of a renal transplant.

Procedure. A number of different radiopharmaceuticals can be used for this procedure (e.g., technetium compounds [Tc-99m] such as technetium pertechnetate, technetium DTPA, technetium glucoheptonate, or I-131-hippuran) and when used, the test title reflects the compound in use.

For the test the patient is placed in a prone position to provide posterior views, but for the evaluation of a kidney transplant, the supine position is used because the implanted kidney is usually placed anteriorly.

A perfusion study is done first. The radionuclide, usually Tc-DTPA, is injected intravenously. The initial images of blood flow are taken (dynamic films, also known as computerized scans) and are followed by images taken at intervals (e.g., 2-minute intervals over a total of 30 minutes).

If a function study is done at the same time, a second radionuclide is administered (usually I-131-hippuran), or this test can be done at a separate time with the same tracer. Measurement of the transit time of the tracer through the kidney while showing absorption of the radionuclide and its excretion is done by placing the detectors or the gamma camera over both kidneys. They monitor uptake and removal of radioactivity. The speed of the uptake and removal are compared with a normal renogram curve either by computer or by individual computation. The radiation counts are plotted over specific lengths of time. Certain curves of excretion are characteristic of certain clinical states, but the findings must be compared with the patient's clinical status and other test results before a diagnosis is made. The renal scans do provide information as to which kidney lacks function or whether the disorder is bilateral. It is a test used as a follow-up after kidney transplantation or any treatment to determine response to the therapy.

IMPLICATIONS FOR NURSING: RENAL SCAN

1. A signed consent form may be required. Check with the nuclear medicine department doing the test
2. Physical preparation
   a. The patient should empty her or his bladder before either the function scan or the combined test
   b. A renal scan should not be scheduled within 24 hours after an IVP
   c. If I-131-Hippuran is to be used, Lugol's solution, 10 drops orally, may be ordered as a blocking agent, usually one-half to 1 hour before the tracer dose is given
   d. For the perfusion and DSMA scans the tracer material will be injected intravenously 2 hours before the scan. This may be done in the nuclear medicine department if renal vascularity is in question
   e. Good hydration, to individual tolerance, is important. Two to three glasses of water before the scan are suggested
   f. Check to determine that any hypertensive medications that the patient has been receiving are withheld
   g. There is possibility of delayed images being done with the DTPA scan
3. Patient education
   a. Explain the steps in the preparation and procedure, and give an adequate rationale for them
   b. The patient should be instructed not to change position during the actual scanning
   c. The patient will need to know which of the different tests she or he will be undergoing
   d. The patient will be seated upright for the procedure, except for the injection
   e. The patient may expect some transient flushing or nausea after the injection
   f. The radionuclides used are very low dose and will be excreted within 24 hours
4. Length of time needed
   a. Function study: About 30 minutes
   b. Perfusion study: About 30 minutes
   c. DSMA: 45 minutes
   d. DTPA/Renal Scans: 45 minutes
   e. Combined renal scan: Approximately 1 hour

K. *Radioisotope Renal/Residual Urine Study*

Purpose. This is a little known and perhaps underused test to facilitate diagnosis and proper management of neurogenic bladder dysfunction. Patients with multiple sclerosis (MS), for example, have three possible urinary dysfunction problems—failure to store, failure to empty, or a combination of both problems (detrusor-sphincter dyssynergia). This study measures residual urine *and* urine flow as well as provides information about the kidney, ureters, and bladder function. As the name implies, it includes a renal scan (see preceding test), as well as measurement of voided urine volume 45 minutes after the test, and scanning for residual volume.

Procedure. I-131-hippuran is given intravenously to a nonfasting, well-hydrated patient. (No bowel preparation is necessary.) The patient is scanned immediately after the injection. Approximately 40 minutes are spent in imaging; 45 minutes after the imaging the patient is asked to void. The residual activity over the bladder is counted and residual volume computed. A minimum bladder capacity of 200 ml is considered necessary for the emptying of a normal bladder. Pathology is more difficult to diagnose when bladder contents are below 200 ml (Holland et al., 1984, p. 190).

IMPLICATIONS FOR NURSING: RADIOISOTOPE RENAL/RESIDUAL URINE STUDY

1. A consent form may be required for the hospitalized patient. The test is often done on an outpatient basis
2. Physical preparation
   a. The test is contraindicated for pregnant women and nursing mothers, so screening of female patients should be done
   b. Check on the presence of active UTIs. If present, the test will probably be deferred because infections usually distort bladder function
   c. No fluid or food restriction applies
   d. Medications may be given on schedule
   e. If the patient is unable to void on request or is incontinent, the department doing the test needs to be informed. This may result in cancelling the test or scheduling a different kind of test
   f. If hydration is to be done orally (MS patients may be hydrated just before the test), the patient should drink several glasses of fluid on the night before and the morning of the test
   g. The department of nuclear medicine will need the following information about the patient before the test
      (1) Any medications being taken
      (2) Level of physical function and degree of disability
      (3) Mental status (will the patient need an attendant during the procedure?)
      (4) Inability to lie either prone or supine for 30 minutes
3. Patient education
   a. Determine what the patient/family already know, its accuracy, and what they want to know *first*. Clarify misconceptions, and start teaching with what is important to the patient and family
   b. Explain about the hydration process and what their responsibility will be, given the need to manage their own fluid intake
   c. Review the steps of the test—particularly the need to return to the department for scanning.
4. Length of time needed: Approximately 2 hours

L. Thyroid Scan

Synonyms: Technetium thyroid scan, iodine thyroid scan, thyroid scintiscan, radioactive iodine uptake test and scan (RAI uptake test/RAIU)

Purpose. The *thyroid scan* (not the RAIU, see the next paragraph) is done to determine the size, shape, and position of the thyroid as well as the presence of nodules. It is useful in diagnosing pathology related to masses in the neck, the base of the tongue, and the mediastinum because thyroid tissue can be found in each of these locations as well as in the thyroid. Scans are most frequently done after nodules of the thyroid have been palpated or gland enlargement is seen—especially asymmetrical enlargement. Scans are also done on persons with no evident thyroid problems but who do have a history of x-ray treatment to the head or neck (e.g., treatment of acne or the thymus gland in 1940 to 1950). Generally, findings are based on "hot" and "cold" spot imaging. The hot spot indicates benign nodules, and the cold spot indicates either cyst formation or malignant nodules. Normal thyroid tissue tends to take up the iodine, whereas cystic or malignant tissue does not.

The *RAIU test* differs from the thyroid scan (see the preceding paragraph) in that the RAIU test provides an indirect measure of thyroid function/activity. It is useful in differentiating hyperthyroidism and hypothyroidism. The outcomes of a RAIU scan are reported much like clinical laboratory tests, which use a reference norm, rather than like diagnostic tests, that is, a certain percentage of uptake in a given length of time is referred to as "normal":

1. Hypothyroid patients have a diminished uptake at all time intervals tested
2. Hyperthyroid patients have a high uptake at 1 and 6 hours after injection of the iodine isotope. Some hyperthyroid patients have uptakes within normal limits, or even low uptakes, at 24 hours because the excessively fast uptake and metabolism will eliminate the test material

Because there is accurate hormonal measurement for both thyroxine (T_3) and triiodothyronine (T_4), the RAIU scan is generally used only in the evaluation of already demonstrated hyperthyroidism or in conjunction with a thyroid scan.

NORMAL REFERENCE RANGES FOR RAIU TEST:

Levels will vary with locale and iodine consumption. Use regional values (Providence Hospital Medical Center, Everett, WA, 1985).

2-hour uptake	1.5–15%
6-hour uptake	4.0–20%
24-hour uptake	6.0–32%

Procedure

Thyroid Scan. The patient is given the radioactive iodine by mouth (usually I-123 because of its short half-life) in the form of a tasteless capsule or liquid. It can be given intravenously but rarely is. Six hours after the isotope is given (only a 30- to 45-minute wait if technetium is used), images of the thyroid are taken, with the patient in a supine position and the neck hyperextended. The use of technetium shortens the waiting time and allows scans to be taken of patients who have had previous gallbladder or IVP x-ray studies.

With findings of any mass on a nuclear medicine thyroid scan, "hot" or "cold," a referral for ultrasound evaluation may be made in order to characterize the mass as being cystic or solid. An aspiration and biopsy is the likely next step if cysts are ruled out. Benign ("hot") nodules usually indicate some degree of hyperthyroidism, which is treated medically if possible, or part or all of the thyroid may be removed. At times surgical removal of a nodule or a lobe of the thyroid may be done for appearance or comfort, but not until after testing for and treating the hyperthyroidism.

RAIU Scan. The patient is given the radioactive iodine (usually I-131 with a longer half-life than I-123) in a liquid-containing capsule of the intravenous form. Two, 6, and 24 hours later—or some similar hour interval—the patient returns to the nuclear medicine department for further imaging and calculation of the percentage of uptake with each image. These measurements are usually taken with the patient sitting up.

Thyroid scans are usually performed by a nuclear medicine technologist.

IMPLICATIONS FOR NURSING: THYROID SCANS

1. Permits are not usually required
2. Patient preparation
   a. Thyroid scan
      (1) A complete history of past exposure (over the last 60 days) to nuclear scanning, use of thyroid suppressive medications, and any drugs that may interfere with iodine uptake (e.g., medications containing iodine) as well as any contrast studies done within the last month is taken, usually by the nuclear medicine department*
      (2) It is also important to verify previous radiation treatments to the head, neck, or chest
      (3) The doctor is responsible for discontinuing treatment with any thyroid medications the patient may have been taking. Sometimes thyroid therapy is not discontinued. If it is discontinued, this is done at different times in different facilities. Generally, treatment with the medications is stopped 3 to 4 weeks before the test, with the exception of iothyronine sodium (Cytomel). Because it has a shorter half-life, Cytomel treatment is discontinued 7 to 10 days before the test. The nurse is responsible to check whether the patient has or has not been taking the drugs and report any discrepancy to the laboratory and physician*
      (4) Food and drink are not restricted unless the patient has been ordered by the physician to eliminate foods high in iodine from the diet. Usually this is done 3 days before the test
      (5) Dentures and any jewelry worn in the area of the scan must be removed to prevent obscuring the scan
      (6) A fast from the midnight before the test may be required. In some facilities a light breakfast is allowed; in others there are no restrictions. Check with the facility in which the test is to be done
   b. RAIU: As for the thyroid scan

---

*Medications that may contain iodine include weight control medications, cough medicine, some oral contraceptives, multiple vitamins, tolbutamide, and some antiseptics. Thyroid suppressants include estrogen, corticosteroids, barbiturates, phenothiazines, aminosalicylic acid, and sodium nitroprusside.

3. Patient education
   a. Check the patient's knowledge level, and then clarify the steps in the preparation and procedure as concisely as needed, with an adequate rationale for each step
   b. With signs or symptoms or a definitive diagnosis of either hyperthyroidism or hypothyroidism, gear the approach to teaching to the patient's attention span and fatigue level (see Sections 1.12 and 7.3.1)
   c. Stress the low dose of radioactivity involved and the especially short half-life of the tracer used in a thyroid scan. If needed, explain the concept of half-life
   d. Be aware of the emotional stress that may be related to a possible diagnosis of malignancy. Research current information as to the treatment and prognosis, if needed. Do not try to answer what is not known with certainty
   e. Explain any medication holds or diet restrictions as necessary
   f. If necessary, expedite laboratory tests of thyroid function (T_3, T_4, T_3 uptake, thyroid-stimulating hormone [TSH]). These are valuable in the interpretation of the images and uptake measurements
4. Posttest care: Any food or fluid restrictions are generally lifted immediately after the test(s) is completed. The physician will reorder medications
5. Length of time needed
   a. Thyroid scan: Approximately 1 hour
   b. RAIU: Approximately 15 minutes for each uptake measurement in addition to scan time if requested (Prekeges, 1986)

17.5 ULTRASOUND DIAGNOSTIC TESTS*

INTRODUCTION

Ultrasound (US) procedures have become more widely used since the 1980s because of their cost-effectiveness, noninvasive nature, and enhanced technical capabilities. In some instances, ultrasound procedures have replaced x-ray and other imaging procedures. In others, ultrasound has become an important adjunct.

Ultrasound examinations are performed by sonographers and are interpreted by a physician called a sonologist. Sonographers are ultrasound specialists, not technicians, who have received specific education and training in the use of ultrasound. Accredited educational programs include both Associate or Bachelor programs.* Sonographers take a national certification examination, administered by the American Registry of Diagnostic Medical Sonographers. On successful completion of the examination they are awarded one of the following titles: registered diagnostic medical sonographer (RDMS), registered diagnostic cardiac sonographer (RDCS), or registered vascular technologist (RVT). Certification provides evidence of competency, which is important in protecting public safety.

---

*Acknowledgment and credit must be given here to Andrea Skelly, BS, RDMS, Assistant Professor and Program Director and Suzanne Adams, BS, RDMS, Assistant Professor of Diagnostic Ultrasound Studies at Seattle University, who went over the text for this section as well as the section on "scans" with remarkable patience, knowledge, and generosity of time and talent. Any errors that may still occur are therefore the responsibility of the author.

Explanation of the Process. The ultrasound (meaning: above the limit of reception by the human ear) used in diagnostic applications is generated by a special probe, more appropriately called a transducer. The transducer can emit sound continuously (referred to as *continuous wave [CW] ultrasound*—See Appendix E for in-depth information about the various kinds of ultrasound), or sound can be emitted in "bursts," or pulses (referred to as *pulsed ultrasound*). Pulsed ultrasound is the basis of *ultrasound imaging.* A burst of sound is emitted from the transducer and is reflected from various tissues, organs and/or vessels in the body. The reflected sound, called an echo, is processed by the machine to produce an image. Different tissues (organs and vessels) reflect sound differently: some produce bright echoes; others produce weak echoes, and fluid-filled structures typically produce *no*, or few, echoes. This reflected wave, then, contains information about the tissue that, when analyzed appropriately, yields diagnostic information in form of an image. Ultrasound travels very well through fluid (e.g., urine, amniotic fluid, ascites). It does not travel well through bone or air. The majority of sound is reflected back to the transducer, and very little of it goes beyond the bone or air to produce an image of the structures below. (This explains why ultrasound is not good at evaluating bowel or lungs. It also explains the purpose for some of the patient preparation before ultrasound examinations, e.g., a full bladder.)

Purpose. US is used not only for imaging but also to guide invasive procedures (e.g., biopsy, aspirations, scentesis) and assist during surgery.

Doppler ultrasound yields information about blood flow characteristics. Blood flow velocities and direction can be assessed in various vessels (arterial and venous), as well as within the heart or across valve areas, which helps assess the severity of disease. Doppler also provides evidence of cardiac tamponade. Doppler testing can be correlated with information obtained via cardiac catheterization. However, the Doppler/echo evaluation can be sufficient for clinical decision making, and the patient may not need to have a cardiac catheterization.

Further information available from the sonogram relates to cardiac enlargement, effusions, aneurysms, tumors, chamber enlargement, and wall thickness. Valve and valve motion are observed, and valve function evaluated. Doppler provides information on flow velocities across valves, shunts [e.g., ventricular septal defect (VSD), patent ductus arteriosis (PDA)], and strictures (e.g., coarctation of the aorta), and gives direct evidence of leakage of valves.

Doppler evaluation of abdominal vessels is frequently done to determine vessel patency, direction of flow, and evidence of organ perfusion, and/or destruction.

Because a thin layer of air exists between the transducer and the patient's skin, an "acoustic couplant" (a hypoallergenic, viscous, water-soluble, nonstaining gel that is produced under several brand names), is used to eliminate this air space. The use of water baths as an air seal is cumbersome, although effective, and limited to a very few portions of the body (e.g., neck, testes).

Advantages of Ultrasound. For the most part, ultrasound is noninvasive, emits no ionizing radiation, can often be performed at the bedside, and is easily repeated. It does require some physical preparation of the patient. No adverse effects have been demonstrated in humans. Current data indicate that the benefits to patients of the prudent use of diagnostic ultrasound outweigh any risks (American Institute of Ultrasound in Medicine).

GENERAL NURSING IMPLICATIONS RELATED TO ULTRASOUND TESTING

1. A permit is usually not required
2. Process
   a. The patient is usually placed on a table in a position that makes the area to be examined accessible
   b. A coupling agent will be placed on the area to be examined
   c. The transducer is placed on the skin in the area prepared. It may be moved or left stationary. There is no sensation other than the gentle touch of the transducer
   d. Depending on the examination and the patient, the patient may be required to hold her or his breath while the imaging is being done
3. Physical preparation (see also specific tests)
   a. The request form must include pertinent patient history and laboratory values, as well as the examination to be done. It must also specify diagnostic concerns (e.g., rule out biliary obstruction, or rule out appendicitis)
   b. The patient should wear clothing that will allow easy exposure of the area to be imaged
   c. Any dressing in the area of interest should be removed if practical. A notice of any dressings to be left in place should be sent with the patient to the ultrasound department
   d. Inform the ultrasound department about any type of isolation, oxygen flow rates, or the presence of any drainage systems
   e. Be sure there is sufficient intravenous fluid to last through the full examination, or make arrangements to see that a bag or bottle can be hung during the test
4. Patient education (see also specific tests)
   a. Determine the patient's level of knowledge, and provide information as needed, clearly, concisely, and with adequate rationale
   b. If a child is to have an US test, a practice session on breath holding may be useful. It can easily be made into a game
   c. Reinforce the benign and painless aspects of the test. (Be aware and accepting of the anxiety engendered by any testing)
5. Posttest care: The coupling gel will be wiped off. There are no examination-related strictures on the patient's activities of daily living unless ultrasound has been performed in conjunction with an invasive procedure such as a biopsy.
6. Length of time needed: One half to one and one half hours for single tests. Will take longer if done in conjunction with multiple tests, which is not unusual. (Dudley and Searle, May 1992 [all pages])

17.5.1 Specific Ultrasound Tests

A. Complete Abdominal Examination

Synonyms: Abdominal sonogram

Components examined: Gallbladder, liver, pancreas, spleen, kidneys, aorta, intravenous cholangiogram (IVC), biliary system, and epigastric vessels. Ultrasound evaluation for appendicitis is becoming more frequent. It may be ordered as an abdominal ultrasound in men, a pelvic ultrasound in women

---

Explanation of the Test. Doppler (see Appendix E for a definition of Doppler) evaluation of abdominal vessels is frequently done to evaluate vessel patency, direction of blood flow, evidence of destruction, and organ perfusion.

Evaluation of abdominal lymph nodes and any fluid that may be present (e.g., ascites) is also routinely done as part of a complete abdominal examination.

Many institutions will use conventional and color Doppler (see Appendix E) to evaluate hepatic, renal, and epigastric vessel blood flow, depending on the disease states to be evaluated and the clinical question to be answered. This may extend the time needed for the examinations.

IMPLICATIONS FOR NURSING

1. Physical preparation
   a. Food and drink are usually restricted. In some facilities the patient will be kept n.p.o. except for sips of water (given *without* a straw) for 8 hours before the test. In others, the restricted period is for 6 to 12 hours. This is of particular importance for evaluation of the gallbladder and biliary systems
   b. Smoking and gum chewing may be prohibited if the pancreas, spleen, or abdominal aorta are the focus of the test because of the probable ingestion of air with these activities
   c. Fluids, given without a straw, are usually allowed when the abdominal area is being visualized because this often helps reduce gas formation
2. Length of time needed: Variable, 30 minutes to 1 hour, depending on the difficulty of the examination. (Generally all abdominal organs are evaluated, even if only a specific organ is requested. These include kidneys, liver, gallbladder, major vessels, pancreas, biliary system and the spleen)

B. Brain Sonography

Synonyms: Neurosonography, neonatal neurosonography

Explanation of the Test. Neurosonography *primarily* evaluates intracranial anatomy and pathology in the preterm infant. In these patients sonography is used for the evaluation of intracranial hemorrhage, periventricular leukomalagia, hydrocephalus, and ventricle size. It works particularly well in infants and sometimes in children up to 2 years because of the open suture line and fontanelles of the skull. It can also be used to monitor shunt function and determine the positions of midline brain structure. In utero, or the neonate, it evaluates congenital malformations of the brain, as well as associated neural tube abnormalities.

Sonographic imaging of the brain is rarely done in other patient populations because of the overlying skull (ultrasound cannot penetrate bone). It is, however, used frequently in the operating room, once part of the skull has been removed, to enhance localization of intracranial masses for the surgeon.

Doppler evaluation of cerebral blood flood (transcranial doppler [TCD]) may be performed as part of the workup for stroke or TIAs. TCD is performed through the suture lines of the skull.

IMPLICATIONS FOR NURSING

1. Physical preparation: See also "General Nursing Implications Related to Ultrasound Testing"
   a. Preterm infants: No specific preparation. However, the nursing staff may be asked by the sonographer to assist in moving fragile infants for the study. It is important to keep the infant warm during the procedure
   b. For Transcranial Doppler (TCD), in some instances, the hair may be cut or the scalp shaved to obtain better visualization. This is not routinely done and avoided if possible
2. Patient education
   a. Parents of infants should be given a full description of the examination prior to the test
   b. The patient must remain motionless during the test
   c. For preterm infants the test is usually done at the bedside
3. Posttest care: Unless the patient's condition contraindicates it, the hair will be washed to remove the coupling gel
4. Length of time needed: Variable, usually about 30 minutes

C. Echocardiogram

Synonyms: Cardiac echogram, heart sonogram, echocardiography, "echo"

Explanation of the Test Process. Echocardiography (including Doppler) is *very* important in the evaluation of congenital cardiac abnormalities, usually being the first procedure done to evaluate them. The structural and hemodynamic information provided by the tests assists in pre- and postoperative assessment of patients. Principles of pediatric echocardiography are used to assess congenital cardiac abnormalities *in utero* during a fetal echocardiogram.

Performed by a cardiac sonographer, a complete echocardiogram consists of an M-mode study, a two-dimensional (real-time) study, and Doppler evaluation (see Appendix E for definitions and explanations of these terms).

Echocardiography information has become part of the routine evaluation of valvular and ischemic cardiac disease. The combination of cardiac echogram and heart sonogram provides information about the anatomy, size, and motion of cardiac structures, which, in turn, complements information about the flow of blood through the heart gained from the use of continuous-wave (CW) Doppler, pulsed-wave (PW) Doppler, and color Doppler. The three types of tests are a routine part of the evaluation as each provides a specific piece of information. The heart images well because it is blood (i.e., fluid) filled. Information from echocardiography is now more routinely used in the operating room to guide surgical repair of valves as well as to evaluate residual regurgitation after repair, or replacement, of a valve. It can also be used to guide thoracentesis in patients with pericardial effusion.

Echocardiography is now also routinely used in the operating room to guide surgical repair of valves and to evaluate residual regurgitation after repair or replacement of a valve.

Stress Echocardiography

Explanation of the Test. Stress echocardiography is performed by a cardiac sonographer in patients at risk for myocardial infarction. The heart's response to exercise is similar to its response to other stressors. The stress imposed is the use of a treadmill, bicycle, or certain drugs (e.g., nitroglycerin, pyrophosphatase). The heart's response to exercise is evaluated to identify myocardial ischemia. (See also "Cardiac Scans," Section 17.4.1.C, "Thallium Scans.") Stress echocardiography is more sensitive in identifying myocardial ischemia than is ECG testing because wall motion abnormalities, which can be seen with echocardiography, occur *before* changes in the S-T segment of the ECG are apparent. As in cardiac scans, the patient's blood pressure, heart rate, and ECG are monitored throughout the study.

Transesophageal Echo (TEE)

Explanation of the Test. TEE is used in patients with surgical scars or lung disease with an obscured "window" for imaging transthoracically. An endoscopic probe with an ultrasound transducer is placed in the esophagus. This allows for a more detailed evaluation of the atrial septum, atria, atrial appendages, and other structures that may not be well visualized from the throat. In infective endocarditis, TEE allows for better evaluation of right heart vegetation.

In patients with mitral valve replacement (and/or of other valves), the degree of leakage is often better assessed with TEE. TEE is also used in the operating room to assist with assessment of valvular repairs or replacement.

IMPLICATIONS FOR NURSING

1. Patient preparation: Usually done in the endocardiography laboratory. The patient may be lightly sedated. A topical anesthetic is sprayed in the throat prior to insertion of the probe to assist insertion and prevent regurgitation
2. Posttest care: Depending on the degree of sedation, the patient should be closely monitored by the staff or a responsible family member until fully alert
3. Length of time needed: 1 to 1½ hours

D. Eye Sonograms

Synonyms: A-scan, axial length scan, orbit sonogram

Definition of the Test. An eye sonogram is frequently used before introcular lens insertion when the measurement of exact eye length is essential. The axial length scan provides this measurement. It also is especially helpful when no other visualization of the eye is possible because of opacities. It is used to identify and evaluate tumors and homorrhage or retinal detachment, as well as other ocular problems.

IMPLICATIONS FOR NURSING

1. Physical preparation (See "General Nursing Implications Related to Ultrasound Testing"): The patient should be assessed for sensitivity to local anesthetics and the ultrasound department notified of any positive findings

2. Patient education
   a. Topical anesthesia will be applied as eye drops to allow the eye to be touched with the transducer, or a water bath may be used for the test, which can eliminate the need for drops
   b. There are three ways the test can be done. In the first method, now rarely done, the eye is immersed in an eye bath, and the transducer can be gently placed in contact with the corneal surface. The transducer can be placed in the water but not contacting the eye at all. The third method of testing is done through the closed eyelid. In any of these procedures there should be no sensation on the surface of the eye, and the process should not be uncomfortable
3. Posttest care: The anesthesia of the eyeball will gradually disappear. The patient should be instructed not to touch or rub the eye until sensation returns
4. Length of time needed: The examination to determine eye length can be completed in as little as 10 minutes. Testing to differentiate pathologies of the eye can take up to 1 hour

E. Gynecologic Sonograms (Pelvic)

Synonyms: Pelvic sonogram, pelvic echogram, ultrasound pelvic examination (includes localization of intrauterine device [IUD])

Explanation of the Test. The preparation and procedure for this sonogram is the same as that given for the obstetric sonogram (next section), except that it is extremely important in the gynecological examination that the woman has a full bladder at the time of the exam so that pelvic structures may be visualized. The major difference between the obstetric and the gynecologic examinations is the medical concern(s) for which the tests are done. The gynecologic sonogram aids in:

1. The diagnosis and evaluation of the nongravid uterus and its adenexa (ovaries and tubes)
2. The identification and characterization of pelvic masses (e.g., cysts, tumors)

Pelvic sonograms may also be ordered

1. To evaluate the appendix in suspected cases of appendicitis in women
2. Routinely in fertility studies to assess ovarian stimulation and to assist with the timing of procedures done around the time of ovulation

In many facilities the name used to identify the sonogram remains the same, regardless of the purpose in evaluating the lower abdominal contents. In all such examinations an "acoustic window" (see Appendix E for definition) to the pelvis is provided by a full bladder, and/or the presence of amniotic fluid. Frequently, if evaluation of pelvic structures is inadequate with the full bladder technique (i.e., transabdominally), a transvaginal (also called endocanitary) ultrasound may be performed. A special transducer (covered with a latex barrier) is inserted into the vagina. This allows for better visualization of pelvic structures in most patients.

F. Obstetric Sonograms

Synonyms: OB sonogram, complete OB sonogram

Purpose. Ultrasonography provides probably the safest known diagnostic tool for the pregnant woman or the woman in her childbearing years. It emits no ionizing radiation and is noninvasive. However, an obstetric ultrasound should be done *only* when medically indicated. Determination of fetal sex and procurement of a picture of the baby for Mom and Dad are *not* generally considered valid reasons for doing the exam. Ethical and legal concerns make videotaping the pregnancy for the parents an inappropriate action.

Uses. The situations in which ultrasonography is recommended as beneficial for this population are:*

1. Estimation of gestational age for patients with uncertain clinical dates or verification of dates for patients who are to undergo scheduled elective repeat cesarean delivery, indicated induction of labor, or other elective termination of pregnancy
2. Estimation of fetal growth in conditions of severe preeclampsia, chronic hypertension, chronic renal disease, severe diabetes mellitus, or other complications of pregnancy where fetal growth is the measure that indicates the impact of the condition on the fetus and guides pregnancy management
3. Vaginal bleeding of undetermined etiology during pregnancy
4. Suspected multiple gestation, which may alter pregnancy management
5. Adjunct to amniocentesis for guiding the needle, assisting fluid recovery, and preventing fetal harm
6. Significant uterine size/clinical date discrepancy to permit accurate dating and detect conditions such as oligohydramnios and polyhydramnios, multiple gestation, intrauterine growth retardation, and fetal anomalies
7. Adjunct to special procedures (e.g., fetoscopy, intrauterine transfusion shunt placement, in vitro fertilization, embryo transfer, or chorionic villi/fetal umbilical blood sampling) for instrument guidance and safety
8. Suspected ectopic pregnancy
9. Adjunct to timing and repair of an incompetent cervix (cerclage)
10. Suspected fetal death
11. Serial surveillance of fetal growth or status with uteral congenital anomalies (e.g., bicornate uterus) or significant leiomyomas
12. Localization of intrauterine contraceptive devices
13. Ovarian follicle development surveillance in the treatment of infertility
14. In high-risk pregnancies, biophysical evaluation for fetal well-being after 28 weeks of gestation (amniotic fluid, fetal tone, body movement, breathing movement, heart rate patterns)
15. Observation of intrapartum events (e.g., version/extraction of second twin, manual removal of placenta)
16. Suspected polyhydramnios or oligohydramnios to confirm the diagnosis and/or identify the cause

(continued)

---

*As determined by the Consensus Development Conference cosponsored by the National Institute of Child Health and Human Development, the Office of Medical Applications of Research, the Division of Research Resources, and the Food and Drug Administration.

17. Suspected abruptio placentae
18. Adjunct to external version (breech to vertex position)
19. Estimation of fetal weight or presentation in premature labor or rupture of membranes
20. Gestational age of fetus in the presence of an abnormal serum alpha-fetoprotein (AFP) value
21. Follow-up of identified placenta previa or fetal anomaly
22. History of previous congenital anomaly
23. Serial evaluation of fetal growth in multiple gestation
24. Evaluation of fetal condition in late registrants for prenatal care
25. Suspected hydatidiform mole (signs and symptoms include hypertension, proteinuria, ovarian cysts, or failure to detect fetal heart tones by Doppler after 12 weeks of gestation)

Findings

1. The presence of amniotic fluid enhances the reflection of sound waves in this test
2. Fetal age is determined either by measuring the baby's size, crown to rump before 12 weeks, or by measurement of the head, abdomen, femur, and other structures after that time.
3. The most common request for obstetric ultrasounds is to evaluate fetal size. Such evaluation (fetal growth/size) is routinely done by using serial measurement of the head, abdomen and femur, compared with the mother's serum estriol and clinical parameters. (See Table 15–2, "Tests of Gonadal Function.")
4. Transvaginal ultrasound may be used in the first trimester to obtain more accurate fetal measurement, verify fetal cardiac activity, and rule out ectopic pregnancy
5. Growth retardation is determined by the use of serial measurements of the head, abdomen, and femur compared with the mother's serum estriol measurement and clinical parameters
6. In utero diagnosis of fetal congenital anomalies, such as polycystic kidney, anencephaly, and hydrocephaly are also possible

---

IMPLICATIONS FOR NURSING

1. Physical preparation: See also "General Nursing Implications"
   a. The patient will be asked to take a quart or more of water 45 minutes to 1 hour before the scheduled test. She will be asked *not* to void until after the test
   b. If the patient is n.p.o., several methods of filling the bladder can be used
      (1) If receiving intravenous fluids, the intravenous delivery can be speeded up for an hour before the examination (or more, depending on the client's hydration)
      (2) A Foley catheter can be inserted and used to fill the bladder with sterile water or normal saline in a retrograde fashion. The nurse is responsible for inserting and clamping off the catheter. If a catheter is already in place, it should be clamped off before the patient is to be tested.
   c. If ectopic pregnancy is suspected:
      (1) A beta subunit hCG test (see 15.1.5.1, "Tests for Risk Populations") should be ordered by the physician to correlate with the ultrasound

(2) A rapid pregnancy test to verify the pregnancy should also be obtained before the ultrasound is ordered

(3) The patient should be kept n.p.o. in case of possible surgery

2. Patient education

a. For this test a full bladder is imperative in the first trimester and with a condition of placenta previa. The bladder will push the bowel out of the way of the uterus, providing an acoustic window, thereby allowing visualization otherwise not possible. A full bladder also enhances the transmission of sound waves and acts as a useful marker to compare and evaluate changes in other pelvic structures. This information needs to be conveyed to the patient in as clear a way as possible to promote maximum compliance with an often uncomfortable state

b. The client should be assured that the only discomfort during the test will be that of the full bladder and possibly the supine position usually required

c. The benign nature of the testing method should be stressed for the psychological comfort of the patient

d. If the patient has concerns related to the safety of the test, refer these concerns to the sonographer for authoritative answers

e. Transvaginal ultrasound is often used in the first trimester to obtain more accurate measurements of the fetal pole; to rule out ectopic pregnancy, and to verify fetal cardiac activity

f. A translabial ultrasound may be used to evaluate cervical length and placenta previa, especially in the third trimester

3. Length of time needed: 30 minutes to 1 hour

G. Renal Sonograms

Synonym: Kidney sonogram

Explanation of the Test. A renal sonogram is most often done as part of the abdominal ultrasound. Doppler evaluation of renal perfusion may be performed as part of the examination, as in patients with renal transplants, and correlated with clinical laboratory tests (e.g., blood urine nitrogen [BUN], creatinine) and nuclear medicine studies (see Appendix E for a definition of the term Doppler). A baseline evaluation documenting renal size, echogenicity, and perfusion should be done within a few days after surgery. With color doppler (see Appendix E for definition), and by evaluation of characteristics of the Doppler Wave Form, renal arteriole stenosis can be detected and renal perfusion qualitatively evaluated. Duplex scanning (see Appendix E) of the transplanted kidney is used to evaluate for resection in many centers. Evaluation of any fluid collections related to the procedure is also done. Biopsy of transplanted kidneys is usually done with ultrasound guidance. (It is becoming more common for kidneys to be transplanted together with a pancreas.)

IMPLICATIONS FOR NURSING

1. Physical preparation: See also "General Nursing Implications Related to Ultrasound Testing"

a. Some facilities require that the patient be kept n.p.o. for at least 6 hours before the scheduled test. Check with the ultrasound department where the test is to be done. The patient should be as well hydrated as possible

b. If a renal biopsy is planned during the echogram, a surgical permit is required, and laboratory tests related to blood clotting and so on should be ordered and reviewed before the echogram

2. Patient education
   a. The patient may be in a prone, supine, or decubitus position for the test, depending on the visualization afforded
   b. During the test the patient will be asked to breathe deeply several times. This causes the kidney to move down into the abdomen slightly, thereby increasing visualization of the upper pole of the kidney

3. Length of time needed: Usually from 30 to 45 minutes

H. Thyroid Sonograms

Synonym: None

Explanation of the Test. A thyroid sonogram assists in determining the size of the thyroid lobes, in differentiating between the presence of a cyst or tumor formation, and, less frequently, in following the response to treatment such as validating the decreased size of the thyroid after antithyroid medication administration.

IMPLICATIONS FOR NURSING

1. Patient preparation: See "General Nursing Implications Related to Ultrasound Testing." There are no specific preparations for a thyroid sonogram
2. Patient education
   a. The patient lies supine on the table with a pillow under his or her shoulders to hyperextend the neck and maximize visualization of the thyroid. Coupling gel is applied to the neck in the area of the thyroid, and the transducer will be applied to the skin. An older, rarely used approach used a water-filled vessel that conformed to the shape of the neck. Coupling gel was applied to it. The transducer was then placed on the waterbag instead of the skin. The water bag provides a regular surface for the transducer and, therefore, better contact without air "leaks" that would block the sound waves
   b. The test may be done in conjunction with a nuclear medicine thyroid scan (see Section 17.5.1.K)
3. Length of time needed: 30 minutes

I. Breast Sonograms

Synonyms: Sonomammogram, ultrasound of the breast (often listed in the category of "small parts ultrasound")

Explanation of the Test. Ultrasound is especially useful in the detection of small tumors (less than ¼ in. in diameter) and is particularly helpful in the assessment of tumors or cysts of dense breast tissue. It differentiates well between cysts and tumors of the breast, and it is the diagnostic tool of choice in the pregnant woman. Because malignancies of the breast tend to grow rapidly during pregnancy, their close evaluation is imperative. Ultrasound can penetrate a silicone prosthesis in the breast, which can conceal abnormalities from a radiographic study. It can show other difficult-to-visualize breast areas such as that close to the chest wall. Ultrasound is rapidly becoming a more routine examination of the breast. Its use increases diagnostic accuracy when coupled with mammography and provides an option for the patient who should not be exposed to radiation.

Ultrasound is now used more frequently to localize breast masses for biopsy and, more routinely, to aspirate cysts (for either diagnostic or therapeutic purposes). It has some advantages over mammography, especially when lesions are lateral, not well seen on mammogram, or difficult to feel. Ultrasound is rapidly becoming a more routine examination of the breast. Its use increases diagnostic accuracy when coupled with mammography and provides an option for the patient who should not be exposed to radiation.

IMPLICATIONS FOR NURSING

1. Patient preparation: See also "General Nursing Implications Related to Ultrasound Testing"
   a. This test is more likely to be done on an outpatient basis, so a printed explanatory sheet given to the person at the time the appointment is made would be most useful
   b. She should be told to wear a two-piece outfit to facilitate breast exposure for the examination
   c. As with mammography, some facilities request that no deodorants, powders or perfumes be worn the day of the test
   d. It is important for any mammography films to be available in the ultrasound department for identification of the area in question and for comparison. If there are no mammography films, then a report from the referring physician locating the area in question (i.e., where the lump was felt, its size, etc.) should be on hand
2. Patient education: The most commonly used procedure includes three simple steps:
   a. The patient is asked to lay supine on the examination table
   b. Gel is applied to the breast(s)
   c. The transducer is placed on the gel, moving over the area of the thyroid
3. Length of time needed: Approximately 30 minutes

J. Vascular Doppler

Synonyms: Doppler ultrasonography, Doppler sonography, vascular ultrasound Doppler, peripheral vascular Doppler

---

Purpose. Vascular Doppler helps evaluate blood flow in the arms, legs, neck, and abdomen. Either veins or arteries are evaluated for patency and lesions (see Appendix E for a definition of the term Doppler). Pulsed C Wave (PC) and color Doppler are routinely used in the evaluation of vessels. Veins are assessed for deep-vein thrombosis primarily, whereas arterial occlusion is more likely to have multiple causes.

IMPLICATIONS FOR NURSING

1. Physical preparation: See "General Nursing Implications Related to Ultrasound Testing." If vessels are to be evaluated in the abdominal region the patient must be kept n.p.o. for 6 to 8 hours. Otherwise, there is no specific preparation

2. Patient education
   a. The patient will need to know the general process to be able to better cooperate with the testing. The test is performed by a vascular sonographer
   b. Peripheral vein evaluation
      (1) The probe will be placed over the vein(s) in question
      (2) At intervals the patient will be asked to take a deep breath, hold it, and bear down (Valsalva's maneuver) while the lower extremities are being examined. This allows the tester to check changes in venous flow. Normally, the flow will decrease on inspiration and increase with expiration. Abdominal compression with Valsalva's maneuver should then eliminate that variation
      (3) Upper extremities are checked as the tester occludes the vein by manual pressure and checks with the Doppler throughout. Manual pressure can be used in checking the legs as well. In both cases, upper and lower extremity evaluation, the increase in blood flow (augmentation) after constriction is carefully recorded
      (4) Several sites are tested
   c. Peripheral arterial evaluation
      (1) Always done bilaterally
      (2) BP measurement is taken on the arm where the Doppler is to be used
      (3) The transducer will be placed on several sites along the artery (arteries) being studied for data collection
      (4) If lower extremity occlusive disease is suspected, a BP cuff will be inflated around the calf and then the thigh while Doppler readings are taken. The wave forms and sounds will be analyzed later
      (5) The same process can be followed in the arms, if needed, with the BP cuff occluding arterial flow at the forearm and the upper part of the arm. The patient will also be asked to extend and flex the arm as the test is repeated. The tests may be repeated a third time with the patient sitting
   d. Carotid artery evaluation
      (1) The patient is supine, with a pillow if desired
      (2) Manual compression is applied to the vessel being examined after its original pressure is recorded by Doppler. Changes in flow are recorded, later to be analyzed in comparison to the norm
   e. Evaluation of abdominal and renal vessels is described in Sections 17.5.1.A and G
   f. Evaluation of impotence is done by evaluating penile blood flow

3. Length of time needed: Depending on how many vessels are studied, from 20 to 30 minutes, up to 1½ hours

K. "Small Parts" Ultrasound Procedures

1. Prostate Ultrasound

Explanation of the Test. Sonographic evaluation of the prostate is done using a special endocavitary probe inserted into the rectum. As with endovaginal ultrasound (see Section 17.5.1.E, "Gynecologic Sonogram"), a latex barrier covers the probe. A special probe attachment allows for simultaneous biopsy of prostate tissue during ultrasound evaluation.

Prostate size, echogenicity, and the presence of any masses are indicators for testing. Ultrasound characteristics of the prostate suggestive of abnormality can be verified through biopsy.

Patient Preparation. None other than positioning and explaining what is to be done. Decubitus position is used for this test.

2. Testicular Ultrasound

Explanation of the Test. Ultrasound is often the first procedure used to evaluate the testes. The patient is placed in a supine position and gel applied directly to the testes and scrotum. The probe may be covered with a cellophane barrier.

Testicular mass, size, and echogenicity are indicators for testing. The use of the Doppler allows the evaluation of perfusion to the testes. Complications related to testicular torsion can be assessed.

All structures can be evaluated, such as the epididymis, presence of a spermatocele, varicocele, abscess, and so on, are determined by ultrasound. There is no special patient preparation.

3. Rotator Cuff Evaluation. Often, before an arthrogram is ordered, an ultrasound test of the rotator cuff is done. Tears in muscles that comprise the rotator cuff can be seen with ultrasound, which can eliminate the need for the arthrogram.

17.6 ELECTRODIAGNOSTIC TESTS*

The tests included in this section are based on the presence of electrical potential in human cellular structure. The cell membranes are selectively permeable to ion distribution and, in health, maintain the ability to respond to a stimuli by changing permeability to transmit the excitation (in the case of muscle and neural fibers) throughout the tissue fiber and to return to the beginning state. The response to a stimuli is called the *action potential* or *evoked action potential* of the cell membrane. Its return to the beginning state is known as the *resting potential*. How well electrical stimulation-response (*conductance*) of a cell or group of cells making up an organ or structure is carried out as compared with a norm of the functions being investigated is particularly useful in the investigation of muscular and neural function.

Some but by no means all of the most frequently used tests based on investigation of cellular response to stimuli are included here.

17.6.1 Impedance Plethysmography

Synonyms: IPG, impedance phlebograph, plethysmographic venous study

---

*The ECG was purposefully omitted because of the need for and the availability of in-depth information on that particular test. Cursory coverage in this text was felt to be a disservice to the reader.

Explanation of the Test. Impedance plethysmography (IPG) differs from other tests presented in this section in that only conduction of electrical stimulation, not tissue response to stimulation, is looked at.

IPG has been the primary noninvasive test for deep venous thrombosis. The use of ultrasound may be sufficient in many cases, however. It is nonpainful and easily repeated, both for screening and follow-up after therapy. IPG is most reliable when detecting proximal obstructive clots and less sensitive to distal, nonobstructive clots. It is more accurate than Doppler (see Section 17.5.1.J), 95 to 100 percent compared with 90 percent, but less accurate, although safer, than a venogram (see Section 17.3.2). The test is based on the fact that the amount of blood in the leg determines electrical conductance—the more blood, the better the conductance and the less the electrical resistance. More blood can be expected to be found in a leg with an obstructed vein.

Procedure. With the patient recumbent, a plethysmograph sensor is placed on the leg and the blood volume recorded by passing a low-frequency electrical current through the leg. A large leg cuff is then placed high on the thigh and inflated to 50 to 60 mm Hg, which occludes venous but not arterial blood flow and which will increase electrical conductance in the normal leg. A second recording is done distal to the cuff. The recording is in graphic form, similar to an ECG tracing. The outcomes are compared with a normal tracing. With normal, unobstructed flow, the release of the cuff would cause venous emptying with a concurrent drop in the conductance of the leg. With venous obstruction, there would be little, if any, change in conductance whether the cuff is inflated or not. The obstructing thrombus causes a maximally blood filled leg by itself.

IMPLICATIONS FOR NURSING: IMPEDANCE PLETHYSMOGRAPHY

1. No permit is required
2. Physical preparation: None
3. Patient education
   a. Provide needed information about the procedure of the test along with an adequate rationale
   b. Assure the patient that the procedure is painless and safe
   c. To help ensure an accurate test, the patient should be instructed to
      (1) Maintain light, even respirations (without sighing or deep breathing). Deep, sustained breaths increase venous volume, and full expiration decreases it because of the changes in intraabdominal pressure on the major vessels
      (2) Keep the leg muscles relaxed; tense muscles increase venous volume by preventing emptying. The legs will be positioned slightly flexed and outwardly rotated for this same purpose and should be kept in that position, but it should also be comfortable for the patient. The patient should ask for an opportunity to change leg position when needed and/or for analgesia if experiencing pain
   d. The patient's legs may also be elevated to 30° to 35° to promote venous drainage
   e. There will be at least two, possibly three wraps on the leg being examined. One, the pressure cuff, will be high on the thigh. The other(s) will be wrapped loosely on the calf
   f. The pressure cuff will be inflated for 45 seconds to 2 minutes and then rapidly deflated
   g. Three to five tracings per leg may be taken, and both legs are usually tested
4. Length of time needed: 30 to 45 minutes

17.6.2 Electromyograph

Synonyms: EMG, electromyography

Explanation. Skeletal muscle at rest has little electrical activity; with contraction there is a marked increase in electrical activity, and it displays a characteristic, progressive "recruitment" pattern of motor units. Reflex electrical activity secondary to needle insertion normally stops within 2 to 3 seconds. Prolongation of this activity is seen in some myopathies.

Findings from testing are compared with normal patterns for amplitude, configuration, duration, and sound as well as whether they are all firing at a regular rate and rhythm. The audio signal also has characteristic tones and levels. Evidence of spontaneous, involuntary electrical activity recorded while a muscle is at rest generally indicates some neuromuscular abnormality.

Purpose. The EMG test, along with electroneurography (Section 17.6.3), provides one of the best means of diagnosing myopathies and neuropathies (e.g., muscular dystrophies, myasthenia gravis, myotonias, and primary nerve lesions such as amyotrophic lateral sclerosis, multiple sclerosis (MS), and traumatic injury). It is often used before a myelogram (see Section 17.2.11) because it is less threatening and less painful. The test is used to detect and measure the electrical discharge (action potential) originating in a skeletal muscle. Thin needles (25 to 27 gauge), one-half to 3 inches long are inserted percutaneously into the muscle to pick up the electrical discharge. This discharge can be monitored by an amplified (1 millionfold) audio signal and a cathode ray oscilloscope display screen. The visual display can be photographed for later review and the audio portion taped. The data collected are usually processed by computer.

Procedure. Depending on the muscle or muscles to be examined, the patient may be supine or seated. The muscle(s) to be tested is positioned so as to be at rest. A reference and a ground electrode are placed under and on the patient, in that order. A thin needle is inserted in small increments into the muscle. The insertion should cause minimal discomfort unless the needle is placed near a terminal nerve. This can be very painful, and the needle will be removed at the first evidence of pain. Muscle response to pain falsifies the findings. The needle is attached by wires to the recorder's sensing device. Several sites may be tested.

IMPLICATIONS FOR NURSING: ELECTROMYOGRAPH

1. A permit is usually required
2. Physical preparation
   a. There is rarely any restriction of food or drink. Some facilities may restrict stimulants (coffee, tea, cola, cigarettes) for 2 to 3 hours before the test
   b. Clothing should be such as to allow easy access to the muscles to be tested
   c. Assess for a history of bleeding disorders or the use of anticoagulants. Report any positive findings because their presence may contraindicate testing
3. Patient education

a. Assess the patient's knowledge and learning needs about the test, and supply concise instruction as needed by the patient

b. Children may be given a mild sedative, but sedation is rarely required for adults and it can falsify findings

c. Stress the small size of the needle and that it is Teflon coated for frictionless insertion

d. Explain that muscle relaxation will help speed the test and ensure accurate results

e. The only expected aftereffects are those of muscle soreness, which can be effectively treated with mild analgesia such as aspirin

4. Length of time needed: This depends on the number of muscles/muscle groups to be tested. The average for one extremity is from 60 to 90 minutes. More extensive testing can last up to 4 hours. This usually includes electroneurograph testing as well (see the next section)

17.6.3 Electroneurography

Synonyms: ENG, motor conduction studies, nerve conduction velocity (NCV)

Explanation of the Test. An ENG traces a nerve impulse from one site to another and determines actual electrical conduction in the nerve. In this test the electrical impulse is provided by an outside source rather than that naturally occurring in the nerve pathway. The speed with which the impulse travels is measured and compared with a norm.

Purpose. ENG along with EMG (see the preceding section) provide one of the best means for diagnosing myopathies and neuropathies. ENG is used in suspected cases of peripheral nerve disorders (e.g., neuropathy of diabetic, alcoholic, or nutritional disorders; peroneal palsy; compression or trauma [nerve entrapment]) as well as for certain endocrine disorders that affect nerve function (e.g., hyperthyroidism). As with the EMG, this test is preferred in an early diagnostic workup. Motor conduction studies may be helpful when nerve damage is doubtful but some atrophy or motor weakness exists.

Procedure. Two pair of electrodes are used: one pair stimulating and one pair recording—either disk-type surface electrodes or ring-type surface electrodes for toes or fingers. A stimulator provides an electrical impulse to the nerve to be tested while regulating the impulse's intensity (up to 300 volts), duration, (0.1 to 1.0) millimeters (ms) and frequency (usually one pulse per second). The nerve to be tested is stimulated at various points along its course. The response is recorded at the end point, and the *latency* (the time from each stimulation point to its response) of the response is measured on the oscilloscope in milliseconds. Conduction velocity, in meters per second, is then computed by taking the distance between the two points of stimulation (in millimeters) and dividing that by the difference in their latencies. The outcome is compared with normal values for the nerve segment being tested.

Normal Conduction Times (most frequently used tests)

- Ulnar and median nerves   50–60 mm/s
- Lateral popliteal nerve   45–55 mm/s

IMPLICATIONS FOR NURSING: ELECTRONEUROGRAPHY

1. A permit is usually required
2. Physical preparation: As for EMG, Section 17.6.2
3. Patient education: As for EMG except:
   a. The patient will experience a slight discomfort when electrical stimulation is applied. The patient should tell the test operator when she or he feels anything
   b. The amount of electricity used for muscle stimulation is very small. The sensation should be even less uncomfortable than experiencing a slight "static shock"
4. Length of time needed: As for EMG (preceding section). ENG usually takes longer than EMG; however, they are most frequently done together

---

17.6.4 Electronystagmography

Synonyms: ENG is often used, but can easily be confused with electroneurography (see preceding test)

Explanation of the Test. Electronystagmography makes a permanent record of eye movements at rest and in response to specific stimuli. It defines the occurrence of persisting nystagmus or its total absence when the norm would be its presence. Nystagmus is the involuntary repetitive eye movement in response to stimulation of the vestibular-ocular reflex. A *temporary* nystagmus is a normal response on head turning, rapid spinning of the whole body, or running a tape measure before the subjects' eyes when they are in a fixed focus on the center point of the tape (optokinetics). These nonpathological responses abate rapidly, however. Persistent nystagmus is considered pathological. It can be caused by a lesion in the centers of innervation or along the pathways to the centers innervating the vestibular system, the brain stem, or the cerebellum. This test registers changes in the electrical field around the eyes when nystagmus is induced. The change in the electrical potential is fed to a unit that amplifies and records it.

Purpose. Electronystagmography is a technique for monitoring nystagmus and is used, along with other tests, to help identify the cause of vertigo. (*Vertigo* is defined as a sense of rotation or movement of self or one's surroundings as opposed to *dizziness,* which is defined as a feeling of movement *within* one's head, i.e., light-headedness, a sensation of unsteadiness.) The test can also help confirm the presence of a lesion in the CNS or specific areas of the peripheral nervous system and provide an indication of the lesion's location. It is most often used when caloric testing of the activity of the labyrinths alone is inconclusive.

Procedure. Electrodes are taped to the skin around the eyes. Various procedures are then used to stimulate nystagmus (e.g., pendulum tracking, head position changes, gaze position changes, caloric tests). Depending on how the nystagmus is to be elicited, the patient may be seated or lying down. The room is usually darkened, or the patient is asked to close his or her eyes. Blinking can mimic nystagmus on the recorder and invalidate the results. Several recordings are made, both at rest and with different head positions and other stimuli. Often, the last evocative test is that of water calorics, with small amounts of warm and/or cold water placed in the ear canals. The patient's nystagmus responses are then compared with expected normal responses and will be reported as "normal," "borderline," or "abnormal." Abnormal findings are described and the possible location of the lesion given (i.e., peripheral, central, nonlocalized). Central lesions may be the result of demyelinating disease, tumors, or ischemia (Hamilton, 1986, pp. 624–625).

IMPLICATIONS FOR NURSING: ELECTRONYSTAGMOGRAPHY

1. A permit is not always required
2. Physical preparation
   a. The patient is usually asked to abstain from caffeine, alcohol, and tobacco for 24 to 48 hours before the test and to eat only a light meal before the test
   b. Eye makeup should not be worn
   c. Nursing assessment, with appropriate documentation and referral, should be done of the patient's
      (1) Recent signs and symptoms, especially related to balance, dizziness, vision, hearing, tinnitus, upper respiratory conditions, and occurrence of asthma
      (2) Physical mobility as related to the ability to perform the exercises included in the testing (e.g., freedom of neck movement, standing strength, and balance)
      (3) Presence of cerumen in the ear canals. This is usually removed before the test
3. Patient education
   a. Provide the patient/family with information as to the purpose and procedure of the test(s) and what will be expected of him or her during the test. Explain that she or he will be given specific instruction on what to do and when to do it throughout the test. Patient cooperation is vital to obtain valid results and prevent a need to repeat the test(s)
   b. Some nausea or dizziness may accompany parts of the testing procedures, but the patient will be given time to recuperate, if necessary, between tests
   c. No risk is involved, but the results are *not always* conclusive
4. Length of time needed: Depending on the number of tests used to elicit nystagmus and the ability of the patient to cooperate with the testing, the test can last from 30 to 90 minutes

---

17.6.5 Electroencephalogram

Synonym: EEG

Explanation of the Test. The EEG is a graphic recording of the electrical activity of the brain in specified bilateral, cortical areas. The making of the graph is based on much the same technique as the ECG, that is, the use of sensors (either applied as subdural needles [rarely used due to increased risk of AIDS contamination], attached with a contact paste or jelly, or affixed with collodion) to help pick up and record the electrical impulses of the brain. The brain's electrical impulses are much weaker than those of the heart and require amplification to be recorded. There are four basic wave patterns (see Table 17–2) that are recorded, the alpha waves being the most common ones found in the healthy adult.

TABLE 17–2. BRAIN WAVES

Type of Wave	Origination	Comments
Alpha: 8–13 cycles/second (c/s). Most adult brain waves are alpha occipital	Primarily in the occipital areas	Blocked by environmental stimuli (visual, thought, noise, touch) and by anxiety and apprehension
Beta: >13 c/s with low amplitude	In the frontal and central brain areas	Blocked by visual stimuli (open eyes), thought, anxiety/apprehension, and excitement
Theta: 4–7 c/s, low amplitude. Common in children. Only 5% of tracing in the adult		Normal with drowsiness in the adult, otherwise considered abnormal. Helpful in locating the site of a lesion when produced in one area only. Does not help identify the type of lesion
Delta: Slow waves <4Hz		

Data from Hickey, 1981; and Miller & Keane, 1983.

Purpose. The EEG is used to study brain function, to evaluate cerebral disease, and to assist in the diagnosis of some neurological disorders such as specific types of seizure disorders, head injury, encephalitis, and meningitis; and some metabolic disorders such as affect the liver or kidney, the brain such as strokes, CNS infections (e.g., encephalitis, abscess); and/or degenerative disorders, such as Alzheimer's disease, Parkinson's disorder, or head trauma. Considerable sophisticated knowledge and skill are required to interpret the test accurately. One of its important uses, evolving out of both ethical and legal concerns, is to confirm brain death—a widely used legal criterion for physiological death, especially for patients maintained on cardiac or respiratory assistive devices. An EEG is used primarily to *support*, rather than make, a diagnosis because abnormalities may not always be present to appear on the graph as with epilepsy, which may or may not have an abnormal tracing between seizures or may show an "epileptic" pattern without any history of seizure disorder. The test can be used, however, to effectively differentiate functional from organic brain disorders (Hickey, 1981, p. 102).

Procedure. An EEG is usually done in a small, quiet (soundproofed if possible) room, with the only window ideally being that which provides the person operating the test visibility of the patient. The patient is placed either in a bed or in an adjustable lounging chair. Sixteen to 24 electrodes are attached to the scalp in specific locations. These are affixed with the aforementioned conduction materials. (Collodion—which is very difficult to remove—has been the standby in the past. Other pastes, gels, and waxes have been developed that are easier to remove. Subdural needles cause some fairly minor discomfort while being placed.) Once the sensors are affixed, a baseline recording is done. Depending on the information needed, further testing may be and usually is done. One type of test done is sometimes referred to as "stress testing" or "activation procedures." It has similarities to the ECG procedure but with very different "stressors." The stress (or stimulation tests) are frequently used in the following order:

1. *Hyperventilation:* Breathing rapidly through the mouth for 3 to 5 minutes. The serum pH is increased to approximately 7.8, which increases nerve cell excitability and stimulates the seizure pattern of brain waves in susceptible persons. The recording is contin-

ued until the wave pattern returns to baseline values. This test is useful in suspected absence (petit mal) seizures but may not be performed on the patient with bullous emphysema because of the potential for severe respiratory problems

2. *Photostimulation (a.k.a. Visual evoked potential):* A flickering light is focused on the eyes, which may be either open or closed. This also stimulates the seizure pattern of brain waves in susceptible persons and should not be used in testing them. The recording is continued until it returns to baseline values. This test is used when generalized seizures of either the absence or myoclonic type are suspected

3. *Sleep EEG:* This test is done to detect abnormal brain waves that occur more frequently or only during sleep as found in frontal lobe epilepsy (Pagana & Pagana, 1992, p. 112). Recordings are done while the patient is falling asleep, while asleep, and while waking. If necessary a hypnotic sedative is given to promote sleep; but the recordings are much more valid if sleep can be natural (see Table 17–2).

IMPLICATIONS FOR NURSING: ELECTROENCEPHALOGRAM

1. A permit may be required, especially if needle electrodes are to be used
2. Physical preparation
   a. Medications such as anticonvulsants, stimulants, tranquilizers, and depressives alter the brain wave pattern and can suppress abnormal patterns. They are usually withheld for 24 to 48 hours before the test. The patient record should accompany the patient to the test area to provide primary information (what medicines taken, when, what dosage) for example, Pavilon, a neuromuscular blocking agent, used to paralyze infants respiration, who will then require mechanical ventilation. Hyperventilation may not be performed when the patient has advanced bullous emphysema as it can cause severe respiratory problems
   b. Dietary intake that is stimulating (e.g., coffee, tea, colas) is withheld for 24 hours before the test
   c. A certain amount of sleep deprivation can be helpful in ensuring good results from the test, especially if a sleep EEG is to be done. In this case the patient may be kept awake through the night, if possible. Generally for all EEGs, a late bedtime the night before the test, early rising the morning of the test, and no naps before the test are considered good preparation as the patient is more likely to relax during the test and even possibly sleep
   d. Hair should be free of oil, hair spray, any clips or pins, and "corn row" braids must be combed out before the test
   e. Breakfast is important in preventing hypoglycemia, which can invalidate the test findings
   f. The record should accompany the patient to provide primary information (e.g., medication names, dosage, when last taken)
   g. Premature infants on Pavilon or other blocking agent while using mechanical ventilation, must have complete records when brought for an EEG
3. Patient education
   a. Explain the purpose and procedure of the test in as much detail as your assessment of the patient/family learning needs, readiness, and ability to learn indicates to be necessary and helpful
   b. Assure the patient and family that there is no pain or discomfort associated with the test (unless scalp needles are to be used, and then discomfort is limited to the insertion only and is relatively minor). Also assure the patient that she or he will receive no electrical current or "shock" and that the flow of electricity is *from* the patient, *not* from the machine to the patient
   c. Explain the need to restrict movement during the test, but only during the time the recordings are being taken. The patient will be able to talk to the test operator if necessary and will be told when

to relax, close his or her eyes, and remain still and when it is all right to move. Even blinking and swallowing can alter the recording

4. Posttest care
   a. The usual medication regimen will be resumed. The patient may need reassurance that the elimination of an anticonvulsant medication for 24 hours rarely interferes with seizure control
   b. Because conductive jel is still sometimes used instead of the newer water-soluble conductive paste, to achieve good electrical contact and to keep the sensor in place, a shampoo is usually given as soon as possible after the test
   c. The test is often done on an outpatient basis. The patient will need to be accompanied to his or her home
   d. No alcohol should be taken after the test for 12 hrs
5. Length of time needed: This is variable (from 40 minutes to 2 hours, average 1½ hrs), depending on the need for and success of a sleeping EEG and on the ability of the patient to cooperate during the testing

17.7 NEWER DIAGNOSTIC MODALITIES

17.7.1 Magnetic Resonance Imaging

Synonyms: MRI, nuclear magnetic resonance (NMR), magnetic resonance angiography (MRA).

Definition.* Magnetic resonance imaging (MRI) is a diagnostic scan based on the magnetic behavior of protons (hydrogen nuclei). It uses safe magnetic fields, radio waves, and computer technology to "see" internal organs and soft tissue. It presents more complete, detailed images of certain body areas than any other imaging modality.

Explanation of the Test. MRI is a noninvasive, diagnostic, imaging process that does not require patient exposure to ionizing radiation (as with x-ray and computerized tomography [CT]). It is based on the spinning motion of specific elements present in biological tissue (e.g., hydrogen, carbon, nitrogen, oxygen, fluorine, sodium, phosphorous), all of which have an odd number of protons in their nuclei and are, therefore, magnetic-resonance (MR) active. Usually, hydrogen nuclei are used in MR imaging because of their abundance in humans and because they contain only a solitary proton that resonates only at radio frequency.

The proton spins, inducing a magnetic field all around it. Such protons can interact with an externally applied magnetic field, which can be "MR active" (Westbrook & Kaut, 1993, pp. 1–3).

Procedure. MRI uses a large, very strong magnet in the shape of a tube. The "bore" of the tube is the central opening into which the patient is placed, called the magnet. When a patient is within the bore of the magnetic resonance scanner, the hydrogen nuclei (protons)

*Particularly heartfelt thanks is directed to Kenneth Reger, MD, who not only instructed the author about the purpose, process, and use of tomography and magnetic resonance imaging with "live" demonstrations, discussion, provision of pertinent literature about the purpose, process and use of tomography and magnetic resonance imaging, but also reviewed and responded to the material written on the subjects. For this kindness and generosity, the author will always be grateful.

within the patient align parallel (pointing in the same direction) to the magnetic field in the imager. The alignment of protons emit measurable radiofrequency that can be detected electronically.

With the application of computer-generated short pulses of radiofrequency waves, the protons are tipped out of their magnetic alignment, causing them to resonate (spin) in a uniform pattern. When radiofrequency waves are stopped, the atoms realign in a uniform pattern with the magnetic field. As they realign, they emit tissue-specific signals based on their realignment time and water content of the nuclei (relative proton density). These signals are monitored, processed, and displayed in high-resolution image by the MRI computer. Normal cells produce signals different from those of abnormal cells, by which normal cells are identified from abnormal ones when the final image is developed. The presence of bone does not obstruct the view. There is no exposure to x-ray (ionizing) radiation (Thompson, et al., 1993, p. 1306).

Purpose. MRI's uses continue to expand. It is a sensitive detector of edema, hemorrhage, blood flow, infarcts, and tumors and can detect a variety of neurologic disorders of the central nervous system (CNS) (e.g., malignancies, degenerative disorders such as Alzheimer's disease, brain edema, spinal cord edema, herniated discs, ischemic-infarcted areas, arteriovenous malformation, congenital anomalies, hemorrhagic areas). It clearly differentiates various types of soft tissues (bones, fat, muscle) and readily defines structures of the musculoskeletal and internal systems. It is not hampered by the presence of bone, deleting it from view if normal. Blood flow allows specific visualization of vessels (MRA).

Intravenous contrast agents can be, and are used, with MRI in selected instances. Paramagnetic contrast substances (e.g., gadolinium [Gd] chelates, a heavy metal that crosses the blood–brain barrier) have a positive effect on the local magnetic field, increasing the signal density of protons (Thompson et al., 1993, p. 1396; Westbrook & Kaut, 1993, pp. 245, 247).

ADVANTAGES OF MRI: (See Table 17–3)

1. Many blood vessels appear as dark lumens if there is a rapid blood flow, providing a natural contrast
2. Imaging can be done directly in the transverse, sagittal, coronal, and complex planes
3. There is no known patient risk if serial studies need to be done
4. There is no risk of ionizing radiation from the procedure

DISADVANTAGES OF MRI:

1. Cost: Expense, still a major negative factor, both to the consumer and the provider. However, it is cost-effective if used appropriately
2. Low availability in rural areas
3. Danger of metallic injury
4. Claustrophobia
5. Not all MRI sites have been able to include the newer, larger MRI unit which accommodates individuals well over 200 pounds in weight. However, there is usually one such unit in each metropolitan area.

TABLE 17–3. ADVANTAGES AND DISADVANTAGES OF MRI

Advantages	Disadvantages
Increased natural soft-tissue contrast	High cost
	Slow scan time; requires a cooperative patient (see the last two disadvantages for causes)
Decreased bone artifact	Aneurysm clips or other implanted metal devices are a contraindication for the test
Increased contrast between flowing blood and vessel walls	Unable to visualize calcium
Can be synchronized with cardiac cycle, i.e., gated (see Section 16.5.2, "Cardiac Scans")	Procedure causes claustrophobia
Noninvasive	Lungs difficult to image because of chest wall motion and proton density
No use of contrast media, therefore no allergic reactions	Abdominal structures difficult to image because of movement
Can be used on women of childbearing age	Effect on fetus not known, thus not used on pregnant women

Data from Iezzoni, Grad, & Moskowitz, 1985; and Mezrich, 1985.

6. The use of contrast media, while an important tool in radiology, poses risks. Minor reactions (nausea, vomiting, hives) occur in about 5 to 10 percent of patients. Major reactions (laryngeal edema, bronchospasm, cardiac arrest) occur in about 1:3000 patients. Contrast-induced renal failure, while usually mild and reversible, also can pose major risks, especially for those with pre-existing renal disease such as diabetics with high-serum creatinine levels (Wall & Futerman in Detmer et al., 1992, p. 191).

IMPLICATIONS FOR NURSING

The referring physician, the professional and lay staff of the imaging center (to include the MRI technician and the physician in charge), and the staff nurse (if the patient is hospitalized) all share responsibility for the safety and well-being of all individuals who may enter the MRI room where a very strong magnetic field exists
1. No permit is needed
2. Physical preparation: none
3. Patient preparation
    a. Provision of safety: Individual being scheduled for an MRI must be given explicit assessment and direction to prevent the presence of ferrous metal items in the test room. Before the scan, printed instructions as to what substances and items can or cannot be safely brought into the scanning room are usually given to the patient and his/her family
        (1) Because of the risks involved, no one may enter the "Magnet Room" (the room containing the MRI equipment) if they are wearing or carrying ferromagnetic objects. Most ferromagnetic metal objects tend to become airborne projectiles in the presence of a strong magnetic field, such as that produced by MRI, causing injury to the person or damage to the MRI scanner. Metal that is ferromagnetic may be found in any of the following items:
            (a) Belt buckles (cloth-covered buckles may have ferrous metal base)
            (b) Bra or girdle with metal hooks and/or underwire support

(c) Coins
(d) Glasses
(e) Hairpins/barrettes
(f) Hearing aid
(g) Jewelry
(h) Keys
(i) Magnetic strip (e.g., credit or bank cards), although not a source of danger to the equipment or the people involved, are themselves altered so as not to be useable after exposure to MRI
(j) Metal bra hooks
(k) Metal zippers/buttons
(l) Paper clips
(m) Pens/pencils
(n) Pocket knife
(o) Pocket scissors or nail clippers
(p) Safety pins
(q) Sanitary belt
(r) Watch
(s) Wallet/money clip

(2) Potential or absolute contraindications to use of MRI: In most cases, the presence of ferrous metalic implants in the patient (as well as the individual who may accompany the patient) contraindicates imaging. Many metalic implants, when placed in a magnetic field, cause serious effects, such as torque, heating, and imaging artifacts. However, identification of the type of metal used for the implant may allow MRI in cases where nonferrous metal was used. MRI-compatible implants and protheses are currently available and in use. Older implants tend to be of ferrous metal. Identify the presence of implants that are absolute contraindications for use with MRI:

(1) Inner ear implants (cochlear)
(2) Electronic implants (e.g., a cardiac pacemaker, epidural stimulator, transcutaneous electrical nerve stimulator, insulin pump). Among many electronic implants, even the lowest strengths (10 G) can be sufficient to cause signal deflection, programming changes, or conversion of the pacemaker to an asynchronous mode. Electrical current and heat can be generated, creating burns as well as implant dysfunction
(3) Blood vessel surgical clips (e.g., brain aneurysm clips). The type of clip needs to be identified. Recent investigation proved the use of titanium clips safe for MRI
(4) Hip prosthesis (a large implant that tends to become heated under MRI). Most are imaged without problems however, but distort images in the region
(5) Ocular (eye) implants tend to be attracted to the MRI magnetic field and activated.

Other devices that can or may contraindicate the use of MRI have been found to include:

(1) Ferrous foreign bodies (especially in sheet metal workers with metal fragments or slivers in or around the eye) that could move or be displaced, causing injury to the eye or surrounding tissue
(2) Presence of bullets, pellets, or shrapnel in the body. Most have proven to be nonferrous, but extreme caution is urged in any imaging, and knowledge of the item's location within the body is imperative to evaluate its potential for harm. (Greatest risk of ferrous ammunition lies in that produced out of the United States, or by the U.S. military.)
(3) Halo vests that are *not* nonferrous or nonconductive
   • Can deflect and dislodge the halo
   • Cause heating within the halo rings
   • Cause electrical arcing
   • Cause artifactual problems, making imaging useless
   Nonferrous/nonconductive halo vests are available commercially
(4) Carotid artery vascular clamps: Only the presence of a Dopper-Blaylock carotid artery clamp is believed to be a contraindication for MRI as it presents a large attractive response to the magnetic field

(5) Other devices that can be impaired by MRI include: dental implants, neuro or bone growth stimulators, cardiac defibrillators, drug infusion pumps, and most ventilators (respirators)

b. Management of claustrophobia: Because the patient is enclosed within the bore of the scanner, and in the case of brain/head scans, the head is within the center of the scanning tube, claustrophobic response is not unusual. Newer scanners with large, open bores at both ends can make the patient feel less restricted, may allay some claustrophic response. However, it is imperative that the patient remain absolutely still during the scan, which adds to the sense of restriction and anxiety. Some patients require sedation. General anesthesia is not usually practical as most respirators and monitors cannot be in the strong magnetic field

Pre-test preventative measures:

(1) Without directly mentioning the potential of claustrophobia (claustrophobia can be created by its mention alone), try to determine its likelihood

(2) Alleviate anxiety by:

(a) Providing opportunity to see the room and equipment that will be used for imaging, both up close (when not in use) and from an adjoining room during use, if possible

(b) Suggesting and encouraging the presence of a relative or friend during the test who can stay in the room and maintain verbal or physical contact with the patient. The patient must remain still

(c) Stressing the availability of verbal communication with the radiologist or technologist during pauses in testing

(d) Providing a mirror so that the patient can see out of the imager

(e) Especially during a head scan, using a thin head pillow (or none at all) so that the patient's head is farther from the upper arch of the imager bore, if this is comfortable and possible

(f) Suggesting that the patient close his or her eyes or cover them with a paper towel or a blindfold to decrease the sense of enclosure

(g) After checking with the radiologist, offering the patient the option of being brought out of the imager between each imaging sequence, especially in long procedures and those that enclose the patient's head as well as body

(h) When great apprehension is noted, or expected, sedation before the test is strongly recommended, especially when the patient's head is being imaged, as well as for the very young child

(i) Sedation is also strongly recommended for the patient who has painful and/or multiple injuries

4. Length of time needed: Usually 30 to 60 minutes, but can be longer

17.7.2 Tomography

Synonyms: Laminogram/laminography, planigrams/planigraphy, polytome, stratiogram/stratiography

Tomography is any one of several noninvasive techniques of roentgenography (x-ray). It is especially designed to show detailed images of body structures in a preselected plane (layer) of tissue in a two-dimensional view. It produces a film that represents a detailed cross section of tissue structure, by blurring images of all structures in other planes and by eliminating superimposed dense structures, that can hide defects in standard x-ray. This feature is particularly useful in the identification of space-occupying lesions. The imaging is more detailed than standard x-ray and can eliminate the need for many other tests.

Tomography is more costly than x-ray. Multiple settings may be necessary for tomography to discover a lesion within tissue. It also requires a special radiographic apparatus that moves in a linear or polydirectional fashion while filming. The film moves in the opposite direction.

DEFINITION OF TERMS:

1. *Tomogram.* A special type of x-ray image that images the bones, organs, or tissues at a specific level or particular depth
2. *Tomography.* Any of several noninvasive special techniques of roentgenography (x-ray) in which the x-ray tube moves during an exposure, obtaining detailed images of structures in a selected plane of tissue and blurring images of structures in all other planes
3. *Computerized axial tomography (CAT Scan).* Tomography where transverse planes of tissue are swept by a pinpoint radiographic beam that circles or partially circles around the body part and where computerized analysis of variance in x-ray absorption produces a precise reconstructed image of that area. This technique has a greater sensitivity in showing the relationship of body structures than conventional radiography and has revolutionized diagnostic studies of the brain and many other parts of the body. Newer procedures allow imaging in many planes (axial, sagittal, coronal)
4. *Positron.* A positron is defined as a particle possessing a positive charge but that has the same mass as a negative electron (Reger, 1994; Clayton, 1981, pp. 1140, 1465)

A. Computerized Tomography

Synonyms:[a] Computed tomography (CT scan), computerized axial tomography (CAT scan), computerized axial transverse tomography (CATT scan)

---

[a]The original CT scanner was called an EMI after the name of the company producing it, the Electrical Musical Industries Scan.

Explanation of the Test. The primary purpose for the use of CT scans is to picture, or image, the structure and characteristics of tissue within body organs, such as a small cavity within a mass, e.g. the brain, liver, lung, and so on. It detects, among other things, bleeding, blood clots, tumors, infection, and abscesses.

CT scanning utilizes tomography and traditionally produces *two-dimensional (2-D) axial views,* or "slices," of body structures. Usually, scanning slices are obtained from top to bottom of the part(s) being scanned. At the same time as the scan information is acquired, the image is also displayed on a video screen and stored on computer tape, or disc, then recorded on an x-ray film. This hard copy film usually contains multiple images that are much sharper and much more detailed than conventional x-rays (radiographs). Radiologists interpret the images and plan the specific scanning techniques.

Purpose

1. CT is used in Hodgkin's disease to visualize lymph nodes and organs in difficult-to-evaluate areas (e.g., internal mammary, subdiaphragmatic, mesenteric nodes, and pulmonary parenchyma)

2. CT has been found to be as accurate as angiography in looking at specific vasculature abnormalities. It can distinguish between types of aortic dissection but does not identify aortic insufficiency or clear extension in the coronary artery branches.
3. CT has been found to provide a better view of abdominal viscera than MRI and is able to demonstrate retroperitoneal hemorrhage and other masses, including metastatic cancer in the liver, mesentery, adrenal glands, or pelvis (see Table 17–4)
4. High-resolution CT of the lung can detect emphysema when other tests are unable to do so
5. Although often the imaging test of choice, CT scans are contraindicted for pregnant women because they use x-ray (ionizing radiation)

ADVANTAGES OF CT SCANS:

1. Many scans can be done rapidly and are, therefore, useful in urgent diagnostic studies
2. CT scans can show calcium deposits and acute hemorrhage better than MRI scans
3. High resolution is not needed
4. The process is noninvasive

Procedure

Head Scan (Cerebral CT). The patient should be informed that the following process and possible body responses will or can occur:

1. The patient is placed on the scanner table in a supine position. The head must be perfectly still during the scan. It will be held in place by a cradle with an elastic strap that is applied around the head or some such mechanism to help the patient keep the head still during the test

(continued)

TABLE 17–4. INDICATORS FOR ABDOMINAL IMAGING

Angiography: Acute mesenteric ischemia and infarction

Barium enema: Colonic volvulus; diverticulitis (suspected or mild); intussuseption; obstructing colon carcinoma; uncomplicated ileitis or Crohn's disease

Computerized tomography (CT): Abcesses; abdominal sepsis; bowel ishemia (nonemergent); diverticulitis, ileitis, and Crohn's disease (advanced/severe/or complicated); febrile illness with no obvious infectious source; intramural bowel hemorrhage; left upper quadrant pain not due to ulcer; pancreatitis (severe or complicated, gallstone panceatitis); perforation and bowel obstruction when plain films are inconclusive; retroperitoneal involvement; suspected pancreatic cancer

MRI: Indications for CT in patients with allergy to contrast, numerous in vivo clips (metal and older than 2 weeks), or barium-filled intestines from diverticulitis from earlier workups

Plain films: Bowel obstruction (especially small bowel); gastrointestinal perforation; renal stones

Real-time ultrasound: Appendicitis (depending on operator experience); gallstone disease; hydronephrosis; pancreatitis (uncomplicated); pelvic pain in women; upper right quadrant pain; renal stone disease when used with renal scintigraphy)

Upper GI series: Esophageal diseases other than acute bleeding, including esophagitis; suspected ulcer disease; upper abdominal symptoms with radiographic free air

Data from Jeffrey et al., with permission.

2. The head of the table will be moved into the opening of the scanner (a large circular structure with a large central open space)
3. The table may be moved slightly during the scan, but the patient must remain still
4. The only sensation the patient will have is that of sound, the hum and click of the x-ray mechanism
5. The patient will be able to talk to the technician in the control room through an intercommunication system between scans, but must remain still while the scan is being done
6. Contrast medium, if used, will be injected intravenously over a 2-minute period. The patient should be informed of the expected physical responses to the contrast material, which can include: warmth and flushing of the face and head, metallic or salty taste, and, perhaps, transient nausea. Severe allergic responses are rare. Newer iodine contrast agents are safer but costly and are often used with patients having allergic histories, asthma, diabetes, or severe cardiopulmonary disease. These iodine contrast agents generally cannot be used in patients with renal failure, even if mild
7. The patient should be informed that the amount of x-ray exposure is small and can be less than that of a regular chest film

Body Scan. Generally the same as the head scan with the following differences and additions:

1. The patient is placed supine on the scanner table with a waist strap to help him or her maintain the position
2. The table moves into the scanner, usually feet first, leaving the head free except when the scan is of the head
3. Inform the patient that he or she may be asked to hold his or her breath at intervals during the procedure to eliminate motion artifact
4. The scan process can be used to do a biopsy. The suspect area will be identified on a scan. Placement of a biopsy needle will be done (under local anesthesia, if needed) outside the scanner. The patient will be returned into the scanner and the biopsy needle placement checked. Again, outside the scanner, the specimen will be taken
5. The amount of radiation exposure to the patient is less than with a series of regular x rays

---

IMPLICATIONS FOR NURSING: CT SCANS

1. A permit (or consent) is usually required for most head or body scans, particularly if a contrast medium is to be used
2. Patient preparation
   a. The patient will almost always be n.p.o. for some period before a CT test, but these periods vary with the type of test and with the laboratory doing the test. *Check the protocol in use.* The following are protocols followed at many sites:
      (1) n.p.o. 3 to 4 hours before the test if contrast medium is to be used, or this is *not known*
      (2) For tests in the morning, n.p.o. 8 hours before testing. Small sips of water are usually allowed up to 2 hours before the test
      (3) Late afternoon or evening testing, full liquid breakfast with sips of water as in (2)
      (4) Medications are usually allowed up to 2 hours before testing
   b. Obtain the weight of grossly obese patients, and inform the CT department. (Most scanners accommodate individuals up to approximately 290 lbs., although some scanners are larger)

    c. Check for any history of iodine sensitivity (shellfish, previous contrast studies) if a contrast medium is to be used or if medium to be used is not known. Inform the CT department immediately of previous sensitivities or allergic responses

    d. Check orders or protocols about the possible need for a heparin lock or for starting an IV infusion before the test

    e. Notify the imaging department if the patient:

      (1) Is diabetic

      (2) Has had any recent barium studies

      (3) Has any physiological needs (e.g., oxygen)

      (4) Has any kidney disease, especially renal failure

      (5) Is allergic to iodine

3. Patient education

    a. Explain the steps of test preparation, and process clearly and simply, with a rationale for each

    b. A head scan is particularly difficult for the person with any tendency to claustrophobia (see also "Implications for Nursing," Section 17.7.1, "MRI"). Do *not* stress the potential problem unless the patient brings it up. In all cases, be sure the patient knows that verbal communication with the person doing the test is available throughout the test and that anything that causes apprehension may be discussed, preferably during scanning breaks. Assure the patient that he or she can be removed from the scanner if necessary, even if the test is not completed. Problem-solve with the patient to determine how he or she usually copes, or best copes, if apprehension is evident

    c. If cost is a concern, inform the patient/family of the cost saving factors of the test compared with the multiple tests it will replace

    d. If a contrast medium is to be used, make sure that the patient knows the early signs or symptoms of physical response (usually flushing of the face, a metallic taste in the mouth, and, less frequently, slight nausea, all experienced for only 1 or 2 minutes). Adverse or allergic responses, such as shortness of breath, tightness in the throat, or facial swelling should be reported at onset. An oral antihistamine may be given to allay the response. *Delayed* allergic responses to contrast medium include headache, skin rash, urticaria, or vomiting and should be reported on discovery. Both early and delayed responses should be reported at onset

4. Test-specific patient preparation

    a. Head scans

      (1) Remove any hair clips, pins, jewelry, hair pieces, hearing aids, eye glasses, or contact lenses to prevent interference with scan visualization

      (2) A mild sedative or tranquilizer may be ordered pretest to

        (a) Decrease anxiety, especially that caused by claustrophobia

        (b) Alleviate discomfort in the neck or back

        (c) Help the patient remain still during the test

    b. Body scans: As for the head scan, with the following differences and additions

      (1) If a *biopsy* is planned, check for history of sensitivity to local anesthetics or of blood clotting disorder

      (2) Check with the imaging department for specific requirements. (For example, a *stomach scan* may require inflation by high-fluid intake before testing. A GI scan may involve the following: low-residue diet and or bowel preparation to decrease or remove bowel flatus; glucagon given to decrease peristalsis, metoclopramide (Reglan) given to increase stomach transit time. For a gynecologic examination a tampon may be placed in the vagina as a marker.)

      (3) Determine that there have been no barium studies within 3 to 4 days before the test

      (4) For abdominal scans, an oral contrast medium is usually given, sometimes the evening before, at least 8 hours before the test is to be done, or the morning of the test

5. Posttest care

    a. Provide fluids, and explain the need for increased fluid intake, if not contraindicated, to flush the system of contrast material and provide fluid replacement

    b. If iodine has been injected, check for signs of *delayed sensitivity* (e.g., hives, weakness, tremors, severe diarrhea), and report reactions. Administer any ordered antihistamines or steroids, explaining their purpose. *Severe allergic reactions*, for which emergency drugs should always be available, include dyspnea, hypotension, itching, palpitations, tachycardia, or urticaria

c. The patient can usually return to his or her usual diet and fluid intake if no further tests are to be done and to normal activity immediately

6. Length of time needed: Varies with the area or number of areas being scanned: 1 to 1½ hours, maximum—usually 15 to 30 minutes. If a contrast medium used, 30 minutes to one hour. Usually, body scans take the longest, head scans the least time. If a biopsy is also done, an additional ½ hour to 1 hour is needed

B. *Computerized Tomography Angiogram/Angiography*

Synonyms: CTA, enhanced CT scans

Explanation of the Test. The term *enhanced CT scans* refers to the use of IV contrast materials with CT to highlight structures. This technique has been found to be particularly useful in brain scans and is generally required for CT scanning of retroperitoneal or abdominal areas (i.e., gallbladder, liver, pancreas, spleen).

The term *computerized tomography angiogram (CTA)* refers to the fairly recent use of CT with angiography. At the time of this writing, when compared to MRI, CTA has been found to do its best work in abdominal and pelvic neurovascular imaging, with a relatively small potential for flow-related artifacts. It has also been found to be equally useful, compared to MRI, in thoracic and pulmonary imaging and to be better tolerated by the elderly as it takes less time than MRI angiography, thereby decreasing the period of immobility (Fry et al., 1989, p. 13; Stephens, 1993a, pp. 39–40, 1993b, pp. 31–40).

C. *Three-Dimensional Reconstruction CT Scans*

Synonyms: 3-D computerized tomography, 3-D CT

Explanation of the Test. This is a noninvasive test that provides a real-time moving picture of the body—including soft tissues—demonstrating irregularities in function as well as structure.

3-D CT scanning adds 180° mobility of the scanner around the body, so that multiple horizontal, cross-sectional, or sagittal planes of x-ray are made at various angles. The slices are then serially organized to form a 3-D data set. The special computer hardware allows the data, when computed and displayed, to appear as a single 3-D image with perspective, surface, and depth shading. It is especially useful in craniofacial reconstruction as it can provide an exact template for the construction of a prosthetic device.

The 3-D test generally takes more time than 2-D CT scanning. Therefore, it is currently used only for patients who have been stabilized, *not* in emergency situations. 3-D images can also be reconstructed from data sets but are often limited because of motion between the separate 2-D images. 3-D images have been found to be particularly useful in planning reconstruction of severe fractures with multiple fracture gaps (i.e., pelvic, spinal, or craniofacial fractures), as well as in planning surgery of brain tumors.

Purpose. 3-D computerized tomography is often used in visualization of complex fractures, mostly for surgical reconstruction planning purposes and except for certain kinds of acute spinal trauma, it is not expected to replace other two dimensional axial slices. The current primary use is in visualization of complex fractures for the purpose of surgical repair planning. The rapid data acquisition (scanning) provides a real-time image of the body as it works, showing irregularities in function. It is not, however, expected to replace the 2-D axial slice (see Section 17.7.2.A, "Computerized Tomography"), except for certain kinds of spinal trauma. The test is also currently emerging as a very promising tool for diagnosis of coronary artery disease (CAD) with a high negative predictive value (i.e., prediction of the absence of coronary artery disease).

ADVANTAGES OF 3-D TESTING:

1. All information gathered during scanning is kept in a primary data base, which prevents having to rescan
2. Spiral scanning shortens total scan time (to less than 14 minutes versus usual 30 minutes), which is especially helpful for patients in pain
3. When displayed on a video screen, the images can be rotated in any direction, to "see" from any direction
4. Detects very narrow fractures (as small as 0.5 mm)
5. Helps surgeons see and understand the 3-D nature of fractures (e.g., rotational component of complex fractures)
6. Provides useful models for reconstruction, analysis of translation, compression, and distraction components of unstable spinal injuries

D. Positron Emission Tomography*

Synonyms: PET, emission computed tomography (ECT), emission CT scan

Explanation of the Test. (See "Definition of Terms," Section 17.7.2.) Relatively noninvasive, PET scans include a computerized tomography technique that allows examination of metabolic activity within body structures. It combines the use of conventional nuclear diagnostic techniques with computerized tomography (CT). Cross-sectional tomographic slices of tissue that have concentrated positron-emitting isotopes are displayed by the computer. The test is relatively noninvasive (Gupta and Frick, 1993, p. 35).

Purpose. PET allows for the measurement of function and metabolism in both normal and diseased body tissues, with particular effectiveness in determining blood flow to the brain or heart. PET imaging has better resolution than other nuclear medicine procedures (Gupta and Frick, 1993, p. 235).

---

*A *positron* is defined as the antiparticle of an electron, a particle having the same mass as a negative electron but possessing a positive charge (Thomas, 1981, p. 118).

Specific uses include:

1. Brain activity or damage measurement in (Corbett, 1992, p. 543)
    a. Alzheimer's disease
    b. Dementia (type differentiation)
    c. Epilepsy
    d. Hypoperfusion
    e. Persistent migraine headaches
    f. Parkinson's disease
    g. Strokes
2. Cancer (See also Section 17.8.2.E, "PET-FDG")
    a. To guide therapeutic management decisions
    b. Staging
    c. To localize biopsy sites
    d. To evaluate treatment for recurrence (tumor uptake index)
3. Heart disease
    a. Hypoperfusion; ischemia
    b. Myocardial infarction (acute)
    c. First 72 hours

Procedure. A specific biochemical substance is tagged with a specific radionuclide that emits positrons. The substance is injected into the bloodstream or inhaled as a gas.

The PET scanner monitors the emissions of positive electrons (positrons). The time needed for uptake and elimination of the tracer (radionuclide) is measured. Computer processing produces color-coded images indicating the intensity of the specific organ's metabolic activity (Kee, 1991, p. 256).

Commonly used radiotracers (isotopes) with a short half-life produced by cyclotrons for PET imaging include compounds labeled with isotopes of carbon 11 (usually used with heart scans), oxygen 15, fluorine 18, and nitrogen 13 (Gupta and Frick, 1993, p. 236). (See also Section 17.7.2.E, "PET-FDG" on cancer scanning.)

There are risks of allergic reaction in the use of IV contrast materials. Assess for potential to, or history of allergic reaction and, if present, inform those doing the test prior to its start.

Time Needed. Dependent on the area being scanned and the early findings of the scan.

E. Positron Emission Tomography with F-18 Fluorodeoxyglucose

Synonym: PET-FDG

Explanation of the Test. Despite the dramatic increase in the ability to identify structural alterations caused by cancer (e.g., PET and MRI imaging), our ability to stage, assist in treatment planning, or monitor the disease is still limited. F-18 fluorodeoxyglucose (FDG), a glucose analog, has been used as a PET radiopharmaceutical to trace glucose metabolism. It is ultimately trapped intracellularly as FDG-6-phosphate, which has a very slow rate of breakdown (dehosphorylation). This is of special importance in the processes of staging, treatment planning, and monitoring cancer response to therapy. Cancer cells have been found to show a high rate of glycolysis (both aerobic and anaerobic) in malignant tumor cells. The level of glycolysis available through this test can be used to characterize a neoplasm as benign or malignant.

Tumor cells have also been linked to increased activity of glycolytic enzymes (e.g., hexokinase, phosphofructokinase, and pyruvate dehydrogenase).

Purpose

1. Combination of PET and FDG provides a way to assess a tumor's glycolytic rate because images of total FDG activity represent relative rates of glycolysis. The rate of tumor growth is related to the magnitude of glycolytic rate increase and vice versa. Assessment of the glycolytic rate can characterize a neoplasm as benign or malignant
2. To help quantitate changes in response to treatment (a glycolysis decrease indicates a decrease in tumor size). It is believed that PET with FDG estimates the extent of viable tumor mass
3. To characterize a soft-tissue neoplasm as benign or malignant (with a high rate of accuracy (e.g., almost 100 percent with pulmonary nodules). A malignancy is usually related to intense increase in FDG uptake
4. To assist in treatment planning and monitoring of lung cancer. It complements radiographic methods to evaluate response to treatment
5. To more accurately predict change in tumor volume than CT scans
6. May be able to provide early information on the presence of chemotherapy-resistant tumor cells line, frequently true in lung cancer
7. Demonstrates increased sensitivity and predictive accuracy over CT testing in colon cancer. In recurrence of colorectal tumor after resection, it may be helpful in differentiating a tumor from scarring or infection (more specific, sensitive, and accurate than PET alone)
8. Obviates need for biopsy to detect tumor recurrence in genitourinary cancer
9. Clearly differentiates high- and low-grade glioma in intracranial neoplasm. The tumor uptake of FDG provides correlation with length of patient survival. It picks up cerebral necrosis after chemo- or radiotherapy and differentiates between cerebral necrosis and residual or recurrent tumor

Procedure. (See Section 17.7.2.D, "Positron Emission Tomography.") In contrast with PET, the radionuclide-tagged biochemical use is FDG.

DISADVANTAGES:

1. Evaluation of larger body regions is limited because of the PET scanner's limited axial view
2. At present, there is decreased sensitivity in detection of small foci of tumors in radiation-damaged or necrosed tissue
3. High cost, despite the test's potential to prevent reoperative procedures

---

IMPLICATIONS FOR NURSING

As the use of PET-FDG is still in a somewhat experimental state, there are few specific nursing implications. The client and family will be fully informed about the process and expectations of the test by researchers. (See also Section 17.8.2.D, "Implications for Nursing.") (Gupta and Frick, 1993, pp. 235-254)

F. Single Photon Emission Tomography

Synonym: SPECT

Definition of the test. SPECT is a tomographic technique closely related to PET. It employs a tomographic principle, imaging with common, conventional radionuclides that are commercially available, and does not require an on-site cyclotron, as is true in PET imaging. It is widely used in cardiac evaluation (ischemia), bone imaging, and brain perfusion studies (Corbett, 1992, p. 544).

DISADVANTAGES. As the name implies, the technique of SPECT looks only at one photon (i.e., gamma ray).

ADVANTAGES. SPECT is less costly and more available than PET. Its use for organ scans has increased in conventional radionuclide studies, in turn increasing their sensitivity, specificity and usefulness (Berkow, 1992, p. 2548).

17.7.3 Biomagnetic Imaging

Synonym: Magnetic source imaging

Explanation of the Test. This is a method to record magnetic fields created by electrical activity inside the brain. The test makes use of a technology, used by the U.S. military to track magnetic fields produced by submarines, called superconducting quantum interference devices (SQUIDS).

Procedure. A sensor unit is placed close to the skin surface of the head or body, depending on the area to be monitored. (At this time, only electricity of the brain is monitored in the one physiological test actually in use, although many aspects are being studied.) A sensor unit is placed close to the skin surface of the head. It picks up the biomagnetic fields in the area. The SQUIDS unit can then convert these to electrical signals that are amplified and displayed on a computer screen. The technique is much like that used in doing an ECG or an electroencephalogram. The cost of the imaging unit is high, similar to that of an MRI or PET scan.

Purpose. The test had been developed to observe and define the source area of epileptic spikes with the aim of surgically treating the disease by removal of minimal brain tissue. Possible future uses include imaging for diagnosis and/or treatment of:
1. Migraine headaches that have distinguishable brain wave patterns
2. Alzheimer's disease
3. Strokes
4. Psychiatric disorders (e.g., depression, schizophrenia) (Phillips, P., 1990, pp. 31, 50)

Part

V

THERAPEUTIC AND TOXIC SUBSTANCES

Therapeutic drug monitoring has become an essential part of medical management of illness. Some treatment requires the use of medications with potential for toxicity. At times that potential is significant. Some medications have a very narrow therapeutic range requiring careful monitoring to provide adequate therapeutic levels without undertreatment or overdosage. Drug dosage to provide optimal therapeutic effect varies widely among individuals and therapeutic agents. With some drugs, the dosage schedule is best monitored by correlation of the dosage with the steady-state concentration in the blood rather than usual therapeutic range (Henry, 1991). This brings up the need to monitor patient response as well as the blood drug levels.

In the past, drug monitoring was done primarily by observation of the patient for effects of the drug. Because of the narrow range of effectiveness of some drugs and individual variation in response to medication, undertreatment or toxic response was not uncommon. Because of the level of difficulty involved in checking serum drug levels, the process was often limited to assessing for environmental toxins. As the technology expanded and simplified, the number of drugs that could be measured increased, and detection of foreign substances in the blood even at very low levels became possible.

In an effort to provide effective therapy with safety, many drugs are now almost routinely measured, especially in the critically ill patient and the hospitalized patient just beginning a course of treatment. The patient being given digoxin for the first time is an example of almost routine measurement of blood levels until the therapeutic range has been reached.

Drug levels are usually monitored for one of the following reasons:

1. Diagnosis of poisoning. Includes exposure to known poison; exposure to an unknown substance that may be a poison; disease of undetermined cause in which poisoning must be ruled out (Olson & Dreisbach, 1987, p. 1005)

2. Estimation of the therapeutic margin (index) for the individual (i.e., individual rate of drug metabolism)
3. Investigation of unexpected patient response to medication
   a. Relationship to patient compliance
   b. Patient variation in drug absorption, use, and excretion
   c. Effects of drug interaction with other medications
   d. Effects of organ disease (e.g., severe liver disease, gastrointestinal disease, renal disease)
   e. Cause of drug toxicity when several drugs are given concurrently
4. Obtaining reason for therapeutic failure
5. Obtaining baseline values after therapeutic response occurs to establish the relationship of a patient's blood drug level to the accepted therapeutic range (Ravel, 1989)

E I G H T E E N

ANALYSIS OF
THERAPEUTIC AND
TOXIC SUBSTANCES

18.1 PURPOSES OF TESTING

1. To determine whether the dosage being administered has reached recognized levels of therapeutic effectiveness
2. To determine whether the dosage needs to be adjusted upward to reach therapeutic levels or downward to prevent toxicity and yet maintain therapeutic levels
3. To determine possible toxicity resulting from environmental contaminants as a cause for otherwise unexplained signs and symptoms

Tables 18–1 through 18–6 give toxic and normal and/or therapeutic levels of nontherapeutic intoxicants, cardiac drugs, anticonvulsants, miscellaneous drugs, tricyclic antidepressants, and sedative/hypnotics, respectively.

RELATED NURSING IMPLICATIONS

1. If the toxicity is secondary to a drug being self-administered by the patient, check on compliance (i.e., is the drug being taken at the proper dosage and at the right time, and are instructions about food intake related to the time of drug administration being followed?)
2. If compliant, or the medications are being given by health care workers in a carefully supervised environment, look at
   a. Total body function compared with the route of administration, absorption, use, and excretion. For example, if the drug is absorbed through the small intestine, has the patient been having diarrhea or a history of malabsorption? If the drug is metabolized by the liver, is there a history of cirrhosis or evidence of jaundice? If the drug is excreted by the kidney, are fluid intake and output balanced?
   b. Other medications being taken concurrently for possible drug interactions or competition
   c. Serum albumin levels if the drug is bound to albumin in the body for metabolism or transport
3. If a blood level of a drug is to be determined, the laboratory will need to know several things besides the name of the drug to be assayed
   a. The patient's age

---

b. The time of the last dose before specimen collection

c. How the medication is being given (oral, intramuscular, intravenous, dermal patch, inhalation)

d. Purpose of the test (e.g., possible toxicity, no response to medication, determination of therapeutic level)

e. All the medications being given concurrently. Some medications may compete for protein-binding sites with the drug being assayed, which would increase the amount of free (nonbound) drug fraction in the blood, the fraction that is metabolically active. The drug assay measures the *total* drug level, bound and unbound. Without information as to other medications in use, the results may be misleading

4. Be aware of physiological or pathophysiological states that can alter either protein binding (e.g., hypoalbuminemia) or inhibit or potentiate the action of the therapeutic agent being given (e.g., hypokalemia, increasing digoxin effect, or hyperkalemia decreasing the digoxin effect because of competition between digoxin and potassium for binding sites)

5. Knowledge of the metabolism of the drug being given is most useful in interpreting blood levels of the drug. Although the nurse is not responsible for such interpretation, she or he can make more knowledgeable decisions as to when the doctor needs to be informed quickly, if she or he has the knowledge (e.g., time of peak effect, given the route of administration; serum half-life; site of metabolism in the body; length of time needed to reach a "steady state" in the blood; and the therapeutic level)

6. If environmental intoxication is suspected, the nurse can be instrumental in assessing for a past history of probable exposure and signs and symptoms experienced to date as well as doing necessary patient teaching for future self-care in the prevention of a recurrence or management of problems related to the intoxication

TABLE 18–1. NONTHERAPEUTIC INTOXICANTS

Drug Name	Normal Level	Toxic Level	Comments
Aluminum (Al)	0–10 µg/L	>10 µg/L	Possible cause of dialysis encephalopathy in chronic renal failure patients. Possible cause of Alzheimer's disease in nonrenal patients
Arsenic (As)	6–20 µg/dl (blood)	—	Samples must be collected in a metal-free container
	≤0.1 mg/L (0–100 µg/L) (urine)	0.1 mg/L/24 hr 200 µg/L/24 gr urine >800 µg/L/24 hr^a urine	Urine testing is the method of choice because arsenic rapidly enters tissue protein
	0.1 µg/g (hair)	0.1–0.5 mg/100 gm (hair) Up to 3 mg/100 g^a (hair)	Nails and hair are used to check chronic arsenic poisoning. Nails need to grow for 6–9 mo after acute exposure before being used for testing; hair should grow for 2 wk after acute exposure
	0.1 µg/g (nails)	>0.1 µg/g (nails)	Urine can be collected as a random specimen, or as a 24-hr sample
Lead (Pb)	0–50 µg/dl	>50–80 µg/dl	Possible to see symptoms at levels over 30 mg/dl (blood)
	(0.01–0.08 mg/dl (whole blood)	>0.10 mg/gl	City dwellers tend to have higher levels than rural populations
	0–100 µg/dl/24 hr (urine)	>0.15 mg/dl/24 hr	Most lead poisoning is chronic
			Total body lead levels are not necessarily indicated by blood levels
Mercury (Hg)	0–7 ng/ml (blood)	>7 ng/ml	Lethal effects are dependent on adequate kidney function, which clears inorganic Hg. The gastrointestinal tract clears 90% of organic Hg
	0.20 µg/L/24 hr (urine)		Chronic exposure leads to Hg accumulation in the brain and decreased cognitive function
			Blood levels are not necessarily a true reflection of total body levels
			The specimen to be checked must not touch metal

^{a}Acute toxicity.
Data from Ravel, 1989; SHMC, 1984.

TABLE 18–2. CARDIAC DRUGS: THERAPEUTIC AND TOXIC LEVELS

Drug Name	Normal Range	Therapeutic Level	Toxic Level
Digoxin (Lanoxin)	0	0.5–2.5 ng/ml	>3.0 ng/ml (2–6 ng/ml range)
Digitoxin (Crystodigin, Purodigin)	0	11–23 ng/ml	26–35 ng/ml
Disopryamide (Norpace)	0	2–5 µg/ml	>6 µg/ml
Lidocaine	0	1.4–6 µg/ml	>6 µg/ml
Procainamide (Pronestyl)	0	4–8 µg/ml (levels with N-acetyl procainamide [NAPA], 10–30 µg/ml	8–16 µg/ml (levels with NAPA, 25–30 µg/ml)
Propranolol (Inderal)	0	20–85 ng/ml	>150 ng/ml
Quinidine (Duraquin, Quinaglute)	0	2–5 µg/ml	>10 µg/ml
Verapamil (Isoptin, Calan)	0	2–4 µg/ml(100–300 ng/ml)	>5 µg/ml

Data from Govoni & Hayes, 1985; McFarland & Grant, 1982; and SHMC, 1984.

Metabolism in the Body	Comments
Half-life: 32 hr Peak level: 30–90 min after administration Plateau: 6–8 hr after administration	Maintaining levels depends on the kidney's ability to excrete the K^+ and Ca^{++} in the blood Overlap between therapeutic and toxic levels makes careful assessment of clinical signs and symptoms, electro-cardiograms(ECGs), and laboratory data extremely important
Half-life: 5–7 days Peak level: 12–24 hr Plateau: 2 days	Action, effects much the same as digoxin but with slower onset and peak effect, and longest half-life, thus used on maintenance Metabolized by the liver; only 8% excreted in urine, thus safer in renal failure
Half-life: variable, 4–10 hr Peak level: 1–2 hr Plateau: 1.5–8.5 hr	Oral antiarrhythmic, similar in action to quinidine and procainamide. Used to suppress/prevent premature ventricular contractions (PVCs). Not used in uncompensated congestive heart failure (CHF), hypotension (unless secondary to arrhythmia), or hypokalemia. Patients are usually digitalized before use Toxic effects include hypoglycemia, agranulocytosis, jaundice Side effects: dry mouth, hypotension, photosensitivity, dizziness, and blurring of vision
Half–life: 2 hr Peak level: intravenous (IV) 10–90 s; intramuscular (IM), 5–15 min Plateau: 5–20 min	Neurotoxic Used for ventricular arrhythmias, rapid control Liver disease interferes with metabolism of drug; kidney disease with excretion of the drug Hypersensitivity reactions possible
Half-life: 3 hr Peak level: variable, 1–2 hr after oral Plateau: 2.2–4 hr (with NAPA, 6–11 hr) Steady state: 11–20 hr (with NAPA, 30–50 hr)	NAPA is a metabolite of procainamide that is produced at different rates in each patient. It adds its own antiarrhythmatic effect Used with ventricular arrhythmias Toxic effects include allergic reactions, bone marrow depression
Half-life: 3–4 hr Peak level: 1–1-1/2] hr IV peak, 15 min after administration Plateau: 6 hr IV, 3–6 hr	Excreted primarily in urine and 0–5% in feces, thus prolonged action in kidney dysfunction Crosses placenta and blood–brain barrier Antiarrhythmic, antihypertensive Can cause profound bradycardia, decreased central nervous system (CNS) function, hypoglycemia in diabetics
Half-life: 4–6 hr Peak level: oral (sulfate), 1 hr after dose; oral (gluconate) 5 hr after dose Trough level: Just before next dose gluconate maintenance dose, 2–3 times each day; sulfate maintenance dose, every 6 hr, 3–4 times each day Plateau: variable Steady state: 20–35 hr	Used to decrease atrial excitability (e.g., atrial fibrillation) Unpredictable rhythm abnormalities and need to be monitored when drug is being started. Hypersensitivity response often a feeling of faintness/fainting (quinidine syncope) because of decreased cardiac output Primarily cardiotoxic Have on hand molar solution of lactate vasoconstrictors/catecholamines for severe hypotension
Half-life: 4 min, initial; terminal phase, 2–5 hr Peak level: 10–15 min Plateau: 6 hr	Antiarrhythmic, used with atrial arrhythmias. Also effective as a vaso-dilator and can therefore decrease blood pressure, relieve angina Adverse reactions occur most often with IV administration, in the elderly, or those with impaired renal function Side effects: severe hypotension, bradycardia or severe tachycardia, pruritis, abdominal discomfort/nausea, constipation Not given in severe CHF; given with caution with many other cardiac drugs (e.g., digitalis, procainamide, and quinidine) and in hepatic or renal dysfunction

Data from Tilian et al., 1979; Widmann, 1983.

TABLE 18–3. ANTICONVULSIVE DRUGS: THERAPEUTIC AND TOXIC LEVELS

Drug Name	Normal Range	Therapeutic Level	Toxic Level
Carbamazepine (Tegretol)	0	4–10 µg/ml	15 µg/ml
Ethosuximide (Zarontin/Succinimide)	0	4–100 µg/ml	150 µg/ml
Phenylethylmalonamide (PEMA), a primidone metabolite	0	5–25 µg/ml	?
Phenobarbital (Luminal)	0	15–40 µg/ml	50 µg/ml
Phenytoin (Dilantin/5-diphenylhydantoin)	0	10–20 µg/ml	20 µg/ml
Primidone (Mysoline)	0	5–17 µg/ml	15 µg/ml
Valproic acid (Depakene)	0	50–100 µg/ml (adults) 50–200 µg/ml (children)	200 µg/ml

Metabolism in the Body			Comments
	Adults	Children	
Half-life:	6–18 hr	2–4 days	Highly bound to plasma protein; excreted in urine and feces, thus effect prolonged with renal dysfunction
Peak:	6–18 hr	6–18 hr	
Plateau:	10–30 hr	8–19 hr	Used for the same convulsive disorders as phenytoin but with fewer side effects
Steady state:	30–42 hr		
(when given three times/day)			Also used in temporal lobe epilepsy and tonic-clonic seizures
			Can be used alone or with other anticonvulsant drugs
Half-life:	20–60 hr		Used primarily in control of petit mal (absence) seizures
Peak:	1–4 hr		Early signs of overdose are headache, drowsiness, or hyperactivity and ataxia
Steady state:			
Adults:	8–12 days		
Children:	6–10 days		
Half-life: 24–45 hr (depends on degree of metabolism of parent drug)			Primidone is metabolized by the liver into PEMA and phenobarbital
Peak: depends on parent drug metabolism, as for half-life			Use of phenytoin (Dilantin) will enhance the metabolism of primidone and increase phenobarbital levels
Steady state: 24 hr			
Half-life: 72–144 hr			Although ordinarily 50 µl/ml is a toxic level, with chronic treatment, therapeutic levels increase and may approach 50 µg/ml without toxicity
	Adults	Children	
Peak:	6–18 hr	6–18 hr	
Steady state:	11–25 days	8–15 days	Used to elevate seizure thresholds
			Side effects: sedation (tolerance increases over time), confusion, or marked excitement (in elderly)
			Overdose: respiratory depression, oliguria, pupil constriction
	Adults	Children	Phenytoin requires longer periods of time for elimination once blood levels reach 10 µg/ml
Half-life:	7–42 hr		
Peak:	4–8 hr	4–8 hr	Blood used for checking levels should be drawn at least 4 hr past the last dose or just before the next dose
Plateau:	18–30 hr	12–22 hr	
Steady state:	4–6 days	2–5 days	Used to control grand mal and psychomotor seizures
			Overdosage causes nystagmus, ataxia, slurred speech, and confusion
			Can cause hyperglycemia, anemia, and hypocalcemia
	Adults	Children	Most effective when given with phenobarbital
Half-life:	3–24 hr		Used to control grand mal, psychomotor, and focal seizures
Peak:	2–4 hr	2–4 hr	Cautious use with chronic lung disease and hepatic or renal dysfunction
Plateau:	3.3–12.5 hr	4–6 hr	
Steady state:	16–60 hr	20–30 hr	Increases need for vitamin D; may impair calcium, folic acid, and vitamin B metabolism
			Linked to neonatal hemorrhage; pregnant women using primidone (Mysoline) need prophylactic vitamin K for 1 mo before and during delivery
	Adults	Children	Therapeutic levels are delayed in patients with liver disease
Half-life:	8–12 hr		Can impair use of phenobarbital and increase its serum level
Peak:	0.5–1.5 hr	0.5–1.5 hr	Used to control absence seizures, and with other agents, used to treat generalized seizures
(wide individual variation, 1–4 hr)			
Plateau:	8–15 hr	6–15 hr	Causes false-positive urine ketone result
Steady state:	40–75 hr	30–75 hr	Prolongs bleeding time, decreases platelet count, and white blood cell (WBC) count
			Crosses placenta; enters breast milk

Data from Govoni & Hayes, 1985; McFarland & Grant, 1982; Ravel, 1989; SHMC, 1984; Tilkian et al., 1987; and Widmann, 1983.

TABLE 18–4. MISCELLANEOUS DRUGS: THERAPEUTIC AND TOXIC LEVELS

Drug Name	Normal Range	Therapeutic Level	Toxic Level
Acetaminophen (Tempra/ Tylenol/Robigesic)	0	10–26 µg/ml	26 µg/ml
Alcohol	0	0.10 g/dl (legal definition of intoxication)	Lethal level: 0.36–0.40 g/dl (350–400 mg/dl)
Cyclosporine	0	100–200 ng/ml (trough)	300 ng/ml
Salicylates (aspirin/Arthropan Mobidin/Salsprin Uracel)	0	Serum: Antipyretic: 20–100 µg/ml Analgesic: 20–100 µg/ml Antiinflammatory: 100–250 µg/ml Urine: 0–50 µg/ml (adult level; may be toxic in children)	300 µg/ml (20–25 mg/dl) Lethal level (adults): 30–35 mg/dl
Secobarbital (Seconal)	0	1–5 µg/dl (10–40 µg/ml for persons with seizure disorders)	>7 µg/ml (150-250 mg/dl) Lethal level: 10 µg/ml (350–400 mg/dl)
Theophylline or aminophylline[a] (Bronkodyl, Theo-Dur Somophyllin-DF)	0	10–20 µg/ml	>20 µg/ml Lethal level: 20–25 µg/ml

[a]Therapeutic action of Aminophylline is dependent on its theophylline content (Govoni & Hayes, 1985, p. 59). The same test is usually done on both aminophylline and theophylline, and the therapeutic, toxic, and lethal levels are the same.

Metabolism in the Body		Comments
Half-life:	1–3 hr	Blood for testing is best drawn just before the next dose
Peak:	$\frac{1}{2}$–1 hr	Excreted in urine
Plateau:	1–5 hr	Overdosage leads to hepatotoxicity, which may be nonsymptomatic in the early stages
		Signs and symptoms of acute overdosage (3–4 hr after ingestion): anorexia, nausea, vomiting, dizziness, lethargy, generalized weakness, diaphoresis
		Monitor hepatic, renal, and hematopoietic function with high dosage or long-term treatment
Half-life:	Variable	5% or 10% alcohol (ETOH) in 5% dextrose in water is used to inhibit premature labor and can be used to provide calories for metabolic needs. Most frequent therapeutic use is to prevent delirium tremens in the emergency surgical patient who is an active alcoholic
Peak:	Variable	
Plateau:	Variable	
		Trough levels are used for measurement 1 hr before next dose is due
		Used to depress T-cell function, thus prevent graft rejection (bone marrow, kidney, heart/lungs, liver)
		A rash accompanies renal toxicity
Half-life:	Dose-dependent	Many false positives in urine testing
Peak:	1–2 hr	Usual adult dose of 600 mg aspirin = serum levels of 50–70 µg/ml
Plateau:	2–4 hr (adults)	Dose of 100 mg/kg body weight = serum concentrations of 200–300 µg/ml
	2–3 hr (children)	Early signs of toxicity: tinnitus, increased respiratory rate and depth leading to respiratory alkalosis. Metabolic acidosis occurs at levels of 450–750 µg/ml

Metabolism in the Body			Comments
Half-life: 20–28 hr			A CNS depressant
Peak:			45–75% bound to plasma proteins
Oral/rectal: 15–30 min			If used for the elderly, usual dose may cause confusion/excitement
IM: 7–10 min			Has sedative and hypnotic effect
IV: 1–3 min			Dose in acute convulsive episodes is 3–5 mg/kg, given IM
Plateau:			
Oral/rectal: 3–5 hr			
IM: ? 30–45 min			
IV: 15 min			

Metabolism in the Body	Adults	Children	Comments
Half-life:	3–8 hr	1–8 hr	Action prolonged in liver disease, with half-life prolonged by as much as 60 hr
		(newborns: 17–45 hr)	Toxic effects: CNS stimulation, cardiac arrythmmias
Peak:			Used for prophylaxis and symptomatic relief of bronchial asthma and treatment of bronchospasm in chronic bronchitis and emphysema
Oral	2–3 hr	—	
Slow release	3–6 hr	—	Early signs of toxic effects: nausea, vomiting, diarrhea, insomnia, headache, marked hypotension
IV	15 min	—	
Steady state:	15–40 hr	5–40 hr	Smoking reduces the half-life. Cessation of smoking may precipitate toxic level if dose not reduced
			Caffeine is an important active metabolite in neonates

Data from Govoni & Hayes, 1985; McFarland & Grant, 1982; Ravel, 1984; SHMC, 1984; Tilkian et al., 1987; and Widmann, 1983.

TABLE 18–5. TRICYCLIC ANTIDEPRESSANT TOXICOLOGY SCREEN (SERUM)

Drug Name	Normal Range	Therapeutic Range (ng/ml)	Toxic Level (ng/ml)	Half-Life (hr)	Steady State (day)	Peak (hr)
Amitriptyline (Elavil)[a]	0	120–250	500	17–40	4–8	4–8
Desipramine (Norpramin/Pertofrane)	0	20–160	500	12–54	2.5–15	2–8
Imipramine (Tofranil)[b]	0	150–250	500	9–24	2–5	1–2
Nortriptyline (Aventyl)	0	50–150	500	30–90	4–19	4–8
Protriptyline (Vivactyl)	0	70–260 (approximately)	Not available	50–198	>10	6–12
Doxepin (Sinequan)	0	150–250	Not available	8–36	2–8	2–6

[a]Amitriptyline is metabolized to the active metabolite compound nortriptyline. Effective and toxic levels given are the *sum* of imipramine and desipramine concentrations.
[b]Metabolized to its active metabolite desipramine. Effective toxic levels given are the *sum* of imipramine and desipramine concentrations.
Adapted from Swedish Hospital Medical Center, Laboratory of Pathology (1984). *Laboratory Procedure Manual.* Seattle: SHMC, with permission.

TABLE 18–6. SEDATIVE, HYPNOTIC, TRANQUILIZER TOXICOLOGY SCREEN (SERUM)

Drug Name	Therapeutic Range (µg/ml)	Toxic Range (µg/ml)	Action
Amobarbital (Amytal), intermediate acting	1–5	>10	Sedative, hypnotic
Butabarbital (Butisol), intermediate acting	1–5	>10	Sedative, hypnotic
Chlordiazepoxide (Librium)	0.1–3.0	>3	Antianxiety
Diazepam (Valium)	0.5–2.5	>3	Antianxiety
Glutethimide (Doriden)	0.5–2.5	>10	Sedative
Mebrobamate (Equinil, Miltown)	5–20	>30	Antianxiety
Methaqualone (Quaalude)	~5	>5	Sedative, hypnotic
Methyprylon (Noludar)	~10	>30	Hypnotic
Pentobarbital (Nembutal), short acting	0.1–1.0	>10	Sedative, hypnotic
Phenobarbital (Luminal),[a] long acting	0.1–1.0	>50	Sedative, hypnotic
Phenytoin (Dilantin)[a]	10–20	>20	Anticonvulsive, sedative, hypnotic
Secobarbital (Seconal),[a] long acting	0.1–1.0	>10	Sedative, hypnotic

[a]See also separate test information for these drugs.
Adapted from Swedish Hospital Medical Center, Laboratory of Pathology (1984). *Laboratory Procedure Manual.* Seattle: SHMC, with permission.

A P P E N D I X   A

ANION GAP

Synonyms: "R" factor, delta gap

(Metheny & Snively, 1983, p. 72)

Purpose. The anion gap is used as an aid in determining the cause of metabolic acidosis based on laboratory values frequently at hand (i.e., measurements of plasma sodium [Na], chloride [Cl], bicarbonate [HCO_3], and in some methods, potassium [K]).

Definition. The computed difference between the sum of plasma sodium concentration (alone or with potassium, see "Purpose") and the sum of chloride and bicarbonate concentrations, which looks at the electrical neutrality balance between the ions

Process. The anion gap is calculated by using the following formula:

$$[Na^+] + [K^+] \text{ (if used)} - [Cl^-] + [HCO_3]$$
$$\text{(Cations} - \text{Anions)}$$

(If the sum of the anions is greater than the sum of the cations, consider a laboratory error)

Reference Range:[a] 8 to 16 mEq/L (without measuring [K^+]);
  8 to 20 mEq/L (measuring [K^+])

---

[a]As a rule of thumb, values less than 8 or greater than 17 are considered abnormal. (According to Porth [1986, p. 452], the highest normal level—even adding in K^+—would be 16 mEq/L). According to Metheny and Snively (1983, p. 73), any metabolic acidosis at or below the 16-mEq/L level would be due to inorganic acids. (Volatile anions are not useful in the calculation. When the concentration of unmeasured anions initially increases, bicarbonate is displaced, and the blood pH drops, which stimulates respiratory compensation with increased respiratory rate and depth and results in volatile acid blowoff.) Levels greater than 16 mEq/L indicate an excellent chance of acidosis due to increased organic acid levels. Levels equal to or greater than 20 mEq/L are almost surely due to increased organic acid levels.

Metabolic Acidotic States with Anion Gap in Normal Range. This is due to an accumulation of inorganic acids, which is related to

1. Primary decrease in bicarbonate level (e.g., severe diarrhea)
2. Accumulation of chloride-containing acids (e.g., HCl, NHCl) as with ureteroenterostomy (Metheny & Snively, 1983, p. 73)

3. Impaired acid excretion (e.g., mild renal insufficiency)
4. Renal tubular acidosis
5. Hyperalimentation due to increased cation content of amino acids

Metabolic Acidotic States with Increased Anion Gap Levels

1. Exogenous acid accumulation: methanol, ethylene glycol, salicylates, methyl ethylene, alcohol, paraldehyde
2. Endogenous acid accumulation as in severe renal failure with PO_4, SO_4, and proteinate retention
3. Diabetic ketoacidosis
4. Lactic acidosis secondary to decreased blood pressure/tissue hypoxia

APPENDIX B

PHYSIOLOGICAL RESPONSE TO STRESS AND RELATED LABORATORY CHANGES

Besides the mechanisms specifically related to providing extra glucose in times of stress, the following physiological changes that cause variation in laboratory findings occur:

1. The spleen contracts, which forces increased numbers of RBCs into circulation (hemoconcentration with increased RBC count, hemoglobin concentration, and hematocrit).
2. Bronchi dilate so that air can be moved more easily in and out of the lung (hyperventilation—respiratory alkalosis, decreased Pco_2).
3. The hypothalamus produces corticotropin-releasing factor (CRF), which stimulates the release of stored adrenocorticotropic hormone (ACTH), which in turn stimulates the release of glucocorticoids (increased plasma cortisol) (Frohlich, 1976).
4. Glucocorticoids foster the fat mobilization (increased levels of free fatty acids [FAAs]) as well as glucagon production and release, which accounts for the increased serum glucose level.
5. During stress, there is a reduction in lymphatic tissue, including the spleen, noted in item 1, and the thymus; this means fewer lymphocytes in circulation.
6. The eosinophil concentration is also reduced in the circulating blood for reasons that are not yet clear.
7. Antidiuretic hormone (ADH) is released by the pituitary causing fluid retention, and if the extracellular volume (ECV) is decreased, aldosterone is released and sodium reabsorbed, which causes further water conservation (potential dilutional hyponatremia, potassium loss, increased serum bicarbonate, decreased sodium and chloride, potential metabolic alkalosis).
8. Urinary output is decreased during and after stress (concentrated urine).
9. There is a net catabolic effect from these hormonal responses that causes muscle loss, weight loss, and an increased serum urea nitrogen concentration (BUN) (Harvey et al., 1986).
10. The generalized response to stress may be less effective if called upon during the night. The diurnal rhythm of adrenocorticosteroid output is diminished during the night (MacBryde & Blacklow, 1970).
11. Because cholesterol is a precursor in the formation of adrenocorticol hormones, cholesterol levels increase in the blood (cholesteremia).
12. The white blood count increases despite the decrease in lymphocytes and eosinophils because of retention of polymorphonuclear cells within the vascular system.

A PPENDIX C

DIALYSIS DISEQUILIBRIUM SYNDROME

The cause of the disequilibrium syndrome is thought to be the rapid removal of urea from the bloodstream, with its accompanying removal from the brain being at a slower rate. This leads to a reverse osmotic gradient that pulls water into the brain and causes cerebral edema—hence the signs and symptoms of headache, nausea, vomiting, and a rise in blood pressure. The coil dialyzer (rarely seen in use at present) removes urea more rapidly than do other types of dialyzers, and the use of this machine has been linked with the occurrence of the syndrome. It is also found to occur most frequently in acutely ill individuals with excessively increased serum urea nitrogen levels. Only occasionally has this syndrome been observed in patients who have undergone previous prolonged periods of uneventful dialysis. Thus, at risk is the person first starting hemodialysis.

The condition is treated primarily by the physician by a change in dialysate (increased glucose concentration in the dialysate has been found helpful in preventing the syndrome [Czaczkes & De-Nour, 1978, pp. 56–58]) or a change in the length or frequency of dialysis. A change in the type of dialyzer is indicated if a coil machine has been used. Also, the use of anticonvulsants before dialysis is felt to prevent the syndrome (Harrington & Brener, 1973, pp. 140–141).

Appendix D

Information on Laboratory Reporting Units

UNITS OF MEASUREMENT

Term	Definition	Abbreviation
Attagram	10^{-18} (quintillionth)	a
Centigram	10^{-2} (hundredth)	c
Decaliter	10 L	Not used in reporting laboratory values
Deciliter	1/10 L or 100 ml	dl
Femtoliter	10^{-15} liters	fl
Gigameter	10^{-9} (huge)	G
Gram	Basic weight unit of metric scale: 15,432 grains	Gm, gm, G, or g[a]
Hectoliter	10^{2} (hundredth)	hl
International unit	Number of moles of substrate converted per second under defined conditions (Henry, 1991)	IU
Megacuries	10^{6} (large/1 million)	MCi
Microgram	One millionth (10^{-6}) of a gram or 1/1000 (10^{-3}) of a milligram	µg[a] or mcg
Micromicrogram or picogram	10^{-12} grams	pg[a] or µµg
Milli-International Unit	1/1000 IU	mIU
Millimicrogram	1/1000 (10^{-3}) microgram or 10^{-9} grams	mµg
Micrometer or micron	10^{-6} meters	µm
Nanogram	10^{-9} grams	ng[a] or nµg
Picogram	10^{-12} (trillionth)	P
Teracuries	10^{12} (monster/trillion)	T

Note: Suprascript positive numbers (e.g., 10^{2}) are multiplication factors designating "times the unit" specified by the root to which it is joined. Negative multiplication factors (e.g., 10^{-2}) are indicated by the suprascript minus sign.
[a]Suprascript a (e.g., g[a]) indicates the abbreviation used in this book when more than one abbreviation is given for a term.

Unit conversion

$$1 \ dl \quad = \quad 100 \ ml$$
$$1 \ mg/dl \quad = \quad 1 \ mg/100 \ ml = 1 \ mg\%$$

g/L   = g% × 10
1 IU/ml   = 83.3 ng/ml
1 mIU/ml = 0.08 ng/ml
1 ng/ml   = 12 MIU/ml

SI Units (Le Systeme International d'Unités). Many possible changes in terminology for units of measurement are proposed in the SI system. The purpose of such change would be to provide common, unambiguous language worldwide for all sciences, not just the biological sciences. Adoption in the United States has been slow, but some of the units are in use in many laboratories (e.g., substitution of millimole [mM] for milliequivalent [mEq]).

A rationale of the need for change is well depicted in this sample by Dr. R. Conn (1991).

- *Present reporting system:* 1.0 g of hemoglobin
    Combines with 1.37 ml of oxygen
    Contains 3.4 mg of iron
    Forms 34.9 mg of bilirubin
- *SI reporting:* 1.0 mmol of hemoglobin
    Combines with 4.0 mmol of oxygen
    Contains 4.0 mmol of iron
    Forms 4.0 mmol of bilirubin

Some serious disadvantages exist in converting from one reporting system to another, aside from the effort involved in becoming familiar with the new terminology and its meaning. For example, some changes would require the development of new instruments for measurement. An everyday example affecting nursing would be the need for a different way to measure blood pressure externally. The present sphygmomanometer is based on a pressure measurement of milliliters of mercury. It would have to be converted to a measurement derived from the basic units of time in seconds, length (distance) in meters, and mass in kilograms.

Listed below are some possibly helpful "rules" or "conventions" that have grown up around the conversion to the SI measurements (Conn, 1991; Powsner, 1984).

1. No periods are used after SI symbols (e.g., mmol) and no *s* is added to plural usage
2. Long numbers are divided by a half-space rather than a comma (e.g., 6,660,000 would be written 6 660 000)
3. Compound prefixes are not used (e.g., picogram rather than micromicrogram)
4. Multiples and submultiples progress in steps of 3 (e.g., 10^3 or 10^{-3})
5. In reporting temperature the degree sign (°) is omitted (e.g., 38C rather than 38°C)
6. The "continental" spelling of words ending in *-er* is used (e.g., metre, not meter)
7. All measurement reports are to include five pieces of information
    a. The system (e.g., plasma)
    b. The component (e.g., sodium)
    c. The kind of quantity (e.g., concentration of substance)
    d. The value (e.g., 138)
    e. The value's unit (e.g., mmol/L)
8. The component must also be very specifically named (e.g., total serum bilirubin rather than serum bilirubin)

APPENDIX E

HISTORY AND EXPLANATION
OF SPECIFIC DIAGNOSTIC TESTS

X-RAY (ROENTGENGRAMS)

X rays are any electromagnetic radiation in the short range of 0.1 to 100 angstroms (nm). When such rays are passed through the human body, their penetration is affected by the density of the substances on which they are focused. Air is the least dense substance in the body, the rays penetrate it fully and leave a dark image on the film plate. The less penetration that occurs, the lighter, or whiter, the image will be. Thus, bone will appear white, water will appear a little grayer, fat darker still, and air will be totally black on the developed film. These contrasts produce "shadow pictures" outlining body structures.

The biological effect of 1 rad of radiation varies with the types of radiation being used. All types of radiation have the same biological effect when measured in roentgen-equivalent-man units (rem). Humans receive environmental exposure each day—from the sun, television, or cosmic rays, for example. If diagnostic x ray is added, it is important that it be used judiciously, ample protection being provided to client and health care worker alike such as the use of lead shields over areas not being x-rayed to prevent "scatter" radiation, limiting the amount of exposure time for each film, and exposing only the subject—others should leave the room in which the x ray is to be done. The "permissible" level of radiation per year is held to be 5 rem or 5000 mrem/yr. Workers in x-ray areas wear x-ray-sensitive badges (the badge changes color when a predetermined REM/RAD exposure level is reached) or audible "beepers" (that beep when the preset REM/RAD level is reached).

DIGITAL SUBTRACTION ANGIOGRAPHY

Digital subtraction refers to the conversion of a fluoroscopic image to digital form and its storage as a matrix. Subsequent views are converted to digital form by subtracting the first image of the object. This leaves only what has changed as the contrast medium flows into and through the area or what is blocked. Digital radiography has an increased ability to visualize soft tissue, organs, vascular structure, and blood flow and volume. Because of this ability it is used extensively with angiograms and is particularly valuable in procedures such as balloon angioplasty. It results in a view of the arteries with almost everything else in the area blocked out. Each view can be recalled for review and stored on magnetic tape or video disks.

RADIONUCLIDES, RADIOISOTOPES, AND RADIOPHARMACEUTICALS

The term *radionuclide* is often used interchangeably with *radioisotope*, but they are not interchangeable. Radioisotope refers to a radioactive (unstable) form of one specific element. Radionuclide refers to *any* radiopharmaceutical (an element with a nucleus that has been made radioactive). The basis for nuclear testing is the administration of a radionuclide that is used or processed by the body part to be imaged. Because there are only a few naturally occurring radioactive elements (e.g., uranium, radium, thorium), nonradioactive substances are made radioactive by bombarding their nuclei with subatomic fragments in a nuclear reactor, or a cyclotron, which makes the elements unstable (i.e., radioactive). Synthetic radioactive elements have certain advantages over naturally occurring ones. They can be purified so as to produce only gamma rays, which penetrate more deeply than do the alpha and beta rays. The half-life of the element may be markedly decreased because the material used has a natural tendency toward a stable rather than an "excited," unstable, radioactive state.

ULTRASOUND

Sound is a form of acoustic or mechanical energy and is vastly different from x rays, microwaves, and radiowaves.

Sound travels through a medium by a mechanical motion within the medium (e.g., for hearing to occur, the eardrum physically moves as a result of the mechanical action of air molecules). One physical characteristic of sound is frequency.

Frequency is generally expressed in hertz (Hz) or in cycles per second. Audible sound is in the frequency range of about 20 Hz to as high as 20,000 Hz (or 20 kilohertz [kHz], kilo corresponding to 1000).

Diagnostic imaging devices use frequencies that are more than 50 times higher than audible sounds and range from 1 to 10 MHz (million Hertz or megahertz). Such high frequencies are required to generate detailed, high-resolution images.

The sonographic imaging devices used today developed from much earlier work in submarine detection with sonar (SOund NAvigation and Ranging) techniques developed mainly after World War II. The principle on which these devices are all based is the transmission of a pulse of sound and receiving an "echo" from an object along the path the sound was directed. By "counting" the lapse of time between the generation of the pulse and the reception of the echo, the distance to the object can be determined. It can be roughly compared with the echo heard by a yodeler, which is a reflection of the yodeler's sound. The longer it takes to be heard by the yodeler, the farther away the "echoing" surface is.

Definition of Terms Used in Ultrasound Diagnostic Testing. Ultrasound diagnostics continue to develop. Because of this, terminology is changing rapidly and can be very confusing to the uninitiated. It can be doubly confusing to the patients, who may rely on the health care worker for at least part of their own information, if the health care worker is also uninformed. The best approach would be to refer questions to the sonographer. In the absence of that option, the following definitions are included in the hope they may prove useful:

1. **Sonographer.** An individual trained in the performance of diagnostic ultrasound imaging, or Doppler, and having primary responsibility for the examination. Sonographers are certified (The American Registry of Diagnostic Medical Sonographers [ARDMS] primarily) in a variety of specialties (e.g., obstetrics/gynecology, adult cardiac ultrasound, abdominal ultrasound)

2. **Sonologist.** A physician trained in the interpretation of sonograms and sonographic studies. Cardiologists, radiologists, vascular surgeons, and obstetricians may obtain advanced training in the interpretation of ultrasound in their specialties

3. **Sonogram.** (See also "Ultrasonogram," item 9). Generally refers to the ultrasound examination and/or the hardcopy pictures produced on film or videotape

4. **Scan.** Used in many different diagnostic test procedures; can be used as a synonym for sonogram or refer to a single ultrasound image or series of images

5. **Acoustic window.** An area where sound can pass freely to allow for the evaluation of structures below. It will not decrease the strength of the sound (attenuate) and will bypass air-filled areas (e.g., a full urinary bladder for evaluation of ovaries, adnexa, and uterus)

6. **Neurosonology.** The use of ultrasound to evaluate intracranial anatomy

7. **Ultrasound diagnostics.** A word derived from ultrasonics. *Ultrasonics* is the term defining which field of science that deals with very high frequency sound. The word *ultrasound* is used as a general term to encompass and identify any diagnostic test using sound waves with frequencies above the range of human hearing

8. **Ultrasonography.** The medical/diagnostic technique using the principles of ultrasonics as a diagnostic aid

9. **Ultrasonogram.** The record made of an ultrasound examination; may be produced in many forms, such as photographs of A-mode or B-mode (see items 19 and 20) tests that are taken from an oscilloscope screen, single emulsion copies of images that have been displayed on a cathode ray tube (CRT), videotapes or sensitive paper prints of M-mode (see item 21) tests, audiotapes of Doppler vascular scans

10. **Echography.** A rarely used term, once used interchangeably with ultrasonography

11. **Doppler effect.** (also known as the Doppler principle, Doppler shift, Doppler shift principle). This speaks of the relationship of the apparent frequency of waves (e.g., light/sound/radio) to the relative motion of the wave and the position of the observer/listener. The frequency increases as the two approach and decreases as they move apart. For example, the Doppler principle is the reason a listener hears different pitches as sound approaches and passes, like that of a train whistle or an ambulance siren passing. The pitch heard depends on how fast the sound is being emitted and whether it is coming toward the listener (high frequency) or going away from the listener (low frequency)

12. **Doppler ultrasound.** The use of ultrasound waves and the Doppler effect to evaluate moving body structures (heart, blood vessels, and fetal monitoring). In this case the sound is emitted by the transducer at a certain frequency. Continuous-wave ultrasound (see item 15) is aimed at the moving object (e.g., a red blood cell). As it comes toward the sound wave, the sound is reflected at a different frequency. The difference between the frequency emitted and that reflected (the Doppler shift) is proportional to the velocity of the movement and tells how fast the red blood cell is moving. Continuous-

wave ultrasound continuously samples and thus, assesses the highest velocities present so that gradients can be determined. If using pulsed-wave ultrasound (see item 16), only one burst of sound is out at any one time, and time can be counted to calculate distance; thus, the location of a structure can be determined

13. **Color Doppler ultrasound.** Assigns a different color to the blood in relationship to its speed and direction

14. **Doppler "noise".** When a doppler examination is being done, the sound of the blood makes a "noise" that gives information as to the condition of the arteries and veins (Montgomery & Lieckti, 1991, p. 75)

15. **Continuous-wave Doppler** (CW Doppler, CW, continuous-echo Doppler). Ultrasound waves are produced continuously. This is the most used form of Doppler wave; it is used to check pulses to determine the patency of peripheral vessels, evaluate the normalcy of the fetal heart signal, or detect the regurgitant jet in the fetal, pediatric, and adult heart. It yields information about high-speed jets of blood and can determine pressure gradients

16. **Pulsed-wave Doppler** (PW Doppler). Ultrasound energy is emitted in short pulses. Between pulses, the distance and the time taken by the pulse to reach various structures and return are measured. Volume size can also be measured. It provides single-point sampling of depth location (the depth of tissues from which the "echoes" emanate) but works fairly slowly, which is called a "low sampling rate"

17. **PW/HPRF** (high-pulse repetition frequency, rapid sampling). A newer form of PW Doppler that overcomes its low sampling rate (Bommer, 1984)

18. **MG Doppler** (multigate; flow imaging Doppler). Another newer form of Doppler that images blood flow by selecting and displaying information from multiple points simultaneously (Bommer, 1984)

19. **A mode** (amplitude modulation). Uses an oscilloscope to display the strength or weakness of an echo as a vertical spike with respect to distance, similar to an electrocardiogram (ECG). It is used mainly to help the sonographer set various equipment parameters and is only used as the primary display method in very specific applications to a limited degree

20. **B mode** (brightness modulation). The strength or weakness of an echo is displayed as a dot of a certain brightness. Strong reflectors such as bone produce bright dots. During an ultrasound examination, a series of B-mode dots creates a picture of the anatomy in a specific plane of a section—a sonographic tomogram. The image is viewable on a TV screen. In such an image, there is a range of dot brightnesses (from very bright to very weak) that is seen as various shades of gray. This display of gray shades is referred to as a *gray scale* and provides better differentiation of tissue density on the picture produced

21. **M mode** (motion modulation). Used to evaluate the moving parts of the heart (e.g., the valves) and uses the B-mode dots aligned according to the valves' anatomic position. A strip chart passes over the dots. When a valve moves (opens and closes), the dots corresponding to the valve move, which leaves a tracing on the strip chart similar to that of an ECG except that there are multiple markings. The motion of the moving valve is recorded on the paper or can be watched on an oscilloscope. Stationary areas are shown as straight lines, moving areas as wavy lines

22. **Real-time imaging** (2-D, two-dimensional real-time imaging). Uses the series of B-mode dots that compose the sonographic tomogram. It is done with a scanner capable of a rapid scanning (e.g., 30 frames per second) and produces a product similar to a motion picture of heart valve action or fetal movements, for example. It takes a number of "frames" in a very short amount of time. The term *2-D* usually refers to the application of real time in cardiac evaluation or other uses referred to as "real time" (e.g., obstetrics, abdominal views). *Real time* is an electronic term that can be roughly defined as the display of anything exactly at the time of the request for the display

The full potential of ultrasound imaging depends heavily on the expertise of the sonographer or sonologist. He or she must have a thorough knowledge of the physical principles and instrumentation of ultrasound in addition to aspects of its clinical application to decrease the acoustic exposure of the patient while not compromising the efficacy of the examination.

APPENDIX F

DIAGNOSTIC SCREENING OF THE ASYMPTOMATIC ELDERLY

According to McCue (1987), routine medical screening of the elderly patient (i.e., a reasonable battery of laboratory tests coupled with careful history taking and physical examination) is more likely to detect "significant or treatable disease" than in younger persons. As he sees it, the goal of such screening is to detect problems (not just diseases) that compromise the older person's ability to maintain independent function and the quality of his or her life (McCue, 1987, p. 23).

The following "diseases" are listed to be specifically screened for:

1. Endocrine disorders: Hypothyroidism, estrogen deficiency
2. Gastrointestinal: Constipation, chewing and swallowing difficulties
3. Musculoskeletal disorders: Osteoporosis, skin manifestations of gout, muscle weakness and atrophy, tremor
4. Neoplasms: Prostate, breast, genitalia, lung, skin, gastrointestinal
5. Neurosensory: Cataracts, glaucoma, deafness, impacted cerumen, tinnitus, vertigo, focal weakness
6. Podiatric disorders: Corns, calluses, nail problems (e.g., thickening), dry and/or unsightly skin
7. Pulmonary: Obstructive lung disease, tuberculosis
8. Urinary dysfunction: Nephrosclerosis, obstructive disease, incontinence, decreased levels of creatinine clearance
9. Vascular disorders: Hypertension, vascular insufficiency—coronary, cerebral, peripheral (McCue, 1987, p. 24)

Common "problems" of the elderly as identified by McCue are:

1. Exercise limitations related to arthritis or stiffness, back pain, chest pain, dizziness, fear of falling, foot problems, leg pain, trouble breathing
2. Self-concept changes related to new "lumps or bumps," sexual dysfunction/dyspareunia, skin changes, urinary incontinence
3. Alteration in comfort and/or decreased nutritional status related to change in bowel habits/constipation, trouble with teeth, trouble with chewing/swallowing, abdominal pains
4. Cognitive impairment related to trouble sleeping, fainting spells/falls, dizziness, forgetfulness, intermittent neurological symptoms (McCue, 1987, p. 24)

Routine yearly laboratory tests suggested as helpful for all elderly in meeting the aforementioned goal are:

1. For *all* elderly
   a. Hemoglobin or hematocrit (nutritional anemias)
   b. Stool for occult blood (cancer of the colon, diverticulitis)
   c. Serum creatinine (age-related loss of nephrons)
   d. Urine dipstick and observation of gross appearance (nephrosclerosis)
   e. Mammography (female) (cancer)
2. Tests to be done based on past history or present signs/symptoms
   a. Serum thyroxine (T$_4$)
   b. Erythocyte sedimentation rate
   c. Cholesterol
   d. Chest film
   e. Tuberculosis skin test
   f. Office spirometry (McCue, 1987, p. 32)

An important aspect of routine screening is a thorough social assessment. McCue provides an excellent tool for that purpose (1987, p. 41) that covers finances, social support systems, daily routine, and the physical environment.

APPENDIX G

NORMAL FLORA AND UNUSUAL OR ABNORMAL FLORA BY SITE

Site	Normal	Abnormal or Unusual
Body fluids and blood (i.e., pleural, synovial, bile, etc.)	Sterile (rarely contaminated with a few diphtheroids or *Staphylococcus epidermidis*)	Potentially any organism
Cerebral spinal fluid	Sterile	Any organism
Ear		
Outer	*Staphylococcus epidermidis* Diphtheroids Micrococci *Bacillus* species	*Pseudomonas aeruginosa* *Staphylococcus aureus* Beta-hemolytic streptococci *Haemophilus influenzae* *Escherichia coli* coliforms[a]
Inner	Sterile	As above

Eye	Small numbers of
	    Staphylococcus epidermidis
	 Streptococcus viridans group
	 Diphtheroids
		Staphylococcus epidermidis
		 Streptococcus pneumoniae
		 Haemophilus influenzae
		    (*Haemophilus aegyptius*)
		 Pseudomonas aeruginosa
		 Streptococcus viridans group
		 Beta-hemolytic streptococci
		 Neisseria gonorrhoeae
		 Acinetobacter species
		 Chlamydia group

Lung (brushings, needle aspirates)	Scant oral flora (*Streptococcus viridans*, plus diphtheroids, *Staphylococcus epidermidis*)	*Staphylococcus aureus* Beta-hemolytic streptococci *Pseudomonas* species Coliforms (particularly *Klebsiella, Enterobacter*) *Haemophilus influenzae* Acid-fast bacilli

[a]*Coliforms:* Term to describe a group of gram-negative bacteria that are non-spore-forming, facultative anerobes such as *Escherichia coli, Klebsiella-Enterobacter* group, *Proteus, Morganella, Hafnia,* etc., which are found ubiquitously in human and animal environs, occasionally occurring in water, on vegetation, etc.

From Harris, P. C. (1980, summer). Interview and written table of microorganisms. Everett, WA: General Hospital of Everett, with permission.

Site	Normal	Abnormal or Unusual
		Fungi *(Coccidioides, Aspergillus, Penicillium)*
		Yeasts *(Cryptococcus,* diphasic fungi)
		Pneumocystis carinii
		Legionella pneumophila and other legionnaires'-like organisms (TexKL, WIGA)
		Anerobic bacteria
Lower respiratory tract (expectorated sputum, endotracheal suction)	See "Upper respiratory tract"	As listed in the next section
Upper respiratory tract: throat, nasopharynx, mouth	*Streptococcus viridans*	Beta-hemolytic streptococci, especially group A, occasionally groups C, F, G
	Staphylococcus epidermidis	
	Scant to occasional *Staphylococcus aureus*	*Staphylococcus aureus*
	Some beta-hemolytic streptococci	*Corynebacterium diphtheriae*
	Micrococci	*Haemophilus influenzae* and occasionally *Haemophilus parainfluenzae*
	Diphtheroids	
	Neisseria species	*Candida albicans* (if heavy)
	Occasional coliforms	Fusiforms and spirochetes in synergy (Vincent's disease)
	Anaerobic gram-negative and gram-positive bacilli and cocci	*Neisseria meningitidis*
		Neisseria gonorrhoeae
		Bordetella pertussis
		Pasteurella multocida
		Branhamella catarrhalis
Skin	*Staphylococcus epidermidis*	Beta-hemolytic streptococci
	Diphtheroids (other than *Corynebacterium diphtheriae*)	*Staphylococcus aureus*
		Corynebacterium diptheriae
	Bacillus species	Some fungi
	Streptococcus viridans	Heavy *Candida albicans*
	Coliforms	*Staphylococcus epidermidis* (in stitch abscess)
	Saprophytic yeast and fungi	
	Micrococci	*Pasteurella multocida* (in cat or dog bites)
		Anaerobic streptococci plus aerobic or facultative organisms in decubiti
Urogenital sites; bladder urine (clean voided)	Occasional to scant lower urethral contaminants (*Staphylococcus epidermidis,* diphtheroides, other skin microflora)	Greater than 100,000 organisms/ml of urine; usually a single type, but occasionally mixed infection
		Escherichia coli
		Klebsiella species
		Enterobacter species
		Proteus mirabilis
		Indole-positive *Proteus*
		Enterococci (fecal streptococci)

Site	Normal	Abnormal or Unusual
		Staphylococcus saprophyticus and other *Staphylococcus epidermidis* *Ureaplasma urealyticum* Cytomegalovirus *Chlamydia* group Rarely, *Salmonella* species, pneumococci Yeasts (*Candida, Torulopsis*)
Catheterized urine	Sterile	Same as above, but counts of 10,000/ml or less may be significant
Urethra	As noted with clean-voided urine	*Neisseria gonorrhoeae* *Hemophilus influenzae* *Gardinerella vaginalis* *Ureaplasma urealyticum* *Trichomonas vaginalis* *Candida albicans* Others from clean-voided list
Vagina	Lactobacilli *Staphylococcus epidermidis* Micrococci Coliforms Occasional group B beta-hemolytic streptococci Mixed anaerobic gram-negative and -positive bacilli and cocci Enterococci Occasional *Candida*	*Neisseria gonorrhoeae* *Haemophilus influenzae* *Gardinerella vaginalis* (when associated with "clue" cells) Herpes virus *Chlamydia* *Mycoplasma* species *Ureaplasma urealyticum* *Staphylococcus aureus* Heavy growth of group B beta-hemolytic streptococci *Trichomonas vaginalis* *Candida albicans*
Cervix	Scant amounts of normal vaginal organisms	*Neisseria gonorrhoeae* *Haemophilus influenzae* *Streptococcus pneumoniae* All others listed for vagina (Significant anaerobic gram-negative bacilli such as *Bacteroides bivius, B. disiens, B. fragilis,* and *B. melaninogenicus* as well as anaerobic gram-positive cocci; anaerobic flora may reflect pelvic inflammatory disease, may be assessed only if cervical culture is taken with special procedures to decontaminate cervical os; best ruled in as pathogens through culdocentesis procedure)

Site	Normal	Abnormal or Unusual
Wounds, abscesses	Surface wounds (i.e., decubiti) as for skin	As for skin
	Deep wounds: Sterile	Many organisms, including but not limited to: *Staphylococcus aureus* Beta-hemolytic streptococci *Pasteurella multocida* Occasionally *P. multocida* and noncholera vibrios Coliforms of all types Viridans streptococci groups Anerobic gram-negative bacilli and cocci, especially *Bacteriodes fragilis, B. melaninogenicus* *Clostridium perfringens* *Clostridium tetani* Other *Clostridium* species *Actinomyces* species Parasites from liver and bowel abscesses
Stool	Coliforms such as most strains of *Escherichia coli* *Klebsiella, Enterobacter, Proteus,* etc. Fecal streptococci Many different anerobic and microaerophilic organisms Yeasts Some types of parasites (*Endamoeba coli*) Occasional *Pseudomonas* and *Acinetobacter* species	*Campylobacter fetus,* sp. *jejuni* *Salmonella* species *Shigella* species *Arizona* species Some strains of *Escherichia coli* Some strains of *Proteus mirabilis* *Yersinia enterocolitica* *Yersinia pseudotuberculosis* *Clostridium difficile* with cytotoxin *Staphylococcus aureus* (enterotoxic) Enterotoxin-producing *Escherichia coli* *Clostridium perfringens* Enteroviruses (e.g., rotavirus, Norwalk agent) Parasites such as *Giardia lamblia, Endamoeba histolytica, Trichuris, Ascaris*

APPENDIX H

SOMOGYI REACTION

The *Somogyi reaction* is the name applied to a situation in which a diabetic demonstrates glycosuria in response to an *overdosage* of insulin rather than a lack of insulin. This paradox is understandable when the pathophysiology is explained.

Briefly, the pathophysiology is as follows: Hypoglycemia, resulting from an insulin overdosage occurs during sleep—often around 2 AM. The individual is unaware of the early subjective symptoms. A hormonal response to the hypoglycemia occurs and stimulates those hormones that counter hypoglycemia (epinephrine, cortisol, and perhaps growth hormone). In response, the blood glucose level rises at a rapid rate as the level of plasma insulin falls, which leads to an 8 AM glycosuria. Despite the administration of too much insulin, the interpretation is often insufficient insulin, and a cycle is produced.

APPENDIX I

CDC-UNIVERSAL PRECAUTIONS IN USE, 1994

Precautions when handling blood and body fluids should be consistently used for *all* patients, especially those in emergency care settings in which the risk of blood exposure is increased and the infection status of the patients is usually unknown.

1. All health care workers should use appropriate *barrier precautions* to prevent skin or mucous membrane exposure when contact with blood or other body fluids is anticipated:
   a. Gloves used for:
      (1) Touching blood, body fluids, mucous membranes, surfaces soiled with blood or body fluids
      (2) Touching nonintact skin of all patients
      (3) Handling items or surfaces soiled with blood or body fluids
      (4) Performing venipuncture and other vascular access procedures
   b. Gloves should be changed after contact with each patient
   c. Masks and protective eyewear should be worn during procedures likely to generate blood or other body fluid droplets to prevent exposure of mucous membrane
   d. Gowns or aprons should be worn during procedures likely to generate splashes of blood or other body fluid
2. Skin surfaces contaminated with blood or other body fluids should be washed immediately and thoroughly. Hands should be washed immediately after gloves are removed
3. Precautions to prevent injuries caused by sharp objects (needles, scalpels, etc.) should be taken:
   a. During procedures
   b. When cleaning used instruments or handling sharp instruments after procedures
   c. When disposing of used needles. Needles should *not* be manipulated by hand (e.g., recapped, purposely bent or broken by hand, removed from disposable syringes)
   d. When disposing of used sharps (e.g., needles or scalpel blades), place them in a puncture-resistant container, kept as near as is possible to their place of use, for transport to reprocessing area
   e. Reusable large-bore needles should be placed in a puncture-proof container for transport to the reprocessing area (CDC, 1988, pp. 372–381)
4. Limit the need for mouth-to-mouth resuscitation (saliva has not been implicated in HIV transmission but can contain blood) by keeping materials for emergency ventilation available in all areas where they could be predicted to be needed (e.g., mouthpieces, resuscitation bags)

5. Health care workers who have exudative lesions or weeping dermatitis should not give any direct patient care nor handle patient care equipment until the condition clears

6. Pregnant health care workers are not known to be at greater risk of contacting HIV infection than nonpregnant workers. Should the mother contact HIV during pregnancy, the child is at great risk at the time of delivery (perinatal infection). Because of this risk, pregnant health care workers should be especially familiar with and strictly adhere to precautions to minimize the risk for their infant (CDC, Aug. 1987, MMWR Supp., pp. 55–65).

These guidelines, if adhered to, eliminate the need for the isolation category of blood and body fluid precautions. Isolation precautions (enteric, all body fluids [AFB]) may be necessary and should be used if infectious diarrhea or tuberculosis are suspected or diagnosed (CDC, 1988, pp. 372–381).

Other precautions for specific areas of practice are available from the Centers for Disease Control (Atlanta, Georgia, 30333), such as invasive procedures (surgery, etc.); dentistry; autopsy/morticians services; dialysis; sterilization and disinfection.

Appendix J

Centers for Disease Control Definition of AIDS (1990)

Acquired immunodeficiency syndrome (AIDS) is an aggregate of signs, symptoms, and illnesses resulting from a compromised immune system. A diagnosis of AIDS requires the definitive or presumptive diagnosis of one or more "indicator disease" and, depending on certain criteria, may or may not require laboratory evidence of HIV infection. The following outline is used by physicians in the United States and most developed countries to arrive at AIDS diagnosis.

1. A diagnosis of AIDS can be made if laboratory evidence of HIV infection has been established and a definitive diagnosis of *any* of the following indicator diseases has been made—regardless of the presence of other causes of immunodeficiency.
   a. Candidiasis of the esophagus, trachea, bronchi, or lungs
   b. Coccidioidomycosis, disseminated
   c. Cryptococcosis (extrapulmonary)
   d. Cytomegalovirus disease of an organ other than the liver, spleen, or lymph nodes in a patient older than 1 month
   e. Herpes simplex virus infection causing a mucocutaneous ulcer (e.g., in eyes, nose, mouth, and/or genitoanal area) that persists for more than 1 month; or bronchitis, pneumonitis, or esophagitis caused by herpes simplex virus in a patient older than 1 month
   f. Histoplasmosis, disseminated
   g. HIV encephalopathy; also called subacute encephalopathy due to HIV; also referred to as HIV dementia or AIDS dementia complex (ADC), which is clinically defined as a disabling cognitive or motor dysfunction interfering with the patient's occupation or activities of daily living, or loss of behavioral development milestones in the absence of a concurrent illness or condition
   h. Isosporiasis with diarrhea persisting longer than 1 month
   i. Karposi's sarcoma
   j. Lymphoma (primary) of the brain
   k. Lymphoid interstitial pneumonitis (LIP) and/or pulmonary lymphoid hyperplasia affecting a child under 13 years of age
   l. Mycobacterial (other than *Mycobacterium tuberculosis*) disease, disseminated
   m. *M. tuberculosis* disease, extrapulmonary (may have concurrent pulmonary involvement)

    n. Non-Hodgkin's lymphoma

    o. *Pneumocystis carinii* pneumonia

    p. Progressive multifocal leukoencephalopathy

    q. Salmonella septicemia, recurrent

    r. Toxoplasmosis of the brain in a patient older than 1 month

    s. Any combination of at least two of the following bacterial infections within a 2-year period affecting a patient less than 13 years of age; septicemia, pneumonia, meningitis, bone or joint infection, or abcess of an internal organ or body cavity caused by haemophilus, streptococcus, or other fever-inducing bacteria

2. A diagnosis of AIDS can be made if laboratory evidence of HIV is positive and any of the following indicator diseases is diagnosed *presumptively*. (A presumptive diagnosis is generally made in situations in which the patient's condition does not permit the performance of definitive testing).

    a. Candidiasis of the esophagus

    b. Cytomegalovirus retinitis with loss of vision

    c. Karposi's sarcoma

    d. Lymphoid interstitial pneumonitis and/or pulmonary lymphoid hyperplasia affecting a patient less than 13 years of age

    e. Mycobacterial disease, disseminated

    f. *Pneumocystis carinii* pneumonia

    g. Toxoplasmosis of the brain in a patient older than 1 month

3. A diagnosis of AIDS can be made if laboratory evidence of HIV infection is *lacking* or *inconclusive but* also if a definitive diagnosis of any of the following indicator diseases is made, provided other known causes of immunodeficiency are ruled out:

    a. Candidiasis of the esophagus, trachea, bronchi, or lungs

    b. Cryptococcosis, extrapulmonary

    c. Cryptosporidiosis with diarrhea persisting longer than 1 month

    d. Cytomegalovirus disease of an organ other than the liver, spleen, or lymph nodes in a patient older than 1 month

    e. Herpes simplex virus infection causing a mucocutaneous ulcer that persists longer than 1 month, or bronchitis, pneumonitis, or esophagitis affecting a patient older than 1 month

    f. Karposi's sarcoma affecting a patient less than 60 years of age

    g. Lymphoma of the brain (primary) affecting a patient less than 60 years of age

    h. Lymphoid interstitial pneumonitis and/or pulmonary lymphoid hyperplasia affecting a patient less than 13 years of age

    i. *Mycobacterium avium* complex or *M. kansasii* disease, disseminated

    j. *Pneumocystis carinii* pneumonia

    k. Progressive multifocal leukoencephalopathy

    l. Toxoplasmosis of the brain in a patient older than 1 month

4. A diagnosis of AIDS can also be made when laboratory evidence of HIV infection is negative if all other causes of immunodeficiency are excluded and the patient has had either a definitive diagnosis of *P. carinii* pneumonia or has a definitive diagnosis of any of the indicator diseases of AIDS and CD_4(T4) cell count less than 400/mm³ (Centers for Disease Control, 1987, Aug. 14, pp. 43–63)

The definition of AIDS was to be expanded on April 1, 1992, to include all HIV-infected adults and adolescents (over age 13) with CD_4 cell counts of 200/mm^3 or less. The change was postponed, and the controversy as to perceived, probable, or potential problems with the planned definition of AIDS being based on cell counts has not been settled at this writing. Supporters of the change claim that the current list of AIDS-defining illnesses excludes many debilitated people from vitally needed financial benefits; the change would help many people get vital care and benefits, especially women with gynecological conditions not on the current list of illnesses that define AIDS. Detractors note that, although the new system provides a simplified method for diagnosing AIDS (a direct measure of immune dysfunction), no provision had been made to provide for medical coverage and financial help that would be needed for the expected increase in the ranks of AIDS-diagnosed people. The need for an adequate number of, and ready access to, laboratory facilities that do lymphocyte phenotyping is also seen as a problem. Distribution of government funds based on the number of AIDS patients cared for was seen to widen the gap between those facilities that are well endowed and the "have-nots."

Reporting of AIDS cases, which has been done anonymously through state health departments, would now fall to primary care physicians, and patient anonimity could be lost. There is also concern for an expected loss of vital scientific and public health data about AIDS with decreased data surveillance of opportunistic diseases. Many people with the required CD_4 counts, but with negative ELISA and Western Blot tests, would be classified by the diagnosis of AIDS despite being able to work and having no other known symptoms or signs (CDC Postpones New Definition of AIDS, 1992. Pfieffer, 1992, pp. 26–27, 30).

APPENDIX K

TERMINOLOGY AND DEFINITIONS RELATED TO RECENT TESTING METHODS

(*Note:* Terminology primarily used in ultrasound diagnostic testing is in Appendix E.)

Assay. Determination of the purity of a substance or the amount of any particular constituent of a mixture

Episomes. Plasmids that may become integrated into the chromosome or that can exist autonomously as well as be integrated within the chromosome

Genetic engineering. Laboratory study of genes

Genetic recombination. Transfer of genetic information in humans

Immunofluorescence. A method of determining the location of an antigen or antibody in a tissue section or smear, using a specific antibody or antigen labeled with a fluorochrome

    Direct method. Fluorochrome chemically linked to a specific antibody

    Indirect method. A labeled antiimmunoglobulin that binds to the specific antibody is used

Plasmid DNA. Any extrachromosomal self-replicating genetic element of a cell. In bacteria, circular DNA molecules that reproduce themselves and are thus conserved apart from the chromosome through successive cell divisions

Recombinant. A new cell that results from genetic recombination (noun). Pertaining or relating to such cells or individuals (adjective)

Recombinant DNA. Laboratory alteration of genes, most frequently by combining the DNA of two or more different organisms

Restriction endonucleases. Enzymes that cleave (cut) plasmid DNA at a specific nucleotide sequence (restriction site). Any group of compounds obtained by hydrolysis of nucleic acid

REFERENCES

Aach, R., Hirschman. S.Z., & Holland, P.V. (1992, August 15). The ABCs of viral hepatitis. *Patient Care, 26,* 34–38, 40, 44–46, 49–50.

Abrams, W. B., & Berkow, R. (Eds.) (1990). *The Merck Manual of Geriatrics.* Rahway, NJ: Merck.

Ackley, A., & Gocke, D. J. (1980). Viral hepatitis. *American Family Physician, 29,* 156–162.

Acute renal failure. (1987). In J. Da Cunha (Ed.), *Patient teaching.* (pp. 352–354). Springhouse, PA: Springhouse Corporation.

Adams, S., Skelley, A. (1993).

Admission stool guaiac: Should it be routine? (1992, September). *Emergency Medicine, 24,* 109–110.

Advances in medical imaging. (1985, July). *Science and Technology for the Executive, 3.*

Ahlquist, D., McGill, D., Schwartz, S. et al. (1985). Fecal blood levels in health and disease: A study using HemeQuant. *New England Journal of Medicine, 312,* 1422–1428.

AIDS: A progress report. (1986, January). *Science and Technology for the Executive, 3–4.*

AIDS Update: Part 1. (1985, November). *The Harvard Medical School Health Letter, 10,* 1–4.

AIDS Update: Part 2. (1985, December). *The Harvard Medical School Health Letter, 10,* 2–5.

AIDS Update: Necrosis factor's potential in AIDS therapy suggested. (1990, February). *Medical World News, 31,* 37.

AIDS virus gets new name amid feuding. (1987, May 26). *Medical World News,* 14–15.

Albert, M. (1987). Health screening to promote health for the elderly. *Nurse Practitioner, 12,* 42, 44, 48, 50–52, 55–57.

Allport, S., & Havron, D. (1980, January). Patients' own tagged leukocytes find infection site. *Medical Tribune, 21,* 1, 18.

American Academy of Pediatrics. (1986). *Report of the Commission on Infectious Diseases.* Elk Village, Ill: American Academy of Pediatrics.

American Cancer Society. (1983, August 3). News service release. New York, NY.

Anabar, M., & Schersten, T. (1985). Diagnostic imaging: A generic overview. *International Journal of Technology Assessment in Health Care, 1,* 3, 740–744.

Anderson, D. M. (Ed.). (1989). *Dorland's pocket medical dictionary, 24th ed.* Philadelphia, PA: Saunders.

A new prenatal screening program. (1987, February). *Harvard Medical School Health Letter, 12,* 6–8.

Antibody tests promise better diagnosis of herpes simplex infection. (1983, March 14). *Medical World News*, 133–134.

Are CT scans necessary after head injury? (1992, January 15). *Emergency Medicine*, 24, 173–174.

Aronchick, J. (1984). Imaging decisions: The solitary pulmonary nodule. *Diagnosis*, 6, 23–24, 26, 30, 34.

Barnes, A. (1987). Adverse reactions to blood transfusions. In R. E. Rakel (Ed.), *Conn's current therapy* (pp. 361–366). Philadelphia: Saunders.

Bauman, D. J. (1980). Creatine phosphokinase isoenzymes and the diagnosis of myocardial infarction. *Postgraduate Medicine*, 35, 103–106, 109–112, 115–116.

Baumgarten, A. (1986). When to assay for alpha-fetoprotein. *Diagnosis*, 8, 93–96, 101, 104.

Beck, W. S. (1983). *Human design*. New York: Harcourt Brace Jovanovich.

Belsey, R. E., Mulrow, C. D., Sox, H. C., Jr. (1993, May). How to handle baffling test results. *Patient Care*, 27, 63–68, 71–72, 74–76.

Bender, B. S., & Quinn, T. (1984). What to know about AIDS detection. *Diagnosis*, 6, 61–63, 66, 69–70, 73, 76.

Bennett, J. A. (1985). HTLV-III AIDS link. *American Journal of Nursing*, 85, 1086–1089.

Bennett, R. M. (Ed.). (1986). Proceedings of a symposium on the fibrositis/fibromyalgia syndrome: Current issues and perspectives. *The American Journal of Medicine*, 81, 1–115.

Bennett, R., Smythe, H. A., Wolfe, F. (1992, March). Recognizing fibromyalgia. *Patient Care*, 26, 211–218, 223, 227.

Benson, A. (Infection Control Nurse Specialist). (1985, September 10). Opinion expressed in Question/Answer Session at Swedish Hospital Medical Center, Seattle, WA: (Tape available at SHMC Instructional Media Center).

Berkow, R. (editor-in-chief) (1992). *The merck manual of diagnosis and therapy*. Rahway, NJ: Merck.

Berman, L. B., & Vertes, V. (1973). The pathophysiology of renin. *Clinical Symposia*, 25, 1–35.

Bessen, H. (1993, July). Averting aortic catastrophes. *Emergency Medicine*, 25, 57–58, 63, 67–68, 70, 74.

Bickerstaff, E. R., & Small, J. (1982). *Neurology for nurses* (2nd ed.). Baltimore: University Park Press.

Bienenstock, H. (1980, April). Arthritis: Diagnostic guide. *Hospital Medicine*, 27–28, 35.

Birnie, D. J., Knipping, A. A., van Rijswijk, M. H. et al. (1992, December). Psychological aspects of fibromyalgia compared with chronic and nonchronic pain. *Journal of Rheumatology*, 18, 1845–1848.

Blacklow, R. S. (1983). *MacBryde's signs and symptoms* (6th ed.). Philadelphia: Lippincott.

Blainey, C. (1986). Diabetes mellitus. In M. L. Patrick, S. L. Woods, R. F. Craven et al. (Eds.), *Medical surgical nursing: Pathologic and pathophysiologic concepts* (pp. 1028–1052). Philadelphia: Lippincott.

Bleicher, J. M., & Lacko, A. G. (1992, May). Physiologic role and clinical significance of reverse cholesterol transport. *Journal of the American Osteopathic Association*, 92, 625–631.

Bodinski, L. H. (1987). *The nurse's guide to diet therapy* (2nd ed.). New York: Wiley.

Bommer, W. (1984). Ultrasound update, part 2. Echocardiography: Choosing the right equipment. *Diagnosis*, 6, 137–139, 142–143, 146–147.

Bonacini, M. (1991, November). Chronic viral heptatitis: From B to D. *Cortlandt Forum*, *4*, 124–128, 131.

Borucki, M. (1992, August). Overshadowed by AIDS, other STDs continue to skyrocket. *The DO*, *33*, 77–82.

Boschert, S. (1993). Firefly Gene's bright future in T.B. testing. *Family Practice News*, *43*, 4.

Bradley, W. A. & Murakami, D. (1993, December). MRI insights. *Diagnostic Imaging*, *15*, 63–65.

Bradley, W. A., Brunzell, J. D., Ginsberg, H. N., LaRosa, J. C., Shonfeld, G. (1992). The emerging role of triglycerides. Special Report on Atherosclerosis; Supplement, *Family practice news*, *22*, 7–9.

Bragg, D. G., & Dodd, G. D. (1987). Imaging in cancer: State of the art. *Ca: A Cancer Journal for Clinicians*, *37*, 131–132.

Broder, S., & Karp, J. E. (1992, March/April). The expanding challenge of HIV-Associated malignancies. *Ca-A Cancer Journal for Clinicians*, *92*, 69–73.

Brown, E. J. (1984). Coronary disease? Answers from nuclear testing. *Diagnosis*, *6*, 106–110, 113–114, 117–120.

Brucker, M. C., & MacMuller, N. J. (1987). Chorionic villus sampling. *Nurse Practitioner*, *12*, 34–36, 40, 42.

Brunner, E. M., & Davis, J. S. (1980). Systemic lupus erythematosus. In H. F. Conn, & R. B. Conn (Eds.), *Current diagnosis* Vol. 6 (pp. 1123–1127). Philadelphia: Saunders.

Brunner, L. S., & Suddarth, D. S. (1988). *Textbook of medical-surgical nursing* (6th ed.). Philadelphia: Lippincott.

Burdash, N. & Fernandes, J. J. (1992, August). Hepatitis testing update. *Journal of the American Osteopathic Association*, *98*, 1028, 1037–1038.

Burke, M. D. (1979). Low sodium: Delusion, depletion or dilution. *Lab 79*, *2*, 40–44.

Burke, M. D. (1980a). Cholesterol, triglycerides, and lipoproteins studies: Strategies for clinical use. *Post Graduate Medicine*, *35*, 263–66, 269, 273.

Burke, M. D. (1980b). Hypertension: Strategies for laboratory diagnosis. *Post Graduate Medicine*, *35*, 77–81, 84–85.

Burrell, L. O. (Ed.). (1992). *Adult nursing in hospital and community settings*, E. Norwalk, CT: Appleton & Lange.

Bush, D., Hemphill, L., & Kappagoda, C. T. (1992, September). More than meets the angiogram. Special Report on Atherosclerosis; Supplement. *Family Practice News*, *92*, 14.

Byrne, C. J., Saxton, D. J., Pelikan, P. K., & Nugent, P. M. (1981). *Laboratory tests: Implications for nurses and allied health professionals*. Menlo Park, CA: Addison-Wesley.

Cameron, J. S., Russell, A., & Sale, D. (1976). *Nephrology for nurses: A modern approach to the kidney* (2nd ed.). New York: Medical Examination Publishing Company.

Caprini, J. A. (1976). *Bleeding problems: Diagnosis and treatment*. Hagerston, MD: Harper & Row.

Carnevali, D. L., & Patrick, M. (Eds.). (1979). *Nursing management for the elderly*. Philadelphia: Lippincott.

Carr, G. S., & Gee, G. (1986). AIDS and AIDS-related conditions: Screening for populations at risk. *Nurse Practitioner*, *11*, 25–26, 29, 32–34, 36, 41–42, 44, 46, 48.

Carrol, H. F. (1986). Letters. *Medical World News*, 4.

Carter, H. B., Pearson, J. D., Metter, J. et. al. (1992, August). Rise in serum PSA: A good clinical marker for prostate cancer. *Modern Medicine, 60,* 105–106.

Cascino, T. (1987). Brain tumors. In R. B. Rakel (Ed.), *Conn's current therapy* (pp. 785–787). Philadelphia: Saunders.

Catalona, W. J. (1991, November). The touted PSA screen. *Cortlandt Forum, 4,* 139.

Centers for Disease Control. (1992, April). Postpones new definition of AIDS. *Medical World News, 33,* 11.

Centers for Disease Control. (1992, May 8). Guidelines for the performance of CD4+ T-cell determinations in persons with human immunodeficiency virus infection. *MMWR, 41,* 1–16.

Centers for Disease Control. (1987a, August). Recommendations for prevention of HIV transmission in health-care settings. *MMWR,* (Suppl.) *36,* 115–125.

Centers for Disease Control. (1987b, August, 14). Revision of the CDC surveillance case definition for acquired immunodeficiency syndrome. *MMWR, 36,* (suppl. no. 1S), 4s–6s.

Centers for Disease Control. (1988, June). Universal precautions for prevention of transmission of human immunodeficiency virus, hepatitis B virus, and other bloodborne pathogens in health-care settings. *MMWR, 37,* 372–381.

Children's vaccine initiative aims to simplify immunization schedule. (1992, September). *Family Practice News, 22,* 25.

Christian, C. L. (1980). Managing arthritis: Three guides to differential diagnosis (DDx), lab, tests, and drugs. *Modern Medicine, 48,* 18–23.

Clark, R. G. (1975). Manter and Gate's essentials of clinical neuroanatomy and neurophysiology (5th ed.). Philadelphia: F. A. Davis.

Cohen, S. M., Kenner, C. A. & Hollingsworth, A. O. (1991). *Maternal, neonatal, and women's health nursing.* Springhouse, PA: Springhouse Corporation.

Collins, R. D. (1975). *Illustrated manual of laboratory diagnosis: Indications and interpretations* (2nd ed.). Philadelphia: Lippincott.

Colt, H. G., & Harrell, J. H. (1992, September). Diagnostic thoracoscopy: New look at an old technique. *Journal of Respiratory Diseases, 13,* 1246–1248, 1251, 1254, 1257–1258.

Conn, H. F., & Conn, R. B. (Eds.). (1985). *Current diagnosis* (Vol. 6). Philadelphia: Saunders.

Conn, R. B. (Ed.). (1991). *Current diagnosis—8.* (8th ed.). Philadelphia, PA: Saunders.

Conn, R. B. (1987). Laboratory reference values of clinical importance. In R. B. Rakel (Ed.), *Conn's current therapy* (pp. 1013–1027). Philadelphia: Saunders.

Conway-Rutkowski, B. (1982). *Carini and Owens' neurological and neurosurgical nursing* (8th ed.). St. Louis: Mosby.

Cooper, C. (1992, September). Puzzle of AIDS-like syndrome without HIV far from solved. *Family Practice News, 22,* 3, 55.

Corbett, J. V. (1992). *Laboratory tests and diagnostic procedures with nursing diagnosis* (3rd ed.). E. Norwalk, CT: Appleton-Lange.

Corey, L. (1991, November). Hepatitis B-induced myalgia? *Cortlandt Forum, 4,* 98.

Corraling a New Cancer Marker. (1986, June). *Medical World News,* 131.

Crawford, E. D. (1992, April). Cancer consultation: Can PSA be used in screening for prostate cancer. *Primary Care & Cancer, 12,* 57–58.

Cunha, B. A. (1992, September). Case studies in infectious disease: Kawasaki disease. *Emergency Medicine, 24,* 209–10.

Cyr, D. (1986, July). (Personal correspondence), Seattle University, Department of Allied Health, Ultrasound.

Damrow, T. (1986, June 27). (Personal Interview), Communicable Disease Laboratories, Washington State Social and Health Services. Seattle.

Davidsohn, I., & Henry, J. B. (Eds.). (1969). *Todd-Sanford clinical diagnosis by laboratory methods* (14th ed.). Philadelphia: Saunders.

Davidson, A. J., & Hartman, D. S. (1987). Imaging strategies for tumors of the kidney, adrenal gland, and retroperitoneum. *Ca: A Cancer Journal for Clinicians, 37*, 151–164.

de Gruttola, V. (1987, April). AIDS: Where is it taking us? *HMS (Harborview Medical Center) Health Letter*, 5–7.

Department of Pediatrics, Section of Neonatal Biology, UCSF Medical School. (1984, February). The jaundiced newborn. *The Newborn Follow-up.*

Detmer, W. M., McPhee, S. J., Nicoll, D. & Chou, T. M. (1992). *Pocket guide to diagnostic tests.* Appleton & Lange, E. Norwalk, CT.

DeVoe, S., & O'Shaughnessy, R. (1984). Clinical manifestations and diagnosis of pregnancy induced hypertension. *Clinical Obstetrics & Gynecology, 27*, 4, 836–853.

(1986) *Diagnostics: Textbook edition.* (2nd ed.). Springhouse, PA: Springhouse Corporation Book Division.

Dialogues in medicine. (1985). *Laboratory Medicine, 16*, 489–492.

Doctor to doctor: who to vaccinate. (1992, August). *Medical World News, 33*, 8-13.

Dodd, G. D. (May/June 1992). American Cancer Society guidelines on screening for breast cancer: An overview. *Ca: A Cancer Journal for Clinicians, 42*, 177–180.

Dodge, W. T. (1985, September 10). *AIDS: How do we protect ourselves?* Paper presented at the Swedish Hospital Health Care Professionals Conference, Seattle.

Doenges, M. E., Jeffries, M. F., & Moorhouse, M. F. (1984). *Nursing care plans: Nursing diagnosis in planning patient care.* Philadelphia: F. A. Davis.

Dudley, M., & Searle, R. (1992, May). The Swedish Hospital Medical Center medical imaging manual. Seattle, WA. (Unpublished, House Organ).

Dx Literature Summaries. (1981). Uterine abnormalities on ultrasound point to DES exposure. *Diagnosis, 9*, 88.

Emmons, J., & Courter, P. (1985). Towards control of chlamydial infections. *Nurse Practitioner, 10*, 15–22.

Engler, M. B., & Engler, M. M. (1986). The hazards of magnetic resonance imaging. *American Journal of Nursing, 49*, 650.

Entman, S. S., & Richardson, L. D. (1983). Clinical applications of the altered iron kinetics of toxemia. *American Journal of Obstetrics & Gynecology, 146*, 568.

Epstein, B. E., & Hanks, G. E. (July/August 1992). Prostate cancer: Evaluation and radiotherapeutic management. *Ca: A Cancer Journal for Clinicians, 42*, 223–240.

Farese, R. V. (1980, April). How to make sense out of the new thyroid tests. *Medical Times*, 95–98, 103, 106.

Faulkner, W., King, J. W., & Damm, M. (Eds.). (1968). *Handbook of clinical laboratory data.* Cleveland, OH: McDaniel Rubber Co.

Fawcett, R., & Singston, B. H. et al. (1991, September). Use of western blot and enzyme-linked immunosorbent assays to assist in the diagnosis of lyme disease. *Pediatrics, 88*, 465–470.

FDA Drug Bulletin. (1985). Bethesda, MD: FDA.

Felver, L. (1986). Acid-base balances and imbalances. In M. Patrick, S. Woods, R. Craven et al. (Eds.), *Medical-surgical nursing: Pathophysiological concepts.* Philadelphia: Lippincott.

Ferris, D. G., & Martin, W. H. (1992, May). A comparison of three rapid chlamydial tests in pregnant and nonpregnant women. *Journal of Family Practice, 34,* 593–597.

Fife, K. H., & Corey, L. (1984). Viral agents: Herpes simplex virus, cytomegalovirus, hepatitis A and B. In K. K. Holmes, P. P. Mardh, P. F. Starline, & P. J. Wiesner (Eds.), *Sexually transmitted diseases* (pp. 829–856). New York: McGraw-Hill.

Finn, Albert F., Jr. (1992, September). Allergy and inflammation: Diagnosing and managing bronchial asthma, Part 2. *Emergency Medicine, 24,* 47–50, 56, 58.

Fischbach, F. (1984). *A manual of laboratory diagnostic tests* (2nd ed.). Philadelphia: Lippincott.

Fischl, M. A., & Dickinson, G. M. (1987). Acquired immunodeficiency syndrome (AIDS). In R. E. Rakel (Ed.), *Conn's current therapy* (pp. 31–39). Philadelphia: Saunders.

Flu vaccine greatly underused in high-risk groups. (1992, September). *Family Practice News, 22,* 20.

Follow-up and feedback. (1984, January). *The Harvard Medical School Health Letter, 9,* 7.

Fracchia, J. A. (1992, May). How can the family doctor most effectively screen for prostate cancer? *Primary Care & Cancer, 4–5:28.*

Frawley, T. F. (1971). Cushings's syndrome. (Monograph). *The Clinician-1: The Adrenal Gland, 37–53.*

Frey, M. A. B., Merz, M. P., & Hoffler, G. W., (1992, May). Effect of breakfast on selected serum and cardiovascular variables. *Aviation Space Environmental Medicine, 63,* 370–374.

Frohlich, E. (Ed.). (1988). *Pathophysiology: Altered regulatory mechanisms in disease* (2nd ed.). Philadelphia: Lippincott.

Fry, R. D., Fleishman, J. W., & Kodner, I. J. (1989, November). Cancer of the colon and the rectum. Clinical Symposia 41:11:2–32. Diagnosis in Symptomatic Patients. 41:11:13–16. Screening. 41:11:29–31.

Galen, R. S. (1979). Best test to launch diagnosis of MI. *Diagnosis, 1,* 35–42.

Gambert, S. R. (1992, June 30). The crucial prostate exam. *Emergency Medicine, 24,* 25–26, 33–35, 39–40.

Gambrell, Jr. R. D. (1992, April). Progestogens and postmenopausal women. *The Female Patient, 17,* 33–34, 36, 45–47, 52–53.

Ganong, W. F. (1987). *Review of medical physiology* (13th ed.). E. Norwalk, CT: Appleton & Lange.

Genital herpes vaccine gets through early test with good antibody effect. (1983, March 14). *Medical World News,* 136.

Gerlin, A. (1992, October). Rash decisions over lyme disease. *Cortland Forum, 5,* 82J,M,N.

Gershon, A. A. (1991, November). Herpesviruses. *Emergency Medicine, 23,* 105–106, 109–110, 115.

Giesser, B., & Sheinberg, L. C. (1983). Better tests for the MS workup. *Diagnosis, 5,* 43–44, 48, 52.

Gilboa, R. (1992, September). Hyperkalemia hypertreatment? *Emergency Medicine, 24,* 11.

Ginsberg, H. N., Brudley, W., & Murakami. (1993, December). MRI insights. *Diagnostic Imaging, 15,* 63–65.

Gitnick, G. (1981). *Perspectives on viral hepatitis, part 1: Non-A, non-B hepatitis.* N. Chicago: Abbott Laboratories, Diagnostics Division.

Gnauck, R., Macrae, F., & Fleisher, M. (1984). How to perform the fecal occult blood test. *Ca: Cancer Journal for Clinicians, 34,* 134–145.

Goodgold, J. (1980). Neuromuscular disorders: How electrodiagnostic studies can help your patients. *Diagnosis, 2,* 34–40.

Goodman, C. E., Lange, R. L., Waxman, J., & Weiss, T. E. (April, 1980). Ankylosing spondylitis in women. *Archives of Physical Medicine and Rehabilitation, 61,* 167–170.

Gorman, C. (1992, August). Invincible AIDS. *Time: The Weekly Newsmagazine, 140,* 29–34.

Govoni, L. E., & Hayes, J. E. (1985). *Drugs and nursing implications* (5th ed.). E. Norwalk, CT: Appleton-Century-Crofts.

Graham. (1986, July 5). (Personal Interview), Research Fellow, University of Washington, Medical School. Seattle.

Gregg, M. B. (Ed.). (1987, August). Recommendations for prevention of HIV transmission in health-care settings. *Centers for Disease Control, Morbidity and Mortality Weekly Report, Supplement, 36,* 11s–12s.

Gregg, M. B. (Ed.). (1988, June). Update: Universal precautions for prevention of transmission of human immunodeficiency virus, hepatitis B virus, and other bloodborne pathogens in health-care settings. *Centers for Disease Control, Morbidity and Mortality Weekly Report, 37,* 375–382.

Greisheimer, E. M., & Wiedman, M. P. (1972). *Physiology and anatomy* (9th ed.). Philadelphia: Lippincott.

Grenadier, E., Alpan, G., & Palant, A. (1980, March). CPK and CPK-MB in myocardial infarction and ischemia. *Practical Cardiology, 6,* 107, 110–111.

Groer, M. W., & Shekleton, M. (1983). *Basic pathophysiology: A conceptual approach* (2nd ed.). St. Louis: Mosby.

Groth, M. L., & Hurewitz, A. N. (1992). Diagnosing and managing bronchial asthma, Part 1: The Diagnosis. *Emergency Medicine, 24,* 31–32, 37–40.

Gump, F. (1980). Acid-base evaluations: Are venous samplings still useful? *Diagnosis, 4,* 50–58, 62–63.

Gupta, N. C., & Frick, M. P. (1993, July/August). Clinical applications of positron-emission tomography in cancer. *Ca: A Cancer Journal for Clinicians, 43,* 235–254.

Guyton, A. C. (1982). *Human physiology and mechanisms of disease* (3rd ed.). Philadelphia: Saunders.

Haffner, S. M., Valdez, R. A., Hazuda, H. P. et al. (1992, June). Prospective analysis of the insulin-resistance syndrome (Syndrome X). *Diabetes, 41,* 715–722.

Hahn, A. B., Barkin, R. L., & Oestreich, S. J. K. (1982). *Pharmacology in nursing* (15th ed.). St. Louis: Mosby.

Hall, J. (1993, Winter). (Personal Telephone Interview), Embryonic Defect Research, Woodinville, WA: CellPro Co.

Halverson, S. G., & Graham, S. (1986). Infectious and inflammatory diseases affecting reproductive function. In M. Patrick, S. Woods, R. Craven et al. (Eds.), *Medical surgical nursing: Pathophysiologic concepts* (pp. 1499–1523). Philadelphia: Lippincott.

Hamburger, J. I., & Hamburger, S. W. (1985). A practical approach to thyroid nodules. *Diagnosis, 7,* 30–32, 35, 38.

Hamilton, H. K. (Ed.). (1986). *Diagnostics* (2nd ed.). Springhouse, PA: Springhouse Corporation.

Hamilton, H. K. (Ed.). (1983). *Diseases*. Springhouse, PA: Springhouse Corporation.

Handsfield, H. H. (1988). Safe sex guidelines: Mycoplasma and chlamydia infections [Questions and Answers]. *Journal of the American Medical Association, 250*, 2022.

Handsfield, H. H., et al. (1986). Criteria for selective screening for chlamydia trachomatis infection in women attending family planning clinics. *Journal of the American Medical Association, 248*, 1730–1734.

Harborview Medical Center. (1987). *Infection control policy*. Unpublished manuscript, Seattle, WA.

Harper, H. A., Rodwell, V. W., & Mayes, P. A. (1979). *Review of Physiological Chemistry* (17th ed.). E. Norwalk, CT: Appleton-Century-Crofts.

Harris, P. C. (1980, Summer). (Interview and written table of microorganisms), General Hospital of Everett, WA.

Hartung, G. H., & Squires, W. G. (1980). Exercise and HDL cholesterol in middle-aged men. *The Physician and Sports-Medicine, 8*, 74–79.

Harvard Medical School. (1987, February). A new prenatal screening program. *Harvard Medical School Health Letter, 26*, 6–8.

Harvard Medical School. (1984, January). Follow-up and feed-back. *The Harvard Medical School Health Letter, 9*, 9.

Harvey, A. M., Johns, R. J., McKusick, V. A. (Eds.). (1988). *The principles and practice of medicine* (22nd ed.). E. Norwalk, CT: Appleton & Lange.

Harrington, J., & Brenner, E. (1973). *Patient care in renal failure*. Philadelphia: Saunders.

Haughton, V. M. III. (1987). Examining the spine with CT. *Diagnosis, 9*, 90–94.

Haughton, V. M. III. (1987). MRI to assess spinal cord diseases. *Diagnosis, 9*, 103–106, 108.

Hazzard, M. E. (1979). *Critical care nursing: Nursing outline series*. Garden City, NY: Medical Examination Publishing.

Hearn, J. A., Ba'albaki, H. et al. (1992, May). Usefulness of serum lipoprotein (a) as a preditor of restenosis after percutaneous transluminal coronary angioplasty. *American Journal of Cardiology, 92*, 736–739.

Hedayati, H. (1992, June). Lyme disease. *Journal of the American Osteopathic Association, 92*, 755–760, 763–765.

Heitkemper, M., & Brubacher, L. (1986). Nursing strategies for common gastrointestinal problems: Nursing diagnosis, interventions, evaluation. In M. Patrick, S. Woods, R. Craven et al. (Eds.), *Medical-surgical nursing: Pathophysiologic concepts* (pp. 1153–1182). Philadelphia: Lippincott.

Heitkemper, M., & Martin, D. (1986). Infections and inflammatory gastrointestinal disorders. In M. Patrick, S. Woods, R. Craven et al. (Eds.), *Medical-surgical nursing: Pathophysiologic concepts* (pp. 1208–1242). Philadelphia: Lippincott.

Hekelman, F., & Ostendarp, C. (1979). *Nephrology in nursing: Perspectives of care*. New York: McGraw-Hill.

Henry, J. B. (Ed.). (1991). *Todd-Sanford-Davidsohn: Clinical diagnosis and management by laboratory methods* (18th ed.). Philadelphia: Saunders.

Hepatic enzymes—up without symptoms. (1989, March). *Emergency Medicine, 21*, 69–70, 73.

Hepatitis B vaccine for children and adolescents? (Doctor to Doctor). (1992, August). *Medical World News, 33*, 38.

Hepatitis B: The sneaky virus. (1992, September). *Hyppocrates, 6*, 7, 9.

Hepatitis C: A potential perinatal menace. (1992, September). *Emergency Medicine, 24,* 231–232.

Herpes shedding during remission. (1992, July). *Emergency Medicine, 24,* 77, 81.

Hickey, J. (1981). *The clinical practice of neurological and neurosurgical nursing.* Philadelphia: Lippincott.

HIV-2 appears far less transmissible than HIV-1. (1992, September). *Family Practice News, 22,* 9.

Hoffart, N. (1986). Acute renal failure. In M. Patrick, S. Woods, R. Craven et al. (Eds.), *Medical-surgical nursing: Pathophysiologic concepts* (pp. 1198–1239). Philadelphia: Lippincott.

Holland, N. J., Wiesel-Levison, P., Miller, G., & Giesser, B. S. (1984, August). Radioisotope studies of neurogenic bladder in multiple sclerosis. *Journal of Neurosurgical Nursing, 16,* 188–192.

Holloway, N. M. (1979). *Nursing the critically ill adult.* Menlo Park, CA: Addison-Wesley.

Holmes, K. K., Mardh, P. A., Sparling, F., & Wiesner, P. J. (1984). *Sexually transmitted diseases.* New York: McGraw-Hill.

Home cholesterol kit cleared for use. (1993, May). *The Female Patient, 18,* 61.

Honing interpretation of thallium heart scans. (1992, January). *24,* 70, 73.

Hoofnagle, J. H. (1981). *Perspectives on viral hepatitis: Part 2: Types A and B viral hepatitis.* N. Chicago: Abbott Laboratories Diagnostics Division.

Hook, W. C., & Fernandes, J. J. (1992, April). Human immunodeficiency virus testing. *Journal of the American Osteopathic Association, 92,* 485–486, 496–498.

Hopkins, R. R. (1984). The role of the primary care physician in screening for colorectal cancer. *Ca: A Journal for Clinicians,* (Journal insert), *34.*

Horton, B. (1992, Fall). (Personal Telephone Interview), Seattle, WA: Odessa Brown Children's Clinic.

Horwitz, C. A. (1980). Laboratory diagnosis of rheumatoid disease. *Postgraduate Medicine, 35,* 193–195, 198–200, 203.

Howard, R. B., & Herbold, N. H. (1982). *Nutrition in clinical care* (2nd ed.). New York: McGraw-Hill.

How is the diagnosis of lyme disease made? (1992, January). *Cortlandt Forum, 5,* 198.

How is lyme disease transmitted? (1992, January). *Cortlandt Forum, 5,* 197.

How should CNS lyme disease be evaluated? (1992, January). *Cortlandt Forum, 5,* 200.

How useful is laboratory testing in lyme disease? (1992, June). *Cortlandt Forum, 5,* 199.

Huff, B. B. (Ed.). (1986). *Physicians' desk reference for nonprescription drugs* (6th ed.). (pp. 726–729).

Huff, B. B. (Ed.). (1986). *Physicians' desk reference for nonprescription drugs* (7th ed.). (pp. 733–734).

Human T-lymphotropic virus type III: Abbott HTLV-III EIA. (1985, February). Chicago: Abbott Laboratories, Diagnostics Division.

Hurley, D. (1992, September). On the trail of a diabetes cure. *Medical World News, 33,* 16–17.

Iezzoni, L. I., Grad, O., & Moskowitz, M. A. (1985). Magnetic resonance imaging. *International Journal of Technology Assessment in Health Care, 1,* 481–498.

Image of acute aortic dissection. (1992, September 15). *Emergency Medicine, 24,* 67–68, 71–72.

Inner Vision. (1987, April). *UCSF Magazine, 10,* 2–17.

Insulin pumps. (1992, April). *Modern Medicine, 60,* 42.

Interpretation of abnormal laboratory values in older adults. (1993, January). *Journal of Gerontological Nursing, Part I, 19,* 41–44.

Interpretation of abnormal laboratory values in older adults. (1993, February). *Journal of Gerontological Nursing, Part II, 19,* 35–40.

Jacobson, H. G. (Ed.). (1988). Magnetic resonance imaging. *Journal of the American Medical Association, 259,* 2132–2138.

Jacobson, H. G. (Ed.). (1988). Positron emission tomography in oncology. *Journal of the American Medical Association, 259,* 2126–2131.

Jeffrey, R. B. Jr., Novelline, R. A., & Ros, P. R. (1992, August). Fast track imaging in abdominal pain. *26,* 107–110, 119, 122, 125–126, 129–130, 132–134, 137–140.

Jenks, S. (1987, May). HIV positive: Where do you go from here? *Medical World News, 28*–32, 37–38, 40–41.

Jensen, M., Duncan, R., & Bobak, I. (1984). *Maternity care: The nurse and the family* (3rd ed.). St. Louis: Mosby.

Jensen, D., & Koff, R. S. (1992, December). Abnormal liver tests, what next? *Patient Care, 92,* 143–145, 149–150, 155–158, 163, 167–170.

Johnson, E., Perez, G., & Slim, J. (1986, June). AIDS tests in office practice. *Medical Aspects of Human Sexuality, 20,* 44, 50, 59, 63, 66.

Jones, D., Dunbar, C. F., & Jirovec, M. I. (Eds.). (1982). *Medical surgical nursing: A conceptual approach* (2nd ed.). New York: McGraw-Hill.

Kagan, L. W. (1979). Renal disease: A manual of patient care. New York: McGraw-Hill.

Kayes, S. A. (1986). *Diagnostics* (2nd ed.). Springhouse, PA: Springhouse Corporation.

Kee, J. L. (1990). *Laboratory and diagnostic tests with nursing implications* (4th ed.). E. Norwalk, CT: Appleton & Lange.

Kelley, M. A. (1985). *Nursing diagnosis source book: Guidelines for clinical application.* E. Norwalk, CT: Appleton-Century-Crofts.

Kessler, H. B. (1984). Imaging decisions: Evaluation of pancreatic cancer. *Diagnosis, 6,* 19–21, 24.

Kilgore, C. (1992, September). Debate on cholesterol screening in chidren is still far from over. *Family Practice News, 92,* 15.

Kinney, A. B., & Bloun, M. (1979, September, October). Effect of cranberry juice on urinary pH. *Nursing Research, 28,* 287–290.

Kintzel, K. C. (1977). *Advanced concepts in clinical nursing* (2nd ed.). Philadelphia: Lippincott.

Kirn, T. (1988). Dimensional magnetic resonance cardiac imaging shows initial promise. *Journal of the American Medical Association, 259,* 2194–2195.

Klein, J. S., Gamsu, G., & Webb, W. R. et al. (1992, March). University of California, San Francisco, and University of British Columbia, Vancouver: High-resolution CT diagnosis of emphysema in symptomatic patients with normal chest radiographs and isolated low diffusing capacity. *Radiology, 13,* 182, 817–821.

Klein, L. W., Lee, G., Salter, L. F., & Yock, P. G. (1992, September). The future of interventional cardiology. Special Report on Atherosclerosis; Supplement, *Family Practice News, 92,* 3–6.

Korones, D. (1992). Detecting less common pediatric anemias. *Family Practice Recertification, 14,* 38, 41–44, 47, 49–52.

Kritz, F. (1992, June). PSA plus rectal exam may detect most prostate tumors. *Medical World News, 33,* 28, 30.

Krupp, M. A., Schroeder, S. A., & Tierney, L. M. (1987). *Current medical diagnosis and treatment 1987*. E. Norwalk, CT: Appleton & Lange.

Kucera, K., & Efrusy, M. E. (1992, August). Hepatitis C: A clinical review. *Journal of Osteopathic Medicine, 6*, 20–23.

Kunin, C. (1987). *Detection, prevention and management of urinary tract infection* (4th ed.). Philadelphia: Lea & Febiger.

Kyba, F. N., Ogburn-Russell, L., & Rutledge, J. N. (1987). Magnetic resonance imaging: The latest in diagnostic technology. *Nursing 87, 17*, 45–47.

The lab., drugs and nursing implications: Tapes 1–12. (1979). (cassette recordings). Chestnut Hill, MA: Health-Care Education Programs of America.

The lab., drugs and nursing implications: Workbook. (1978). Chestnut Hill, MA: Health-Care Education Programs of America.

Laboratory of Pathology of Seattle. (1991, January). Laboratory procedure manual. Seattle, WA: (Unpublished, no pagination).

Lab tests for seizures: Low yield, high cost. (1992, September). *Emergency Medicine, 24*, 197–198.

Lamb, J. O. (1984). *Laboratory tests for clinical nursing*. Bowie, MA: Brady.

Langer, R. D., Criqui, M. H. & Reed, D. M. (1992, March). Lipoproteins and blood pressure as biological pathways for effect of moderate alcohol consumption on coronary heart disease. *Circulation, 85*, 910–915.

Larsen, G. (1981). Chewing and swallowing. In N. Martin, W. B. Holt, & D. Hicks (Eds.), *Comprehensive rehabilitation nursing* (pp. 173–185). New York: McGraw-Hill.

Larson, E., & Edwards, W. F. (1986). Are the elderly at increased risk of infection? If so, why? *Journal of Gerontological Nursing, 12*, 17–21.

Larson, S. M. (1981, Spring). Monoclonal antibodies for diagnosis and therapy: A new frontier in immunology. *University of Washington Medicine, 8*, 4.

Larson, W. G., Felmar, E., Molina, M. M., Edwards, G. (1992, July). The problematic papanicolaou smear. *The Female Patient, 17*, 31–34, 37–39.

Lasersohn, J. T. (1989, January). Lyme disease in western Washington. Informational Mailing.

Laws, E. R. Jr., & Kamal, T. (1993, September/October). Brain tumors. *Ca: A Cancer Journal for Clinicians, 43*, 263–271.

Lehman, B. (1987, July 15). Lactose intolerance may not require avoiding all dairy foods. *The Seattle Times*. p. E 3.

Leibovitch, E. R. (1992, June). A systematic approach to managing the patient with hyperlipidemia. (Interview of Reagan Bradford, Sr.) *Modern Medicine, 60*, 80–84, 87–90, 93.

Leibovitch, E. R. (1992, October). Chronic hepatitis infection: Keys to work-up and treatment. *Modern Medicine, 60*, 10:56–58, 65–69.

Lenes, B. A. (1987). Therapeutic use of blood components. In R. E. Rakel (Ed.), *Conn's current therapy* (pp. 356–361). Philadelphia: Saunders.

Leung, D. Y. M. (1991, November). Recognition and treatment of kawaski disease. *Family Practice Recertification, 13*, 30–32, 41–44, 47–50.

Levine, G. M. (1987). The malabsorption syndromes. In R. E. Rakel (Ed.), *Conn's current therapy* (pp. 401–411). Philadelphia: Saunders.

Levy, R. I. (1980, May). Hyperlipoproteinemia and its management. *The Journal of Cardiovascular Medicine, 5*, 435–442, 444–447, 452.

Lewellen, T. K. (1981, Winter). Digital imaging or don't nybble when you can byte. *University of Washington Medicine, 8,* 15–21.

Lewis, S. M., & Collier, I. C. (1992). *Medical surgical nursing: Assessment and management of clinical problems* (3rd ed.). St. Louis, MO: Mosby Year Book

Lithium as a granulopoietic agent. (1979). *Current Prescribing,* 25–32.

Littrup, P. J. (1992, June). Prostate cancer screen: Follow PSA with ultrasound. *Modern Medicine, 60,* 38.

Liver function tests in blunt trauma. (1991, November). *Emergency Medicine, 23,* 87, 90.

Loken, S. (1986). Giardiasis: Diagnosis and treatment. *The Nurse Practitioner, 11,* 20, 21–22, 26, 28, 30, 32.

Low HDL, high risk. (1989, January). *Diagnosis, 11,* 9.

Low incidence of AIDS transmission in health care settings cited. (1987). *Family Practice News* 15–31.

Lucci, J. A., & Berman, M. L. (1992, May). Improving the accuracy of the pap smear. *Emergency Medicine, 24,* 87–88, 91–92, 95.

Luckmann, J., & Sorensen, K. C. (1987). *Medical-surgical nursing: A psychophysiologic approach.* Philadelphia: Saunders.

Lusby, G., & Schietinger, H. (1983, August). *Infection precautions for people with AIDS.* Unpublished manuscript, San Francisco General Hospital; Shanti AIDS Residence Program; San Francisco General Hospital Medical Special Care Unit, and Bay Area APIC AIDS Resource Group.

Lutwick, L. I. (1980). Principles of antibiotic use in the elderly. *Geriatrics, 5,* 54–56, 58–60.

Lyme disease update. (1992, August). *University of California at Berkeley Wellness Letter, 8,* 1–2.

Lynch, P., Jackson, M. M., & Gilmore, D. S. (1986). Isolation practices: How much is too much or not enough? *Asepsis: The Infection Control Forum, 8,* 2–5.

Macbryde, C. M., & Blacklow, R. S. (1979). *Signs and symptoms: Applied pathologic physiology and clinical interpretation* (5th ed.). Philadelphia: Lippincott.

Mammograms' benefit in younger women questioned. (1993, May). *The Female Patient, 18,* 47.

Managing urinary incontinence in women. (1992, July). *Patient Care, 92,* 79–82, 87–90, 93–94, 97, 100–101, 105–106, 108.

Mangal, R. K., Geary, W. L., Robichaux, A. G., & Lassen, A. H. (1992, May). Hepatitis B screening during pregnancy. *The Female Patient, 17,* 48, 51–52.

Marchette, L., & Holloman, F. (1985, November). A first-hand report on the new body scanners. *RN,* 28–31.

Mardh, P-A. (1984). Bacteria, chlamydiae, and mycoplasmas. In K. K. Holmes, F. Sparling, & P. J. Wiesner (Eds.), *Sexually transmitted diseases* (pp. 829–856). New York: McGraw-Hill.

Marks, R. G. (1980). NIH panel urges wider use of amantadine in Influenza A. *Current Prescribing,* 55, 58.

Martin, D. (1992, Fall). (Personal Telephone Interview), Seattle, WA: Fred Hutchison Cancer Research Center.

Martinez-Lavin, M., Vaughn, J. H., & Tan, E. M. (1979). Autoantibodies and the spectrum of Sjögren's syndrome. *Annals of Internal Medicine, 97,* 185–190.

Mazzaferri, E., & Manalo, M. (1984). The solitary thyroid nodule. *Diagnosis, 6,* 54–50, 63–64, 69, 77.

McCance, K. L., & Huether, S. E. (1990). *Pathophysiology: Clinical concepts of disease processes.* St. Louis, MO: Mosby.

McCormick, K. B. (1986). Assessment of neurological function. In M. Patrick, S. Woods, R. Craven et al. (Eds.), *Medical-surgical nursing: Pathophysiologic concepts* (pp. 837–849). Philadelphia: Lippincott.

McCue, J. (1987). Routine medical screening of the relatively asymptomatic elderly patient. *Geriatric Medicine Today, 6,* 23–24, 26–27, 30–32, 41, 44–45.

McFarland, M. B., & Grant, M. M. (1982). *Nursing implications of laboratory tests.* New York: Wiley.

McGill, A. T., & Ruben, F. L. (1992, September). There's no time like *now* to prepare for influenza. *The Journal of Respiratory Diseases, 13,* 1231–1233, 1237–1238, 1243–1244.

McGowan, E. (1980). Blood component transfusion therapy. *Continuing Education for the Family Physician, 12,* 37–40.

McIntosh, H. (1992, April). News from NCI: The search for tumor markers continues. *PSA-Primary Care & Cancer, 12,* 49–50, 55.

McKenna, W. R., & Sparling, P. F. (1985). Sexually transmitted diseases: Changing patterns of infection. *Diagnosis, 7,* 66–72, 75, 78–79, 82, 85.

McNamara, M. T., Higgins, C. B., Schechtmann, N. et al. Detection and characterization of acute myocardial infarction in man with use of gated magnetic resonance. *Circulation, 71,* 717–721.

Meizner, U. (1993, May). Percutaneous umbilical blood sampling: A unique modality for fetal assessment. *The Female Patient, 18,* 103–106.

Mellilo, K. D. (1993, January). Interpretation of abnormal laboratory values in older adults. *Journal of Gerontological Nursing. Part I, 19,* 39–45.

Mellilo, K. D. (1993, February). Interpretation of abnormal laboratory values in older adults. *Journal of Gerontological Nursing. Part II, 19,* 35–40.

Menacker, S. J. (1992). Take advantage of HBV vaccination, in consultations and comments. *Consultant, 32,* 20–22.

Merange, S. G. (1984). Imaging decisions: When pulmonary embolism is suspected. *Diagnosis, 6,* 17–19, 22, 26, 35.

Merrit, C. (editor-in-chief), Carroll, B. A., Mittelstaedt, C. A. & Nyberg, D. A. (1992). *Yearbook of ultrasound: 1992.* St. Louis, MO: Mosby Year Book.

Metheny, N. M., & Snively, W. D. (1983). *Nurses' Handbook of Fluid Balance* (4th ed.). Philadelphia: Lippincott.

Mettlin, C. G., Jones, G., Averette, H., Gusberg, S. B., & Murphy, G. P. (1993, January/February). Defining and updating the American Cancer Society guidelines for cancer-related checkup: Prostate and endometrial cancers. *Ca: A Cancer Journal for Clinicians, 43,* 42–46.

Mezrich, R. (1983). Fitting magnetic resonance into the workup. *Diagnosis, 5,* 31, 35–36.

Miale, J. (1972). *Laboratory medicine: Hematology* (6th ed.). St. Louis: Mosby.

Middleton, D. B. (1985). Identification, education, compassion. *Diagnosis, 7,* 9.

Milhorn, H. T., Jr. (1980). Understanding arterial blood gases. *American Family Physician, 29,* 12–120.

Miller, B., & Keane, C. B. (1983). *Encyclopedia and dictionary of medicine, nursing, and allied health* (3rd ed.). Philadelphia: Saunders.

Miller, H. C. (1992, May). Does rectal exam raise PSA? *Cortland Forum, 5*, 24.

Minshaw, B. H. (1979). Assays and antimicrobial susceptibility. *Drug Therapy, 9*, 79–83, 87–88, 91, 95–96.

Montgomery, M., & Lieckti, P. J. (1991). *A nursing guide to diagnostic imaging*. Rutand, VA: Health and Allied Science Publishers.

Montgomery-Rice, V., & Leach, R. E. (1993, May). New options for the diagnosis and treatment of ectopic pregnancy. *The Female Patient, 18*, 31–32, 34–35, 38, 43, 46.

Morrow, S. F. (1986). Gonadal Hormones. In H. K. Hamilton (Ed.), *Diagnosis* (2nd ed.), (pp. 184–194). Springhouse, PA: Springhouse Corporation.

Moss, G. (1977). Postsurgical decompression and immediate elemental feeding. *Hospital Practice, 2*, 73–82.

Mountcastle, V. B. (1980). *Medical Physiology* (14th ed.). St. Louis: Mosby.

Mowad, J. J. (1979). Pyuria: Guide to management. *Hospital Medicine*, 34–37.

Multiple sclerosis vaccine promising. (1992, May). *The Female Patient, 18*, 53.

Murphy, G. P. (1993, March/April). Benefit and cost of prostate cancer early detection. *Ca: A Cancer Journal for Clinicians, 43*, 134–149.

Nadler, J. P. (1992, May). HIV in your practice. *Emergency Medicine, 24*, 133, 137–138, 141–144, 153.

Nadolny, M. D. (1980). Infection control in the hospital: What does the infection control nurse do? *AJN, 80*, 430–431.

Nasal calcitonin, lyme vaccine appear promising. (1992, August). *Modern Medicine, 60*, 30–31.

Nash, D. T. (1989, January/February). Should we bother older patients about elevated cholesterol levels? *Senior Patient, 1*, 59–60, 63.

National cholesterol education program expert panel on blood cholesterol levels in children and adolescents. (1992, May). Highlights of the Report of the Expert Panel. *American Family Physician, 45*, 2127–2135.

Nelson, K. (1993, June). Role of gadopentetate dimeglumine in patient management. *MRI Perspectives*, (MRI program handout Berlex Laboratories), 1–5.

Nettleton, M. D., & Jones, R. B. (1987). Chlamydia infections: Whom should you test? *Diagnosis, 9*, 58–59, 63, 65–66, 71.

New diagnostic tool: Lasers. (1985, December). *Science and Technology for The Executive*, p. 7.

New drugs/Drug news. (1980, June). *Drug Therapy, 10*, 21–23, 27.

Noble, R. C. (1986, September). Herpes update: Detection, therapy, and prevention. *Medical Aspects of Human Sexuality, 4*, 60, 64, 66–68.

Noble, R. C. (1984). Urethral discharge—Which culprit? *Diagnosis, 6*, 97–100.

Nord, H. J. (1992, October). When the fecal blood test is positive. *Emergency Medicine, 24*, 238, 242–244.

Nordin, D. (1980, Spring). (Written comments). Everett, WA.

Occupational Health and Safety Program of the Washington State Nurses Association. (1986, November). *Position on AIDS. WSNA Community Health Newsletter*.

Office of Research, Reporting, and Public Response. (1983, October). *Understanding the Immune Response*. Bethesda, MD: National Institute of Health.

Older maternal age may reduce the risk for IDDM in children. (1992, September). *Family Practice Recertification, 14*, 120.

Olds, S. B., London, M. L., & Ladewig, P. A. (1988). *Maternal-newborn nursing: A family-centered approach* (3rd ed.). Menlo Park, CA: Addison-Wesley.

Olson, K. R., & Dreisbach, R. H. (1987). Poisoning. In M. A. Krupp, S. A. Schroeder, L. M. Tierney (Eds.), *Current diagnosis and treatment*. E. Norwalk, CT: Appleton & Lange.

Ozuna, J. H. (1986). Nursing strategies for common neurological problems. In M. Patrick, S. Woods, R. Craven et al. (Eds.), *Medical-surgical nursing: Pathophysiologic concepts* (pp. 850–871). Philadelphia: Lippincott.

Pagana, K. D., & Pagana, T. J. (1992). *Mosby's diagnostic and laboratory test reference*. St. Louis, MO: Mosby Year Book.

Pagana, K. D., & Pagana, T. J. (1982). *Diagnostic testing and nursing implications: A case study approach*. St. Louis: Mosby.

Paparone, P. (1992, September). There is no standard approach to lyme disease: Your management must be individualized. *Modern Medicine, 60*, 95–99, 102.

Patient information 7: Cerebral CT scan. (1984). *Diagnosis, 6*, 64.

Patient information 10: Intravenous pyelography. (1984). *Diagnosis, 6*, 89.

Patient information 11: Mammography. (1984). *Diagnosis, 6*, 51.

Patient information 14: Nuclear scanning. (1984). *Diagnosis, 6*, 181.

Patient information 18: Sigmoidoscopy. (1987). *Diagnosis, 9*, 143.

Patient information 27: Lung scan. (1985). *Diagnosis, 7*, 41.

Patient information 31: Magnetic resonance imaging. (1987). *Diagnosis, 9*, 142.

Patrick, M., Woods, S., Craven, R. et al. (Eds.). (1986). *Medical surgical nursing: Pathologic and physiologic concepts*. Philadelphia: Lippincott.

Paulus, D. D., Jr. (1984). Guidelines for using mammography. *Diagnosis, 6*, 40–45, 49–50.

Paulus, D. D., Jr. (1987). Imaging in breast cancer. *Ca: A Cancer Journal for Clinicians, 37*, 133–150.

Pedley, C., & Bloomfield, R. (1992, September). Hypertension in diabetes: Factors that influence therapeutic choices. *Consultant, 32*, 108–110, 112–113.

Penicillin is out for gonorrhea. (1992, June). *Cortlandt Forum, 5*, 142.

Pepper, G. (1985). Oral acyclovir (Zovirax): Major or minor miracle. *Nurse Practitioner, 10*, 50–51.

Permutt, M. A. (1980). Is it really hypoglycemia? If so, what should you do? *Medical Times, 109*, 35–43.

PET: Predicting bypass success. (1986, September). *Medical World News*, 25.

Peters, I. (1987, February 17). *How sexuality issues affect clinical–patient interaction in STD visits*. (Presented at Harborview Medical Center).

Peterson, C. M., Koenig, R., Jones, R. et al. (1977). Correlation of serum triglyceride levels and hemoglobin A_{1c} concentrations in diabetes mellitus. *Diabetes, 27*, 507–509.

Pfieffer, N. (1992, May). AIDS guidelines: Why were they postponed? *Medical World News, 33*, 26–27, 30.

Phillips, P. (1991, January). CT wins favor in CAD diagnosis. *Medical World News, 32*, 26.

Phillips, P. (1992, July). Antioxidants on trial to reduce CAD. *Cortlandt Forum, 5*, 244–245.

Phillips, P. (1990, February). Biomagnetic imaging joins lineup. *Medical World News, 31*, 50.

Phillips, S. F., & Von Weiss, D. L. (1992, March). When cholesterol levels are too low. *Patient Care, 26*, 24.

Phipps, W. J., Long, B. C., & Woods, N. F. (1983). *Medical surgical nursing: Concepts and clinical practice* (2nd ed.). St. Louis: Mosby.

Pien, F. (1991, April). Therapeutic imperatives for gonorrhea, chlamydia, herpes simplex, and syphilis. (Periodical). 59, 41–42, 45–48, 53.

Pillitteri, A. (1985). *Maternal-newborn nursing: Care of the growing family* (3rd ed.) (pp. 324–327). Boston: Little, Brown.

Planned Parenthood of Seattle—King County. (1986, June). Chlamydia.

Planned Parenthood of Seattle—King County. (1986, June). Expected outcome/goals of STD counseling.

Planned Parenthood of Seattle—King County. (1986, May). Five steps in helping patients with their feelings surrounding past or present STD's.

Planned Parenthood of Seattle—King County. (No date). How sexuality issues affect clinical—patients interaction in STD visits.

Planned Parenthood of Seattle—King County. (No date). *No one can afford to ignore STDs (sexuality transmitted diseases).* Unpublished Pamphlet.

Plumer, A. L. (1982). *Principles and practice of intravenous therapy.* Boston: Little, Brown.

Plus two other sexually transmitted diseases. (1986, March 14). *Medical World News.* 133.

Polish, L. B., Bauer, F. et al. (1992, March). Nosocomial transplantation of hepatitus B virus associated with the use of a spring-loaded finger-stick device. *New England Journal of Medicine, 326,* 721–725.

Pollner, F. (1986, June 9). Antibody acts as AIDS self-defense weapon. *Medical World News.* 21.

Polycystic kidney disease underdiagnosed in primary care. (1992, September). *Family Practice News, 92,* 43.

Pope, T. L., Jr., & Chen, M. Y. M. (1992, September). Imaging the acutely painful shoulder. *Emergency Medicine, 24,* 122–126, 133–134, 136, 139.

Porth, C. M. (1986). *Pathophysiology: Concepts of altered health states* (2nd ed.). Philadelphia: Lippincott.

Posner, J. B. (1993, September/October). Brain tumors: Advances in Neuroimaging. *Ca: A Cancer Journal for Clinicians, 43,* 261–262.

Powsner, E. R. (1984). SI quantities and units for American medicine. *Journal of the American Medical Association, 79,* 1737–1741.

Prchal, J. T. (1980). Red cell enzymes: An overview. *Continuing Education for the Family Physician, 12,* 41–42, 44, 49–50.

Prekeges, J. (1986, July). (Personal correspondence), Seattle University Department of Allied Health, Nuclear medicine.

Price, S. A., & Wilson, L. M. (1992). *Pathophysiology: Clinical Aspects of Disease Processes* (4th ed.). St. Louis, MO: Mosby.

Pritchard, J. A., & McDonald, P. (1984). *William's Obstetrics* (17th ed.). E. Norwalk, CT: Appleton-Century-Crofts.

Providence Hospital Medical Center of Everett, WA, Clinical Laboratory. (1985, July). *TDx drug levels: Controls and ranges: Therapeutic and alarm levels.* Unpublished manuscript.

Quinn, T. C., Groseclose, S. L., & Spence, M. et al (1992, May). HIV in Baltimore: So goes the nation. *Patient Care, 26,* 9:252.

Rakel, R. E. (Ed.). (1987). *Conn's current therapy.* Philadelphia: Saunders.

Rapid chlamydia tests not advised for low-risk patients. (1986, June 9). *Medical World News*, 51–52.

Rapid diagnostic test for chlamydia infection. (1992, May). *American Family Physician, 45*, 2335.

Ravel, R. (1989). *Clinical laboratory medicine: Application of laboratory data* (5th ed.). St. Louis, MO: Mosby.

Rapid Diagnostic Test for Chlamydial Infection. (1992, May). *American Family Physician, 45*, 2335.

Recommendations for immunization for HTLV-/LAV-infected children. (1986, November). *Community Health Nursing Interest Group Newsletter.* 9.

Recommend commercial insect repellents to help ward off lyme disease. (1992, August). *Modern Medicine, 60*, 23.

Reger, K. (1994, Spring). (Personal Interview), Tour of imaging laboratory: Reviewer of MRI and CT sections. Renton, WA.

Reis, G. L., Kuntz, R. E., Silverman, D. I. et al. (1992). Effects of serum lipid levels on restenosis after coronary angioplasty. *American Journal of Cardiology, 68*, 1431–1435.

Ricker, D. M., Rohde, R. et al. (1992, July). Can complement C4 be dropped as serologic assay for lupus activity. Citation in *Journal of Musculoskeletal Medicine, 9*, 52.

Ring, A. M. (1969). *Laboratory correlation manual*, Springfield, IL: Charles C. Thomas.

Robinson, L. (1984, September). Acquired immunodeficiency syndrome (AIDS)—An update. *Critical Care Nurse, 4*, 75–82.

Robinson, S. B., & Demuth, P. L. (1985). Diagnostic studies for the aged: What are the dangers? *Journal of Gerontological Nursing, 11*, 7–9.

Roitt, I. M. (1977). *Essential Immunology* (3rd ed.). Oxford, England: Blackwell.

Rokosky, J. S., & Shaver, J. (1982). Fluid and electrolyte balance. In S. Underhill, S. Woods, E. Sivarajan, & C. J. Halpenny (Eds.), *Cardiac nursing* (pp. 83–100). Philadelphia: Lippincott.

Role of oat bran in cholesterol reduction. (1992, May). *American Family Physician, 45*, 2317–2318.

Rose, C. D., Fawcett, P. T., Singsen, B. H. et al. (1991, September). Use of western blot and enzyme-linked immunosorbent assays to assist in the diagnosis of lyme disease. *Pediatrics, 99*, 465–470.

Rosenberg, N. (1992, June). Test identifies lyme disease earlier. *Medical World News, 33*, 27.

Rosenblum, L., Darrow, W., & Witte J. et al. (1992). Sexual practices in the transmission of hepatitis B virus and prevalence of hepatitis delta virus infection in female prostitutes in the U.S. *JAMA, 267*, 2471–2481.

Rothschild, B. M. (1990, May-June). Diagnosing and treating fibrosis and fibromyalgia. *Geriatric Consultant*, 26–28.

Rubin, R. (1985). Thromboembolism: Warning signs and work-up strategies. *Diagnosis, 7*, 98–103, 108–109.

Sabiston, D. C., Jr. (Ed.). (1981). *Davis-Christopher textbook of surgery: Biological basis of modern surgical practice*. Philadelphia: Saunders.

Safai, S., Diaz, B., & Schwartz, J. (1992, March/April). Malignant neoplasms associated with human immunodeficiency virus infection. *Ca: A Cancer Journal for Clinicians, 42*, 74–95.

Salmond, C. E., Beaglehole, R., & Prior, I. A. M. (1985). Are low cholesterol values associated with excess mortality? *British Medical Journal, 290*, 422.

Sampliner, R. E. (1992, January). Tracing the source of a child's liver disease. *Consultant, 32*, 15–18.

Sanford, J. P., Sande, M. A., & Gilbert, D. N. (1992). *The Sanford guide to HIV therapy.* Dallas, TX.

Sanford, J. P., Sande, M. A., Gilbert, D. N., & Gerberding, J. L. (1992). The Sanford Guide to Antimicrobial Therapy, Inc. Dallas, TX.

Sauerbrunn, B. J. L. (1971, January). Radioisotope organ imaging in tumor diagnosis and management. *American Family Practice, 3*, 86–98.

Saul, T. G. (1987). Acute head injuries in adults. In R. B. Rakel (Ed.), *Current therapy* (pp. 776–782). Philadelphia: Saunders.

Saxon, S. V., & Etten, M. J. (1987). *Physical change and aging* (2nd ed.). New York: Tiresias Press.

Schacter, J. (1978). Chlamydial Infections. *New England Journal of Medicine.* 298, 428–435, 490–495.

Schacter, J., & Dawson, C. R. (1978). *Human Chlamydial Infections.* Little, MS: PSG Publishing.

Schneider, K. D. (1978). Prenatal care. In M. Duxbury, & P. Carroll (Eds.), *Primary care of the pregnant woman: Laboratory tests.* (Series 2, Module 1). White Plains, NY: March of Dimes Birth Defects Foundation.

Schoen, E. J. (1992, May). Childhood cholesterol screening: An alternative view. *American Family Physician, 45*, 2179–2182.

Schutzer, S. E. (1992, May). Diagnosing lyme disease. *The American Family Physician, 45*, 2141–2156.

Schwenk, T. L. (1992, May). Fibromyalgia and chronic fatigue syndrome: Solving diagnostic and therapeutic dilemmas. *Modern Medicine, 60*, 50–53, 55, 59–60.

Scipien, G., & Barnard, M. V. (Eds.). (1983). *Comprehensive pediatric nursing* (3rd ed.). New York: McGraw-Hill.

Scoggin, C., & Sahn, S. A. (1980). The common cold—A few new tricks that make the going easier. *Modern Medicine, 48*, 28–33.

Sees much room for improvement in hepatitis C detection. (1992, September). *Family Practice News, 92*, 11.

Seitz, J. F., & Giovanni, M. et al. (1991, October). Elevated serum gastrin levels in patients with colorectal neoplasia. *Journal of Clinical Gastroentrology, 13*, 541–554.

Silverman, S. L., & Mason, J. H. (1992, July). Measuring the functional impact of fibromyalgia. *Journal of Musculoskeletal Medicine, 9*, 15–17, 22–23.

Serridge, M. S. (1980). The anemic patient. *Family Practice Recertification, 1*, 44–47, 50–52.

Sexuality update: Test for chlamydia at least once a year. (1986). *Medical Aspects of Human Sexuality, 20*, 8.

Sharpe, G. (1980). Mixed connective tissue disease: Diagnosis and treatment. *Continuing Education for the Family Physician, 12*, 33–40.

SHMC, Laboratory of Pathology. (1984, May). New RBC parameter—RDW. Unpublished manuscript, *Newsletter.* Seattle: SHMC, 1.

SHMC, Radiology Department. (1985, April). *Radiology services manual.* Unpublished manuscript. Seattle: SHMC.

Skelly, A. C. (1986, 1994, July). (Personal notes, correspondence, and interview). Seattle University, Department of Allied Health, diagnostic ultrasound.

Smith, M., & Bernat, J. L. (1985). Should you order electromyography and electroneurography? *Diagnosis, 7*, 125–130.

Smythe, H. (1986). Tender points: Evolution of concepts of the fibrositis/fibromyalgia syndrome. *American Journal of Medicine, 81*, 2–6.

Sochurek, H. (1987). Medicine's new vision. *National Geographic, 171*, 2–41.

Sodeman, W. A., Jr., & Sodeman, T. M. (Eds.). (1982). *Pathologic physiology: Mechanisms of disease* (7th ed.). Philadelphia: Saunders.

Soltis, B. (1979). Fluid and electrolyte imbalance. In W. J. Phipps, B. C. Long, & N. F. Woods, (Eds.), *Medical surgical nursing: Concepts and clinical practice* (pp. 327–357). St. Louis: Mosby.

Sorenson, K. C., & Luckmann, J. (1979). *Basic nursing*. Philadelphia: Saunders.

Spencer, R. T. (1973). *Patient care in endocrine problems*. Philadelphia: Saunders.

Steere, A. C. (1992, August). Distinguishing lyme disease from its look-alikes. *Emergency Medicine, 24*, 28, 30, 33–34, 41–42, 44.

Stephens, T. (1993, December). Roundtable: MR, CT Vie for honors in vascular imaging. *Diagnostic Imaging, 15*, 37–40.

Stephens, T. (1993, December). Imaging news: Surgeons visualize trauma using 3-D reconstructions. *Diagnostic Imaging, 15*, 15–16.

Stern, W., & Schulman, H. (1985). Ultrasound update, part 1: Doppler for the primary care physician. *Diagnosis, 7*, 123–124, 127, 130, 134.

STD risk should trigger tests. (1986, June 9). *Medical World News*. 52.

Strickland, D. A. (1990, February). Biomagnetic imaging joins lineup. *Medical World News, 31*, 50–51.

Strickland, D. A. (1991, February). Self monitoring skills spotty. *Medical World News, 32*, 17.

Stroot, V., Lee, C., & Barrett, C. A. (1984). *Fluids and electrolytes: A practical approach* (3rd ed.). Philadelphia: F. A. Davis.

Sumida, S. E., & Mullarkey, M. (1979, Spring). Antinuclear antibodies; characterization and clinical applications. *Bulletin of the Mason Clinic, 33*, 25–32.

Sussman, A. (1984, April). (Letter to Eastside Medical Laboratory.) *The Voice*.

Swedish Hospital Medical Center (SHMC), Laboratory of Pathology. (1984). *Laboratory procedure manual*. Unpublished manuscript. Seattle, SHMC, 1984.

Thomas, C. L. (Ed.). (1981). *Taber's cyclopedic medical dictionary*. (14th ed.). Philadelphia, PA: F.A. Davis Company.

Thompson, J. M., McFarland, G. K., Hirsch, J. E., & Tucker, S. M. (1993). *Clinical nursing* (3rd ed.). St. Louis, MO: Mosby.

Thompson, W. M. (1987). Imaging strategies for tumors of the gastrointestinal system. *Ca: A Cancer Journal for Clinicians, 37*, 165–185.

Thorn, G. W. (1971). Adrenal Corticol Hypofunction. *Clinician-1: The Adrenal gland, 1*, 23–34.

Three-dimensional imaging. (1992, September). *American Family Physician, 46*, 964.

Tietz, N. W. (Ed.). (1990). *Clinical guide to laboratory tests*. (2nd ed.). Philadelphia: Saunders.

Torosian, M. (1992). Cancer consultations: What further work-up for this CEA of 25.3? *Primary Care & Cancer, 12*, 26.

Treseler, C. (1993–94). Resource on infectious disease. Issaquah, WA.

Treseler, P. (1993–94). Reviewer of DNA section. Issaquah, WA.

Treseler, P. (1992, July). DNA probe. Unpublished Manuscript.

Troutman, M. E., Blend, M. J., Kniaz, J. L., & Efrusy, M. E. (1980). Antigen and antibody testing in viral hepatitis A and B. *Osteopathic Physician*, *7*, 35, 39–41.

Tucker, E. S., & Nakamura, R. M. (1980). Laboratory studies for the evaluation of systemic lupus erythematosus and related disorders. *Laboratory Medicine*, *11*, 717–726.

Turck, M. (1980). Urinary tract infections. *Hospital Practice*, *5*, 49–58.

Ulrich, S. P., Canale, S., & Wendell, S. (1986). *Nursing care planning guides: A nursing diagnosis approach.* Philadelphia: Saunders.

Underhill, S. Woods, S. Sivarajan, E. S., & Halpenny, C. J. (Eds.). (1982). *Cardiac nursing.* Philadelphia: Lippincott.

United States Department of Health and Human Resources, National Institute of Health, Division of Research, National Institute of Child Health and Human Development, and Radiological Health Division of the Federal Drug Administration. (1984, February). *Imaging in pregnancy.* Washington, D.C.: U.S. Printing Office.

University of California, Berkeley. (1985, July). Wrap-up: Cholesterol. *Wellness Letter*, 4–5.

University of California, San Francisco. (1987, April). Inner vision. *UCSF Magazine. 9*, 2–17.

University of Washington, Department of Obstetrics and Gynecology. Chorionic villus sampling (CVS) patient information sheet. Unpublished manuscript.

University of Washington Hospitals. (1985, Spring). New imaging tools improve diagnosis, treatment of head tumors. *Synapse*, 5.

Update. (1985, July). Imaging MI damage. *Diagnosis*, *7*, 14.

Update. (1984, May). NMR detects chronic heart disease. *Diagnosis*, *6*, 14.

Uszler, M., & Hiss, J. M., Jr. (1986a). Nuclear tests—1986 update. *Diagnosis*, *8*, 49–53, 56.

Uszler, M., & Hiss, J. M., Jr. (1986b). Nuclear tests—1986 update. *Diagnosis*, *9*, 49–53, 56.

Vogelzang, N. (1991). The touted PSA screen. *Cortlandt Forum*, *4*, 139.

Vogl, G., Miller, M., & Esluer, M. (1985). *Mosby's manual of neurological care.* St. Louis: Mosby.

Vvlaanderen, E. (1992, July). Cholesterol management: Risks and realities. *Cortlandt Forum*, *5*, 172, 175–176, 179–182, 185.

Wait 20 minutes to ensure accurate cholesterol readings. (1992, July). *Modern Medicine*, *60*, 31.

Wallace, D. J. (1993, July). Practical answers to your clinical questions. *Journal of Musculoskeletal Medicine*, *10*, 14.

Wallach, J. (1992). *Interpretation of diagnostic tests. A synopsis of laboratory medicine* (5th ed.). Boston: Little, Brown.

Wallack, J. J., & Bialer, P. A. (1992, January). Physicians and nurses' attitudes towards AIDS patients and their care. *Primary Care & Cancer*, *12* 53–56.

Ward, J. D. (1987). Acute head injuries in children. In R. E. Rakel (Ed.), *Conn's current therapy* (pp. 782–787). Philadelphia: Saunders.

Watson, J. E. (1979). Medical surgical nursing and related physiology. Philadelphia: Saunders.

WSNA (Washington State Nurses' Association). (1986, March). *Community Health Newsletter.* 8.

Wenig, P. (1980). Diagnosis and treatment of rheumatoid arthritis. *Osteopathic Annals*, *8*, 17–19, 22–25, 29, 33–35, 38–40.

Westbrook, C., & Kaut, C. (1993). *MRI in practice* (1st ed.). Boston, MA: Oxford Blackwell Scientific Publications.

Whaley, L. F., & Wong, D. L. (1991). *Nursing care of infants and children* (4th ed.). St. Louis: Mosby.

Wheeler, L. A. (1984). Maternal assessment; Urine evaluation: Blood pressure. In M. L. Duxbury, B. S. Raff, & P. Carrol (Eds.), *Prenatal care* (Series 2, Module 2, Parts A and B), (pp. 1–2). White Plains, NY: March of Dimes Birth Defects Foundation.

Wheelis, R. F. (1979). Making sense of coagulation tests. *Bulletin of the Mason Clinic, 33,* 1–9.

Which surgical tests are worthwhile? (1992, Oct. 15). *Emergency Medicine, 24,* 88–89.

Widmann, F. (1983). *Clinical interpretation of laboratory tests* (9th ed.). Philadelphia: F. A. Davis.

Wilson, R. A. (1992). Viral hepatitis: Diagnosis and treatment. Lecture Notes, unpublished.

Winchell, H. S. (1981). Radioactive tracers in medicine. *Hospital Practice, 6,* 49–60.

Wolfe, T. (1985). *Pregnancy induced hypertension.* Unpublished manuscript lecture notes for Maternal Child Nursing course, presented at Seattle University School of Nursing.

Worley, R. J. (1984). Pathophysiology of pregnancy induced hypertension. *Clinical Obstetrics and Gynecology, 27,* 831–835.

Yost, J. (1992, October). Serologic testing only part of lyme disease. *Diagnosis, 92,* 1218–1219.

Yulsman, T. (1992, February). Blood lipids reconsidered. *Medical World News, 33,* 35, 37.

Zoler, M. (1986, June 9). Monoclonal antibodies: On the verge of therapeutic reality? *Medical World News,* 93–94, 99, 102, 105–108.

INDEX